Pharmacy Management in Canada

Pharmacy Management in Canada

K. W. Hindmarsh, Editor-in-Chief

Edited by:
Michael S. Jaczko
Alan Low
Jason Perepelkin
Kevin W. Hall
Roderick A. Slavcev
Rita E. Winn

DAYLE ACORN, CANADIAN FOUNDATION FOR PHARMACY, PUBLISHER

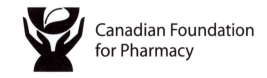

Canadian Foundation
for Pharmacy

The Canadian Foundation for Pharmacy
5809 Fieldon Road
Mississauga, ON L5M 5K1

Production management by
Brush Education Inc.
www.brusheducation.ca

Cover and interior design: Carol Dragich, Dragich Design

Library and Archives Canada Cataloguing in Publication
Pharmacy management in Canada / K.W. Hindmarsh, editor-in-chief; edited by Michael S. Jaczko, Alan Low, Jason Perepelkin, Kevin W. Hall, Roderick A. Slavcev, Rita E. Winn, Dayle Acorn.
Includes bibliographical references and index.
Issued in print and electronic formats.
ISBN 978-1-55059-644-1 (pbk.).—ISBN 978-1-55059-645-8 (pdf).—ISBN 978-1-55059-646-5 (mobi).—ISBN 978-1-55059-647-2 (epub)

1. Pharmacy management—Canada.   I. Hindmarsh, K. Wayne, editor   II. Canadian Foundation for Pharmacy, issuing body
RS100.4.C3P55 2015   615.1068   C2015-900709-7   C2015-900710-0

We acknowledge the financial support of the Government of Canada through the Canada Book Fund for our publishing activities.

Canadian Heritage   Patrimoine canadien

Contents

I. BUSINESS ENVIRONMENT – THE CANADIAN PHARMACY LANDSCAPE
Section Editor: Roderick A. Slavcev

II. ANALYSIS AND PLANNING
Section Editor: Alan Low

III. LEADERSHIP, MANAGEMENT, ENTREPRENEURSHIP AND PERSONAL EFFECTIVENESS
Section Editor: Kevin W. Hall

IV. FINANCIAL MANAGEMENT FOR YOUR PRACTICE
Section Editor: Michael S. Jaczko

Editorial Board

Authors

The *Pharmacy Management in Canada* Editorial Board would like to thank the following experts for their contributions to the textbook.

Zubin Austin, BScPhm, MBA, MISc, PhD; Professor, Leslie Dan Faculty of Pharmacy, University of Toronto

J. Reddy Bade, B.Sc.Pharm, Certified Diabetes Educator, Certified to Administer Medication by Injection; Shoppers Drug Mart 2401

Susan E. Beresford, BScPharm; Pharmacy Manager; ADAPT Moderator

Michael Boivin, Rph.; Pharmacist Consultant, CommPharm Consulting Inc., Barrie, ON

Todd A. Boyle, PhD; Professor and Canada Research Chair in Quality Assurance in Community Pharmacy, Gerald Schwartz School of Business, St. Francis Xavier University

Rene Breault, BScPharm, PharmD; Clinical Assistant Professor, Faculty of Pharmacy and Pharmaceutical Sciences, University of Alberta

Anita Brown, Bsc Pharm, Certified Diabetes Educator, Additional Prescribing Authorization, Certified in Patient Care Skills; Shoppers Drug Mart 2401

Bob Brown, Bsc Pharm; Owner Associate, Certified to Administer Medication by Injection; Shoppers Drug Mart 2401

Rick Brown, B.Sc.Pharm.; President, Innovative Pharmacy Solutions Inc.

Billy B. Cheung, R.Ph., B.Sc.Phm.; Region Director, Pharmacy & Strategic Initiatives, Pharmasave Ontario

Rubin Cohen, CA, CPA

Mark Coulter, BA, MIR, CHRP; Director, Organizational Development & Talent Acquisition, Rexall

Della R. Croteau, RPh, BSP, MCEd

David Cunningham, CPA, CA, LPA, CMA, BMath (Hons.)

Bryan Davis, BSc, MBA

F.A. Derek Desrosiers, BSc(Pharm), RPEBC, RPh; Director, Pharmacy Practice Support, British Columbia Pharmacy Association; President, Desson Consulting Ltd.

R. Mark Dickson, BSc(Pharm), MBA

Alan Dresser, B.Sc., B.Ed., BSP, MBA

Atul Goela, BSc. Phm., RPh

Kelly A. Grindrod, BScPharm, PharmD, MSc; Assistant Professor, School of Pharmacy, University of Waterloo

Lisa M. Guirguis, BSc Pharm, MSc, PhD; Associate Professor, Faculty of Pharmacy and Pharmaceutical Sciences, University of Alberta

P. A. Neena Gupta, B.A. (Hons.), LL.B., LL.M.; Partner, Gowling Lafleur Henderson LLP

Jill Hall, BScPharm, ACPR, PharmD; Clinical Assistant Professor, Faculty of Pharmacy and Pharmaceutical Sciences, University of Alberta

Kevin W. Hall, B.Sc.Pharm., PharmD, FCSHP; Clinical Associate Professor, Faculty of Pharmacy and Pharmaceutical Sciences, University of Alberta

Certina Ho, RPh BScPhm MISt MEd; Project Lead, Institute for Safe Medication Practices Canada; Lecturer, Leslie Dan Faculty of Pharmacy, University of Toronto; Adjunct Clinical Assistant Professor, School of Pharmacy, University of Waterloo

John T. Hunt, LL.B., LL.M., CFP, CLU

Michael S. Jaczko, BSc. Phm., RPh, CIM® (Chartered Investment Manager); Partner and Portfolio Manager, K J Harrison & Partners Inc., Toronto, ON

Stacy Johnson, B.Sc.Pharm; Director of Pharmacy Professional Services, Pharmacy Department, Safeway Operations, Sobeys Inc.

Leigh Jones, Loss Prevention Coordinator, Shoppers Drug Mart, Eastern Ontario

Harold Lopatka, PhD; Executive Director, Association of Faculties of Pharmacy of Canada

Alan Low, BSc.(Pharm.), PharmD., RPh, ACPR, FCSHP, CCD; Clinical Associate Professor, Faculty of Pharmaceutical Sciences, University of British Columbia, and Manager, Reimbursement and Medical Affairs, Servier Canada

Carlo A. Marra, BSc(Pharm), ACPR, PharmD, PhD, FCSHP; Professor and Dean, School of Pharmacy, Memorial University of Newfoundland

Ron McKerrow, BSc (Pharm), MBA; Principal, Concilio Consulting

Jeff Morrison, MA; Director of Government Relations and Public Affairs, Canadian Pharmacists Association

Vesna Nguyen, BSc (Pharm), MBA, PhD

Jason Perepelkin, BA, BComm, MSc, PhD; Assistant Professor of Social and Administrative Pharmacy, University of Saskatchewan

Tracey Phillips, B.Sc.Phm, MBA; Owner, Westport Village Pharmacy

Ron Poole, Risk Management Consultants of Ontario (RMCO) member

Meagen Rosenthal, PhD, MA, BA, University of Alberta

John Shaske, BSc(Pharm), ACPR, RPh

Jody Shkrobot, B.Sc. Pharm.

Roderick A. Slavcev, PhD, MBA, MSB, C.Biol; Assistant Professor, School of Pharmacy, University of Waterloo

Mike Sullivan, RPh, BSP, MBA; President, Cubic Health Inc.

Roger Tam, B.Sc.Phm., LL.B., R.Ph.; Vice-President, Legal, Hoffmann-La Roche Ltd.

David Toner, Loss Prevention Coordinator, Shoppers Drug Mart, Burnaby, BC

David Town, H.B.A., CHRP; President, Your Leadership Matters Inc.

Aleksandra Trkulja, BScPharm, Additional Prescribing Authorization, Certified to Administer Medication by Injection, Certified in Travel Medicine, Certified in Patient Care Skills; Shoppers Drug Mart 2401

Nicole W. Tsao, BSc(Biol), BSc(Pharm), MScPharm; Faculty of Pharmaceutical Sciences, University of British Columbia

Ross T. Tsuyuki, BSc(Pharm), PharmD, MSc, FCSHP, FACC; Professor of Medicine and Director, EPI-CORE Centre/COMPRIS, Faculty of Medicine and Dentistry, University of Alberta

Dr. Kishor M. Wasan, R.Ph, PhD, FAAPS, FCSPS, FCAHS; Professor and Dean, College of Pharmacy and Nutrition, University of Saskatchewan

Kyle John Wilby, BSP, ACPR, PharmD; Assistant Professor, College of Pharmacy, Qatar University

Bill Wilson, BSP; Director of Pharmacy, Mount Sinai Hospital; Lecturer, Leslie Dan Faculty of Pharmacy, University of Toronto

Grant Alexander Wilson, BComm, MSc; PhD Candidate, College of Pharmacy and Nutrition, University of Saskatchewan; Marketing Manager at a genetics company

Rita E. Winn, RPh, B.Sc.Phm; COO and General Manager, Lovell Drugs Limited

Mark N. Wiseman, B.Sc., M.Env.Sci., LL.B.

Anne Marie Wright; President, Elements Strategy Inc., *Transforming Healthcare from the Inside Out*

Reviewers

Through a double-blind process, each chapter was reviewed by two external reviewers. The *Pharmacy Management in Canada* Editorial Board would like to thank the following experts for their feedback.

Andrew Ashenhurst, Corporate Counsel, Walmart Canada Corp.

Zubin Austin, BScPhm, MBA, MISc, PhD; Professor, Leslie Dan Faculty of Pharmacy, University of Toronto

Sandra A. Aylward, B.Sc. (Pharm), R-PEBC, R. Ph; Vice-president, Professional and Regulatory Affairs, Lawtons Drugs & Sobeys Pharmacy

Keith Bailey, B.Sc. (Pharm), MBA

Bertrand Bolduc, B. Pharm., MBA, ICD.D.; Chair and co-owner, Galenova Inc./Gentès & Bolduc Pharmacists Inc.

Allan Braido, RPh, BScPhm, BSc

Fred Bruns, R.PH., B.Sc.Phm.; Chief Operating Officer, Medical Pharmacies Group Limited

Sal Cimino, B.Sc.Phm., R.Ph.; Director, Pharmacy Services, Green Shield Canada

Joel Clark, CFA; Partner and Portfolio Manager, K J Harrison & Partners Inc.

Rose Dipchand, B.Sc. (Chem.), B.Sc. (Pharm.)

Roy Dobson, BScPharm, MBA, PhD; Associate Professor, College of Pharmacy and Nutrition, University of Saskatchewan

Lisa M. Guirguis, BSc Pharm, MSc, PhD; Associate Professor, Faculty of Pharmacy and Pharmaceutical Sciences, University of Alberta

Jason Heath, Certified Financial Planner; Managing Director, Objective Financial Partners

David S. Hill, Ed.D., FCSHP; Professor, College of Pharmacy and Nutrition, University of Saskatchewan, Saskatoon, SK

Ryan Itterman, R.Ph., B.Sc.Pharm.; Regional Director, Pharmacy Services, Alexandra Marine & General Hospital and Huron Perth Healthcare Alliance

Lowell C. Johnstone, B.Sc.Pharm., MBA; Director of Pharmacy Services, PharmaChoice

Nancy Kleiman, BSP, MBA; Pharmacy Practice Liaison & Instructor, College of Pharmacy, University of Manitoba

Trent Lane, BSP; National Director, Pharmacy Innovation, Pharmasave Drugs (National) Ltd.

Johnny Ma, R.Ph., B.Sc.Phm.; President, Mapol Inc.

Charles MacQuarrie, B.Comm, MBA; President, MacQuarrie's Pharmasave

Jeffrey G. May, B.Sc. Pharmacy; Sr. Director, Healthcare Operations, Target Canada

Carole McKiee, R.Ph., B.Sc.Phm., FASCP

Colleen J. Metge, BSc (Pharm), PhD

Dean Miller, BSc Phm (Alberta); Past Chair, Ontario Pharmacists Association, Ontario Pharmacy Council, VP Business Development and Government Relations Remedy'sRx

Allan Mills, PharmD., FCSHP; Director of Pharmacy Services, Trillium Health Partners

Marshall Moleschi, R.Ph., B.Sc.(Pharm.), MHA; Registrar, Ontario College of Pharmacists

Andrea Murphy, BScPharm, ACPR, PharmD; Associate Professor, College of Pharmacy, Dalhousie University

Emily Lap Sum Musing, RPh, BScPhm, MHSc, ACPR, FCSHP, CHE, FACHE; Executive Director, Pharmacy, Clinical Risk and Quality, University Health Network; Associate Professor (status only), Leslie Dan Faculty of Pharmacy, University of Toronto

Jeff Nagge, PharmD, ACPR; Clinical Pharmacist, Centre for Family Medicine; Clinical Assistant Professor, School of Pharmacy, University of Waterloo

Michael Nashat, PharmD; Executive Director, OnPharm Inc.

Susanne Priest, BScPhm, RPh, MBA

Roberta (Bobbi) Reinholdt, B.Sc.PHM; Founder, Amberwood Retail Strategies

Bob Ross, CPA, CA; President, Quoddy Bay Management Inc.

Anne Snowdon, RN., PhD; Professor and Chair, International Centre for Health Innovation, Ivey Business School, Western University

Judith A. Soon, R.Ph., ACPR, PhD, FCSHP; Assistant Professor, Faculty of Pharmaceutical Sciences, University of British Columbia

J. Peter Spence; Partner, Harrison Pensa LLP

Gerry Spitzner, Founder and Principal Consultant, pharmacySOS.ca

Barbara Sproll, BScPharm; Medication Safety Pharmacist, Winnipeg Regional Health Authority

Jake J. Thiessen, PhD; Founding Director, School of Pharmacy and Health Sciences Centre, University of Waterloo; Professor Emeritus, Leslie Dan Faculty of Pharmacy, University of Toronto

Patrick Thomas, C.A.; CFO, Redtail Pharmacies Ltd.

Liz Tiefenthaler, B.S.; University of Wisconsin, President, Pharm Fresh Media

Isabelle Tremblay, B.Pharm., MBA; Consultant

Angie Wierzbicki, BScPharm, MBA; Group Director of Pharmacy, Sobeys-Safeway Operations

David T. Windross, R.Ph., B.Sc.Phm., FCSHP; Vice President External Affairs, TEVA Canada

Acknowledgements

The Editorial Board would like to express our appreciation to the 56 contributing authors and 41 reviewers who volunteered their time and expertise to make this textbook a uniquely Canadian quality educational tool.

We would also like to recognize the Board of Directors at the Canadian Foundation for Pharmacy (CFP) who put the capital at risk to make this project a reality. Without their vision, this project would not have been completed today. Under the direction of Dayle Acorn, they saw the need for this textbook in the pharmacy community, and provided the much needed support. Since 1945, the Canadian Foundation for Pharmacy has fulfilled its mandate of advancing the profession of pharmacy. Through the Innovation Fund, CFP has supported a number of research projects that are focused on demonstrating the value that pharmacists can contribute to the Canadian health care system. We hope that this textbook will also contribute to the advancement of the profession by helping to develop the next generation of pharmacists.

As well, we would like to extend our gratitude to Christine LeBlanc as Managing Editor for keeping this project moving and grounded in sound editorial context. We would like to thank Brush Education, who provided the steady guidance required of a publisher to see this project to completion.

Supporting the Foundation were a number of companies and individuals who very generously provided **unrestricted educational grants** to support this project.

PRINCIPAL BENEFACTORS

GREEN SHIELD CANADA ($25,000)
Established in 1957 by five pharmacists, Green Shield Canada (GSC) is Canada's only national not-for-profit health and dental benefits specialist. Our reason for being is the enhancement of the common good so we seek out innovative ways to broaden the availability of health care services, including drug programs, to all Canadians. As innovators in benefit plan management, we established Canada's first pre-paid drug plan in 1957 and developed the technology selected as the platform for the following provincial health care plans:
- Ontario Drug Benefit Program
- Régie de l'assurance maladie du Québec
- BC Pharmacare
- Newfoundland and Labrador Prescription Drug Program

GSC's Pharmacy Services Team has led the benefits industry in finding innovative solutions to drive drug program sustainability. Partnerships with pharmacy in areas like smoking cessation and cardiac disease management have shown how patient health can be improved through creative cross-industry collaboration. We are proud to support educational initiatives like this textbook and value our continued relationship with the pharmacy community.

McKESSON CANADA ($25,000)

McKesson Canada believes strongly in the contribution pharmacists make to the delivery of quality health care in Canada. This value is expressed by the emphasis we place on our family of independent pharmacy banners, including the Medicine Shoppe, Proxim, and one of Canada's oldest and largest network of independent community pharmacies, Guardian and I.D.A.

As part of a global organization, McKesson Canada is able to leverage learnings from our pharmacy partners in Europe and South America through our Celesio business, and Health Mart in the US. These learnings are part of the competitive advantage we offer independent pharmacies here in Canada.

McKesson's family of pharmacy banners offer independent pharmacists an infrastructure that supports owners with marketing, merchandising, procurement and professional services, ensuring the sustainable growth of independent pharmacy.

McKesson Canada is proud to support community pharmacy, and is pleased to be part of this important textbook.

PHARMASCIENCE ($20,000)

Pharmascience is a leading manufacturer of generic drugs in a wide range of therapeutic categories, with more than 1400 dedicated employees. We are dedicated to lifting the burden of both pharmacists and pharmacy students alike and we believe that this textbook will be a great tool to help develop skills required to successfully manage a pharmacy practice.

DESANTE CANADA ($15,000)

Desante Financial Services Inc. is a leader in the Canadian health care market, focused on providing financing solutions to health care professionals. Desante Financial, in conjunction with its sister company Maxium Financial, is one of Canada's largest privately held finance companies with a portfolio in excess of $1 billion and more than 55,000 customers. Both Desante and Maxium have earned a reputation for their innovative lending solutions and are proud of their ability to build long-term relationships.

ONTARIO PHARMACISTS ASSOCIATION ($10,000)

The Ontario Pharmacists Association (OPA) is committed to evolving the pharmacy profession, and advocating for excellence in practice and patient care. As Canada's largest advocacy organization, and continuing education and drug information provider for pharmacists, the Association represents pharmacy professionals across Ontario. By leveraging the unique expertise of pharmacy professionals, enabling them to practise to their fullest potential, and making them more accessible to patients, OPA is working to improve the efficiency and effectiveness of the health care system.

PATRONS OF THE FOUNDATION ($5,000)

Jeffrey Robb, Turner Drug Store Ltd., London, ON (in memory of Glen Robb)
Alberta Pharmacists Association (RxA)
Allied Pharmacists Inc.
AstraZeneca Canada

BC Chain Drug Stores
Pharmasave Drugs (National) Ltd.
Safeway Pharmacy
Shoppers Drug Mart
TEVA Canada

FRIENDS OF THE FOUNDATION ($1,000)

AdhereRx, Toronto, ON and Sunshine Coast, BC
Canadian Society of Hospital Pharmacists, Ottawa, ON
Jones Healthcare, London, ON
LEO Pharma, Toronto, ON
Lovell Drugs, Oshawa, ON
Manitoba Society of Pharmacists, Winnipeg, MB
Remedy's Rx, Markham, ON
Shoppers Drug Mart National Associates Alumni

In addition to the corporations above who generously supported this initiative, there were a number of individual pharmacists who answered the personal call to leave a legacy. Their generous support of the project is greatly appreciated.

Elaine Akers, Peterborough, ON
Carolyn & Neil Bornstein, Newmarket, ON
Rick & Sandy Brown, Aurora, ON
Aubrey Browne & Dalia Salib, Toronto, ON
William & Barbara Coon, Muskoka Medical Centre Pharmacy, Muskoka, ON
Roger Daher, Lefko Pharmasave #794, Toronto, ON
Ryan Fullerton, Brown's Guardian Pharmacy, Walkerton, ON
Ivan Ho, Kennebacasis Drugs, Rothesay, NB
Sheila Kemp, Aikenheads Pharmacy, Renfrew, ON
Claudia McKeen, Ottawa, ON
Carole & Michael McKiee, Toronto, ON
Esmail Merani, Carleton Place Drugmart IDA, Carleton Place, ON
Marshall Moleschi, Toronto, ON
Gerry Morelli, Bird-Mor Drugs Ltd., Hamilton, ON
Brian Mulvihill, Jane Mulvihill and Joan Weise, in memory of Thomas Mulvihill, Pembroke, ON
Frank Murgic, Sunshine Drug Ltd., Windsor, ON
Rob Parsons, Ingersoll Pharmasave, Ingersoll, ON
Balu Patel, Balu's Guardian Pharmacy, Stirling, ON
Linda Prytula, Burlington, ON
Dom Ricciutto, Ingersoll Pharmasave, Ingersoll, ON
Mark F. Scanlon, Mather & Bell IDA Pharmacy, Peterborough, ON
The Simpson Family, Niagara on the Lake, ON
Mac & Linda Sparrow, Burlington, ON
Roxanne Tang, Markham, ON

Dr. Jake Thiessen, Unionville, ON

Scott Wilton, Collingwood, ON

David & Cathy Windross, Toronto, ON

Rita Winn, Peterborough, ON

Karen Wolfe, Toronto, ON

David Yurek, Health Centre Pharmacy, St. Thomas, ON

Marita Zaffiro, Marchese Health Care, Hamilton, ON

Dr. J. Gordon Duff (in memory), Professor Emeritus, College of Pharmacy, Dalhousie University, Halifax, NS

Introduction

Welcome to *Pharmacy Management in Canada*. The Canadian Foundation for Pharmacy is proud to present a new all-Canadian textbook, authored and reviewed by experts with years of experience in pharmacy management. This book provides pharmacists and pharmacy students with a rich resource of information. With the ever-changing scope of practice for pharmacists and the need for maintaining clinical expertise, often management issues are not given the same dedicated focus. While management issues are a required part of the academic programs in Canada, overwhelmingly managers from community and hospital environments find graduates from pharmacy schools not well prepared for management issues.

This is the first Canadian pharmacy management textbook since 1998 and covers many more areas and in more depth. The textbook features 12 sections: Business Environment; Analysis and Planning; Leadership, Management, Entrepreneurship and Personal Effectiveness; Financial Management for Your Practice; Risk Management; Operations; Quality Control, Quality Assurance and Continuous Quality Improvement; Human Resources Management; Developing, Implementing and Managing Clinical Pharmacy Services; Organizational, Business and Professional Communications; Marketing, Promotion and Customer Service; and Business Plans.

Our Editorial Board is a real cross-section of experts from across Canada and they put together a resource that represents pharmacy practice in the twenty-first century. It has been indeed my pleasure to work with this group of dedicated individuals from both academia and practice.

I congratulate the Canadian Foundation for Pharmacy for leading this initiative. I do hope the learning objectives of each chapter will provide a guide to the usefulness of each chapter and the Canadian content will be appreciated by all those who use this valuable resource.

K. W. Hindmarsh, PhD, FCSFS, FCAHS, FFIP
Editor-in-Chief

I. BUSINESS ENVIRONMENT – THE CANADIAN PHARMACY LANDSCAPE

CHAPTER 1

Industry Analysis: The Past, Present and Future

Roderick A. Slavcev, *PhD, MBA, MSB, C.Biol; Assistant Professor, School of Pharmacy, University of Waterloo*

Learning Objectives

- Introduce some of the key issues influencing and impacting the profession.
- Introduce the current state of pharmacy industry and new developments.
- Describe trends in pharmacy and plotting the future.
- Understand the importance of environmental analysis as part of the strategic management process.

Pharmacy as an industry in Canada is in a state of redefinition and reorganization that will increasingly force changes to previously existing business models in the retail sector. Demographic and political pressures are influencing the industry to add value to the previous business model, largely driven by drug distribution, and to impart clinical access to an aging and health care intensive population. Increasing competition in the industry is forcing smaller players such as independents to differentiate their businesses and find niche markets, particularly in underserviced regions.

The effective understanding of these trends and navigation of these dramatic changes requires understanding the forces at work. The chapters in this section identify and explain critical management tools used to analyze a firm's external environment. Pharmacy is an important contributing segment in sustaining health care in Canada, but it will require adequate managerial training to rise to the challenge and to seize the countless opportunities afforded by this versatile profession.

WHERE ARE WE?

Pharmacy, like any industry, is subject to external macro-environmental (see Chapter 2: Macro-environmental Analysis) and micro-environmental (see Chapter 3: Micro-environmental Analysis) forces and trends that influence the dynamics of the profession and supporting business model(s). Current trends of demographics and health care expenditure in Canada threaten the future sustainability of Canadian health care. At present, approximately 15% of the Canadian population is over the age of 65,[1] costing our health care system an estimated (2013) $5,988 per capita[2]; this accounts for 11.2% of gross domestic product (GDP). The number of 65+ seniors in our population is growing at about 3.5% per year and by 2036, Canada's seniors will likely comprise close to one-quarter of the Canadian population,[1] with health care expenditures estimated at almost $7,000 per capita just by 2016.[3] Complemented by an estimated 10% reduction in the national workforce by this time,[1] public health care spending is estimated to comprise up to 100% of total revenues in some Canadian provinces, based on the past 10-year trends.[4] These projections indicate a rather disturbing trend where costs begin to outpace revenues and suggest that without action, the sustainability of Canada's universal health care system will be severely compromised for the next generation. Moreover, it makes drugs (drugs might be cocaine and marijuana), which currently comprise 16.3% of health care costs ($34.5 billion), second only after hospitals (30%) and closely followed by physicians (15%),[5] a natural target for health care expenditure control policies that impact manufacturers and pharmacies alike.

Health care technologies have been, and will likely continue to serve as, a strong target for public cost reduction measures, both through legislation and by exertion of government buyer power. As such, reduced prices for medicines paid for by ministries of health are an expected continuing legislative trend. At present, 70% of health care spending is funded by the public purse and recent provincial/territorial measures to curb spending are successfully managing to reduce the growth rate of health care costs (only 2.6% in 2013).[6] Canada's prices for generics are among the highest in the world, and in light of the impending funding crisis, provincial/territorial measures to cut costs in health care are necessary and have in some cases been sudden and volatile. At the time of this book's writing, British Columbia leads cost-cutting measures by limiting the price reimbursed to pharmacies for generics to 20% that of brand. Québec and Ontario are close behind at 25% with all other provinces/territories either at or moving toward a minimum of 35%.[7] The trend and direness of the situation suggest that the onslaught of price-cutting will continue to get progressively deeper. In addition, pressures on the federal government Patented Medicine Pricing Review Board (PMPRB) to control brand drug prices in Canada for new medicines will further threaten drug reimbursement for retailers. Unity between provinces/territories to expand and increase their buyer power can be expected to increase. From a market forces perspective, the provincial/territorial government strategic alliance, Pan-Canadian Pricing Alliance (PCPA), imparts massive volume-driven purchasing power for publicly funded medicines. It has already conferred a national 18% reimbursement rate for the top six generics and can be expected to continue to impose its buyer power to drive down the price provinces/territories pay for generic and brand name medicines.[8]

Such pricing pressure also places a great deal of constraint on generic manufacturers that are less willing to offer discounts in the form of rebates to pharmacies without sufficient purchasing volume (see Chapter 10: Change Management). This particularly affects pharmacies in provinces/territories where rebates are still legal but undoubtedly impacts large chains with high purchasing power far less than independents that rely on rebates to reduce operating costs. Pharmacies currently generate more than half of their revenues from the sale of brand medications which, due to the upcoming patent expiration of many medicines in 2015 (referred to as a "patent cliff"), will further impact the bottom line of pharmacies after this point. For further consideration is the effect that preferred pharmacy networks (PPNs) in the Canadian market may have on pricing, creating a situation in which Canadian retailers become selective over which manufacturers' products appear on their formulary and affecting the willingness of pharmaceutical manufacturers that make brand-name medications to pay for listings, which they have not done to date.

On the positive side, the market for drugs (medications) is increasing which, despite current antagonistic trends, will likely keep the drug distribution business model healthy, but within a remodelled industry. At present, 62% of seniors on public drug programs use 5 or more drug classes and 29% of individuals aged 85 and older use 10 or more.[9] As the baby boomer population continues to retire, the 3.5% per year[1] increase in Canada's senior population, in combination with extended lifespans, will undoubtedly stimulate the growth of prescriptions and patient use of medicines. In addition, as personalized medicines and expensive biologics continue to rejuvenate the pipelines of brand manufacturers, future prices for both brand and generic drugs will raise prices, likely increasing revenues from drug distribution of retail pharmacies. In combination, these trends may provide enough demand to continue to fuel growth despite the countervailing forces, but with a few important caveats.

First, Ministry concerns over health care sustainability will undoubtedly continue to drive drug prices lower by both legislative and buyer power strategies as substantial cost growth threatens the sustainability of universal health care in all provinces/territories. Second, the market for drug distribution services, while likely still in the late stages of growth, is maturing and will continue to increase competition within the industry (see Chapter 3: Micro-environmental Analysis). Third, as industry rivalry continues to increase, primarily from one-stop shop stores and online drug distribution services that offer pharmacy as more of a convenience than a high-quality service, cost pressures will favour only those with the scale (large chains) to cut costs and remain competitive. Thus, while growth will likely continue, smaller players such as independents, with higher operating costs, are more likely to be usurped by chains to continue to expand scale and reduce costs.

The general retail pharmacy business model primarily relies on drug distribution as a driver of revenue, although attempts to differentiate by growing the front store through medical supplies, food and cosmetic goods, etc., have met with varying degrees of success. Recent trends to take advantage of increased scope of clinical activities and to increase offerings of very basic clinical services to customers are meeting customer demand, but those pharmacies that have successfully differentiated usually serve niche markets, while others' attempts to extend into this realm are rivalled by larger suppliers that are increasingly offering a service in combination with dispensing activities. These offerings are not vastly different between suppliers, commoditizing the product offered to customers, and commodity suppliers competitively fight for share of the market on price rather than any other value-creating dimensions.

Moreover, recent increases to enrollment capacity for several Canadian pharmacy programs continue to expand supply listing the pharmacist as the fastest-growing health care professional at a rate of more than 4%,[10] contrasted against the reducing growth rate of pharmacies (<0.7%).[11] The laws of economics dictate that increasing the supply of pharmacists relative to the demand for their currently practised services will reduce the market price for this service, negatively impacting profits for owners and wages for traditional pharmacist services.

WHERE DO WE NEED TO GO AND HOW DO WE GET THERE?

The adept manager endeavours to predict future trends, influence where possible and adapt the firm as necessary. At present, cost-effective improvements to health care translate to increasing the scope for frontline health care professionals and a trend in this direction is certain to persist, at least for the near future—a challenge that may well be best accepted by pharmacists, but in advanced clinical roles that redefine and capitalize on the value the profession may offer in improving access to cost-effective health care. The scope of clinical activities pharmacists can perform has expanded quite rapidly and dramatically within the past few years to meet the growing needs of an aging population. Already, in some provinces/territories, pharmacists can prescribe and order/interpret lab tests,[12] which can be expected to be a growing trend given the need for health care access at reduced public cost. This increase in scope shifts the pharmacist from dispenser to clinician, and the profession from an unspecialized service to a specialized practice that addresses growing patient access needs.

While health care professionals may face drastic cost-reduction measures on the horizon, the need for change is evident and strong opportunities can be captured by those who move first in this market and who can effectively manage the change. In addition to conducting a thorough analysis of the external environment, the adept pharmacist manager will also identify the dominant stakeholders (current and future) that impact the industry and firm and assess the economic and social imperatives of each (see Chapter 4: Stakeholder Analysis) as part of the strategic planning process (see Section II: Analysis and Planning). The application of environmental analytical frameworks serves to identify opportunities to improve health care access at a reduced public cost and to protect the sustainability of universal health care rather than compromise it.

For instance, consider that already about half of the population (>16 million Canadians) live with some chronic conditions[13] and incidence is increasing, where 40% of the population suffers from at least one of the seven most common chronic conditions: arthritis, cancer, emphysema or chronic obstructive pulmonary disease, diabetes, heart disease, high blood pressure and mood disorders (not including depression).[14] The continued shift from acute to chronic disease ailments presents strong opportunities for frontline health care professionals to improve a patient's quality of life throughout a full cycle of care. Such a long-term approach to health care would increase customer value, in turn improving brand equity, and reduce competition and the threat of substitute services that could reduce market share (see Chapter 3: Micro-environmental Analysis).

Health care in Canada is a complicated and opaque system, occupied by many players who act in silo in the health care value network (see Figure 1.1). Each player is paid differently and for different tasks and outcomes.[15] Generally, physicians are incentivized by billing for consults and capitation; pharmacists by prescriptions filled and services rendered; insurers by cost reduction; manufacturers by drug sales; governments by balancing health care technology effectiveness with cost, and innovation with safety, public satisfaction, etc. These misaligned incentives translate into wastage of funds paid into the system, or economically speaking, slack[16] that may account for up to 40% wastage in Canada and other Western countries' health care systems.[17]

In this convoluted system, pharmacists offer clinical skills and medication expertise that cannot be duplicated by any other kind of professional. This unique and highly versatile skill set and its expansion is best suited to cross these barriers in health care and interact with doctors and

Figure 1.1

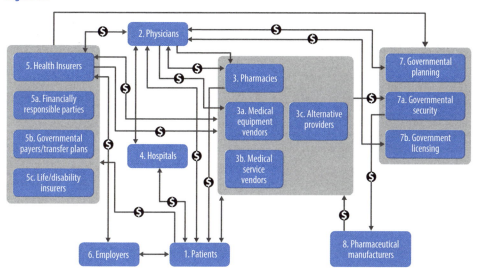

The Canadian Health Care Value Network

patients, government and manufacturers, insurers and manufacturers, clinicians and manufacturers, pharmaceutical and clinical sciences, and of course, science and business. By identifying these opportunities and capitalizing upon them, the opportunities that could await pharmacists are limitless and lucrative and essential to the sustainability of Canada's health care system, especially in light of the growing need for access to health care.

Capitalizing on these opportunities, however, requires a redefinition of the existing pharmacy model and requires the necessary entrepreneurship and management skills to extract maximal value from the pharmacist's competence set. Stated differently, a marriage of intra/entrepreneurship and strategic management skills is required for sustainable value creation, where intrapreneurship refers to project ventures initiated within an existing business. Management entails, in one form or another, the iterative process of analysis of an organization's internal and external environments, a unifying alignment strategy, planning across functional levels of business, understanding how to implement the plans and to keep track of progress, all of which is an ongoing process. The remainder of this section examines the necessary tools and skills to adeptly analyze a firm's environment as the first step in the strategic management process.

The pharmacy industry in Canada is reorganizing according to economic, political and competitive forces acting upon it. Despite growth of future prescriptions, it is the industry's big players that are likely to continue growth in drug distribution operations, which is a maturing and increasingly competitive industry. The expanding scope of pharmacists offers strong opportunities for pharmacists to move from commoditized dispensing services to specialized and differentiable clinical practices. Strategic management skills are critical for today's pharmacist to navigate the dynamic waters of the industry, and not just survive, but compete effectively and sustainably.

REFERENCES

1. Federation of Canadian Municipalities. Canada's aging population: the municipal role in Canada's demographic shift 2013. Available: www.fcm.ca/Documents/reports/FCM/canadas_aging_population_the_municipal_role_in_Canadas_demographic_shift_en.pdf (accessed Nov. 8, 2014).

2. Canadian Institute for Health Information. National health expenditures and MIS reporting 2014. Available: www.cihi.ca/CIHI-ext-portal/Internet/EN/SubTheme/spending+and+health+workforce/spending/cihi01595414000/capita/annum stat (accessed Sept. 15, 2014).

3. solutions E. The Economist Intelligence Unit [Internet]. Eiu.com. 2014. Available: www.eiu.com/index.asp?layout=ib3 Article&article_id=78929792&country_id=1490000149&pubtypeid=1152462500&industry_id=&category_id=775133077 (accessed Sept. 15, 2014).

4. Rovere M, Skinner B. Canada's Medicare bubble: is government health spending sustainable without user-based funding? Studies in Health Policy, April 2011. Available: www.fraserinstitute.org/uploadedFiles/fraser-ca/Content/research-news/research/publications/canadas-medicare-bubble.pdf (accessed Nov. 8, 2014).

5. Canadian Institute for Health Information. Health spending in Canada 2013. Available: www.cihi.ca/CIHI-ext-portal/Internet/en/document/spending+and+health+workforce/spending/release_29oct13_infogra1pg (accessed Sept. 15, 2014).

6. Canadian Institute for Health Information. Canada curbs health spending as expenditures reach $211B. Available: www.cihi.ca/CIHI-ext-portal/Internet/en/Document/spending+and+health+workforce/spending/RELEASE_29OCT13 (accessed Sept. 15, 2014).

7. Blueprint for Pharmacy/Canadian Pharmacists Association. Generic drug pricing – provincial policies Feb. 2013. Available: http://blueprintforpharmacy.ca/docs/resource-items/generic-drug-pricing---provincial-pricing_cpha_feb2013.pdf (accessed Sept. 12, 2014).

8. Canadian Institute for Health Information. National prescription drug utilization information system database – plan information: summary of changes, July 1, 2014. Available: https://secure.cihi.ca/free_products/NPDUIS_SummaryOfChanges2014_EN.pdf (accessed Sept. 12, 2014).

9. Canadian Institute for Health Information. Seniors and prescription drug use. Available: www.cihi.ca/CIHI-ext-portal/pdf/Internet/seniors_drug_info_en (accessed Sept. 15, 2014).

10. Canadian Institute for Health Information. Pharmacists in Canada 2011. Available: www.cihi.ca/CIHI-ext-portal/pdf/Internet/PHARM_2011_HIGHLIGHTS_PROF_EN (accessed Sept. 15, 2014).

11. Calculated from yearly pharmacy data personally communicated from National Association of Pharmacy Regulated Authorities.

12. Blueprint for Pharmacy. Summary of pharmacists' expanded scope of practice in Canada. Available: http://blueprintforpharmacy.ca/docs/pdfs/scope-of-practice-eng-dec-19-2014.pdf (accessed Jan. 29, 2015).

13. Canadian Academy for Health Sciences. Transforming care for Canadians with chronic health conditions. Available: www.cahs-acss.ca/wp-content/uploads/2011/09/cdm-final-English.pdf (accessed Sept. 12, 2014).

14. Canadian Institute for Health Information. Seniors and the health care system: what is the impact of multiple chronic conditions? Available: https://secure.cihi.ca/free_products/air-chronic_disease_aib_en.pdf (accessed Sept. 12, 2014).

15. Slavcev RA. Optimizing healthcare access: through the alignment of economic and ethical imperatives. *Healthc Q.* 2011;14(4):44–6. http://dx.doi.org/10.12927/hcq.2013.22650. Medline:22116565.

16. Ghemawat P. *Commitment.* 1st ed. New York: Free Press; 1991.

17. World Health Organization. The world health report 2000 – Health systems: improving performance. Available: www.who.int/whr/2000/en (accessed Sept. 15, 2014).

CHAPTER 2

Macro-environmental Analysis

Harold Lopatka, *PhD; Executive Director, Association of Faculties of Pharmacy of Canada*

Learning Objectives

- Understand the basics of PEST analysis and why this tool is important.
- Understand how to identify macro-environmental political (P), economic (E), social (S) and technological (T) factors and trends.
- Understand how to conduct a PEST analysis of community pharmacy macro-environment.
- Understand how to synthesize implications of these factors and trends on community pharmacy.
- Understand how to identify key opportunities and threats to community pharmacy from macro-environment.

All organizations, including pharmacy organizations, are affected by external and internal environments. Generally, internal environmental factors are controllable by the organization; for example, employees, capital assets (equipment or facilities), operating systems, policies and products and services produced. External macro-environmental factors are generally not controllable by the organization; for example, legislation, economy, social patterns and technology. These macro-environmental factors impact the pharmacy organization's internal environment, decision making, performance and strategies. The effective manager should be routinely scanning the macro-environment and not be blindsided by unforeseen changes.[1] One such strategic management tool used to identify the impact of changes in the macro-environment is the PEST analysis.

WHAT IS PEST ANALYSIS?

There are several management frameworks for an organization to scan the macro-environment. A well-known framework used in the development of marketing and business plans is the SWOT analysis.[2] Many of the opportunities (O) and threats (T) of the SWOT analysis can be gleaned from a well-conducted PEST analysis. In a PEST analysis, four factors are considered:

- Political: Refers to federal, provincial/territorial or municipal government laws, legislation, regulations and policies. Also includes political stability and the extent to which government provides goods and services.

Figure 2.1

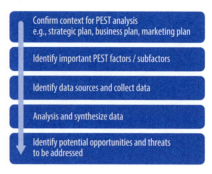

Steps In PEST Analysis

- Economic: Refers to economic growth, interest rates and inflation rates.
- Social: Refers to population growth rate, age distribution and work attitudes. Also includes cultural factors.
- Technological: Health care technology is the application of organized knowledge and skills in the form of devices, medicines, vaccines, procedures and systems developed to solve a health problem and improve quality of lives (World Health Organization definition). This factor refers to the stage of innovation and the rate of technology change.

There are five basic steps in conducting a PEST analysis (see Figure 2.1). First it is important to confirm the context for the PEST analysis. The PEST analysis can be used as a component of plans used in businesses; for example, developing or revising a strategic plan, business plan or marketing plan. The second step is to identify subfactors relevant to support the type of plan being developed (strategic, business or marketing). Table 1 illustrates PEST categories and an example of generic subfactors for each of the PEST categories. The third step in the analysis is to collect information about each of the four factors. This can be done through the collection of data from various data sources; for example, reviewing documents and Internet sites, interviewing experts and general brainstorming with key stakeholders.

After the data collection phase, data analysis is conducted. Relevant opportunities and threats to the organization are identified. The results from the PEST analysis are then used to support management planning and decision making.

PEST ANALYSIS FOR COMMUNITY PHARMACY IN CANADA

The following PEST analysis has been conducted to illustrate how PEST is used as a tool. The perspective taken for the analysis is at a high level on community pharmacy in Canada. This example PEST analysis might be used to support the development or revision of a strategic plan for a national community pharmacy organization.

Initial brainstorming about the community pharmacy industry identified several PEST macro-environmental subfactors. (See the Resources section for a listing of Canadian websites useful

Table 1. Summary of PEST Factors and Generic Subfactors[3]

Political	Social
Government type and stability	Population growth rate and age profile
Freedom of press, rule of law and levels of bureaucracy and corruption	Population health, education and social mobility, and attitudes to these
Regulation and de-regulation	Population employment patterns, job market freedom and attitudes to work
Social and employment legislation	Press attitudes, public opinion, social attitudes and social taboos
Tax policy, and trade and tariff controls	Lifestyle choices and attitudes toward them
Environmental and consumer-protection legislation Likely changes in political environment	Social changes
Economic	**Technological**
Stage of business cycle	Impact of emerging technologies
Current and projected economic growth, inflation and interest rates	Impact of Internet, reduction in communication costs and increased remote working
Unemployment and labour supply	Research and development activity
Labour costs Levels of disposable income and income distribution Impact of globalization Likely impact of technological or other change on the economy Likely changes in the economic environment	Impact of technology transfer

for researching community pharmacy PEST factors.) The subfactors identified were those having a significant impact on one component of the community pharmacy internal environment, namely the outputs produced in community pharmacy; for example, prescription services, over-the-counter (OTC) counselling and patient-focused pharmacist services. The factors and subfactors are shown in Figure 2.2.

POLITICAL FACTORS AND TRENDS

Political macro-environmental factors are important to organizations involved in the delivery of health care services because of our publicly funded health care system in Canada. Political factors can influence the quality, volume and cost of health care services provided. Three subfactors were identified as being significant as political factors: governments, employers and pharmacy organizations.

Health care policy in Canada is not exclusively determined by one order of government. Depending on the nature and scope of the health care issue, it may be addressed by federal or provincial/territorial legislation. Table 2 summarizes key roles and responsibilities of the federal and provincial/territorial governments for health care.[4]

Federal and provincial/territorial roles and responsibilities have been shaped by our Constitution. For more information about federal and provincial/territorial government constitutional responsibilities, see Government of Canada Intergovernmental Affairs.[5]

Figure 2.2

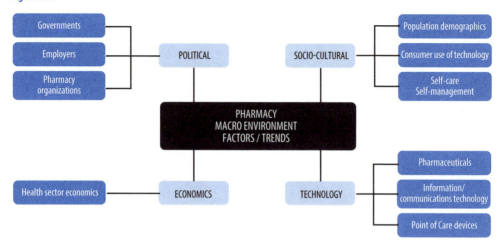

Identify Significant PEST Factors / Subfactors

Table 2. Federal and Provincial/Territorial Government Roles in Canada

Federal Government	Provincial/Territorial Government
Setting and administering national principles for the system under the Canada Health Act	Administration of their health insurance plans
Financial support to the provinces and territories	Planning and funding of care in hospitals and in other facilities
Funding and/or delivery of primary and supplemental services to groups (e.g., First Nations, Inuit, Canadian Forces, veterans)	Services provided by doctors and other health care professionals
Health protection and regulation (e.g., pharmaceuticals and medical devices), consumer safety, disease surveillance and prevention	Planning and implementation of health promotion and public health initiatives
Support for health promotion and health research	Negotiation of fee schedules with professionals Provide and fund supplementary benefits for groups (e.g., prescribed drugs, ambulance costs, hearing, vision and dental care for low-income residents and seniors)*

* Provincial/Territorial governments' role of providing and funding supplementary benefits for low-income and seniors groups is not covered in the Canada Health Act.

Under the Canada Health Act, provinces and territories must provide all insured persons reasonable access to medically necessary hospital and physician services without financial or other barriers. It is important to note that the Canada Health Act does not include medications or pharmacist services used outside of hospitals as medically necessary services. Canada does not have a formal comprehensive national pharmaceutical strategy that addresses the general WHO goals: (a) maximizing access to medicines; (b) ensuring quality of medicinal products;

(c) minimizing costs related to medicines and health care use, and (d) promoting rational use of drugs through prudent use of the health care workforce.[6]

Most of our pharmaceutical policies and planning (relating to both pharmaceuticals and the pharmacy profession) are focused at the provincial/territorial or local level. Individual provincial/territorial drug plan policies dictate eligibility, cost-sharing mechanisms, drug pricing, professional fees, markups, coordination of benefits and restricted/exception drug coverage process.[7] Provincial/Territorial government policies enable provincial/territorial pharmacy regulatory organizations to license and discipline pharmacists (health care professions self-regulation). This includes setting the scope of practice for pharmacists. Recent regulatory changes have expanded pharmacists' scope to include the provision of emergency prescription refills, renew/extend prescriptions, change dosage/formulation, make therapeutic substitution, prescribe for minor ailments/conditions, initiate prescription drug therapy, order and interpret lab tests and administer a drug by injection.[8]

The provinces/territories work collectively on pharmaceutical initiatives through the Council of the Federation.[9] The Council is made up of Canada's 13 provincial and territorial premiers. The Council has been actively taking a coordinated approach to price setting for generic pharmaceuticals and joint negotiations for brand name drugs.

In many instances, the public policy-making process is related to the government's electoral cycle. The following is an illustration of the relationship between the electoral cycle and policy making:[10]

- red zone: In the year leading up to an election, governments tend to avoid making controversial policy decisions.
- orientation year: In the first year following an election, the government usually takes time to get oriented. It has to assess the relative priority of each issue that needs to be tackled.
- activist stage: While government's electoral mandate is still relatively fresh, the government is ready to make major policy decisions. These decisions often tend to shake up the status quo.
- patching and filling stage: Once the major decisions have been made, governments tend to make minor adjustments and less significant decisions.

The influence of private health insurance organizations is significant. In 2013, there were 99 life and health insurers employing 150,000 people and with a combined asset value of $1,280 billion. The industry provides supplementary coverage to more than 23 million Canadians that accounts for about 12% of all health care expenditures in Canada. The 2012 premiums for supplementary health and disability insurance were $30.9 billion. Private health insurance plans offer supplementary plans that provide levels of coverage for non-core health care services not covered by government or public plans including prescription drugs. The majority of Canadians obtain drug benefits through private health insurers. In 2011, private sector life and health insurers paid $10.1 billion for prescription benefits.[11]

Private health insurance coverage varies depending on the plan. Commonly there are partial- and full-coverage plans, with the premiums determined by the extent of coverage. The majority of these plans are offered as group plans through employment. Most group plans are administrative-services-only plans where the employee plan is purchased from the insurance company. The insurance company administers the plan only and does not guarantee benefits. Employers pay for all the plan benefits. Plans usually cover immediate family members (e.g., spouse, children). Deductibles, coinsurance and maximums are common in these plans. In the pharmaceutical component of the plan drug formularies, generics and special-use policies are used to control costs. For large expenditures, the enrollee often requires a predetermination of benefits (where the amount the plan will pay is determined). In situations where both spouses have coverage with different private plans, coordination of benefits occurs between each plan.[12]

The Canadian Life and Health Association has called for reforms to the Canadian patchwork of prescription drug coverage.[13] Concerns were identified about inequitable prescription drug access and drug prices for Canadians, and about the financial sustainability of employer drug plans. The recommendations are primarily directed toward the federal and provincial/territorial governments and they include developing a common national minimum formulary, developing a national, comprehensive, high-cost drug strategy and expanding pharmacists' scope of practice to allow for therapeutic substitution.

Various advocacy and regulatory national and provincial/territorial pharmacy organizations attempt to influence the pharmacy political macro-environment.

The following are the main national pharmacy organizations. The Canadian Pharmacists Association (CPhA) is the main advocacy organization for Canadian pharmacists. Individual pharmacists are members through their provincial/territorial pharmacy advocacy organizations. The CPhA represents pharmacy and pharmacists' interests in discussions with Health Canada and national pharmacy and health organizations. The Canadian Society of Hospital Pharmacists (CSHP) is a voluntary organization focusing on professional issues related to pharmacists practising in hospitals and collaborative health care settings. CSHP develops practice guidelines and conducts educational programs for its members. The Canadian Association of Chain Drug Stores (CACDS) is an advocacy organization for chain pharmacy organizations. CACDS members are community pharmacy organizations (not individual pharmacists). In addition, there are several national for-profit corporations that provide pharmacy and pharmacist services; for example, Rexall, Medicine Shoppe, Loblaw, Sobeys, Shoppers Drug Mart, Walmart, etc. Each of these corporations has a national management infrastructure, and advocacy activities are part of their responsibilities. There is limited coordination of advocacy programs among organizations. The efficiency and effectiveness of national advocacy initiatives are difficult to measure with three national not-for-profit organizations and multiple for-profit corporations advocating for pharmacists and pharmacies. Federal competition legislation limits the effectiveness of national pharmacy organizations participating in discussions about pharmacy reimbursement. The National Association of Pharmacy Regulatory Authorities (NAPRA) is an umbrella organization for provincial/territorial regulatory organizations. Through NAPRA, a national approach is taken toward common regulatory issues.

At the provincial/territorial level, there are separate advocacy and regulatory pharmacy organizations in each province. The pharmacy regulatory organizations are legitimized in provincial/territorial legislation (through provincial/territorial acts and regulations) to self-regulate the profession including both pharmacists and pharmacies. Pharmacists' scope of practice is established through the regulatory body. All practising pharmacists and pharmacies require annual licensure through their respective provincial/territorial regulatory organization. Provincial/Territorial pharmacy advocacy organizations focus their activities on communications, pharmacy reimbursement, pharmacist education and membership benefits. Provincial/Territorial advocacy organizations usually negotiate a memorandum of agreement on pharmacy reimbursement with the provincial/territorial government. Membership in these organizations is usually voluntary and open to pharmacists and pharmacy corporations. Community pharmacists are non-unionized; however, in most provinces/territories, hospital pharmacists are members of health care sciences professional associations (unions). The unions have a major influence over management-worker relationships in hospitals.

In general, pharmacy advocacy organizations attempt to achieve a broad mandate with limited resources, and their overall effectiveness in attaining their mandate is the subject of considerable debate among members. In comparison, the mandate of pharmacy regulatory organizations is narrow and with greater resources, their overall effectiveness is generally greater in achieving their mandate compared to advocacy organizations.

Table 3 summarizes the complex matrix for how and where the responsibilities for Canadian pharmaceutical policy exist.

Table 3. Pharmaceutical System Policy and Planning Responsibilities Across Canada[4]

Policy Levers Employed for Pharmaceutical Policy Planning	Provincial/Territorial/Local	National
Processes for assuring quality, safety, efficacy and cost effectiveness of prescription medicines		Government of Canada (GOC) – Health Canada Pharmaceutical industry Canadian Agency for Drugs and Technologies in Health (CADTH)
Policies for maximizing access to prescription medicines, such as coverage eligibility, cost sharing and formularies	Ministries of Health Employers Local health authorities	
Programs/Strategies for minimizing costs related to prescription medicines and health care use	Ministries of Health Employers Local health authorities	Council of the Federation
Programs/Strategies for promoting rational use of prescription drugs through prudent use of the health care workforce	Ministries of Health Local health authorities Pharmacy corporations	
Processes to ensure quality and effective delivery of pharmaceuticals to population	Distribution organizations (e.g., wholesalers) Pharmacy corporations Local health authorities	Pharmaceutical industry
Setting pharmacy/pharmacist practice standards	Regulatory organizations Professional associations Employers	National Association of Pharmacy Regulatory Authorities (NAPRA) Professional associations
Determining pharmacist scopes of practice	Regulatory organizations	Pharmacy corporations (national)
Processes to ensure quality and effective delivery of pharmacist services to the population	Pharmacy corporations Local health authorities Regulatory organizations	
Determining system financial incentives	Ministries of Health Bargaining agents	
Data collection and monitoring	Ministries of Health Private insurers Pharmacy corporations Research organizations	Canadian Institute for Health Information (CIHI) IMS/Brogan

ECONOMIC FACTORS AND TRENDS

The economics of health care continues to be a frequent topic of conversation among politicians and in the media. In the 10-year period 2001 to 2011, national health care expenditures doubled from approximately $100 billion to $200 billion. The average annual growth rate was 4% over this period. In 2011, total health care expenditures were 11.4% of the gross domestic product (GDP) while in international comparisons, Canada's spending of $5,803 per person placed us in the top quartile of countries (2011 comparison). Public sector accounts for approximately 70% of expenditures and private sector (private insurance, out of pocket) for the remainder. Hospitals and physicians were mainly funded through public sector, and drugs and other professionals through the private sector. A detailed breakdown of health care expenditure information is available for 2011. Total health care expenditures were $200 billion (11.4% of GDP). The breakdown by source of finance is as follows: provincial/territorial government – 65.3%, out of pocket – 14.7%, private health insurance – 11.8%, other public sector – 5.1%, and other categories – 3.1%. The breakdown by use of funds is as follows: hospitals – 29.5%, drugs – 16.5%, physicians – 14.6%, other professionals – 9.8%, other institutions – 10.4%, and other categories – 19.2% (see Figures 2.3 and 2.4).[14]

Figure 2.3

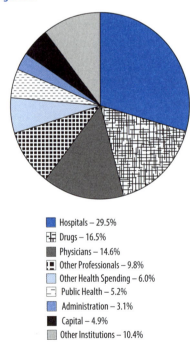

Figure 2.4

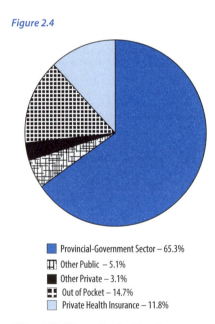

- ■ Hospitals – 29.5%
- ▦ Drugs – 16.5%
- ■ Physicians – 14.6%
- ▣ Other Professionals – 9.8%
- ☐ Other Health Spending – 6.0%
- ⊟ Public Health – 5.2%
- ▨ Administration – 3.1%
- ■ Capital – 4.9%
- ▨ Other Institutions – 10.4%

- ■ Provincial-Government Sector – 65.3%
- ▦ Other Public – 5.1%
- ■ Other Private – 3.1%
- ▦ Out of Pocket – 14.7%
- ☐ Private Health Insurance – 11.8%

What is the Money Being Spent On?

Source: National Health Expenditure Database, CIHI, 2011 Actual Data. Used with permission from the Canadian Institute for Health Information.

Where is the Money Coming From?

Source: National Health Expenditure Database, CIHI, 2011 Actual Data. Used with permission from the Canadian Institute for Health Information.

On average, the provinces/territories spend 40% of their annual budgets on health care. This leaves provinces/territories with the challenge of continuing to fund other important programs and services (e.g., education, social, transportation, etc.), with approximately 60% of their budgets. Future increases in the federal government health care transfers to the provinces/territories have been capped. As a result, the provinces/territories will receive less future federal funding for health care compared to past funding arrangements. This will result in provinces/territories aggressively searching for new approaches to deliver health care in more cost-efficient and cost-effective ways.

Drug expenditures make up the second-largest category of national health care expenditures—$33 billion or 16.5% (2011 data). The sources of funding for national drug expenditures are 63.7% private sector and 36.3% public sector (2011 data). In 2011, 84.6% of total expenditure on drugs was for prescribed drugs and of this portion, 36.3% is public sector and 48.3% is private sector. The remaining 15.4% of private sector drug expenditures is for non-prescription (OTC) drugs. More than half of public drug spending (60.8%) was for a small proportion of individuals (12.7%), where $2500 or more was paid for annual drug costs. Conversely, 6.2% of public drug program spending was for more than half (52.1%), where $500 or less was paid for annual drug costs (see Figure 2.5).[15]

The average annual growth of 10.1% was observed in retail prescription expenditures between 1998 and 2007. The main drivers for these increases were changes in volume and treatment mix effects (attributable to changes in treatment guidelines, increased disease prevalence and the uptake of new drugs). Population growth and aging had a modest impact, and drug price changes had no impact. Three drug categories, cholesterol-lowering drugs, cancer drugs and immuno-suppressants, accounted for roughly one-third of overall growth in drug spending. A substantial

Figure 2.5

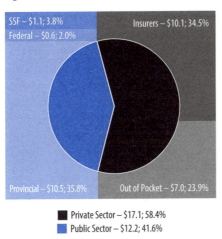

SSF – $1.1; 3.8%
Federal – $0.6; 2.0%
Insurers – $10.1; 34.5%
Provincial – $10.5; 35.8%
Out of Pocket – $7.0; 23.9%

Private Sector – $17.1; 58.4%
Public Sector – $12.2; 41.6%

Prescribed Drug Expenditure by Source of Funding, 2013

Source: National Health Expenditure Database, CIHI, 2013.
Used with permission from the Canadian Institute for Health Information.

number of drug patents are set to expire in the short term and this will result in increased availability of generic drugs. Savings to public and private drug plan expenditures are expected from
the short-term increase in new generic drugs.[16] For the future, the drug classes know as biologics
and biosimilars will dominate pharmaceutical spending.

Health care expenditures will always be in the spotlight even when there are periods of slower
growth rates. Health care expenditures will always constitute a significant proportion of expenditures in relation to all other expenditure categories. The two main stakeholders, governments
and employers, will continue to be pressured to closely monitor and find strategies to reduce the
growth in health care and pharmaceutical expenditures. Expenditures for pharmaceuticals and
for reimbursement to pharmacies/pharmacists will always be under scrutiny. It is unlikely that
any new funds will be made available to fund new programs or volume increases. Increasingly,
we will see governments and employers prioritizing and redirecting funds from one program to
another. Also, there will likely be more scenarios where a public or private sector payer eliminates funding for a program and service and leaves it to clients to pay for the program or service
expense out of their own pocket.

SOCIAL FACTORS AND TRENDS

Through consumer behaviour, social factors impact both the business and practice aspects of
community pharmacy. These factors are important in the consumer decision-making process
for purchasing prescription services, OTC medications and other community pharmacy products and services. The following social subfactors were identified: changing population demographics, increased use of communications technology and consumer interest in self-care/
self-management.

The major population demographic factor that will impact health care and community pharmacy is the increasing proportion of those 65+ years old.[17,18] Canadian statistics show that the
number of Canadians aged 65 and older is close to 5 million (14.8% of the total population). The
number in the 65+-year-old age group has increased 14.1% in the period 2006 to 2011. The
next wave of seniors in the 60- to 64-year-old age group increased 29.1% in the same period.
This trend will continue for another 15 years as the remainder of the baby boom population
age (8.2 million individuals born between the years 1946 and 1965). See the Statistics Canada
population pyramid[19] to visualize the shift in the shape of the Canadian population pyramid for
the period 1921 to 2011 and the growth in the 65+ age category. This group will, on average,
utilize more prescriptions compared to those in earlier generations.

Consumer behaviour is being shaped by the use of communications technology. A 2012
study reported that 84% of Canadians are connected to the Internet and, on average, had 2.6
Internet-capable devices per user. One-half of these Canadians search the Internet before purchase, review sites before buying, search for the best place to buy and buy products online.[20]
These consumer behaviours are being observed in the pharmaceutical sector. Several websites exist for consumers to conduct research about their medications, including comparisons
between medications (e.g., WebMD, RxList, etc.). Community pharmacy corporations have
comprehensive websites with applications including the following: online prescription refills,
transferring prescriptions, information about product recalls, product advertisements, information about pharmacist services, pharmacy locators, loyalty program information, information

about pharmacist clinics including online booking, self-reporting and diarizing of tests (e.g., blood pressure), health self-assessments, secure access to personal medication profile, requests for home delivery, selected online product purchasing, price checkers, online queries and questions, links to other online resources and general information about health.

Consumers and families provide significant self-care for acute conditions and increasing levels of self-management for chronic conditions. Self-care is an under-reported component of our health care delivery system. Most adults consider self-care first for minor ailments. Reports indicate that 81% of adults use OTC medicines as the first response to minor ailments. US consumers make 26 trips per year to purchase OTC products and visit their doctor 3 times per year. It is estimated that 70% to 90% of all illness episodes are addressed with self-treatment. Self-care products are widely available. In the US, there are 54,000 pharmacies and more the 750,000 retail outlets that sell OTC products. Self-care saves the health care system money (estimated in the US that every dollar spent on OTC medicines saves the system $6 to $7). About 89% of consumers believe that OTC medicines are an important component of their overall family health care.[21] Self-management is included in formal chronic disease management programs. Evidence indicates that interventions to support self-management programs of chronic conditions lead to improved outcomes.[22]

TECHNOLOGICAL FACTORS AND TRENDS

Technology is a strong macro-environmental factor impacting community pharmacy. The following technological subfactors are significant to pharmacy: introduction of new pharmaceuticals, medical devices, information and communications technology and automation.

Pharmaceuticals (as a technology) reduce the need for other interventions (e.g., institutional care, emergency care, etc.) and they continue as the most common type of treatment intervention in our health care system. A constant stream of new pharmaceuticals has significantly reduced morbidity and mortality in several conditions (e.g., cancer, cardiovascular, mental health, AIDS, etc.). Many "transformative" drugs and classes of drugs were introduced in the past 25 years. The following is a list of "transformative" drugs/classes and their area of use as identified in one report.[23]

- ACE (angiotensin-converting enzyme) inhibitors (nephrology/cardiology)
- Alglucerase (genetics)
- Anti-VEGF (vascular endothelial growth factor) agents (ophthalmology)
- Bisphosphonates (endocrinology/rheumatology)
- Epoprostenol (pulmonary medicine)
- Fluoxetine (psychiatry)
- HIV protease inhibitors (infectious disease)
- Imatinib (oncology)
- Lovastatin (cardiology)
- Omeprazole (gastroenterology)
- Propofol (anaesthesia)
- TNF (tumour necrosis factor) blockers (dermatology, gastroenterology, rheumatology)
- Sildenafil (urology)
- Sumatriptan (neurology)

Community and hospital pharmacies maintain the supply chain and pharmacists provide patient-focused consultative services over the market life of these and other pharmaceuticals. Pharmacy practice patterns have evolved as new pharmaceuticals/classes have been introduced and as these pharmaceuticals have been added to clinical practice guidelines. For example, current pharmacist standards of practice provide guidance about the pharmacist's roles and responsibilities for the administration of injectable medications and for monitoring compliance for medications that pose risk to patients. Most medications in the biologic class or bio-similar require injection and close monitoring. Chronic medications that are taken for a long duration (e.g., bisphosphonates) require pharmacist monitoring for compliance and risk of adverse events.

There are several sources of information about new or emerging medications. In Canada, the Canadian Agency for Drugs and Technologies in Health (CADTH) is a valuable source for new medications and devices. CADTH is responsible for the common drug review process and the pan-Canadian Oncology Drug Review process. CADTH publishes various reports, reviews and scans about recently approved and emerging drugs and technologies.[24] Walgreens publishes the quarterly *Pipeline Report* on specialty medications that will be approved by the US FDA within a few years. The report is divided into the following subsections: medications to watch, medications recently approved, pipeline medications in phase III trials, new dosage forms in the pipeline and new indications in pipeline. The medications are organized according to the disease or condition where the medication will be used.[25] Prescribing information about the specialty medications in the Walgreens' report can be found through the Daily Med website.[26] Reviews of these information sources provide pharmacists with information to assess practice and business implications, opportunities and threats associated with new and emerging medications and technologies.

The application of new information and communications technologies has been a significant part of pharmacy practice for more than 30 years.[27] The introduction of the personal computer in the early 1980s led to the development and use of pharmacy enterprise systems. These systems were primarily used for prescription processing, drug plan claims adjudication, inventory management and patient record documentation. Beginning in the early 2000s, the development and implementation of electronic health records, including drug information systems, led to upgrades to pharmacy enterprise systems to allow pharmacies to be integrated with the electronic health record. Enterprise systems are being modified to allow pharmacist documentation of patient-focused services provided. This information, along with drug information, is being included within electronic health records. Pharmacy information is being shared with other health care providers, and information from other health care providers is now accessible to pharmacists. Building on current electronic health and medical record platforms, development is now taking place on new e-health applications such as e-prescribing, e-visits, e-views, e-renewal/refills and e-scheduling. The electronic sharing of information with other health care professionals is improving coordination, safety and efficiency of patient-care services.[28]

The introduction of new and improved technologies has significantly impacted and changed retail business practices. For example, technologies such as product procurement software and retail point-of-sale (POS) systems have impacted inventory management. The availability of corporate websites, applications for Internet shopping and interactive voice response systems has changed the dynamics of customer relations. The automation of work processes through robotics has resulted in improvements in quality, safety and efficiency.

The communication technology "telepharmacy" includes videoconferencing using web-based software programs and telephone communications, where communications are two-way. Through the use of this technology, pharmacists are able to remotely provide management or patient-care activities. Telepharmacy is enabling pharmacists to expand services and improve quality and efficiency.

Developments in pharmacy automation began in the 1970s with the addition of electronic tablet counters. In the late 1990s and early 2000s, robotic prescription-dispensing systems, decentralized automated-dispensing cabinets and unit dose medication repackaging systems were introduced. These technologies have been refined over the years, and the devices can be linked to pharmacy enterprise systems. These systems improve efficiency, reduce costs and improve safety and service.

There has been continuous development of point-of-care devices. Point-of-care testing (POCT) is available for blood glucose testing, blood gas and electrolytes analysis, rapid coagulation testing, rapid cardiac markers diagnostics, drugs of abuse screening, urine strips testing, pregnancy testing, fecal occult blood analysis, food pathogens screening, hemoglobin diagnostics, infectious disease testing and cholesterol screening. Patients are using point-of-care devices or apps on smart phones or tablet computers to diarize and transmit test results to health care providers. POCT provides patient-specific current information.[29]

OPPORTUNITIES AND THREATS

Based on the PEST analysis, the following were identified as opportunities and threats for each macro-environmental factor or trend.

POLITICAL OPPORTUNITIES AND THREATS

Until the mid-2000s, macro-environmental impact of the political system on community pharmacy was minimal. The situation changed when provincial/territorial governments independently supported expanded scope of pharmacist practice legislation and implemented community pharmacy reimbursement reforms.

The legislative changes in pharmacist scope of practice vary between the provinces/territories. Preliminary reports from provinces/territories where these changes have been made indicate the impact from these expanded services has been significant to improve patient access and convenience. In provinces/territories where pharmacists administer injections, public access to vaccinations has increased significantly for residents. Similarly, where pharmacists renew/extend prescriptions or change dosage/formulation, the positive impact on patient access and convenience has been significant. It is anticipated that similar results will be observed as the scope of pharmacist practice is expanded in all jurisdictions. For specific information about regulatory reforms (implemented or in progress), see Canadian Pharmacists Association.[30]

The prevailing community pharmacy business model and economic situation was relatively stable until the wave of provincial/territorial government policy changes to prohibit/limit professional allowances, implement generic drug reimbursement price caps, implement brand-name drug product listing agreements and implement alternative reimbursement frameworks to pay for pharmacist patient-focused services. Private drug plans have implemented generic drug reimbursement price caps. The public sector policies significantly reduced community pharmacy incentives related to drug distribution and created incentives for pharmacies to pro-vide patient-focused services. The private drug plan policies reduced incentives related to generic drug distribution. The policy changes have resulted in pharmacy corporations conducting sub-stantial reviews of their business models and business plans. The difference between for-public- and private-sector reimbursement models has required pharmacy corporations to create separate business models and plans for the two sectors.

The following major opportunities are associated with political macro-environmental factors:

- continued refinement and spread of provincial/territorial public policies related to the implementation of pharmacy professional regulatory reforms (expanded scope of pharmacy practice) and the implementation of new alternative payment plans for pharmacist services
- acceptance of new alternative payment plans for pharmacist services in private drug plans and in Health Canada supplemental plans (for First Nations, Inuit, Canadian Forces, veterans, etc.)

The major threats are as follows:

- significant variation and/or limited pharmacists' uptake of the expanded scope of practice frameworks
- limited pharmacy utilization of alternative payment systems (in drug plan budgeting, financial decisions about the drug plan budget are determined annually and previous-year savings cannot be carried forward to next-year budgets)

ECONOMIC OPPORTUNITIES AND THREATS

Health care and pharmaceutical expenditures continue to increase annually and this cre-ates a challenge for provincial/territorial governments in balancing their annual budgets. The increasing share of provincial/territorial expenditures allocated for health care requires further cost-constraint policies so that other non-health provincial/territorial government services and programs can be provided. Similarly, the continued increase in health care and pharmaceutical expenses provides a similar challenge to employers in managing employee supplementary health care benefit programs. As a result, pharmaceutical expenses will always be on the radar screen of public and private drug plan managers, and reimbursement for pharmaceuticals and pharmacy/ pharmacist professional services will continue to be subject to further cost-constraint policies.

The following are major economic opportunities:

- for pharmacy advocacy organizations to develop business cases for public- and private-sector payers about the economic benefits of implementing community pharmacy and pharmacist services
- for provincial/territorial advocacy organizations to seek further revisions to the first-generation alternate reimbursement programs (e.g., definitions of services, adjustments to maximum fees schedules and the establishment of new fee codes for new services)
- for community pharmacy management to continue to be vigilant in searching for cost-efficient and cost-effective pharmacist services and operating systems
- for community pharmacy organizations to develop and implement pharmacist service programs and alternative reimbursement models for non-insured clients (e.g., cash-paying customers) or for clients with discretionary health care spending accounts

The major economic threat is as follows:

- public and private payers implementing cost-constraint policies that will be applied to drug reimbursement and new reimbursement programs for patient-focused pharmacist services (drug plans will not allow for open-ended annual expense budget relating to payments for pharmacist services)

SOCIAL OPPORTUNITIES AND THREATS

Community pharmacy service organizations have a strong record of reacting to changes in consumer needs and behaviour that lead to increased revenues and profit. Where there is a strong business case and the consumer needs and demand for products and services are strong, the industry has responded well (e.g., product categories such as natural health products, immunization programs). Where the business case is weaker, and consumer demand is weak or unknown, the pharmacy service provider's response has been cautious (e.g., provision of medication therapy management). It is anticipated that these pharmacy service organizations will continue to respond to the opportunities and threats associated with social factors and trends.

The major opportunities are as follows:

- There will be a continued demand for pharmacists to provide consultations on minor ailments and self-care conditions (for OTC medications and related health care supplies).
- The demand will increase for well-designed community pharmacy medication therapy management programs (based on self-management principles) to complement general chronic disease self-management programs.
- Increased revenues (and potentially profits) will result from the growth in prescription volumes from the continued growth in the 65-years-and-older population segment.
- The demand will increase for pharmacists to fill the role as an apomediary (professional who stands by and offers Internet guidance and information).

The following are the major threats:

- Community pharmacies will not be able to balance the increased demand for prescription services and maintain the impetus to fulfill the opportunities enabled through the expanded scope of practice frameworks.
- Other health care professionals (e.g., physicians, nurses) will expand their roles in areas such as drug distribution, prescribing, immunizations and medication therapy management.

TECHNOLOGICAL OPPORTUNITIES AND THREATS

Pharmacists are accustomed to the continual introduction of new pharmaceutical products (technologies). Through pharmacy organizational policies and pharmacist continuing professional development, community pharmacies and pharmacists have seamlessly provided these products and the associated services. It is anticipated that this capacity will continue for the constant stream of new pharmaceuticals.

Community pharmacies were early adopters of technology with the adoption of pharmacy computer enterprise systems in the 1980s and automated pharmacy dispensing systems in the 2000s. With the more widespread adoption of technology within the health care system (e.g., electronic health records, telemedicine and mobile devices), a new set of opportunities and threats exists for the integration of these technologies within community pharmacy. The business case for the adoption of the newer technologies has favoured the status quo. It is anticipated that the business case will change when the changes in the pharmacy reimbursement model are considered.

The following opportunities have been identified with technological environmental factors:

- The need/demand for an efficient, reliable and accessible supply chain for distribution of pharmaceuticals directly to the population will continue as an essential role in our health care system. Community pharmacies have carried out this role well, and it positions the community pharmacist to carry out patient-focused activities.
- The scope and pace of provincial/territorial e-health initiatives are changing with more provinces/territories focusing on drug information systems early in the implementation of provincial/territorial electronic health records. This opportunity will allow increased numbers of pharmacists to be supported in expanded scopes of practice and participate in team-based care from access to the electronic health record and e-health initiatives (e.g., e-prescribing, e-refills/renewals, e-visits, e-scheduling).
- Increasing numbers of community pharmacies will upgrade their pharmacy enterprise systems to integrate within provincial/territorial e-health initiatives. This will result in improved work processes for effective documentation of clinical activities from software improvements.
- Increased automation device options (e.g., size, numbers of suppliers) will improve the business case for more community pharmacies to make the decision to acquire and implement automated robotic prescription-dispensing systems.
- With expanded pharmacist scope of practice and reimbursement for patient-focused services, more pharmacists are providing medication therapy management services. A large potential primary health care retail market exists for point-of-care testing devices. The community pharmacy is well positioned to become the lead retailer and expert for these devices in the primary health care setting.

The main threats to macro-environmental technology factors are as follows:

- poor rates of pharmacy uptake of technology (e.g., electronic health records, new types of automation)
- pharmacy regulatory organizations not being able to keep pace with emerging technologies
- pharmacy software developers not being able to make revisions to current pharmacy enterprise system software to support expanded scope of practice

PEST analysis provides a simple and practical framework for managers to examine the complex macro-environment for any organization. The PEST analysis was applied at a high level for community pharmacy organizations.

Three environmental political subfactors were identified as having significant impact on the internal environment of community pharmacy. These subfactors were governments (mainly at the provincial/territorial level), employers (sponsors for private drug plans) and pharmacy organizations (with regulatory and advocacy roles). Provincial/Territorial governments have enabled pharmacy regulatory organizations to implement regulatory reforms to expand the scope of

pharmacist practice. Provincial/Territorial governments and employers have introduced reimbursement policy reforms to reduce financial incentives related to drug distribution. Provincial/
Territorial governments have implemented reimbursement reforms to support pharmacists to
deliver patient-focused services. The main opportunity is for continued refinement and spread
of regulatory reform of pharmacists' expanded scope of practice and alternative payment frameworks. The major threat is that poor uptake by pharmacists of current reforms will occur and
policy makers will reduce their commitment.

One environmental economic factor was identified as being significant, namely the economic
state of Canada's health care system. The trend for continued growth in health care expenditures presents a major challenge for provincial/territorial governments and employers who
are the major funding source and have limits to their budgets. Next to hospital expenditures,
pharmaceutical expenditures continue to grow and be the second-largest expenditure category.
Pharmaceutical expenditures (including payments for pharmacy and pharmacist services) will
be in the spotlight of decision makers because of their growth and their prominence as a key
health care expenditure. Cost effectiveness and efficiency will be an ongoing priority for funding decisions. The opportunities are to refine first-generation alternative reimbursement models, expand alternative reimbursement models to private insurance and continually improve
efficiency and effectiveness of pharmacist services. The major threat is that payers will reduce
budgets for alternative reimbursement programs.

The following were identified as significant social environmental factors: the increasing proportion of the population in the 65-years-old and older age bracket, consumers' high use of the
Internet for buying and consumers' continued high reliance on self-care for minor ailments and
self-management for chronic conditions. The opportunities include additional revenue from
increased prescription volume and reimbursement for pharmacist OTC counselling, a new
role in the provision of drug information and improved uptake of pharmacy-based chronic disease management programs. The threats are the inability to balance and respond to consumer
demands and competition to respond to consumer needs from other health care professionals.

The introduction of new technologies and refinements to existing technologies will continue
to have a major impact on community pharmacy. As a technology and treatment intervention,
pharmaceuticals have had a major impact on health care processes and outcomes. There will be
continual introduction of new breakthrough pharmaceuticals and incremental improvements
to existing pharmaceuticals. Community pharmacy's legitimized role as the primary distributor
of prescription and scheduled drugs to the population will position the industry well to have
greater opportunities than threats relating to the introduction of new pharmaceuticals. New and
improved information and communications technology (e.g., electronic health records, telemedicine and automation) will be introduced to improve efficiency, quality and safety of operating systems and processes. The opportunities are for improved work processes and outputs,
increased capacity to provide pharmacist services and enabling integration within the health care
team. The threats are poor implementation support and incomplete pharmacy adoption.

In conclusion, the principles and concepts of a PEST analysis were described and an example PEST analysis was conducted. The analysis illustrated that each of the four general macro-
environmental factors (political, economic, social and technological) has a significant impact

on the community pharmacy organization. Depending on the complexity of the general factor, there were one to three subfactors associated with each general factor. The collective impact of the community pharmacy macro-environment is highly significant. On balance, there are a similar number of opportunities and threats associated with the four factors and subfactors. The analysis shows that community pharmacy organizations have many potential opportunities to act on and many potential threats to prevent or mitigate. Usually, these opportunities and threats would be considered and addressed through the pharmacy organization's strategic, business and/or marketing plans.

RESOURCES AND SUGGESTED READINGS

Useful Canadian websites for conducting pharmacy PEST analysis:

Canada Health Infoway. Available: www.infoway-inforoute.ca (accessed April 29, 2014).

Canadian Agency for Drugs and Technology in Health. Available: www.cadth.ca. (accessed April 29, 2014).

Canadian Generic Pharmaceutical Association. Available: www.canadiangenerics.ca (accessed Aug. 29, 2014).

Canadian Institute for Health Information (CIHI). Available: www.cihi.ca (accessed April 29, 2014).

Canadian Life and Health Insurance Association. Available: www.clhia.ca. (accessed April 28, 2014).

Canadian Pharmacists Association (CPhA). Available: www.pharmacists.ca (accessed Aug. 29, 2014).

Canadian Society of Hospital Pharmacists (CSHP). Available: www.cshp.ca (accessed Aug. 29, 2014).

Council of the Federation. Available: www.councilofthefederation.ca (accessed April 28, 2014).

Health Canada. Available: www.hc-sc.gc.ca (accessed Apr. 29, 2014).

Health Council of Canada. Available: www.healthcouncilcanada.ca (accessed April 29, 2014).

Industry Canada. Available: www.ic.gc.ca (accessed April 29, 2014).

National Association of Pharmacy Regulatory Authorities. What's New: Pharmacy Technician Bridging Education Program Course and PLAR Exam Schedules. Available: www.napra.ca/pages/home/default.aspx (accessed Aug. 29, 2014).

Patented Medicine Prices Review Board. Available: www.pmprb-cepmb.gc.ca (accessed Aug. 29, 2014).

Public Health Agency of Canada. Available: www.phac-aspc.gc.ca (accessed April 29, 2014).

Rx and D. Ottawa. Rx and D – Canada's Research Based Pharmaceutical Companies, 2014. Available from www.canadapharma. org (accessed Aug. 28, 2014).

Science and Technology. Ottawa: Government of Canada, Industry Canada – Science and Technology, 2014. Available: www. ic.gc.ca (accessed April 29, 2014).

Statistics Canada. Available: www.statcan.gc.ca/start-debut-eng.html (accessed April 29, 2014).

The Conference Board of Canada. Ottawa: The Conference Board of Canada, 2014. Available: www.conferenceboard.ca (accessed April 29, 2014).

REFERENCES

1. Day GS, Schoemaker PJ. Scanning the periphery. Harv Bus Rev. 2005;83(11):135–40, 142, 144–8 passim. Medline:16299966

2. Whittington Goldstone L, Kennedy AK, Clark JS, et al. Developing and evaluating clinical pharmacy services. In: Chisholm-Burns MA, Vaillancourt AM, Shepherd M, editors. *Pharmacy management, leadership, marketing, and finance*. 2nd ed. Burlington, MA: Jones and Bartlett Learning; 2014. p. 199–216.

3. Tools M. *PEST analysis*. London, UK: Mind Tools Ltd; 2014. Available: www.mindtools.com/pages/article/newTMC_09.htm [cited 2014 April 29].

4. Health Canada. Canada's health care system. Ottawa: Government of Canada, Health Canada, 2014. Available: www.hc-sc. gc.ca/hcs-sss/pubs/system-regime/2011-hcs-sss/index-eng.php (accessed April 28, 2014).

5. Affairs I. *The constitutional distribution of legislative powers*. Ottawa: Government of Canada; 2013. Available: http://www.pco-bcp.gc.ca/aia/index.asp?lang=eng&page=federal&doc=legis-eng.htm [cited 2014 April 28].

6. Almarsdóttir AB, Traulsen JM. Studying and evaluating pharmaceutical policy--becoming a part of the policy and consultative process. Pharm World Sci. 2006;28(1):6–12. http://dx.doi.org/10.1007/s11096-006-9011-0. Medline:16810452

7. Canadian Institute for Health Information. National prescription drug utilization information system – NPDUIS database – plan information document. Ottawa: Canadian Institute for Health Information, 2013. Available: https://secure.cihi.ca/free_ products/NPDUIS_SummaryOfChanges_1307_e1.pdf (accessed April 29, 2014).

8. Canadian Pharmacists Association. Summary of pharmacists' expanded scope of practice in Canada. Ottawa: Canadian Pharmacists Association, 2014. Available: http://blueprintforpharmacy.ca/docs/pdfs/scope-of-practice_eng-dec-19-2014. pdf (accessed Jan. 29, 2015).

9. Council of the Federation. Ottawa: Council of the Federation secretariat, 2013. Available from www.councilofthefederation.ca/en/ (accessed April 28, 2014).

10. Long S. Creating pharmaceutical policy. Lecture presented for University of Alberta Pharmacy 494 Fall 2012 Term; 2012 Sep 27; Edmonton, AB.

11. Canadian Life and Health Insurance Association Inc. Industry key statistics. Toronto: Canadian Life and Health Insurance Association Inc. 2014. Available: www.clhia.ca/domino/html/clhia/clhia_lp4w_lnd_webstation.nsf/page/40BC606F18B5CE CE8525780E00664EBE!OpenDocument (accessed Aug. 29, 2014).

12. Canadian Life and Health Insurance Association Inc. A guide to supplementary insurance. Toronto: Canadian Life and Health Insurance Association Inc. 2014. Available: http://clhia.uberflip.com/i/199452 (accessed Aug. 29, 2014).

13. Canadian Life and Health Insurance Association Inc. CLHIA report on prescription drug policy – ensuring the accessibility, affordability and sustainability of prescription drugs in Canada. Toronto: Canadian Life and Health Insurance Association Inc. 2013. Available: http://www.clhia.ca/domino/html/clhia/CLHIA_LP4W_LND_Webstation.nsf/resources/CLHIA_Prescription_Drug_Paper/$file/CLHIA_Prescription_Drug_Policy_PaperEN.pdf (accessed April 29, 2014).

14. Canadian Institute for Health Information. CIHI – national health expenditure trends – 1975–2013. Ottawa: Canadian Institute for Health Information, 2014. Available: https://secure.cihi.ca/free_products/NHEXTrendsReport_EN.pdf (accessed April 29, 2014).

15. Canadian Institute for Health Information. CIHI – drug expenditure in Canada – 1975–2012. Ottawa: Canadian Institute for Health Information, 2013. Available: https://secure.cihi.ca/free_products/Drug_Expenditure_2013_EN.pdf (accessed April 29, 2014).

16. Canadian Institute for Health Information. CIHI – prescribed drug spending in Canada, 2012: a focus on public drug programs. Ottawa: Canadian Institute for Health Information, 2014. Available: https://secure.cihi.ca/estore/productFamily.htm?locale=en&pf=PFC2499 (accessed April 29, 2014).

17. Statistics Canada. Canada year book, 2012. Ottawa: Government of Canada. 2013. Available: www.statcan.gc.ca/pub/11-402-x/index-eng.htm (accessed April 29, 2014).

18. Statistics Canada. The Canadian population in 2011: age and sex. Ottawa: Government of Canada, 2014. Available: http://www12.statcan.gc.ca/census-recensement/2011/as-sa/98-311-x/98-311-x2011001-eng.cfm (accessed Apr 29, 2014).

19. Statistics Canada. Historical age pyramid. Ottawa: Government of Canada; 2011. Available: www12.statcan.gc.ca/census-recensement/2011/dp-pd/pyramid-pyramide/his/index-eng.cfm (accessed April 29, 2014).

20. Business Development Bank of Canada. Mapping your future growth – Five game changing consumer trends. Ottawa: Business Development Bank of Canada, 2013. Available: www.bdc.ca/EN/Documents/analysis_research/Report_BDC_Mapping_your_future_growth.pdf#search=%22mapping%22 (accessed Aug. 29, 2014).

21. Consumer Health Products Association. OTC value – statistics on OTC use. Washington: Consumer Health Products Association, 2014. Available: www.chpa.org/MarketStats.aspx (accessed Aug. 29, 2014).

22. Agency for Healthcare Research and Quality. Patient self-management support programs; an evaluation. Rockville: Agency for Healthcare Research and Quality. Prepared by Rand Health. 2007. Available: www.ahrq.gov/research/findings/final-reports/ptmgmt/index.html (accessed Aug 29, 2014).

23. Kesselheim AS, Avorn J. The most transformative drugs of the past 25 years: a survey of physicians. Nat Rev Drug Discov. 2013;12(6):425–31. http://dx.doi.org/10.1038/nrd3977. Medline:23681007

24. Canadian Agency for Drugs and Technology in Health. Ottawa: Canadian Agency for Drugs and Technology in Health, 2014. Available: www.cadth.ca (accessed Aug. 29, 2014).

25. Walgreens. Quarterly Pipeline Report. Deerfield: Walgreens. 2013. Available: www.walgreens.com/pdf/newsletterreport/Pipeline_Report_4Q2013.pdf (accessed Aug. 29, 2014).

26. US National Library of Medicine. Daily Med. Washington: US National Library of Medicine, 2014. Available: http://dailymed.nlm.nih.gov/dailymed/index.cfm (accessed Aug. 29, 2014).

27. Gomez TA, Norman CM, Chisholm-Burns MA. Pharmacy operations: workflow, practice activities, medication safety, and technology. In: Chisholm-Burns MA, Vaillancourt AM, Shepherd M, editors. *Pharmacy Management, Leadership, Marketing, and Finance*. 2nd ed. Burlington, MA: Jones and Bartlett Learning; 2014. p. 143–62.

28. Canada Health Infoway. Toronto: Canada Health Infoway, 2014. Available: www.infoway-inforoute.ca (accessed April 29, 2014).

29. Publications T. Trimark Publications, 2014. Available: www.trimarkpublications.com/products/Point-of-Care-Diagnostic-Testing-World-Markets.html (accessed May 29, 2014).

30. Blueprint for Pharmacy. Policy changes by region. Ottawa: Canadian Pharmacists Association, 2014. Available: http://blueprintforpharmacy.ca/policy-changes-by-region (accessed April 29, 2014).

CHAPTER 3

Micro-environmental Analysis

Roderick A. Slavcev, *PhD, MBA, MSB, C.Biol; Assistant Professor, School of Pharmacy, University of Waterloo*

Learning Objectives

- Understand industry forces in a pharmacy perspective: rivalry; new entrants; power of suppliers, buyers and substitutes; assessing the attractiveness of an industry.

- Understand distribution versus clinical practice model: competitive positioning and lifecycle analysis; market lifecycle; strategic groups; industry overview.

THE INDUSTRY FIVE FORCES

Chapter 2 examines tools to assess the macro-environment that applies to an industry. The elements of PEST (political, economic, social and technological) analysis identify trends and forces that are not necessarily specific or directed to an industry, but may impart enormous impact and influence upon it. This chapter examines a more granular and microscopic analysis—the industry itself.

An industry can be viewed as a group of firms offering products and/or services that are close substitutes for each other, satisfying the same basic consumer need(s). An essential industry analysis framework was developed in 1979 by Harvard Business School's Michael Porter.[1] Porter is one of the most influential contributors to organizational strategy, and his work on competitive strategy and industry organization is recognized and applied to strategic planning around the world in all industry sectors. Porter's Five Forces Model is an essential industry analysis tool employed to identify industry trends, threats and opportunities, and to assess the overall attractiveness of an industry. The tool identifies potential threats across five essential dimensions within any industry: threat of rivalry caused by existing competition within the industry itself; threat of new entrants; bargaining power of buyers; suppliers; and threat of substitutes. This micro-environmental industry analysis in combination with the PEST macro-environmental analysis paints a picture of the current condition and trends in which an organization exists, and it serves to identify current and/or future opportunities and threats impacting it (see Figure 3.1).

Figure 3.1

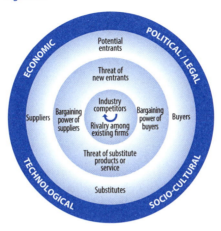

Organization's business landscape including indirect/direct impact by components of PEST analysis outside of the industry and Porter's five identified industry forces acting directly on the industry[1]

Identified threats arising from each of these dimensions can be gauged as low, medium or high to guide the overall assessment of the industry and the organization's position within it. Recognizing the degree to which each of the five dimensions threaten or may threaten an organization permits the proactive development of strategies during the strategic planning process (see Section II: Analysis and Planning) to mitigate these threats where possible, and/or benefit from non-threatening opportunities. This chapter examines the components of the five forces and some simplified examples to illustrate the concepts, but also to apply the framework to pharmacy—contrasting retail pharmacy drug distribution with clinical practice business models. An augmented version of the model was later developed by Sharon Oster in 1995 in her book *Strategic Management for Nonprofit Organizations: Theory and Cases*, deemed to better identify the forces impacting not-for-profit organizations.[2] Although the impact of the public and government is relevant to pharmacy, for the sake of simplicity, this chapter adheres to Porter's original five forces impacting an industry.

FORCE 1: RIVALRY

Rivalry, or the threat of competition, is a critical *force* to consider in evaluating the attractiveness of an industry and an organization's current and future threats and opportunities. Rivalry refers to the degree of competition or supply that can threaten the size of the slice of pie or market share of an organization. Elevated competition drives down the price of a product or service, particularly for undifferentiated goods that are uniform across suppliers, referred to as *commodities*. Firms, in turn, suffer reduced margins and must minimize costs to remain competitive, or increase volume of sales to meet revenue targets.

While the lists that follow, impacting each of the forces, are not exhaustive, they serve to provide a working understanding of the concept impacting an organization. Further itemized explanation of the framework and its components are readily available through several free online sources (e.g., QuickMBA, CGMA 2).

Factors influencing rivalry:

- industry concentration
- product differentiation
- fixed costs
- strategic groups
- product lifecycle positioning

Industry concentration refers to the number of firms possessing the majority of the available market share.[3] The greater the number of players within the industry, the more intense is the expected competition. An industry with a large number of players, where no or few firms possess significant share of the market, is considered to be *fragmented*. Competition intensifies and leads to price wars in fragmented industries, where no one firm can influence the direction of the industry. In such industries, firms compete on price and will undercut each other in the attempt to gain market share from competitors.[4] Restaurants, clothing retail, agriculture and computer hardware are examples of fragmented industries, and firms within compete fiercely on price to gain market share, thereby narrowing margins. In contrast, within industries consisting of a few firms, an *oligopoly*, or where the majority of market share is owned by only a few large firms, the industry is *concentrated* and hence, disciplined with respect to pricing.[5] Due to the few competitors present, firms are less likely to threaten each other's profitability by engaging in irrational price wars, as all players' profitability would suffer in the process. Instead, firms practise discipline and seek to maximize their profitability, engaging in higher and comparative pricing. Contrast this to collusion, the illegal practice of price negotiation and agreement between firms, thereby constituting a *cartel*. Concentrated industries, such as oil and gas and pharmaceutical industries, are comprised of only a few large firms. As such, it is very uncommon to see competitors repeatedly undercut each other on price to gain market share. Instead, firms try to maintain a price that does not hinder market share position and maximizes profit for each. The remarkable degree of discipline practised by oil and gas firms and the fact that this commodity is priced according to global supply and demand leads many to believe that this industry is in fact a cartel and that firms must be engaging in collusion.

Attributes of a product or service that render it more unique or differentiated compared to other substitutes in the market that aim to accommodate the same or similar consumer need(s) benefit from *product differentiation*.[6] For instance, Lululemon is highly differentiated compared to other manufacturers of athletic wear. In addition to high-quality yoga gear, it carries with it a brand strongly contributed to by status, life beliefs, mental and physical health and a sense of belonging, all of which deliver additional customer value. With each purchase comes an experience rather than just a clothing product. These added benefits differentiate Lululemon's products from competitors, thereby offsetting rivalry, since its added features are unique and cannot be imitated to accommodate the exact customer experience despite being a very similar product. In contrast, *commodities*, or products that are generally quite uniform across the industry, are subject to rival on price alone as no additional features are available to offset competition between substitutes. At present in pharmacy, even if services may differ slightly between suppliers, patients may tend to attribute the prescription price to the product rather than the service, compromising efforts to differentiate.

Industries that face high *fixed costs* generally experience heightened rivalry. Fixed costs are simply costs that do not change regardless of the quantity of output. The fixed costs of getting a new drug to market, when considering previously failed products and opportunity costs, may range from approximately $800 million to $1.5 billion.[7] Thus, the first product to market carries that massive fixed cost and is reduced only by maximizing the volume produced, thereby reducing the fixed cost per unit. If an industry suffers from very high fixed costs, as does the pharmaceutical industry, then the need to mass produce to limit fixed cost per unit will increase rivalry in the industry. On the other hand, high fixed costs can also simultaneously serve as a powerful barrier to new entrants (visited later in the chapter). In Canada, price ceilings may help to control costs as drug prices for patented medicines are set by the federal government through the Patented Medicine Prices Review Board (PMPRB).

Retail pharmacy in Canada is becoming increasingly consolidated with 66% market share occupied by the three largest firms within the industry,[8] subjecting the industry to lower levels of pricing discipline. While the pricing of drugs, markup and dispensing fee limits are increasingly legislated by provincial/territorial governments, strategies of waiving co-payment (also known as co-pay), reducing or eliminating dispensing fees altogether are examples of price wars in the attempt to increase market share. Like the medications sold, retail pharmacy is a relatively undifferentiated service that is uniformly offered by other suppliers within the industry (commodity). The lack of uniqueness again serves to increase rivalry, forcing suppliers to compete on price alone. Strategic mergers between larger firms within the industry, also known as *horizontal integration*, can increase scale and reduce costs per unit for the firm, while also concentrating the industry to reduce rivalry. Examples include the major player Katz Group Pharmacies' acquisition of Ontario-based Dell Pharmacies in 2012, and Loblaw's 2013 acquisition of Shoppers Drug Mart, which itself continues to acquire independents.[8] This trend on the drug distribution side of the equation can be reasonably expected to continue, especially in light of poorly performing independents that pose easy acquisition targets. In contrast, pharmacy as a clinical consultative service can be quickly and easily differentiated by quality, specialization, patient experience, service, guarantees, disease prevention, service bundling and ultimately, improved patient health outcomes and quality of life over a cycle of treatment. Such differentiating approaches serve to improve delivered customer value that can come at a premium price and offset rivalry versus retail pharmacy and other clinical specialties alike.

HOW STRATEGIC GROUPS INFLUENCE RIVALRY

A strategic group would be a cluster of companies in an industry that follows similar strategies on the basis of similar endowments. The closer the strategic groups are to each other, the greater the rivalry.

One of the factors in considering rivalry within an industry is the occurrence of what are called *strategic groups*, a term coined by Hunt (1972) who noted the anomaly of a high degree of rivalry in the appliance industry, despite it being relatively concentrated.[9] In essence, strategic

groups are subgroups of competitors within an industry that generally employ the same strategies and business models to compete. This is to say that they possess similar resources and
deploy these resources with similar routines to do what they do best and gain a viable position
within the industry. For instance, for several decades Coca-Cola and Pepsi have occupied the
same strategic group within the beverage industry, increasing rivalry between them. In contrast, brand pharmaceutical firms employ very different strategies compared to generic suppliers and require different resources and capabilities and as such, they occupy different strategic
groups. The importance here is that the further the strategic groups are from each other within
an industry, the lower the rivalry between them. While rivalry is driven in part by the concentration of players within the industry, it is also important to consider the strategic groups
within which they reside. At present, retail pharmacies, while mildly differentiated between
each other, generally occupy the same strategic group. However, pharmacy skills deployed to
create novel business models revolving around clinical consultative practices offer the opportunity to develop unique strategic groups. As such, rivalry between strategic groups would be
reduced and thus, profitability improved.

Market growth, a market's demand for an industry's product/service offerings and an industry's
position within a product's lifecycle can provide essential information in assessing trends of
industry rivalry. The *product lifecycle theory* is a stylized temporal map of an average product or
services demand in the market developed by Raymond Vernon in 1966,[10] depicted in Figure 3.2.
Originally developed to explain international trade shifts in the market, the model is theoretical
in nature and rarely follows exactly the stages shown, but nonetheless serves to conceptually
position a market with respect to its growth or decline trend and predict its influence on rivalry
within the industry (see Chapter 50: Market Segmentation and Strategy).

Take, for example, the evolution of the wireless technologies market. In its embryonic stage,
while most customers were tied to telephone landlines, beepers and other substitutes, wireless
technology providers sought to educate the market of the benefits and improve this disruptive
technology. This stage involved educating about the benefits and increasing exposure to those
who were most likely to adopt the advantages of the technology and co-opt complementary

Figure 3.2

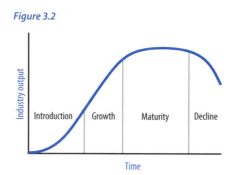

*Influence of Industry/Product
Lifecycle Theory on Rivalry[10]*

goods that would add value to the technology. The number of suppliers at this stage was initially limited. In the growth stage, first movers to the market benefited as new markets were developed and the new technology began to disrupt existing technology, becoming the technology paradigm. During this growth stage, while the exponentially growing market was seeking a cell phone, rivalry remained relatively low due to growing demand that benefited the margins of all suppliers and offset rivalry. However, new suppliers continued to pour into the market to benefit from the rapid growth, incrementally increasing rivalry. Eventually, the market was saturated for cell phones and demand declined. Now, too many suppliers occupied an industry supplying a mature market based *not* on growing customer acquisition of a cellular device, but rather only on replacement. Rivalry for the remaining demand became fierce and as cellular devices increasingly became commoditized, firms generally competed on price alone, shaking out firms that did not possess the scale and could not compete on cost.

Consider the implications of product lifecycle theory on pharmacy and how its position impacts the degree of rivalry within the industry. Pharmacists are currently the fastest-growing group of health care professionals in Canada, at almost 10% since 2012—more than double the growth rate of the Canadian labour force.[11] This growth of professional supply will require equivalent demand growth to employ this skilled labour pool that already faces more than 7% primary registered pharmacist unemployment.[11] This is largely due to the fact that the retail pharmacy growth rate has tapered and exhibits stagnation since 2012.[12,13] If pharmacists continue to primarily follow a product distribution technical service model, this trend suggests an imminent and growing oversupply that would continue to deteriorate the professional wage and commoditize the profession. Moreover, the excess supply suggests a mature market, whereby firms and professionals who cannot adequately compete on cost will be subject to *shake out*, thereby removing competitors who cannot reduce their costs per unit to compete in an industry increasing in rivalry. An increasingly aged population will certainly serve to increase market growth and reduce rivalry and industry restructuring in the meantime, driven by many trends and forces, will certainly favour those firms that possess the scale and cost advantages to capture the future drug distribution market. In addition, expanding scope of services increasingly offered by pharmacists will reduce costs and could instead serve to reinitiate growth by improving access to health care services, thereby reducing rivalry.

FORCE 2: THREAT OF NEW ENTRANTS

To assess the *threat of new entrants* into an industry, it is necessary to investigate and rank the existing barriers to entry. This simply amounts to evaluating how easily a new competitor can enter the industry, thereby adding supply and threatening a firm's market share—in effect making a firm's profit slice of the market pie smaller. Relevant entry barriers that can limit or prevent new entrants into an industry follow next.

Factors influencing new entrants:
- brand loyalty
- experience curve
- economies of scale
- switching costs

- capital requirements
- others

Brand loyalty can offer a powerful barrier to entry when existing players possess a very strong brand.[1] Consider buyers of products from the prominent computing company Apple, Inc. Many customers possess strong loyalty and would be far less likely to adopt a new cell phone, computer or tablet of any other brand. Similarly, patients who have experienced exceptional clinical service, be it from a dentist, physiotherapist, doctor or pharmacist, are less inclined to become a patient of a new entrant due to the loyalty they possess for their current clinical service provider. A strong reputation for clinical or other services confers a strong brand position and provides a barrier to new entrants. Contrast this against pharmacy as a commoditized distribution service for an undifferentiated good (medications). Some medications do themselves benefit from brand loyalty. For example, acetaminophen and ibuprofen are preferred and more trusted in their brand forms of Tylenol and Advil; however, their distribution is rather commoditized and this service, in many cases, does little to establish brand and establish a barrier to new entrants in this capacity. Patients suffering from chronic conditions and on several medications may indeed be far more likely to develop strong relationships with their pharmacists, in turn increasing brand loyalty, but this is more likely to be attributed to a trusted and repeated health care service around the medication rather than the provision of the medication itself.

An organization's *experience curve*[14] relates to cost advantages that can be enjoyed by a firm over time due to operational experience that serves to improve efficiency. Improved efficiency in turn reduces costs and may improve quality compared to a new entrant that would not benefit from this experience and, as such, would be at a cost disadvantage and more poorly positioned to compete. For example, many physicians with a long duration of practice and with extensive patient rosters have devised systems through experience to maximize efficiency without compromising quality of care. This would similarly apply to experienced pharmacies.

Economies of scale can best be described as the ability to minimize the cost for offering a product or service due to increased size, output or scale of operation.[15] This may translate into cheaper materials for production due to bulk buying or mass production, thereby minimizing the fixed cost per unit. Revisiting the drug development example, if the opportunity cost to get a new drug to market is $800 million, then the cost of that first marketed pill would also be $800 million. Again, the fixed cost per pill is reduced with each new pill made—by the second it is $400 million per pill, and by the four millionth it is $200 per pill and so on, thereby reducing fixed cost per unit through mass production. A chain pharmacy with a significant inventory would have lower costs for its products because it is able to buy in high volume or scale. Such economies of scale reduce costs for suppliers and, thus, may allow them to reduce their price as well, creating value for customers. New entrants may not be able to do so if they are entering with smaller scale and, thus, may be less able to compete on cost.

Switching costs pertain to the ease with which a customer may switch from one supplier's product(s) or service(s) to another.[16] Products/Services that are uniform across suppliers (i.e., commodities) may have very low switching costs as fewer time, energy, financial or psychological costs hinder the switch. As such, demand will be closely linked to price and/or convenience. However, consider switching operating systems on a computer. Along with the switch comes necessary understanding and training, transferring of files and programs and perhaps repurchasing of applications for the new system, all of which make the cost of switching quite high. Similarly, consider a dentist or physician who may possess a patient's medical records and provides rapid service due to an established relationship, thereby increasing switching costs. Firms try to increase switching costs to lock in their customers and if these costs can be maintained as high, they in turn serve as a powerful barrier to new entrants as the market is reluctant to switch over to a new competitor's products/services. Retail pharmacy as a drug distribution service, particularly for acute treatment, is arguably quite uniform across suppliers, as are the retailed drugs themselves, making this a commoditized service that may not make switching too difficult and may drive customers to the service that is the most inexpensive and/or convenient. Again, longitudinal provision of medication management services to patients with chronic conditions permits relationship building and brand development that can dramatically increase switching costs.

If the *capital requirements*, or resources, needed for a new entrant are large, then this may also pose a substantial barrier to entry. For example, it would be far less resource intensive to start up a new clinical consulting business than it would be to start an oil refinery or an airline where the capital cost requirements to enter are massive, strongly deterring entrance into the latter industries.

Consider the impact of the discussed barriers to entry on retail pharmacy versus clinical service business models. In its purist form, the former is relatively undifferentiated and does not generate many barriers to entry, apart from perhaps medium to high capital cost requirements, although pharmacists are still able to start new businesses with full financing provided from banks and wholesalers. In contrast, pharmacy as a clinical consultative practice may benefit strongly, depending on quality of service, from most of the noted barriers to entry.

In most Canadian provinces/territories, only pharmacists are legally permitted to open up pharmacies. This, while serving as a strong barrier to entrants, is offset by a growing national supply of pharmacists.

FORCE 3: BARGAINING POWER OF BUYERS

Factors influencing the bargaining power of buyers:
- buyer number
- purchasing volume
- price sensitivity
- brand identity and product differentiation
- switching costs
- backward integration
- others

An industry's *buyers* belong to the downstream industry from that of the firm's being analyzed. For example, the buyers to consider in the textile industry would be clothing manufacturers. Subsequently, clothing retailers would represent the buyers for the clothing manufacturing industry. In the retail pharmacy industry, buyers represent the payers such as insurance companies, provincial/territorial governments and patients who buy the products/services and fuel a pharmacy's revenue stream(s). The more *fragmented* the industry, where the majority of the market share is not owned by a few large companies and no player can influence the actions of the market, then the lower the power or threat of buyers on the organization. As a supplier, a firm has choice and if it does not like the terms of one buyer, then it could negotiate with another. Buyers occupying a fragmented industry are themselves in high competition to outcompete their rivals. This provides an opportunity for the supplying firm to raise its prices due to the low power of its buyers. In contrast, a buyer oligopoly, or a few large buyers possessing the majority of the market share, transfers bargaining power to the buyer and imposes significant threat to the supplying firm.[17] With few buyers to whom to sell, the organization is subject to price-setting by the buyer, with little choice—a situation often referred to in economics as a "hold-up,"[18,19] where a buyer or supplier reaches into the profit stream and "steals" profits (see Chapter 8: Assessing the Critical Attributes of a New Venture).

As buyer-purchasing volume becomes more significant, so therein does the power and the posed threat to the supplier, as large-scale purchasing demands a reduction in price per unit. For a firm, profit is influenced both by margin (selling price minus costs) and by the volume of sales, and while high-volume purchasing is favourable for sales, it comes at the cost of a reduced margin as the price that the buyer would be willing to pay is bargained down. Hence, the greater the purchasing volume of a buyer, the greater the threat it may pose to the supplying firm due to high bargaining power.

Price sensitivity, brand identity and *product differentiation* can be examined together with respect to their influence on bargaining power of buyers.[17] The more unique or *differentiated* a desired product or service may be, the less likely it is that another substitute good supplied by the industry can accommodate the exact same consumer need.[20] This differentiated value may come from its brand identity (a feature that distinguishes a product offering from others in the mind of the consumer) or its unique value proposition. Rolex, for example, occupies the high-end quality position of the watch industry spectrum, which differentiates the firm from other watch manufacturers by both quality and status. This differentiated position detracts power from the buyer, as there are few suitable substitutes for the product. Applied to a health care setting, stellar clinicians are more likely to be revisited and develop the personal brand as top-quality service experts, differentiating them from other providers of similar services. Differentiation here may be driven by improved patient responsiveness, bedside manner or just innovative and/or higher-quality clinical skills that serve to reduce the bargaining power of buyers since the service is difficult or impossible to imitate or suitably substitute. Similarly, pharmacist-differentiating services include specialized services to seniors, compounding centres, biologic specialization, travel pharmacy, mobile pharmacies and others.

Revisiting *switching costs*, how much financial, time, energy and psychological costs are involved in switching to another supplier is yet again relevant—this time in assessing buyer bargaining power. If these costs are high, they would detract power from buyers as they could add costs in terms of difficulty and inconvenience (time and energy costs) and perhaps even additional financial costs. Take, for example, a pharmacy education program. As buyers of a pharmacy program, the switching costs for students to move to another supplier (college or university) is so high in time, energy, psychological and additional financial cost that it removes a great deal of their bargaining power.

Backward integration is a form of vertical integration discussed with strategic planning (see Section II: Analysis and Planning). In short, it is a firm's purchase of a supplier to improve efficiency, improve control and/or relieve supplier threat. This scenario not only may impact the firm's sales to the organization, but also adds to the industry's supply, thereby increasing rivalry in the industry.[17] If this likelihood is high for a buyer, then it increases their bargaining power and, thus, the threat they pose to the organization. Pharmacy chains that supply their own stores, removing wholesalers, have backward-integrated into their supplier's (wholesaler) industry. Shoppers Drug Mart's and Katz Group's attempts to produce their own low-price private generic drug label can be viewed as further vertical (backward) integration, now competing with other drug manufacturers.

The retail pharmacy industry continues to consolidate with Jean Coutu, Katz Group, Loblaw (Shoppers Drug Mart) and other grocery firms controlling most of the Canadian market share.[8] As of 2013, 41.6% of prescription drug spending was financed by the public sector; 34.5% by insurers, of which 60% was covered by the top three insurance companies through provincial/territorial drug benefit plans; only the remaining 23.9% was paid out-of-pocket.[21] These buyers pose significant threat to retail pharmacy through either the consolidated nature of their industries and/or the volume of their purchasing. Furthermore, provincial/territorial governments not only impose strong bargaining power through high-volume purchasing, but also mediate legislation that continues to reduce generic pricing intra- and now inter-provincially/inter-territorially through the Pan-Canadian Pricing Alliance—most recently at 18% that of brand for formulary listings.[22] The pharmaceutical industry has partnered in new and innovative ways since drug reform was introduced into the Canadian retail pharmacy market; it does not appear that the impact of drug reforms has influenced pharmacists to continue to view pharmacy as a good investment.

FORCE 4: BARGAINING POWER OF SUPPLIERS

Factors influencing the bargaining power of suppliers:
- supplier concentration
- specialized inputs
- switching costs
- forward integration
- others

The key considerations in assessing the bargaining power of upstream or downstream business partners are largely the same for buyers and suppliers. Again, the greater the number of suppliers, the lower the threat to the buyer as there is choice and the costs will likely be lower due to the competitive nature of the supplying industry.[17]

The semiconductor industry, for example, is highly concentrated where few players in this industry own the majority of the market share. The semiconductor manufacturer Intel is the largest and, as the industry leader, poses a significant threat as a supplier to the downstream computer manufacturers (buyers) that require Intel products to power their computers. Similarly, in Canada, consider the drug wholesaler industry that supplies pharmacies. They are very few in number, represent a concentrated industry (McKesson currently supplies more than 40% of the Canadian market[23]) and as a result, possess high bargaining power particularly over independent pharmacies. Independents, therefore, possess little room for bargaining manoeuvrability and must generally accept supplier terms and pricing.

Suppliers that offer *specialized inputs* (physical supplies or services) to an organization that cannot be substituted or acquired anywhere else again lessen the organization's bargaining power. Many new biologics are unparalleled in quality or ability to treat disease in a customized manner and as such have no suitable substitutes. Pricing regulations notwithstanding, the provision of a specialized input(s) confers bargaining power to the biologic manufacturer with respect to price.

Here we again revisit *switching costs* that in this context refer to the energy, time and/or financial costs influencing the switch to another supplier. The time, energy and financial ramifications of switching wholesalers, all of which offer similar terms anyway due to their oligopolistic presence in Canada, increase an independent retail pharmacy's reliance on a supplier and hence the threat it poses.

Forward integration is the opposite of backward integration and entails the diversification of an organization into the downstream (buyer's) industry, effectively removing the middleman. When considering the threat of suppliers, the propensity or availability of a firm's supplier to move into their industry may not only threaten the organization's supply chain but also its existing market share through increased competition. Such a scenario was recently envisioned in 2012 by the forward integration of a major wholesaler, McKesson Corporation, into the retail pharmacy market through the purchase of Drug Trading Company Ltd. and Medicine Shoppe Canada Inc. retail pharmacy labels.[24]

Strategic planning aimed at mitigating the threat posed by a supplier may warrant the backward integration of pharmacy retailer(s) into the wholesaler's industry, thereby improving control over supply and eliminating supplier threat, instead threatening the market share of the former supplier.[17] Such a backward integration strategy has been practised by larger chains in Canada and the United States, and while attractive, such a diversification approach does require the necessary core competence to ensure competitiveness in both industries.

An independent retail pharmacy is particularly under significant threat from large and consolidated wholesaler middlemen that increase the firm's costs of inventory and financing and can threaten entry into their market. In contrast, pharmacy as a clinical consultation service business possesses limited suppliers, and whether including partnerships with other health care professionals, lease agreements and/or physical supplies, none of these represent concentrated or otherwise threatening industries.

FORCE 5: THREAT OF SUBSTITUTES

Factors influencing the threat of substitutes:
- switching costs
- product price to performance ratio
- buyer inclination to substitute
- others

Where competitors in a commodity market add supply, thereby decreasing the slice of the market pie that a firm may acquire, substitutes instead serve to decrease demand from that industry.[17] For example, naturopathic medicine offers a holistic therapeutic approach that can be defined as a substitute for conventional orthodox medicine, but at some level of influence reduces demand for orthodox medical services. The threat posed by substitutes can be gauged through several considerations.

Switching costs in the context of substitutes are yet again important to consider governing the ease with which a customer may move from an organization's product offering(s) to a substitute good(s) that similarly meets consumer needs. Take, for example, print publishing. A substitute such as digital e-books, while not identical, would serve to detract demand from print books. The time, energy and financial costs required by the customer to shift from one product to the other while generally satisfying the same consumer needs are arguably relatively low. More relevant to pharmacy, consider the switching costs involved in filling a prescription or picking up allergy medication. There is little involved in this product offering that makes the replacement difficult in terms of time, energy and cost, especially where the service/product is provincially/territorially subsidized in some locations and essentially free to the public. Again, in contrast, consider a value-added clinical relationship between pharmacist and patient that is based on information and cognitive services, and rather focused on chronic disease management through a full cycle of care. The latter offering captures time and energy costs involved in relaying and problem solving, and trust development and record/outcome keeping that may serve to reduce the threat of a customer switching to a substitute for any further related services. Curtailing the threat of substitutes is not a simple task and requires permeating boundaries between the business and substitutes to strategically ally with substitute good providers, thereby preventing the reduction of demand.[12] Take, for example, a collaborative venture comprised of a pharmacist, physician, nutritionist, nurse practitioner and physiotherapist to offer a retail clinic that specializes in cardiovascular disease management and prevention. The strategic alliance may rather increase demand for each of the specialties as customer/patient value is added in their collaborative combination.

Product price to performance ratio involves taking the perspective of a customer in asking, "What do I get for what I pay?" For example, the replacement of a consumer's beeper by a cell phone comes at higher price. Is the enhanced performance benefit derived from the substitute worth it to the customer? With the advent of new biologics, the personalized and value-enhanced performance of some current and pipeline therapeutics possesses exceptional and customized performance profiles, aiming to set prices that still provide an effectiveness-to-price ratio that delivers high customer value to patients.

Last, it is important to consider *buyer inclination to substitute*. Customers with reigning interest in holistic medicine are not likely to switch to orthodox medical practices in the maintenance of their health. Reasons for the inclination to substitute or prevention thereof may be incidental, cultural, religious or other, but they are necessary to identify in assessing the threat from substitutes.

The summation of the five forces industry model serves to provide an indication of current and future forces by which trends may be surmised to guide strategic planning of an organization. Intense rivalry yields a *decline* in industry profits and can in some cases also render an industry inherently unattractive.[1,17]

The five forces impacting the pharmacy industry at present appear to render the current definition of the industry as unattractive and in the process of reorganization. Nonetheless, the opportunities facing pharmacy and pharmacists are many, not only in expanding scope and differentiated services, but also in the management of current and future specialized health technology. Such shifts serve to create patient value, reduce rivalry, redefine suppliers and buyers and limit substitution. As such, redefined forces that are assessed as low threats can be conversely seen as new opportunities to create sustained value.

REFERENCES

1. Porter ME. How competence forces shape strategy. *Harv Bus Rev*. 1979;57(2):137–45.
2. QuickMBA online strategy. Porter's five forces. Available: www.quickmba.com/strategy/porter.shtml (accessed July 31, 2014).
3. Bronzen Y. *Concentration, mergers, and public policy*. New York, NY: Macmillan; 1982.
4. Hill C, Jones G. *Strategic management theory: an integrated approach*. 9th ed. New York, NY: McGraw Hill; 2009.
5. Willlis J, Negbenebor A. *Microeconomics (the freedom to choose)*. CAT Publishing; 2001.
6. Chamberlin E. *The Theory of Monopolistic Competition*. 1st ed. Cambridge: Harvard University Press; 1969.
7. DiMasi JA, Hansen RW, Grabowski HG. The price of innovation: new estimates of drug development costs. J Health Econ. 2003;22(2):151–85. http://dx.doi.org/10.1016/S0167-6296(02)00126-1. Medline:12606142
8. Turk S. Pharmacies and drug stores in Canada: market research report. IBIS World Industry Report 44611CA2014; 2014.
9. Hunt M. *Competition in the major home appliance industry, 1960–1970*. 1st ed.
10. Vernon R. International investment and international trade in the product cycle. Q J Econ. 1966;80(2):190–207. http://dx.doi.org/10.2307/1880689.
11. Canadian Institute for Health Information. Pharmacist workforce, 2012 highlights current trends in pharmacist practice across a variety of demographic, education, mobility and employment characteristics. Available: https://secure.cihi.ca/estore/productFamily.htm?locale=en&pf=PFC2353 (accessed July 31, 2014).
12. Canadian Institute for Health Information. Pharmacist workforce, 2012—provincial/territorial highlights. Available: https://secure.cihi.ca/free_products/PharmacistWorkforce2012HighlightsEN.pdf (accessed July 31, 2014).
13. National Association of Pharmacy Regulatory Authorities. Pharmacist national statistics 2014. Available: http://napra.ca/pages/Practice_Resources/National_Statistics.aspx?id=2104 (accessed July 31, 2014).
14. Wright TP. Factors affecting the cost of airplanes. J Aeronaut Sci. 1936;3(4):122–8. http://dx.doi.org/10.2514/8.155.
15. Sullivan A, Sheffrin SM. *Economics: principles in action*. Upper Saddle River, NJ: Pearson Prentice Hall; 2003. p. 157.
16. Thompson R, Cats-Baril W. *Information technology and management*. 1st ed. Boston, MA: McGraw-Hill; 2003.
17. Porter ME. The five competitive forces that shape strategy. Harv Bus Rev. 2008;86(1):78–93, 137. Medline:18271320
18. Ghemawat P. *Commitment*. 1st ed. New York, NY: Free Press; 1991.
19. Williamson OE. *The economic institutions of capitalism: firms, markets, relational contracting*. New York, NY: Free Press; 1985.
20. Porter ME. *Competitive strategy*. New York, NY: Free Press; 1980.
21. Canadian Institute for Health Information. National health expenditure database, 2013. Available: https://secure.cihi.ca/free_products/Prescribed_Drug_Spending_in_Canada_EN.pdf (accessed July 8, 2014).
22. Busby C, Blomqvist A, Husereau D. *Capturing value from health technologies in lean times*. CD Howe Institute Commentary; 2013. p. 396.
23. Johnston J. Rx distribution sector marked by consolidation, globalization. Chain Drug Rev. 2011;(June):5.
24. McKesson Canada News Release. McKesson Canada; Jan. 30, 2013. Available: https://www.mckesson.ca/news-releases/-/asset_publisher/GzhhvvIpo9IT/content/mckesson-to-acquire-independent-banner-and-franchise-businesses-of-katz-group-canada-inc- (accessed July 20, 2014).

CHAPTER 4

Stakeholder Analysis

Atul Goela, *BSc. Phm., RPh*

Pharmacy does not operate in isolation, but affects and is affected by many stakeholders in Canada's convoluted health care continuum. Successful management and sustenance of competitive advantage require proper understanding of these stakeholders and their economic imperatives. This chapter identifies the most relevant stakeholders to the pharmacy industry and systematically discusses the drivers and trends and how they may influence pharmacy today and in the future.

Learning Objectives

- Make sense of stakeholders and assess their relevance: stakeholder urgency, power and legitimacy.
- Identify key stakeholders and economic imperatives of each: pharmacists; government; physicians, nurses and technicians; manufacturers and wholesalers, academics, third-party payers and pharmacy benefit managers; and patients.
- Identify stakeholder trends, key opportunities and threats.

Health care advancements have allowed Canadians to live longer lives. Between the 1960s and 2010, average life spans increased 11 years for men and 9 years for women.[1] While the benefits of prescription drugs in managing chronic disease and extending life spans are extensive, these benefits are not without significant financial cost. Between 1998 and 2007, retail spending on prescription drugs ballooned from $8 billion to $19 billion—an average increase of 10.1% per year.[2]

These costs are borne by both the public purse and private sectors. Canada spent $33 billion on drugs in 2012, of which $27.7 billion was on prescription drugs; the government sector accounted for $12.3 billion (44.5%) and the private sector (including private insurers as well as individual out-of-pocket expenditures) accounted for the remaining $15.4 billion (55.5%).[3]

Greater pressures can be expected for all stakeholders due to rising rates of chronic disease, innovations in drug therapies and an aging population. The question of sustainability will become a greater issue.

THE DRUG APPROVAL PROCESS

When a new drug is developed, the pharmaceutical company applies to the federal government for a trademark (on the brand name) and patent (on the brand drug molecule). A patent allows a company the right to sell its drug without competition. In Canada, patent protection currently lasts for 20 years, allowing the company time to recoup their research and development costs and funnel further profits into the creation of new drugs.

After a patent expires, other pharmaceutical companies may manufacture and sell generic versions of the brand-name drug. Regardless of manufacturing source, Health Canada requires that all products must meet common requirements for quality, safety and efficacy. For generic drug products, a key prerequisite is that they must be bioequivalent to their brand-name counterparts, meaning the active ingredient(s) must be as pure, dissolve at the same rate, and be absorbed into the body in the same way as the brand equivalent. Although generics must contain the same active ingredient(s) as the brand-name version, non-active ingredients (that provide, shape, colour and taste) may vary.

Government drug plans and private drug plans each have their own formularies (lists of drugs that are eligible for reimbursement). Government plans and private plans also have their own processes for determining which new drugs will be included in their formularies.

GOVERNMENT

The federal government is the largest public sector stakeholder with the most influence. Each level of government has a distinct role to play in Canada's health care system. The federal government provides overarching governance through Health Canada and the Canada Health Act. Meanwhile, the provincial/territorial governments administer health care services and insurance.

The main objective of Canadian health care policy is to make access to health care available to all eligible residents without financial barriers. The Canada Health Act is the federal legislation that governs this publicly funded health care insurance. The Act sets out the terms and conditions the provinces/territories must adhere to in order to receive the federal transfer payments, called the Canada Health Transfer, that fund their health care systems.

Health Canada, through its Therapeutic Products Directorate (TPD), approves and monitors all drugs sold in the country. TPD also administers the Special Access Program that allows physicians, in very special circumstances, to prescribe unavailable or unapproved drugs. As well, the TPD conducts ongoing surveillance of approved drugs. It investigates complaints, monitors adverse events and inspects and licenses production sites. When necessary, TPD also manages recalls.

Although the federal government decides which drugs are approved for sale in the country, insurance coverage of medical devices and drugs is predominantly left to the discretion of the provincial/territorial governments. The federal government does provide prescription drug coverage through various programs for members of eligible groups, including First Nations and Inuit, members of the military, veterans, members of the RCMP and inmates in federal penitentiaries.

To aid in their decision making, the provinces/territories rely on the Canadian Agency for Drugs and Technologies in Health (CADTH), an independent not-for-profit agency funded by the federal and provincial/territorial governments. CADTH evaluates the cost and clinical effectiveness of devices and drugs and makes formulary recommendations for the government drug programs.

Pharmacy and drug coverage is just one part of the much larger health care expenditure for the provinces/territories and decision makers have an economic imperative to ensure the sustainability of the total health care system. Prescribed drugs accounted for 13.9% ($29.3 billion) of the total health care expenditure in 2013. Other major health care expenditures included hospitals (29.6%, $62.6 billion) and physicians (14.9%, $31.4 billion).[4]

Provincial drug reform has led to a massive reduction in the price of generic drugs, which have dropped from historic prices of 85% of the cost of brand-name equivalents, to about 20% to 25% of the cost of brand-name equivalents. This represents significant savings for both government and private sectors.

Provincial/Territorial governments have also found efficiencies through collaboration. In 2003, the 13 provincial/territorial premiers formed the Council of the Federation. One joint initiative of this Council is the Health Care Innovation Working Group (HCIWG) that, in addition to seniors' care, has two other focus areas: pharmaceutical drugs and team-based health care delivery models.

PHARMACEUTICAL DRUGS

As of August 2014, through the Pan-Canadian Pricing Alliance (PCPA), the provinces/territories jointly negotiated significant reductions in the cost of 43 brand-name drugs. As well, 10 commonly used generic drugs were reduced in price (18% of the cost of the brand-name equivalents). Through these two initiatives, HCIWG has achieved combined annual savings of more than $260 million in pharmaceutical drug costs, and these strategies are scheduled to continue for the coming years.[5]

TEAM-BASED HEALTH CARE DELIVERY MODELS

Given growing evidence that health care dollars are wasted when patients receive treatments ill-suited to their needs, HCIWG seeks out opportunities to use team-based models that increase the role pharmacists and paramedics play in providing frontline services.[6]

THIRD-PARTY PAYERS AND PHARMACY BENEFIT MANAGERS

This relationship seems to be the least understood by most pharmacists. In the dispensary, a prescription is processed and, assuming it is covered by the patient's drug plan (public or private drug plan), an amount to be charged to the patient and an amount that will be paid by the plan are generated. But how are these amounts determined?

In the case of private drug plans, the patient is a plan member of an employer-sponsored benefits plan. Part of the benefits plan is the coverage of drugs. The amount or the level of reimbursement of coverage is also stipulated in the employer-sponsored benefits plan that constitutes the plan design. Note: Plan design is a reference to the overall benefits plan and/or elements within the overall benefits plan (plan design of the drug plan component).

Many employer-sponsored benefits plans cover 100% of total prescription costs. Coinsurance, co-payment, dispensing fee caps and deductibles all offer methods for plan sponsors to share portions of the costs with their plan members, resulting in savings for the sponsor, which then are used for other business needs.

The following are some common cost-sharing methods:

- coinsurance: a fixed percentage to be paid by the employer regardless of the total cost for each prescription (For example, the employer may be responsible for paying 90% of the total cost for each prescription, with the remaining 10% of the cost to be paid by the plan member.)
- co-payment: a fixed flat amount to be paid by the plan member regardless of the total cost for each prescription (For example, the plan member may be responsible for paying $5 for each prescription.)
- dispensing fee caps: the drug plans caps (or limits) the amount that will be reimbursed for the dispensing fee (In this case, a fixed amount is paid toward the pharmacist's professional dispensing fee charged on every prescription and the plan member would be required to pay any difference between the capped fee and the dispensing fee.)
- deductibles: a fixed flat amount to be paid over the course of a predefined timeframe (typically annually) by the plan members and/or their dependents before coverage through the employer begins

Such cost-sharing methods are often applied concurrently by plan sponsors. For example, a plan design may incorporate an annual deductible and once met, a coinsurance and dispensing fee limit are applied to each prescription.

Employers work with insurers, brokers and consultants who advise them regarding the benefits plan and associated costs. Plan design affects the cost of the plan; a comprehensive benefits plan with no patient/employee out-of-pocket amounts will cost significantly more for the employer than one that shares costs with employees.

The plan is purchased by the employer through the insurer (e.g., carrier of the insurance policy), who is responsible for ensuring claims are processed and reimbursed to plan members as per the purchased plan design.

Drug claim processing (e.g., adjudication) is one of the functions carried out by a pharmacy benefit manager (PBM)/third-party payer (TPP). The PBM/TPP can be a function carried out by the insurer or can be outsourced to another company by the insurer.

The role of the PBM/TPP is, in part, to adjudicate the claim submitted by the pharmacy and apply the level of reimbursement and any other elements of the plan design to the prescription claim that have been agreed upon by the insurer and employer. As a result, pharmacies' relationships have traditionally been with only the PBM/TPP and/or those divisions within the carriers.

Mechanics of a public plan are similar in some aspects to that of private plans. The biggest difference is the population for which public plans provide coverage. In the case of private plans, coverage is established for the employer's workforce, which is demographically quite different than the population for which governments provide coverage. Governments predominantly serve seniors, social assistance recipients or those with exceptionally high annual drug costs in relation to their annual income. In addition, public drug plan decisions are guided to a greater extent by political factors and the implications to the broader health care budget (see Chapter 17: The Canadian Third-Party Payer Market).

PHARMACY

The cost of drug benefit programs is rising due to rising rates of chronic disease, innovations in drug therapies and an aging population, all of which combine to increase the number of prescriptions being dispensed. If they are to remain sustainable, drug benefit programs have historically implemented cost-containment and cost-sharing strategies.

Generics had been singled out for government reform because of their unusually high historic costs in Canada compared to other countries. However, most recently concerted steps have been taken to rein in these costs. To understand why generics have been so costly, consider the history of generic drugs and their relationship with the profession of pharmacy.

HISTORY OF DRUG REFORM

In the late 1960s, the federal government enacted legislation to limit patent terms, opening the door to generic drug manufacturing. This development soon became a boon for drug benefit plans, particularly in recent years, as the patents of several popular and costly medications have expired.

As a robust generic drug sector grew, another change began on the distribution end. Through the 1970s and 1980s, community pharmacies began consolidating under large chains and banners. Small independent local pharmacies began disappearing, replaced by national titans. With their increased buying power and influence, these large retail chains were able to negotiate lower prices from the manufacturers, thereby creating a gap between the purchase and the maximum reimbursement price; their profit margins grew. The result was a philosophical schism between pharmacy as a retailer and the pharmacist as a health care professional. In the competition for retail shelf space, generics began offering increasingly generous rebates, or allowances, to pharmacies. At 40% to 60% of the invoice price,[7] these rebates and allowances led to artificially higher prices.

As the cost of health care and drug plans rose, provinces, beginning with Québec and Ontario, enacted legislation to limit allowances and set prices for generics. For example, Ontario passed Bill 102 in 2006, which set a firm limit on allowances for retail pharmacies doing business with the Ontario Public Drug Program. Bill 102 also set generic drug prices in the public sector at 50% of brand cost.

IMPACT OF DRUG REFORM ON PHARMACY

Drug reform has been a double-edged sword for pharmacists. On the one hand, it has squeezed their profit margins by capping generic drug costs, limiting or eliminating rebates depending on province/territory. A prescription drug that once cost $100 plus a 10% markup meant that a pharmacy saw a $10 gross profit. Now the same drug costs as little as $18. At an equivalent markup, the pharmacy now sees only $1.80 in gross profit. The limiting or elimination of rebates has further eroded pharmacy margins.

However, new legislation has also benefited the profession by recognizing pharmacists as valuable members of the health care team and widening their scope of practice beyond dispensing medications. These reforms hold the promise of new revenue streams.

In the midst of this evolution, the profession has laid out a Blueprint for Pharmacy[8] that charts its course forward. Looking to the future, pharmacists intend to do the following:

- practise to the full extent of their knowledge and skills as an integral part of emerging health care models
- help patients, caregivers and health care providers better manage drug therapy
- take a prominent role in health care promotion, illness prevention and chronic disease management by promoting more informed and empowered patient decision making
- be compensated in a manner that recognizes their expertise and the complexity of the care they provide

Already, pharmacists have achieved great strides in bringing this vision to fruition. They are taking on vital roles in new health care delivery models that emphasize inter-professional collaboration. For example, many provinces/territories have implemented community practice models wherein general practitioners work in concert with a team of allied health care professionals, including pharmacists, all of whom are a part of the primary care teams.

Drug reform and new legislation have allowed pharmacists to expand their scope of practice. In most jurisdictions, they can now renew and extend prescriptions, provide emergency refills and change drug dosage and formulations. In some jurisdictions, they can make therapeutic substitutions, vaccinate patients, order and interpret laboratory tests, prescribe medication for minor ailments and initiate prescription drug therapy.

Pharmacists are no longer merely just dispensing; decision makers are recognizing the need to compensate their new responsibilities. In its 2012 budget, the federal government recognized pharmacists as health care "practitioners." As a result, all non-dispensing professional fees they charge are exempt from Goods and Services Tax (GST)/Harmonized Sales Tax (HST) (see Chapter 46: Advocacy and Strategic Communications).

PHYSICIANS

In Canada, most physicians operate as independent, self-employed small-business owners. They receive no pension, paid vacations or other benefits and must use their compensation to cover their practice's overhead, the cost of which varies but for most physicians is estimated to range from 25% to 40% of the total operational cost.

PHYSICIAN COMPENSATION

Compensation is negotiated between provincial/territorial governments and physician associations and, therefore, varies greatly from province to province/territory to territory. There are two reimbursement models: fee-for-service (FFS), traditionally the most common form of physician compensation, and alternative payment plans (APP).

In the FFS model, physicians bill provincial/territorial health insurance plans for each procedure, test or clinical service they provide. APP can take the form of a salary or capitation, where the physician is paid an annual fee for each patient on the roster regardless of how much attention a patient needs. Physicians may also be compensated using a blended model.

Increasingly, there has been a move away from FFS and toward greater use of APP. In 1999–2000, alternative models accounted for 10.6% of gross clinical payments. By 2012–2013, they accounted for more than one-quarter (29.3%) of all clinical payments.[9]

APP is better able to compensate for the services physicians provide that go beyond direct patient care, such as emergency medicine, on-call services, teaching and research. It can also attract physicians to practise in rural areas where demand for service is low and unpredictable, making FFS models untenable. APP models also encourage physicians to engage with newer practice models, such as primary team-based medicine and preventative care.

PHYSICIAN SHORTAGE

In a 2010 report, the Canadian Institute for Health Information (CIHI) concluded that the low number of physicians per capita in Canada may be the reason "why Canadians continue to report difficulties in accessing health care when compared to other countries." The United States has 27 physicians per 10,000 people. Most continental European G7 counties have >30 physicians per 10,000 people. In comparison, Canada has merely 19 physicians per 10,000 people. Furthermore, with 22% of physicians currently aged 60 or older, our country is on the cusp of a retirement wave.[10]

The solution may come from the allied health care professions. Through increased multidisciplinary collaboration, mediated by the use of electronic health records (EHR), allied health care professionals, such as pharmacists, could take on new responsibilities, ease physician workload, improve system efficiency and improve patient care.

TECHNOLOGY

In the future, the foundation of patient care will be e-health. A patient's comprehensive health record—including imaging, laboratory results, drug information and medical history—will be electronically available to all health care providers. Electronic access to a patient's complete medical record will aid pharmacists in their newly expanded roles, allowing them to prescribe with greater confidence, administer and record vaccinations and provide more informed counselling on drug interactions.[11]

COLLABORATION

Health care in Canada is evolving from siloed practice to integrated multidisciplinary care, thanks in part to the growing recognition of an expanded role for pharmacists. For example, in a 2005 statement, the College of Physicians and Surgeons of Ontario committed to fostering greater collaboration with the province's pharmacists to improve patient care.[12,13]

PHARMACEUTICAL COMPANIES

The pharmaceutical sector is responsible for the research, development and manufacture of branded and generic varieties of prescription medications and over-the-counter (OTC) drugs, as well as biologics and their generic equivalents, subsequent entry biologics (SEBs). The sector consists of generic drug manufacturers, brand-name pharmaceutical companies, biopharmaceutical small- and medium-sized enterprises (biopharmaceutical SMEs) and contract service providers (CSPs).

In addition to the brand and generic manufacturers previously discussed, biologics and SEBs are an emerging form of therapy. Unlike drugs, which are synthesized from chemicals, biologics are manufactured from biological sources.

Brand-name products make up 76% of all Canadian drug costs and 37% of prescriptions dispensed; generics account for the rest.

The pharmaceutical industry is one of the nation's most innovative yet domestic productions, valued at $7.7 billion in 2011 and on the decline with the average annual growth rate falling by 1.7% since 2004. Research and development (R&D) expenditure is also on the decline. Total business expenditure on R&D by Canadian pharmaceutical companies has fallen below $1 billion since 2011. Between 2001 and 2012, industry R&D dropped by 15.6%. Business models are changing, with more R&D being outsourced. Instead of conducting in-house research, companies are investing their R&D dollars in SMEs, venture funds and partnerships with the CSP sector.

Developing new drugs is cost-intensive. The R&D phase for a new drug averages 12 to 13 years and $605 million (US dollars). In contrast, a generic takes 2 to 3 years and $3 million to $10 million in R&D to prove equivalency.[14]

Pharmaceuticals represent approximately 16% of total health care expenditures for government. Prices of branded drugs (both prescription and OTC) are regulated at the federal level by the Patented Medicine Prices Review Board (PMPRB), an independent pseudo-judicial body operating at arm's-length from the federal government. The PMPRB reviews prices of new brand-name products on the market to ensure they are not excessive. Further complicating the matter are the provincial/territorial governments' recent drug reforms and the role they play in limiting the price of generic drugs. Generic medications that are not included in provincial/territorial formularies are at the mercy of the market and priced according to what the market will bear.

PATIENTS

As the end users of drug therapy and pharmacy services, patients are perhaps the most important stakeholder group. In their expanded roles as counsellors and medication managers, pharmacists must keep in mind that today's patients are more educated and knowledgeable. They are in a better position to be thoughtful users of medication and equal partners in the management of their own health care.

Thanks to the Internet, patients also have greater access to both health information and misinformation, a fact that pharmacists have to mediate when counselling on medication therapies, prevention strategies and chronic disease management. With Canadian life expectancies at 86 years for women and 83 years for men, patients are living longer, thanks in part to medications. Yet, as people live longer, they fall victim to complex diseases. Generally, this factor becomes the basis for major expenditures during the final stage of life.

Tobacco remains a contributor when it comes to ill health. The majority of lung cancer and 17% of all deaths can be attributed to smoking. Pharmacist-administered smoking cessation services may be seen as an important part of a prevention strategy.

Given growing obesity rates (25% of Canadians are considered obese), more chronic long-term illnesses can be expected, such as diabetes (8.7% prevalence in Canada with an additional 1% of Canadians having undiagnosed diabetes), heart disease and cancer.[15] It is likely that pharmacists will become indispensable in prevention services, medication management for multiple co-morbidities and chronic disease management.

A large subset of patient population—the so-called Sandwich generation—is responsible for not just their own health care and drug usage, but those of their elderly parents and young children. So in many cases, pharmacists will counsel not only patients but their intermediaries as well.

Health care is a complex interplay between many stakeholders. Using a pharmacy-centric perspective to describe the evolution of health care, pharmacists are taking on an expanded scope of services that involves greater responsibility, increased collaboration with other allied health care professionals, adoption of technology, recognition from government and opportunities for new revenue streams. Longer life spans, increased disease burden, increased drug costs and the need for public and private sectors to manage costs to ensure sustainability are clear contributors to this evolution. Then there are the patients, who are living longer, are savvier about their health care and are generally taking on more of a partnership role. How do pharmacists engage with today's health care consumer, who was perhaps once just a customer in the days when pharmacists were exclusively dispensing, and now with the ever-changing stakeholder dynamics, are their patients?

REFERENCES

1. Statistics Canada. Life expectancy at birth, by sex, by province (table), last modified 2012–05–31, Toronto: Statistics Canada, 2014. Available: www.statcan.gc.ca/tables-tableaux/sum-som/l01/cst01/health26-eng.htm (accessed Oct. 5, 2014).

2. Canadian Institute for Health Information. *Drivers of prescription drug spending in Canada.* Ottawa: CIHI; 2012.

3. Canadian Institute for Health Information. *Drug expenditure in Canada, 1985 to 2012.* Ottawa: CIHI; 2013.

4. Canadian Institute for Health Information. *Prescribed drug spending in Canada, 2012: A Focus on Public Drug Programs.* Ottawa: CIHI; 2014.

5. Canada's Premiers, and the Health Care Innovation Working Group. Ottawa: Canada's Premiers, 2014. Available: www.canadaspremiers.ca/en/initiatives/128-health-care-innovation-working-group (accessed Oct. 5, 2014).

6. Canada's Premiers, and the Health Care Innovation Working Group. Ottawa: Canada's Premiers, 2014. Available: www.canadaspremiers.ca/en/initiatives/128-health-care-innovation-working-group (accessed Oct. 5, 2014).

7. Grootendorst P, Rocchi M, Segal H, et al. *An economic analysis of the impact of reductions in generic drug rebates on community pharmacy in Canada.* Toronto: Leslie Dan Faculty of Pharmacy; 2008. Available: http://individual.utoronto.ca/grootendorst/workingpapers.htm [cited 2014 Dec. 9].

8. Key blueprint for pharmacy resources. Vision for Pharmacy (June 2008). Blueprint for Pharmacy, 2014. Available: http://blueprintforpharmacy.ca/resources (accessed Oct. 6, 2014).

9. Canadian Institute for Health Information. *Physicians in Canada, 2013: summary report.* Ottawa: CIHI; 2014.

10. Ontario Ministry of Finance. Commission on the reform of Ontario's public services, chapter 5: health. Toronto: Ministry of Finance, 2014. Available: www.fin.gov.on.ca/en/reformcommission/chapters/ch5.html (accessed Oct. 11, 2014).

11. The College of Physicians and Surgeons of Ontario. eHealth. Toronto: The College of Physicians and Surgeons of Ontario, 2014. Available: www.cpso.on.ca/Policies-Publications/Positions-Initiatives/eHealth (accessed Oct. 12, 2014).

12. The College of Physicians and Surgeons of Ontario. Physician working relations with pharmacists. Toronto: The College of Physicians and Surgeons of Ontario, 2014. Available: www.cpso.on.ca/Policies-Publications/Positions-Initiatives/Physician-Working-Relations-with-Pharmacists (accessed Oct. 11, 2014).

13. Canadian Medical Association. Collaborative care. Ottawa: Canadian Medical Association, 2014. Available: www.cma.ca/En/Pages/collaborative-care.aspx (accessed Oct. 12, 2014).

14. Industry Canada. Pharmaceutical industry profile. Ottawa: Government of Canada, 2014. Available: www.ic.gc.ca/eic/site/lsg-pdsv.nsf/eng/h_hn01703.html (accessed Oct. 12, 2014).

15. Canadian Institute for Health Information. Benchmarking Canada's health system: international comparisons. Ottawa: CIHI, 2014. Available: https://secure.cihi.ca/estore/productFamily.htm?pf=PFC2416&lang=en&media=0 (accessed Oct. 13, 2014).

II. ANALYSIS AND PLANNING

CHAPTER 5

Essential Components of a Strategic Plan

Jason Perepelkin, *BA, BComm, MSc, PhD; Assistant Professor of Social and Administrative Pharmacy, University of Saskatchewan*

Dr. Kishor M. Wasan, *R.Ph, PhD, FAAPS, FCSPS, FCAHS; Professor and Dean, College of Pharmacy and Nutrition, University of Saskatchewan*

Learning Objectives

- Describe the main elements of a strategic plan.
- Discuss the rationale and purpose of a strategic plan.
- Describe the strategic planning process.

Strategic planning is a continuous exercise in almost every type of organization, from an independent community pharmacy, to a regulatory authority, to a health region. Strategic plans allow organizations to review where they have been and to strategize about where they would like to be in the future.

Before beginning to draft a strategic plan, it is important to define stakeholders. Stakeholders of an organization are people and/or entities that are affected by, or can affect, the operations and practices of an organization. There are two types of stakeholders: primary (or market) and secondary (or non-market/indirect). Primary stakeholders are those people and entities that engage in economic transactions with the organization as it conducts its operations, while secondary stakeholders are people and entities that do not engage in direct economic transactions with the organization but are affected by or can affect its activities.

Due to the economic nature of interactions between an organization and its primary stakeholders, the stakeholders have sufficient influence on the organization's operations to affect its progress and plans. Some examples of primary stakeholders include customers/patients, employees, suppliers, shareholders and funding agencies (e.g., banks, government, third-party payers). While they do not engage in direct economic transactions with the organization, secondary stakeholders can still influence how an organization operates. Examples of secondary stakeholders include advocacy groups, local communities, unions, competitors and governments.

As an example of stakeholders in pharmacy practice, consider an example of a pharmacist-owner at The Best Pharmacy in Canada, a small, independent pharmacy. The primary stakeholders

Table 1. Rubric of Stakeholder Importance and Influence

		Importance of Stakeholder			
		Unknown	Little/No Importance	Moderate Importance	Significant Importance
Influence of Stakeholder	Unknown				
	Little/No Influence				
	Moderate Influence				
	Significant Influence				

would include the pharmacy's patients/customers, employees (e.g., pharmacists, technicians, assistants, cashiers) and the provincial/territorial drug plan. The owner's spouse, as a silent partner/owner, is also a stakeholder. Secondary stakeholders include the provincial/territorial regulatory authority, patient advocate organizations, prescribing physicians, other health care professionals and local pharmacy competitors.

In preparing the strategic plan, it is important to seek input and feedback from the stakeholders, both primary and secondary, who are identified as having a stake in the organization. When identifying stakeholders, consider the stakeholders' influence on strategy development and execution, and what effect the strategic direction of the organization will have on its stakeholders (e.g., with the start of offering a methadone maintenance program [MMP], identifying what effect this will then have on current patients, the neighbourhood, those requiring methadone therapy, etc.).

Another way an organization can lay out its stakeholders is by creating a table and rating the importance and influence of each stakeholder. Going back to the MMP example, it would be safe to assume the importance of the patient is significant as the addition of an MMP can increase access, while that same patient may have moderate influence over implementation of an MMP due to the perceived stigma attached to patients requiring methadone. Ratings are in four categories: unknown, little/no importance/influence, moderate importance/influence or significant importance/influence (see Table 1).

RATIONALE AND PURPOSE OF A STRATEGIC PLAN

Strategic planning is a means of establishing major directions for an organization or department and helping provide direction for stakeholders. In higher education, those stakeholders include students, employers of graduates, funding agencies and society, as well as internal stakeholders such as faculty and staff. Strategic planning is a structured approach to anticipating the future and "exploiting the inevitable," as well as leveraging strengths. The strategic plan should chart the broad course for the entire organization for a long-term period such as the next five years. It is a process for ensuring that the budget dollars follow the plan rather than vice versa. Strategic planning is not just a plan for growth and expansion. A strategic plan can and often does guide retrenchment and reallocation, while being responsive and incorporating environmental factors and influences.

McConkey[1] said that the essence of strategy is differentiation. What makes this pharmacy different from any other? Pharmacies, like other service organizations, can differentiate themselves based on types of programs/services offered, where they provide goods/services (e.g., at a long-term care home or in the counselling room at the pharmacy), which patients to target/attract and location. Similarly, as part of a larger chain pharmacy organization, a specific pharmacy location involved in strategic planning will identify its unique niche within the organization, but also within the community in which it operates. Without addressing strategic planning for each pharmacy within a chain pharmacy organization, subpar performance may result because of not addressing the needs of the stakeholders of a specific location.

ESSENTIAL COMPONENTS OF A STRATEGIC PLAN

Communication strategy is essential for the effective development and implementation of a strategic plan because it informs all those who will be affected or who will play a role and helps to set appropriate expectations. In developing this aspect of the strategic plan, participants involved in the planning process are informed how they will be involved, their role, who is receiving what information and what to expect next. An effective communication strategy will align efforts and lead to a successful execution of the strategic plan, ensuring that things that must be done a certain way are carried out in that manner.

Strategic planning task force: The development of a core team of organizational leaders is mandatory in the effective creation of a strategic plan. Each task force member should represent a key operational area or department of the organization to ensure the plan has organization-wide input and buy-in. The task force meets regularly with clearly defined deliverables to be presented at each meeting. For example, if developing a strategic plan for a hospital pharmacy, one should consider including pharmacists, technicians/assistants, ward staff, nurses, physicians, dieticians and managers on the task force; one may even consider including patients and/or patient advocates.

Vision statement: An organization's vision statement is simply its road map for the future. The direction of the organization should be broad enough to include all areas of impact but narrow enough to clearly define a path. An example of a vision statement could be, "The vision of the pharmacy is to provide efficient, patient-centred care to improve patient outcomes and reduce waste."

Mission statement: An organization's mission statement is a definition of whom and what it is and what it hopes to do. Often mission statements include core goals and values of the organization. As an example, the Pharmacy Examining Board of Canada's (PEBC) mission is, "To certify the qualifications of Pharmacists and Pharmacy Technicians."[2] This helps inform us about the purpose of PEBC.

Values are the organization's fundamental beliefs in how it operates. Values can provide a guideline for management and staff for acceptable organizational behaviour, and they often relate to the organization's culture.

Goals are broad-based strategies needed to achieve the organization's mission.

Objectives are specific, measurable, action-oriented, realistic and time-bound strategies (SMART) that enable the organization to achieve its goals and support the organization's vision.

Tasks are specific, actionable events that are assigned to individuals or departments. They, too, should be specific, measurable and time-bound.

Implementation strategy: Once the plan has been outlined, a tactical strategy is built that prioritizes initiatives and aligns resources. The implementation strategy pulls all the components of the plan together to ensure there are no missing pieces and the plan is achievable. As a part of the implementation strategy, accountability measures are put into place to ensure successful execution and completion.

Monitoring of strategic plan: During the implementation of a strategic plan, it is critical to monitor success, to challenge planning assumptions and to measure outcomes. When evaluating the successes of a plan, look objectively at the measurement criteria defined in the goals and objectives. It may be necessary to retool the plan and its assumptions if elements of the plan are off track. A strategic plan should be treated as a living document, reviewed and updated regularly to assist an organization to successfully achieve its goals and ensure ongoing organizational success. A strong strategic plan keeps the team focused on the end goal, mapping out who they are, where they are going and how they get there.

Every organization should have a strategic plan in place that has been created to provide direction, alignment and guidance. With changes in the organization, personnel, stakeholders and the environment, strategic plans are revisited and updated to ensure the organization continues to reach the vision in the best possible way.

RESOURCES AND SUGGESTED READINGS

Canadian Council on Continuing Education in Pharmacy (CCCEP). Canadian Council on Continuing Education in Pharmacy strategic plan 2012–2015. Saskatoon, SK: Canadian Council on Continuing Education in Pharmacy (CCCEP), 2012. Available: www.cccep.org (accessed April 12, 2014).

Canadian Pharmacists Association. Canadian Pharmacists Association 2012–2014 strategic plan. Ottawa, ON: Canadian Pharmacists Association, 2012. Available: www.pharmacists.ca/cpha-ca/assets/File/about-cpha/StratPlan2012EN.pdf (accessed April 12, 2014).

College of Pharmacists of British Columbia. Three year strategic plan 2014/15 to 2016/17: quality of pharmacy services to optimize patient outcomes. Vancouver, BC: College of Pharmacists of British Columbia (CPBC), 2014. Available: www.qualitypharmacy.ca (accessed April 12, 2014).

Harrison DL. Effect of attitudes and perceptions of independent community pharmacy owners/managers on the comprehensiveness of strategic planning. J Am Pharm Assoc (2003). 2006;46(4):459–64. http://dx.doi.org/10.1331/154434506778073718. Medline:16913389

Harrison DL. Effect of strategic planning education on attitudes and perceptions of independent community pharmacy owners/managers. J Am Pharm Assoc (2003). 2007;47(5):599–604. http://dx.doi.org/10.1331/JAPhA.2007.06146. Medline:17848349

Harrison DL. Strategic planning by independent community pharmacies. J Am Pharm Assoc (2003). 2005;45(6):726–33. http://dx.doi.org/10.1331/154434505774909652. Medline:16381420

McDonough, RP (2013). Strategic planning to ensure future practice success. Pharmacy Today, American Pharmacists Association. Available www.pharmacist.com/strategic-planning-ensure-future-practice-success (accessed April 12, 2014).

Zellmer WA. *Pharmacy forecast 2014–2018: strategic planning advice for pharmacy departments in hospitals and health systems.* Bethesda, MD: American Society of Health-System Pharmacists Research and Education Foundation; 2013., Available www.ashpfoundation.org/pharmacyforecast, [cited 2014 April 12].

REFERENCES

1. McConkey DD. Strategic planning in non-profit organizations. Health Manage Forum. 1981;2(3):61–76. Medline:10253141
2. Pharmacy Examining Board of Canada. Vision and mission. Available: www.pebc.ca/index.php/ci_id/6382/la_id/1.htm (accessed Oct. 30, 2014).

CHAPTER 6

The Foundations of Building a Successful Strategic Plan

F.A. Derek Desrosiers, *BSc(Pharm), RPEBC, RPh; Director, Pharmacy Practice Support, British Columbia Pharmacy Association; President, Desson Consulting Ltd.*

Learning Objectives

- Describe the importance of an environmental scan and market analysis.
- Describe how to conduct an environmental scan and market analysis.
- Identify important key stakeholders and their involvement.
- List the key components of a strategic plan.
- Describe a process for setting SMART strategic goals for a business.
- List the critical factors in the execution of a strategic plan.

The success of any business can be significantly influenced in a positive manner if that business develops and successfully executes a strategic plan. A strategic plan is about charting a course of where one wants to go, when to get there and how to get there (achieving goals). It is important to be as comprehensive as possible when developing a strategic plan. Trying to make decisions in a context without the benefit of environmental and market information is more likely doomed to failure.

Think about trying to make therapy decisions for patients without knowing anything about them. If some key information is not known about a person such as diagnosis, gender, age, weight, height, family history, kidney function or even other medications the person may already be taking, it would be very difficult to make decisions and set goals of therapy for that patient.

Business is no different. One needs to have a sound understanding of the world around them from both a macro- and micro-perspective. So the question becomes, how does one gather and utilize such information? The key is to conduct an environmental scan and market analysis as the foundation of a strategic plan.

An environmental scan is a broad review of an organization's internal and external environments to identify factors that may be threats to the business today and to future plans, as well

Figure 6.1

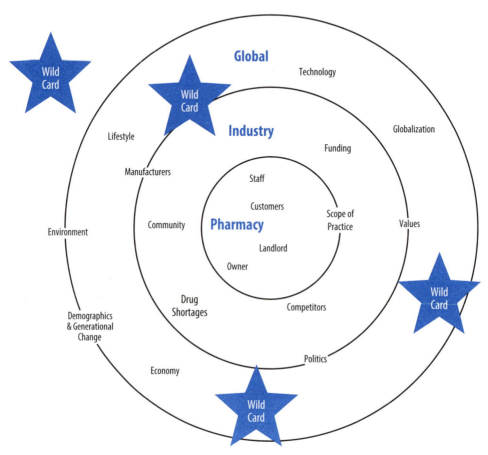

*Concentric Environmental Scanning
(used and modified with permission from Maree Conway October 24, 2014).*

as to detect opportunities that could help the business flourish and grow. Figure 6.1 provides an overview of the types of factors that should be reviewed, and these are discussed in more detail in the Scan section. It is not a totally comprehensive representation of every category to be reviewed; however, remember that the broader the scan, the more information there will be available to make informed decisions later.

As the name suggests, a market analysis is about defining and understanding the market in which the business will operate. It is important to know who will shop at the pharmacy and what their expectations are as customers and patients. It might be helpful to think of the market analysis as a much more specific and focused version of an environmental scan but with a slightly different purpose (as discussed in more detail further on in this chapter).

Building a strategic plan can be a complex and daunting task, but it does not have to be that way. Breaking the process down into key components makes it much more manageable. From a broad perspective, the process order is to scan, interpret the results, make decisions and then implement the plan.

SCAN

The scan should include both internal and external sources and can be completed by a pharmacist or manager, or by a professional business consultant. It is best to try to collect a robust list of trends and emerging issues that could affect the business today and into the future. There is no one single way to conduct an environmental scan and market analysis; however, there are some key features that should be included regardless of the methodology used.

Scanning the environment includes looking at things both internal and external to the business. This process should also include doing a very specific market analysis. Try to identify the bigger forces that will likely have an effect on the way business is carried out and how customers expect to interact with the business and staff.

Figure 6.1 illustrates how some drivers can have a complex relationship with each other while some drivers are the result of pressures exerted by other drivers. Some of these forces can be somewhat predictable while others can appear without warning with an uncertain effect on the industry and the business. Note that many of the terms cross circles; this indicates they can be viewed specifically just in the pharmacy industry or more globally. Focus mainly on those forces within the industry, but do not ignore broader societal trends.

Within an organization, the main concerns will be staff members, key stakeholders such as health care professionals who prescribe, and suppliers. Government is also an important stakeholder for pharmacy. The wild cards depicted in Figure 6.1 are events that are quite unlikely to happen but will have an extremely high and immediate impact if they do occur. Two examples of wild cards are the severe acute respiratory syndrome (SARS) outbreak in Canada between February and September 2003 that resulted in several deaths, and Hurricane Katrina in New Orleans in 2005.

At the global level, pay particular attention to what is happening in the areas of technology, social media, lifestyle, economy, and demographics and generational change. Being aware of the trends and forces in these areas may provide substantial opportunities to differentiate oneself and one's organization by adapting products or services to meet a unique or previously unidentified need. It is about finding a niche that no one else is occupying and setting the organization apart from others so it is seen as a leader; for example, by offering a new service that has previously never been offered in a pharmacy.

Starting from the centre and working outward, one can begin with a scan focusing on issues very specific to pharmacy and gradually broaden the perspective.

ENVIRONMENTAL SCAN

When managing a pharmacy business that is already in existence, the staff and customers are an extremely important source of information. When developing a strategic plan for a new start-up pharmacy that is not open yet, the benefit of consulting staff and customers as a source of information is not an option. However, the staff and customers of competitors could be a great source of information if it can be collected. This is where the use of a professional may be extremely beneficial.

Discussions with staff members to gain their views of the future are an extremely valuable source of information. Remember that employees are in constant contact with customers and likely have a very good understanding of customers' expectations, wants and needs. They will have very strong views about the future of the business and how things can come together when the entire organization works as a team.

There is a variety of methods to collect input from staff members. One can conduct a staff survey or use a suggestion box in the staff room and consider any staff complaints that may have been received. These can be very important in helping guide the business through change.

Customer surveys are another good source of information about what people want and expect from a pharmacy in terms of products and services. When opening a new pharmacy, it is a good idea to ask customers about the nearest competitors and what they feel would be important to offer. Customer feedback is most important in identifying the things that create customer loyalty. Offering the right products and services at the right prices will create customer loyalty, which is critical to the long-term viability of any business (see Section XI for more on marketing).

External scanning should include the broader pharmacy industry to identify trends that could affect the business in the future. There are many good sources of information in this area including provincial/territorial pharmacy associations, national pharmacy organizations and both brand and generic drug manufacturers. The retail pharmacy industry is very dependent on a relationship with government. Therefore, it is vital to have an awareness of government programs, public drug plans and potential changes to legislation and regulation. Provincial/Territorial pharmacy regulatory authorities (colleges of pharmacists), provincial/territorial pharmacy associations, government websites (e.g., Ministry of Health) and the pharmacy's local provincial/territorial political representative (e.g., Member of the Legislative Assembly, Member of Provincial Parliament) can all be great sources of information.

It is also important to know and understand all of the different private third-party payer contracts that one's pharmacy may have in place. Some of these contracts contain restrictions that could jeopardize aspects of a strategic plan. The strategic plan must align with the requirements of such contracts.

An additional source of external information that should be considered is one's colleagues. Other pharmacists and pharmacy owners may provide valuable insight into the profession from a different perspective than any other source. This is also where one can gather ideas that may be incorporated for best practices that may be a good fit for a strategic plan and help achieve goals.

Other health care practitioners who may be stakeholders or colleagues located nearby, such as physicians and nurses, may be useful sources of information not only from their own perspective but also from that of their patients. This too can be very helpful in developing a comprehensive set of data for analysis.

MARKET ANALYSIS

A market analysis is a more specific, focused review that usually includes defining one's customer base and their needs, current gaps in meeting those needs and detailed knowledge of immediate competitors.

A market analysis may be completed before or after the environmental scan. The only time it may be worth conducting the market analysis first is when one is starting a new business. In this case, the market analysis can be critical in assessing the value of a particular location. Many new businesses, including pharmacies, do not succeed despite having solid business plans because they failed to do one thing. That one thing is to ensure the viability of the location and carry out a thorough location analysis identifying the strengths, weaknesses, opportunities and competition in the area.

A market analysis should include a detailed review of the following factors as a minimum:

- assessment of the physical location of the pharmacy, including features such as street access and parking
- complete listing of all competitors, including key services, products and pricing offered by each of them
- assessment of market share of each competitor
- potential customer base, including demographics such as gender percentages, age brackets and income levels

One of the most easily accessible and comprehensive tools for market analysis can be accessed through Pitney Bowes—its PSYTE HD Canada product.[1] It is a geodemographic market segmentation system that provides a plethora of market information based on several data inputs, including the Canadian census base. By defining a specific geographic area using postal codes, one can gain an in-depth insight into the market segmentation of the people living in closest geographic proximity to the business.

The market analysis from this tool will identify the following key information about a specific market:

- demographics including age, marital status, education and household income
- media habits including what they read, how they get their news, type of music they listen to and type of television programs they watch
- leisure activities including sports, hobbies and favourite travel destinations
- shopping habits including favourite retailers and preferred brand of automobile

This information can be invaluable in determining the types of products and services one intends to offer in their pharmacy.

INTERPRET

Properly interpreting and analyzing all the information collected during the scanning process is critical to making good decisions that will form the basis of a strategic plan.

One of the most common and effective methods for analyzing the data collected in a scan is to perform a SWOT analysis. SWOT is an acronym for strengths, weaknesses, opportunities and threats.

Strengths: characteristics of your business that may be viewed as unique or different and are likely to be seen as giving one an advantage over competitors

Weaknesses: characteristics of a business that may place one at a disadvantage relative to competitors

Opportunities: usually areas that if implemented, could provide an advantage over others and thus become strengths

Threats: elements identified in an environmental scan and market analysis that could cause difficulty for a business and threaten its viability and success[2]

Often, many items from the scan can be viewed under more than one of these categories. For example, a pharmacy may not offer free prescription delivery but competitors do. This could be viewed as a weakness and/or a threat. Another example may be that during the environmental scan, some customers may have identified a particular product or product line that their pharmacy does not carry. This could be viewed as a weakness but also an opportunity because there is demand, so plans can be made to stock that product line and begin promoting it.

DECIDE

Once the information collected in the environmental scan and market analysis has been categorized, the next step is to make some decisions about how to use that information in creating a finalized plan.

Before getting down to specific goal setting, it is often useful to develop a vision statement or a statement of distinctive excellence. It is a statement that defines, in one or two sentences, that particular strength of a company that it does very well and sets it apart from its competitors.

To develop a vision or distinctive excellence statement, one needs to determine the organization's competitive strategy. Most companies employ one major competitive strategy. They are either product leaders, customer intimate or operationally efficient. Most organizations are great at one and good at the other two (see Figure 6.2).

Product leaders are always trying to bring superior products to their customers, which in turn often translates into being able to charge premium prices because of the experience their products create for their customers. A good example of a product leader is Apple.

Operationally efficient organizations focus on cost reduction by streamlining processes and procedures. These types of organizations are usually quite centralized and provide a consistent experience from one location to another. Walmart and IKEA are examples of operationally efficient organizations.

Customer-intimate organizations focus on the needs of the customer. These types of organizations tend to be highly service oriented and will adapt quickly to individual customer needs.

Figure 6.2

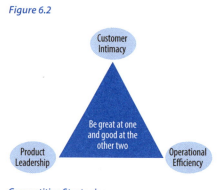

Competitive Strategies

They place a heavy emphasis on building a strong and loyal relationship with their customers. Two examples of customer-intimate organizations are IBM and Amazon.com.

Develop a mission statement once the competitive strategy is clear. The mission statement is simply the reason the organization exists. It is about the purpose of the organization and should encompass all the goals in one broader statement. A mission statement should state who the market is, what is being offered to them and what makes the offering unique. For example, Rite Aid pharmacy's mission statement is, "To improve the health and wellness of our communities through engaging experiences that provide our customers with the best products, services and advice to meet their unique needs."[3] Another pharmacy example of a mission statement is from Walgreens. It states, "To be the most trusted, convenient multichannel provider and advisor of innovative pharmacy, health and wellness solutions, and consumer goods and services in communities across America. A destination where health and happiness come together to help people get well, stay well and live well."[4]

Once the competitive strategy and mission statement are clear, the focus can shift to the details of the strategic plan. It is probably easiest to think of a strategic plan as a set of specific goals that one wants to achieve for the business and a description of how to get there. It is usually advisable to keep the number of goals small. The more goals there are, the more difficult it is to achieve any of them as resources tend to get spread too thin. Two to four goals is a good realistic number. Once one or more of the goals have been achieved, new ones can be added as the plan moves into the future.

The goals should be SMART: specific, measurable, attainable, realistic and timely.

Specific means including things such as who, what, when, where and why in the goals. For example, a general goal might be, "fill more prescriptions"; a specific goal could be, "fill 25% more prescriptions in the next six months than in the past six months."

Measurable means ensuring one has criteria that can be measured toward the achievement of the goal. When progress is measured, it is easier to stay on track and keep focused resulting in a higher likelihood of reaching target dates and numbers. This can be achieved by keeping a scorecard, graph or chart to track progress and displaying it where all staff members can view it.

Attainable means setting goals that can truly be achieved. It does not mean making the goals small and easy but rather making them about the things that are most important to the business. Focus on being able to use the skills, abilities and resources available. Even the culture within a staff group can help make goals more attainable.

Realistic means setting goals that one is motivated to achieve. Lofty goals are fine as long as one is willing and able to work toward them. Feeling motivated and constantly measuring progress usually means the goals are realistic. Sometimes high goals are easier to reach than low ones because one is more motivated and gains significant satisfaction from reaching it.

Timely means setting goals that can be achieved within a reasonable time frame and that will have a positive effect on the business. Most strategic plans look three to five years into the future. Any longer than five years makes it difficult to assess the success of strategies and to make changes to adapt to the changing environment in which the business is operating. That does not mean all the goals should have the same time frame. It is possible to have a goal with a target date for achievement in year one while another goal may take three years to achieve.

Figure 6.3

	Existing Products	New Products
Existing Markets	Market Penetration	Product Development
New Markets	Market Development	Diversification

Ansoff Matrix[5]
(used with permission from QuickMBA.com)

Figure 6.4

Target Scope	Advantage	
	Low Cost	Product Uniqueness
Broad (Industry Wide)	Cost Leadership Strategy	Differentiation Strategy
Narrow Segment (Market Segment)	Focus Strategy (low cost)	Focus Strategy (differentiation)

Porter's Generic Strategies[6]
(used with permission from QuickMBA.com)

Another tool one may find helpful in determining an approach to the market is Ansoff's Matrix. This matrix, depicted in Figure 6.3, can help one decide on a growth strategy; that is, should the business grow by finding new markets (customers) or grow in existing markets with new products and services or with existing products and services?

Another potentially useful tool is Porter's Generic Strategies (as depicted in Figure 6.4). This tool is more directed at finding out whether the position of the business within the industry is about differentiation and uniqueness or cost superiority.

Once decisions have been made about goals, one needs to decide on the strategies that need to be implemented to achieve these goals.

IMPLEMENT

Implementing a strategic plan takes preparation and planning. Involving all staff members is usually a good idea. Everyone has to know and understand what the long-term goals for the business are and what the plan is to get there. Furthermore, they each need to understand their own role and how they will contribute to the achievement of the overall goals for the business.

The potentially most important aspect of the successful implementation of a strategic plan is the full and complete commitment of the business owner and/or senior management team. This aspect is critical because all the other staff members will take their cues from the executive of the organization.

HUMAN RESOURCES INFORMATION

One should constantly communicate ongoing progress and keep employees involved and engaged. This is where a visible scorecard is useful. For example, one may have a chart with each goal or task listed on it and indicated via colours if things are on track. Traffic-light colours work well. Green means things are on track from both time and budget perspectives; yellow means there are some concerns that need attention; and red means serious problems that must be addressed immediately.

Another way to ensure alignment of business activities to goals is by using the balanced score-card. "The balanced scorecard is a strategic planning and management system that is used extensively in business and industry, government, and non-profit organizations worldwide to align business activities to the vision and strategy of the organization, improve internal and external communications, and monitor organization performance against strategic goals."[7]

Stay focused on the goals that have been set for the business. Keep monitoring the environment for changes that may affect the organization and adjust accordingly. A strong strategic plan and good execution could be the difference between business success and failure.

RESOURCES AND SUGGESTED READINGS

Kim WC, Mauborgne R. *Blue ocean strategy: how to create uncontested market space and make competition irrelevant.* Boston, MA: Harvard Business School Publishing Corporation; 2005.

Olsen E. *Strategic planning kit for dummies.* 2nd ed. Hoboken, New Jersey: John Wiley & Sons, Inc; 2011.

Rohm H, Wilsey D, Stout Perry G, et al. *The institute way: simplify strategic planning and management with the balanced scorecard.* Cary, NC: The Institute Press; 2013.

Rumelt R. *Good strategy bad strategy: the difference and why it matters.* New York: Crown Publishing Group; 2011.

Stern CW. Deimler MS, editor. *The Boston Consulting Group on strategy: classic concepts and new perspectives.* Hoboken, New Jersey: John Wiley & Sons, Inc; 2006.

REFERENCES

1. MapInfo. PSYTE HD Canada, Pitney Bowes, 2014. Available: www.mapinfo.com/data-products/psyte-hd-canada/ (accessed July 27, 2014).
2. Internet Center for Management and Business Administration, Inc. Quick MBA.com, strategic management, SWOT analysis, 1999–2010. Available: www.quickmba.com/strategy/swot/ (accessed Nov. 9, 2014).
3. Rite Aid Corp., core values and mission statement, 2001–2014. Available: www.riteaid.com/about-us/mission-statement (accessed Aug. 2, 2014).
4. Walgreens MS. 2014 Available: http://news.walgreens.com/article_display.cfm?article_id=1042 (accessed Aug. 2, 2014).
5. Internet Center for Management and Business Administration, Inc. Quick MBA.com, strategic management, Ansoff matrix, 1999–2010. Available: www.quickmba.com/strategy/matrix/ansoff/ (accessed Aug. 2, 2014).
6. Internet Center for Management and Business Administration, Inc. Quick MBA.com, strategic management, Porter's generic strategies, 1999–2010. Available: www.quickmba.com/strategy/generic.shtml (accessed Aug. 2, 2014).
7. Balanced Scorecard Institute. Balanced scorecard basics, 1998–2014. Available: http://balancedscorecard.org/Resources/About-the-Balanced-Scorecard (accessed Nov. 9, 2014).

CHAPTER 7

The Pharmacist Entrepreneur

Alan Dresser, *B.Sc., B.Ed., BSP, MBA*

Michael S. Jaczko, *BSc. Phm., RPh, CIM® (Chartered Investment Manager); Partner and Portfolio Manager, K J Harrison & Partners Inc., Toronto, ON*

Learning Objectives

- Define what it takes to be an entrepreneur.
- Describe the five roots of entrepreneurial opportunity.
- Identify the common character traits of an entrepreneur.
- Identify the skill sets required for success.
- Identify the key considerations an entrepreneur pharmacy owner/manager needs to identify when considering going into business.

THE EVER-INCREASING CHOICE TO BECOME AN ENTREPRENEUR

More than 500 million people worldwide were either actively involved in a new startup venture or owners of a new business in 2010.[1] Entrepreneurs continue to drive the transformational renewal of economies worldwide. The Canadian retail pharmacy landscape continues to be reshaped as an increasingly larger number of independent pharmacies open their doors every year.

ENTREPRENEURSHIP

The World English Dictionary defines an entrepreneur as, *"A person who sets up a business or businesses, taking on financial risks in the hope of profit."*[2] There is certainly no shortage of successful young entrepreneurs in business today. It is hard to miss business news stories of fast-growing startups from New York City to Silicon Valley, headed by CEOs such as Mark Zuckerberg and Tim O'Shaughnessy. Although without the notoriety, creative minds in the Canadian pharmacy industry continue to demonstrate the power of energetic tenacity and innovation, combined with a sharp eye for business.

ENTREPRENEURIAL FRAMEWORK CONDITIONS

The number of entrepreneurs continues to rise as traditionally labour-intensive large-scale employers decline. Corporate downsizing and dropping pharmacist wage rates due to government pricing pressures and increased supply has led to a rising share of new entrepreneurs in the ages 55 to 64 group.[3] Corporate consolidation, reduction in extended-hours stores and an increasing number of recent undergraduates entering the market are also likely contributors.

MONEY—SOURCES OF CAPITAL IN CANADIAN PHARMACY

One of the most difficult problems in the new venture creation process is obtaining financing.[4] Entrepreneurs have the right personal financial profile to make the leap. This does not mean that only the wealthy can be entrepreneurs. However, financial sacrifices are necessary when starting.

Pharmacy is no stranger to that age-old practice of borrowing from friends and family; it's quite common when it comes to securing the first level of cash required to engage a prospective seller. Better rates or conditions may be possible if the money comes from a family member. However, "less than arm's-length" forms of financing can be fraught with complications, so it is always best to seek advice from experienced advisors and to define repayment terms to avoid misunderstandings and issues.

Countless partnerships (involving two or more owners) are formed for the purpose of pooling their resources, both financial and sweat equity (labour), with a view to purchasing a pharmacy business. This provides an excellent opportunity for both parties to share in the work, the risk and the benefits associated with building a prosperous pharmacy practice. But don't forget—good fences make good neighbours. Before embarking on any sort of partnership, prospective partners should solidify their finances through a properly conceived and constructed shareholders' agreement that describes each partner's commitment and an agreed departure of a partner. (See Chapter 14: Financial Statements and Forms of Business Ownership and Chapter 53: Business Planning to Business Plan for more on partnerships and forms of ownership.)

Another source of money is groups known as angel investors. These are individuals who have significant financial assets and business acumen, who are looking for investments with a relatively higher rate of return. They may often expect an equity position in the pharmacy business they are investing in. They have extensive business experience and are willing to take a risk, albeit for an expected higher rate of return.

Pharmacy entrepreneurs often turn to funds that are readily available from Canada's chartered banks and financial corporations. Bank of Montreal and Scotiabank (in Québec, National Bank and Laurentian) have positioned themselves in the retail-pharmacy industry. Financial companies have also become increasingly prominent as a source of capital for pharmacists. Today's big players include the stalwart Desante and the newcomer Element Capital. Traditional banks and financial corporations each present their advantages and disadvantages. Always get legal and financial advice before signing any financial documents.

KEY BANKING RELATIONSHIPS

When borrowing from a financial institution, there will be terms and conditions that must be met, and when the amount required is completely paid, the business is owned free and clear.

It is important to develop a relationship with the financial entities that may someday finance an acquisition. Start that relationship the moment the prospect of purchasing a pharmacy becomes a possibility. It can be as simple as an introduction to a local banker. Kindling such relationships will provide the comfort that institutions will invariably need to gain confidence in the potential owner and the business plan—before they approve a business loan. From there, the importance of communicating proactively and regularly with the financial institution cannot be overemphasized. Understandably, financial institutions hate surprises. Actively communicate through financial statements all significant changes in the business, good or bad, as they arise. Doing so continues the bankers' hard-earned trust.

Financial institutions expect preparation. This would be evident in sound financial statements and realistic projections (or "pro forma statements"), developed in advance of a meeting. Prepare best-case, worst-case and probable-case projections. Presenting a well-conceived business plan often makes the difference in successfully attaining the desired financing (see Chapter 8: Assessing the Critical Attributes of a New Venture and Chapter 53: Business Planning to Business Plan).

FIVE CS FOR ACQUIRING CREDIT

Practically speaking, lending institutions expect to be repaid any money they loan plus interest. Much of their work (referred to as "loan underwriting") is determining the likelihood that someone will, in fact, repay them. Considering the following five Cs may greatly increase the chance of success: character, capacity, capital, collateral and conditions.

CHARACTER

Lending institutions are assessing. They judge character, integrity, experience, communication skills and the preparedness of a request. They are also judging the business that may be purchased, specifically the cash flow EBITDA (earnings before interest, tax, depreciation and amortization). EBITDA offers an excellent barometer for gauging the ability of a targeted pharmacy business to service a loan and will be looked at closely.

CAPACITY

Repaying (also known as servicing a loan) means paying back a portion of the loan—the principal, plus the interest on the outstanding balance—on a monthly basis.

CAPITAL

Capital refers to the amount of equity (cash) that is put into a prospective business. Financial institutions require varying "paid in capital" amounts, based on the nuances of the specific deal.

COLLATERAL

The assets found in or outside of the business that may be pledged against the loan are known as collateral. It provides one form of security that lenders often require. The banks, in particular, will go to several levels of commitment, including personal guarantees from the buyer, the buyer's spouse and other relatives, and claims on the buyer's house or other assets.

CONDITIONS

Finally, there are the conditions of both the overall pharmacy business/regulatory environment and the local economy of the community in which the store is located. The poorer the conditions, of course, the greater the risk and the less favourable the loan conditions that a prospective buyer may encounter.

THE VENTURE

Tolerance of ambiguity is an important character trait in risk-taking. A person must be able to withstand the fear of uncertainty and potential failure. Michael Sherod, entrepreneur-in-residence at the Neeley School of Business, states, "It all boils down to being able to successfully manage fear."[5] Typical fears experienced by entrepreneurs include the fear of failure.

Before getting involved in a venture such as starting or acquiring a pharmacy, it is of paramount importance that a prospective buyer measure tolerance to risk on different levels. The following six questions need to be answered to really have a better understanding of risk-tolerance level:

HOW MUCH MONEY ARE YOU WILLING TO LOSE?

For many young people, risking money is difficult as they may not have much capital accumulated. Depending on a person's age and family status, there may be much or very little to risk. Pharmacists should remember to always make sure that they will be able to make a living if the venture does not work.

HOW MUCH TIME CAN YOU INVEST?

If a person is young, investing 5 or 10 years in a venture that may go wrong may not be that critical as the experience gained will help in the next venture. However, as a person's career progresses, the more productive years are at risk.

DO YOU HAVE THE SUPPORT OF YOUR FAMILY?

People who are married or in a committed relationship, and especially those with young children, need the unconditional support of their partners to succeed. Other family-member support may be important as well. Many relationships do not last if support is not agreed upon before jumping into the venture.

DO YOU HAVE THE MENTAL/PHYSICAL ENERGY TO SUCCEED?

Many people do not realize how much energy is needed to succeed. Also, if there are other priorities (immediate and extended family, community, sports, training, etc.), time will have to be diverted into the business. Some people stop training and eating well and may end up in a health situation that is difficult. It takes enormous discipline to combine an entrepreneurial project with a healthy lifestyle. Work-life balance will be out of balance for the first five or more years in most cases.

ARE YOU WILLING TO HAVE YOUR REPUTATION DAMAGED?

If the project fails, other people may think (and will likely say) that the entrepreneur is a failure who didn't have what it takes, etc. This will hurt. Entrepreneurs must be strong enough to be able to stand these comments from colleagues, friends or family if they fail.

CAN YOU KEEP YOUR SELF-ESTEEM?

People who are not successful may blame themselves for it even if they have nothing to do with the failure. Before beginning such a journey, they should reflect on themselves and think about how they would perceive themselves if things go wrong. This is important because people most probably want to live a happy life even if a project did not work. Being able to maintain good self-esteem whatever way things go is very important.

Market analysis and the development of a business plan are paramount (see Section XI: Marketing, Promotion and Customer Service and Section XII: Business Plans to guide the new entrepreneur through these processes).

An early decision involves the choice to buy an existing pharmacy business or start a new one (a startup is often referred to as a "greenfield pharmacy"). Having a vision of what to build is an important first step. The ability to spot an opportunity and imagine something where others have not will serve a person well.

There are five roots of opportunity in the marketplace that entrepreneurs can exploit[6]:
- problems the pharmacy business can solve
- changes in laws, situations or trends
- inventions of totally new products or services
- competition (If entrepreneurs can find a way to beat the competition, they can create a very successful business with an existing product or service.)
- technological advances

It can be readily argued that the Canadian pharmacy industry is currently subject to all of the above-mentioned roots of opportunity!

Entrepreneurs have a curiosity that identifies overlooked niches or run-down store operations and that puts them at the forefront of innovation and emerging fields of opportunity. An increasing number of entrepreneurs are choosing to become involved with operating a franchise type of operation such as Shoppers Drug Mart. These opportunities provide a place to learn management skills under the guidance of a main office and require considerably less capital when investing.

CHARACTER TRAITS OF AN ENTREPRENEUR

The most important characteristics of a successful entrepreneur are succinctly identified by Bygrave and Zacharakis as the 10 Ds.[7]
- Dream: Entrepreneurs have a vision of what the future could be like for them and their businesses. More importantly, they have the ability to implement their dreams.
- Decisiveness: Entrepreneurs don't procrastinate. They make decisions swiftly, a key factor in their success.
- Doers: Once they decide on a course of action, entrepreneurs implement it as quickly as possible.
- Determination: Entrepreneurs implement their venture with total commitment. They seldom give up, even when confronted by obstacles that seem insurmountable.
- Dedication: Entrepreneurs are totally dedicated to their businesses, sometimes at considerable cost to their relationships with friends and families. They work endlessly.

Twelve-hour days and seven-day work weeks are not uncommon when an entrepreneur is striving to get a business off the ground.

- Devotion: Entrepreneurs love what they do. It is the love that sustains the entrepreneur, and it is love of their product or service that makes them so effective at selling it.
- Details: The entrepreneur must pay attention to the critical details of aspects of the business to respond to constant changes in the marketplace.
- Destiny: Entrepreneurs want to be in charge of their own destiny rather than dependent on an employer.
- Dollars: Entrepreneurs assume that if they are successful, they will be rewarded. Getting rich is not the prime motivator of many entrepreneurs but often is a significant benefit.
- Distribute: Entrepreneurs distribute the rewards of their businesses with key employees who are critical to the success of the business. This may happen in the form of shared ownership or by way of bonuses.

Experience can only be gained with time. It comes from active patient care service during pre-licensing, internship and working in a variety of practice settings. Each work experience provides a unique perspective, and the student/new practitioner gains knowledge and experience unique to each situation. View every experience within the context of three perspectives: the employee, the patient/customer and the owner/manager.

Aspiring owners should reflect and consider what they would have done and how they would have behaved if they had found themselves in a similar situation. Consider what further information would be needed to make decisions or if what was done and how it was done is acceptable. Accept or take leadership opportunities that present themselves to accelerate obtaining experience. Such an approach forces people to think like an owner/manager. Most entrepreneurs learn on the job and as a result, require an innate ability to be versatile or flexible with planning and changing plans.[8]

Education and support services: Within the courses offered by the professional faculty, take the best of any elective courses required to complete the degree. Taking management and business courses will kickstart someone's thinking like a businessperson. As well, there are offerings by chambers of commerce, provincial/territorial pharmacy associations and corporate management training worthy of consideration. Many young pharmacy entrepreneurs have chosen to take evening business courses at local universities and community colleges to start their business acumen.

Self-confidence: Investors, venture capitalists and business partners require that entrepreneurs be extremely confident about their business practice. Staff members will continue to present challenges and questions that require a firm, confident response, but the greatest confidence is shown when someone admits to not knowing and follows up to find out the answer.

Self-knowledge and emotional intelligence: It is important to take time to reflect and ask tough questions. Entrepreneurs have to ask themselves if they are prepared to do the work; prepared to invest great amounts of time, thought and energy into the business; prepared to delay financial and monetary rewards of a regular job as they work toward entrepreneurial goals. They have to consider if they are comfortable with complexity and uncertainty, if they are aware of the loneliness of ownership and leadership, and if they can prepare themselves to deal with this.

Entrepreneurs must ask themselves if they know their strengths and weaknesses and then plan to accommodate or strengthen these areas. For most, the first few years after graduation should be spent discovering the functions and skill sets they are naturally good at. Are they applicable to this venture? It may be wise, if possible, to hire someone with those compensating strengths to fill in the void.

The fact of the matter is no entrepreneur possesses all the skills and attributes required to ensure an absolute positive outcome.

MARKETS, CUSTOMERS, CLIENTS, PATIENTS

Kenneth B. Elliott, Vice President of Studebaker Corporation (1941), wrote of customers (and patients): *"A customer is not an interruption in our work; he is the purpose of it."*[9]

Early stage questions entrepreneurs should ask themselves include the following: Is there a market for you that shares your vision? What sort of service do you want to provide? As the role of pharmacists continues to evolve, a counselling service or a patient-advocacy service coordinating the patient's care between general practitioners, specialists and community services may be a niche that could be in demand and be possibly profitable. Perhaps a compounding, nutritional or chronic disease-focused pharmacy would be a better fit for the business and your target market. Are there enough customers to make this viable? Is there an underserviced area for a traditional service or perhaps a competitive market with a niche that others are not prepared to enter?

It is important to appreciate that for new ventures, marketing can be particularly challenging (see Section IX: Developing, Implementing and Managing Clinical Pharmacy Services). Developing a clear understanding of an intended market is an essential and ongoing task that contributes to the related tasks of refining the product/service mix and gaining legitimacy.[10]

BUY/NEW

The classic question invariably asked is, "Is it better to buy or build new?" The purchasing of an existing business involves several steps as well as determining the value of goodwill. This is a value of the existing clientele and the likelihood that it will continue to patronize that pharmacy. Owners can depend on sustained cash flow for three months or more, which should give an attentive purchaser time to develop a culture that will attract and maintain a strong client base.

Site location and service selection with a new store (greenfield store) is paramount. A new store will have a slower cash flow and customer base development. Picking a banner program (e.g., IDA, Pharmasave), negotiating a lease, establishing supplier terms, purchasing store fixtures and choosing the proper technology (e.g., pharmacy management system) are some of the early major decisions in either case.

PROCESSES, CONTROLLING OPERATIONS AND TECHNOLOGIES

While motivation, creativity and developing a dream are key components on the path to success, the task of managing operations, technologies and controls is integral to actually achieving success. When considering a new venture, it is important to distinguish between the processes that simply have to be done to a minimum standard from those that could provide a real competitive advantage.[11] Thoughtfully developed systems form the base that allows the employee to meet the needs of customers and patients.

It is true that "the devil is in the details," a well-quoted saying coined by German art historian Aby Warburg.[12] An entrepreneur's chances for success can be dramatically improved by making every repeated step part of a systematic process. Doing so will reduce the chances for errors. When steps are systematized, every employee can provide the same quality service to patrons.

Investing in technology is important. Automation represents a key component of success ensuring processes are repeatable devoid of human variability and error. For example, a point-of-sale (POS) system can combine bookkeeping, inventory control, ordering, selling, cash handling and customer relations processes to provide uniform, systematic performance and function. These automated functions are done much faster and more accurately than humans possibly can and every step has an audit trail.

For a comprehensive review of the details required to properly manage a pharmacy practice/operation, see Section VI: Operations, Section VII: Quality Control, Quality Assurance and Continuous Quality Improvement, and Section VIII: Human Resources.

SURROUND YOURSELF WITH EXCELLENT ADVICE

Entrepreneurs will need legal and accounting assistance early on in their business venture. Doing so saves time, provides experience and ultimately saves money in the end. Ideally, it is best to work with subject-matter experts who have experience in the pharmacy industry as they can often provide timely guidance and decision-making structure along the way.

Supporting the provincial/territorial professional association is a worthwhile investment in one's future as doing so gives voice to the profession and provides advocacy with other industry and government stakeholders.

A cooperative/banner group can be a time- and money-saving decision for the independent owner. Banners and cooperative groups can assist with marketing and provide operational support and buying power with suppliers. It will also provide tools designed to help build the store's profile in the community.

PROFIT

The word *profit* is often cast in a dim light within the context of Canadian health care. The level of profit that is reasonable depends on the type of business. In Canada, retail pharmacies earn profits in the range of 2% to 10%, averaging 5% to 6%.[13] Profit is the return a company or owner receives for providing value to the customer. It is the source of funds for debt payment, business expansion and owner's return on investment.

Profitability as a measure of profit is discussed in further detail in Section IV: Financial Management for Your Practice. Protection of profit is a primary concern of an entrepreneur.

Business-operating surpluses in the early years of ownership are used to service debt and bank loans and later on may serve as a source for business expansion and retirement, both of which greatly contribute to the overall economic health and viability of the Canadian economy.

In conclusion, being an entrepreneur takes a special breed of individual. Self-confidence and an element of risk-taking are often met with significant personal and financial rewards. Furthermore, working for oneself provides the ability to control the work practice environment and shape one's own professional destiny.

REFERENCES

1. Global Entrepreneurship Monitor estimate, GEM adult population surveys. Available: www.gemconsortium.org (accessed Oct. 31, 2014).

2. Entrepreneur definition. Oxford dictionaries. Available: www.oxforddictionaries.com/definition/english/entrepreneur (accessed Oct. 31, 2014).

3. Kauffman index of entrepreneurial activity. Available: www.kauffman.org/~/media/kauffman_org/research%20reports%20and%20covers/2014/04/kiea_2014_report.pdf (accessed Oct. 31, 2014).

4. Hisrich RD, Peters MP, Shepherd DA. *Entrepreneurship.* 8th ed. New York: McGraw-Hill Irwin; 2010. p. 308–15.

5. Sherrod M. Neeley School of Business, Texas Christian University, The 7 traits of successful entrepreneurs. Available: www.entrepreneur.com/article/230350 (accessed April 28, 2014).

6. Mariotti S, Glackin C. *Entrepreneurship.* 2nd ed. New Jersey: Prentice Hall; 2010. p. 16–7.

7. Bygrave WD, Zacharakis AI. *Entrepreneurship.* 2nd ed. Hoboken, New Jersey: John Wiley & Sons, Inc; 2011. p. 53.

8. Awe SC. *The entrepreneur's information sourcebook, charting the path to small business success*: 2nd ed. ABC-CLIO, LLC, 130 Cremona Drive, P.O. Box 1911, Santa Barbara, California 93116–1911.

9. The customer is not an interruption in our work; he is the purpose of it. Quote Investigator. Available: http://quoteinvestigator.com/tag/kenneth-b-elliott/ (accessed Jan. 31, 2015).

10. Blundel R, Lockett N. *Exploring entrepreneurship, practices and perspectives.* Great Clarendon Street, Oxford ox26DP. Oxford University Press; 2011. p. 109–33.

11. *Ibid.,*p136–57.

12. Ancient Wisdom Publications. The devil is in the details. Available: www.andras-nagy.com/wordpress/?p=539 (accessed Oct. 31, 2014).

13. K H Harrison & Partners database, Toronto, ON. Accessed April 28, 2014.

CHAPTER 8

Assessing the Critical Attributes of a New Venture

Roderick A. Slavcev, *PhD, MBA, MSB, C.Biol; Assistant Professor, School of Pharmacy, University of Waterloo*

Learning Objectives

- Understand what are the critical gaps in developing a new venture.
- Learn to effectively assess the critical attributes of a venture and assess business feasibility and managerial competence
  - Critically identifying if the venture is a business
  - Critically assessing if the venture can be managed
  - Identifying the core competence and whether the venture team can do it

---

A well-articulated business plan is undeniably effective in the evaluation of a new project, managerial planning and for investors and lenders. However, there exists a disconnect in entrepreneurship as it is the business plan itself that is used to try to entice funding, while planning is the essential component of a new venture's success and effective management, and what investors are more interested in evaluating. Funding decisions of new ventures are generally influenced by two important considerations: how an entrepreneurial business plan is written and how it is evaluated. Though a venture's quality should ultimately be indicated by its performance, Mainprize and Hindle rather surprisingly found that writing, rating and performance effects of entrepreneurial business plans are highly under-researched topics.[1] As a result, it turns out that venture capitalists and other investors tend to evaluate business plans indiscriminately, while entrepreneurs may write business plans erratically and unpredictably.

Of course, there is no foolproof framework that can ensure a new venture or project's success, but there is a model that shifts the view to specifically address the key questions of a banker or private investor and should dramatically improve a venture's chances of funding and success. Such a model has been developed by Dr. Ronald K. Mitchell, appropriately termed the *New Venture Template* (NVT), and while originally designed for the entrepreneur, the questions addressed are just as relevant to the improvement/screening of an existing venture.[2] The model is based in actuarial science and has conferred a screened new venture success rate of 54%, compared to 17% identified by the more traditional business plan approach.[3,4]

The template follows the methodology of providing an expanded executive summary covering the essentials of the venture to identify critical gaps. This approach is known as the "known attributes" approach and contradicts traditional assumptions that a business plan must be produced before screening can take place. The NVT evaluates a venture or project's essential attributes and addresses Mitchell's three simple yet critical questions: *Is it a business? Can you keep it? Can you do it?* Attributes answering the first of these address market-related issues, while those of the second address resistance to competition and sustainability and the third addresses managerial competence.

Mitchell identified six fundamental gaps that commonly result in the failure of new ventures. The focus of a new venture or even an existing business to address these gaps confers the relevant attributes of high-potential ventures. Specific questions are further identified within each attribute.

The ability of a new venture to cross each gap can be gauged by scoring its performance across each of the 15 questions as either low, medium or high. Mitchell recommends that each be assessed in the order described and that a low score needs to be corrected before continuing on to the next attribute. Of course, it is important to note that scoring is subjective and open to interpretation and as such, the tool is only valuable in assessing new business ideas if it is applied conservatively and honestly.

ASSESSING THE CRITICAL ATTRIBUTES OF A VENTURE

1. IS IT A BUSINESS?

A. Innovation Gap

In crossing the innovation gap, a new venture must ask questions that relate to new economic combinations and a proper and real fit between the product offering (product or service) and the market for which it is intended. A new economic combination was described by Austrian economist Joseph Schumpeter as, "a new value that is imparted to existing resources through innovation."[5] These combinations must be further matched to market need before they possess inherent wealth-generating capacity.

Is it a new combination?

New combinations arise from the correcting of market imperfections arising from either excess supply without demand or excess demand without supply. These form the basis for entrepreneurial discoveries and can be either circumstantially or scientifically generated.[2] A new drug that could cure all cancers, albeit highly unlikely, matches supply to excess demand through scientific invention. In contrast, the formation of at-home clinical care teams represents an innovation that coordinates existing health care professionals with excess demand of at-home patients. A *low* score here suggests that the new venture or project idea is not new to the market and thus, is not innovative. A *medium* score suggests an incremental improvement that may help to deal with or fix a market problem, while a *high* score is indicative of a revolutionary innovation that represents a market need. If a new combination is not present (low score), the venture should not be pursued until this can be corrected. Some potential examples are offered as follows:

- low: A startup that seeks to follow a traditional retail model and provide the same services and products as a large chain pharmacy would likely be categorized as *low* in innovation.
- medium: The same new pharmacy would plan to offer more complementary services such as regular follow-up and a dedicated pharmacist-patient relationship.
- high: A mobile health unit that provides health care services and therapies to rural underserviced areas or people who cannot easily visit the pharmacy or medical clinic may be categorized as high.

Is there a product-market match?

Assessing the degree of a product-market match of a new idea pertains to the inclination of your market to purchase a product or service. Securing purchase orders before entry of the product to the market serves to signify strong product-market match. In contrast, a lack of any purchase orders signifies that a product-market match may not yet be present, threatening the wealth-creating capacity of the new combination. In the case of a low score in this category, the venture or business idea should not be pursued until this insufficiency is corrected. In existing businesses, a low score in this category suggests that future sustainability may be threatened.

It is important to note that traditional business plans generally articulate untested assumptions about the product-market fit, which may often prove incorrect. In his take of the lean startup model,[6] Steve Blanks instead teaches that individuals need to "get out of the building" and speak to potential customers to properly identify the target market and assess the product-market fit of their business idea and test hypotheses regarding their presumed value proposition(s). Potential examples of ratings for this category follow:

- low: a new chain pharmacy sets up in a community where there were only small stores
- medium: the same chain pharmacy that has a drive-through service in a community where the clientele is made up of working, middle-class people who appreciate fast service
- high: a chain pharmacy that has implemented a fully electronic renewal service including automatic renewals and email/SMS alert service, coupled with home or work delivery

B. Value Gap

Determining whether a new venture or business idea creates value requires its examination from two different perspectives. The first is the value of a product offering to the customer or patient, while the second is the value created for the business, which in simple terms can be assessed as the total revenue minus the cost of its generation. Crossing the value attribution gap requires, according to Mitchell,[2] a sequential assessment of the venture's ability to create net buyer benefit (customer value) and adequate margins and volume (business value).

Is there net buyer benefit?

This question addresses a venture's ability to provide net delivered customer value (NDCV), which may be best described as the sum of all the benefits provided by the product or service (functional benefits, service, social) minus the sum of all the costs of attaining that product such as financial, energy and time.[7] If the net value is psychologically assessed by the customer as positive, then the service has created NDCV. A high rating here would leave a customer thrilled with the product and/or service and eager to return, while a low rating would provide a customer perception of getting "ripped off." A medium rating would thus fall between these two extremes. A low rating in this category should preclude further pursuit of the business until corrected by either reducing costs to the customer or increasing/improving the benefits offered. The following potential examples illustrate levels of net buyer benefit:

- low: a local pharmacy with undifferentiated services must lower its dispensing fee to compete with other pharmacies in the vicinity to keep its customers
- medium: a local pharmacy offers disease-prevention programs to its customers for a fee, with several returning customers
- high: a local pharmacy offers personalized follow-ups on a weekly basis, with new product/ services proposals for clients with food/seasonal allergies

Are there margins?

This part of the value equation now shifts to examining profit generation for the business. The margin is simply the profit arising from the revenue generated by a business or service, less the sum of all costs and expenses in generating that revenue in a given period. Competition serves to drive down the price, particularly for undifferentiated products (commodities), reducing margins and forcing suppliers to reduce their costs to remain competitive, or increase volume of sales. While industries will vary in average margins, with some considerably more attractive than others, much of pricing in drug distribution in Canada is regulated by provincial/territorial governments, standardizing margins somewhat and forcing focus on volume and addition of other products and services. If the margins are lower than the industry average, then it may not warrant going forward with the business unless narrow margins can be compensated by sufficient volume (next category). Examples to illustrate margin ratings follow:

- low: a small independent pharmacy offers drug distribution services with higher cost per unit compared to other chain pharmacies in the vicinity
- medium: a small independent pharmacy offers new community-learning sessions for key-demand health topics at a fee and despite being smaller, has met the industry's average margin
- high: the same pharmacy offers compounding services providing its clientele with a higher-margin/highly differentiated product/service offering

Is volume sufficient?

Volume simply refers to the number of sales and refers directly to market demand for your product or service. In industries where margins are particularly thin, adequate volume is essential to generate adequate value to the firm. Volume is generally considered with margins to assess total profit. If volumes are not sufficient to meet profit targets, given the current margin, then the business should not go forward unless either sales or margins can be increased. Ratings can be defined as volume either being deficient, adequate or exceeding necessary sales to meet profit targets.

- low: a chain pharmacy that offers a news service for stomatized patients
- medium: a new chain pharmacy that offers dispills or dosetts services to one of several nursing homes

- high: a pharmacy chain merges with another chain to double its volume sales, thereby far exceeding sufficient volume to meet profit targets

C. Persistence Gap

By this point, it should be clear that the venture or business idea is both innovative and valuable. However, a business idea that cannot persist in value creation over time is nothing more than a fad and is not sustainable into the long-term future. According to Mitchell's model,[2] the comprehensive assessment of a venture's persistence requires investigating three essential principles: repetitive purchasing, long-term need and the availability of resources to sustain the venture. Failure to demonstrate all of these suggests that the business does not have a long-term sustainable outlook.

Is it repetitive?

Quite simply, this question seeks to assess how repetitive is usage leading to replacement (repurchase). A good analogy can be seen in golf, where golf tees are readily used and replaced, less so with golf balls, and less yet with golf clubs. The more often and predictably the product/service is replaced, the less likely it is to become obsolete. If the purchasing is erratic and seldom and rated low in this category, then the venture should not proceed unless ways can be found to increase purchasing frequency. In some cases, this can be achieved by limiting the amount (number of uses) of the product per purchase. Potential examples follow:

- low: a low-cost therapeutic balm lasts one year with repeated usage
- medium: a new vaccine requiring one booster immunizes universally against influenza for five years
- high: a new expensive cocktail of drugs must be taken daily to treat a lifelong viral infection

Is there a long-term need?

This question pertains to the product lifecycle of an offering. If the demand for a product/service will not be demanded into the future, then this will obviously impact the future sustainability of the business. The product lifecycle theory is a stylized temporal map of an average product or services demand in the market developed by Raymond Vernon in 1966.[8] Notwithstanding marketing challenges and strategy, entry at *introductory* and *growth* phases are ideal and suggest greatest potential for long-term need. In contrast, the *mature* and *decline* stages indicate the low-demand replacement phases of the cycle, threatening long-term need, unless the product/service can be redefined/improved to reinitiate growth. If the venture's rating for this criterion is low, then do not continue unless other uses with long-term outlook can be identified or the product/service can be redefined to reinitiate growth. Conversely, a new technology could render the product/service obsolete overnight, indicating the importance of a suitable macro-environmental analysis (see Chapter 2: Macro-environmental Analysis). Potential rating examples for this category follow:

- low: a new diet pill that is a fad
- medium: a new all-protein diet strategy with medium persistence
- high: a "fast health" access centre serving a persistent and growing population need for frontline health care

Are resources sufficient to sustain the venture?

To have reached this point, the proposed or existing venture is innovative, valuable and deemed persistent, suggesting that its wealth-creating capacity will grow. While of course this is desirable, it is essential that the venture possesses access to sufficient growth capital—for services, this may translate to new hires, venues, etc.; for products, this will mean scaling up production capacity and other. Cash flow is a critical consideration in the growth of new ventures, where if financial management is not properly planned, growing success can quickly use up capital and subject the business to insolvency and failure. As such, some form of business plan, whether conventional (see Chapter 53: Business Planning to Business Plan) or the lean startup canvas[9] (see Chapter 53: Business Planning to Business Plan), is a necessary exercise to undertake to ensure that a reasonable and conservative growth strategy and assessment have been conceptualized. A low rating here for a new venture should preclude further pursuit until this deficiency is rectified (additional financing and planning). A low rating for an existing business is a strong sign of danger. Ratings may be perceived as follows:

- low: none or very few resources and/or few sources from which to draw additional resources
- medium: adequate resources with some sources for additional resourcing
- high: abundant resources and sources from which to draw additional resources

2. CAN YOU KEEP IT?

D. Scarcity

The establishment of a new business (idea) that is innovative, valuable and persistent indicates strong wealth-creating capacity for your venture. However, business is not static and where value is created and readily available, competition will soon appear. The scarcity (protection of) attribute relates to the protection of your valuable innovation over time. The competitive landscape of the industry in which a business seeks to exist is very necessary to assess (see Chapter 3: Micro-environmental Analysis) to ensure that its market share is protected. The assessment of this attribute seeks to address protection against additional supply (imitability) that shrinks the business's slice of the market pie and substitutes (substitutability) that can detract demand from your offering, thereby making the pie smaller.

Is it protected against imitability?

There is a variety of strategies to provide excludability to your product or offering. If a relevant option, legal excludability relates to patents, trademarks, copyrights and trade secrets to protect against imitation. However, excludability may also be achieved by first-mover advantages (getting a head start), locking in suppliers, buyers, etc., branding and many other strategies that may prove preferential depending on the nature of the venture and its industry dynamics. For professional consultative services, such as clinical consultations, reputation and quality of service can dramatically impact and differentiate a service as unique capabilities can be much harder to imitate than resources.[10] If a low rating is scored in this category, then the innovation and value-creating capacity will likely be imitated, continually reducing the venture's market share; the business should not be pursued until a strategy is in place to fend off imitators. The threat of imitability is covered in some detail in Chapter 3, captured by Porter's threat of *New Entrants,*[11] which also illustrates the importance of a thorough environmental analysis in the planning of a new venture. Potential examples for ratings of non-imitability follow:

- low: an innovative diabetes pharmacy specialist teaches other pharmacists new interventions and techniques for a fee; upon completion, graduates are certified and are now qualified to teach other pharmacists
- medium: a new venture captures, analyzes and packages provincial health care outcome data for sale to pharmaceutical companies
- high: a new drug is under patent for 20 years with data protection for a minimum of eight years before it is subject to generic manufacture

Is it non-substitutable?

Substitution again limits scarcity for a product or service, not by adding supply, but rather by detracting demand. The threat of substitutes[11] is one of the forces influencing the attractiveness of an industry such as pharmacy (see Chapter 3: Micro-environmental Analysis). It is important to note that approaches that protect against imitability may in some cases not protect against substitutes. For instance, a new drug protected under patent offers no protection against a different molecule that offers the same therapy. Curtailing the threat of substitutes is not easy and requires permeating boundaries between the business and substitutes to strategically ally and prevent the reduction of demand.[12] Understanding what substitutes currently exist and their potential impact on your business is a critical component of environmental scanning and the strategic-planning process. If a venture rates low in this category, further development of the business should not continue. Potential rating examples for non-substitutability are offered:

- low: the drug distribution service provided by a pharmacist can be offered by a nurse practitioner, a registered pharmacy technician and can be automated
- medium: immunization and invasive drug administrations can be offered conveniently by a pharmacist, nurse and (less conveniently) by physician
- high: a specialized cross-disciplinary cardiovascular treatment team consists of a collaborative team including a cardiologist, nurse, pharmacist and nutritionist

E. Non-appropriability Gap

Appropriation is best defined as economic theft. As Mitchell[2] describes, a venture that can demonstrate innovation, value, persistence and scarcity is of great value and is a target of "claim jumpers" who add inefficiency to the supply chain, reducing the size of the pie, and "thieves" who "steal" the venture's profits, reducing the size of the venture's slice. Contending with appropriation is a critical component of the venture's evaluation to ensure that it is not bled dry by waste (slack) in the system and redistribution of profits (hold-up).

Is there no slack?

Slack refers to waste in the supply chain of the product or service, whereby upstream suppliers or downstream customers (note this does not necessarily mean the end user) of the venture are inefficient and pass the cost of this inefficiency onto the venture, thereby reducing the size of the pie.[12] The primary reason for slack in an organization is the misalignment of incentives; if the rating for this category is low, then pursuit of the venture should not continue until this deficiency is rectified. The solution to work toward is to align incentives between suppliers and buyers of the firm (as best as possible) to reduce slack to a minimum. In some cases, this can be accomplished by vertically integrating; for example, gaining control of upstream or downstream supplier and/or buyer positions (such as major players in the oil and gas industry). Alternately, alignment can be achieved by collaboration, as shown by Toyota, that offers and helps to implement its revolutionary Toyota Production System to its suppliers to build operational efficiency for them and hence, Toyota in tandem. The following are examples of prevention-of-slack ratings:

- low: a health care system where drug manufacturers, physicians, hospitals, pharmacists, governments, insurers, etc., are all incentivized differently and act independently of each other
- medium: a health care system with the same players as in the low category, where risk-adjusted outcomes of patients through a full cycle are recorded at all levels of health care, rewarding best health care providers
- high: a competitive risk-adjusted system that rewards innovation, where every player in the health care system is incentivized according to longer-term patient outcomes

Is there no hold-up?

The economic concept of "hold-up"[12,13] refers to the taking of business profits by force and is identified by the *Power of Buyers* and *Power of Suppliers* forces[11] that influence the attractiveness of an industry (see Chapter 3: Micro-environmental Analysis). Powerful suppliers who are few in number can threaten to enter the venture's industry, or they may offer the venture specialized assets critical for business. As such, they possess a strong negotiation position and can force high prices for critical supplies, with few alternative sources, thereby increasing the price that the venture must pay for its critical supplies. Similarly, buyers who are few in number and with either strong purchasing power or high potential to enter the industry can dictate prices, thereby lowering the price they pay for the venture's product/service. A low rating in this category suggests that buyers and/or suppliers will "steal" all the profits of the venture and the venture should not be pursued unless this position can be corrected. Possible solutions to hold-up include solid contracts, negotiation and even a show of strength (posturing). Examples of ratings to prevention of hold-up follow:

- low: a wholesaler supplier to an independent pharmacy dictates price and terms of agreement as there are only a few from which to choose
- medium: a proactive pharmacist offers specialty and bundled diabetic services but still relies on physicians to issue prescriptions
- high: a collaborative and cross-disciplinary team of health care professionals specializing in several disease states possesses many diverse programs and offerings and is paid through membership fees, public and insurance funds

F. Flexibility Gap

This attribute relates to the ability of the venture to deal with uncertain events and manage the risk around such events. No new venture will play out exactly according to the plan, so it is the ability to manage *unplannable* events that becomes a critical attribute for any new or even existing venture. Of course, there is no way of knowing when an event may occur, but this differs from not having any idea about what types of events might occur that impact the venture and the inability to manage such risk. As such, it is imperative to build flexibility into the venture to confer an adaptable organization. Mitchell[2] explains that such events can fall into two categories.

The first relates to events that are expected to occur but where the timing is uncertain; the second relates to an unknown and unpredictable event or unknown consequences arising from it, referred to as ambiguity. To confer adequate flexibility, a new venture must plan for uncertainty and mitigate ambiguity to adequately minimize risk.

Is uncertainty minimized?

This category translates to risk management, where an event is definite to occur but its timing cannot be pinpointed. Mitchell[2] identifies the key risks that a new venture must manage such as a key stakeholder's death, the disintegration of the venture itself due to dispute or other, tax inflexibility and ignorance, or natural disaster. If the venture possesses a low rating in this category, it should not be pursued until this deficiency is corrected. While tax planning should be simple, due to inexperience many new ventures inadequately identify and are unprepared to pay necessary taxes. Contingency planning around the death of a key individual or owner, disputes in advance and acquiring the necessary insurance to protect against disaster can effectively manage risk, building flexibility into the venture. Potential rating examples for uncertainty minimization follow:

- low: a new independent pharmacy, owned by three partners, has taken no steps to plan in case of disputes, death, damage or theft
- medium: the new independent pharmacy has purchased insurance protection against theft/damage and has planned tax issues, but as good friends the partners have found it uncomfortable to discuss a risk management plan around death or dispute
- high: the new pharmacy has a written agreement for all potential anticipated risks

Is ambiguity minimized?

There is, unfortunately, no way to completely eliminate ambiguity as it relates to events that are unknown and unforeseen and that extend beyond that which even trend and industry analysis, or operational management tools, may identify. Dealing with ambiguity requires the foresight that the venture's landscape is dynamic and that the only constant is change itself. As such, fixed homogeneous thinking that may impart great profit to a venture at one point may be the cause of its extinction in the midst of an environmental shift.[14] While it is impossible to prepare for the consequences of environmental shifts, planning decisions made through unstructured groups with heterogeneous composition are conducive to permitting the venture to adapt in turbulent episodes.[15,16] Mitchell[2] suggests that this is best achieved by developing an advisory board comprised of people of different genders, ethnicity and geographic background, and need not necessarily represent the composition of the venture's management team. The venture should not stop in its planning until ambiguity is addressed.

3. CAN YOU DO IT?

Do you have the core competence?

Core competence is defined as "a harmonized combination of multiple resources and skills that distinguish a firm in a marketplace."[17] In addition to being difficult to imitate (note relation to question nine in the template) it should also serve to access several markets and should contribute to delivered customer value of your product or service. In more realistic terms this comes down to assessing the venture's experience and capabilities. Does the team have entrepreneurial and/or industry experience pertinent to the venture? Does it possess the necessary capabilities to routinely deploy its resources to drive the business forward successfully? Again, the venture should not stop in its planning until it possesses a core competence.

Mitchell's template for new ventures focuses a new venture's attention on the greatest gaps generally overlooked by new startups from both the market and managerial perspectives. The new pharmacy venture/project should strive to conservatively and realistically gauge its success by the template's questions to maximize its potential for success and sustainability.

REFERENCES

1. Mainprize B, Hindle K. *Is the quality of entrepreneurial business plans related to the funding decision?* MA: Babson Park; 2003.

2. Mitchell R. *Topic review notes—new venture template.* International Centre for Venture Expertise; 2000.

3. Mainprize B, Hindle K, Mitchell R. Toward the standardization of venture capital investment evaluation: Decision criteria for rating investee business plans. 2002;1–16.

4. Mainprize B, Hindle K, Smith B, et al. Caprice versus standardization in venture capital decision making. J Priv Equity. 2003;7(1):15–25. http://dx.doi.org/10.3905/jpe.2003.320060.

5. Schumpeter J, Opie R. *The theory of economic development.* 1st ed. Cambridge, Mass.: Harvard University Press; 1934.

6. Blank S. Why the lean start-up changes everything. Harv Bus Rev. 2013;91(5):63–72.

7. Kotler P. *Marketing management.* 1st ed. Upper Saddle River, N.J.: Prentice Hall; 2000.

8. Vernon R. International investment and international trade in the product cycle. Q J Econ. 1966;80(2):190–207. http://dx.doi.org/10.2307/1880689.

9. Osterwalder A, Pigneur Y, Clark T. *Business model generation.* 1st ed. Hoboken, NJ: Wiley; 2010.

10. Barney J. Firm resources and sustained competitive advantage. J Manage. 1991;17(1):99–120. http://dx.doi.org/10.1177/014920639101700108.

11. Porter ME. The five competitive forces that shape strategy. Harv Bus Rev. 2008;86(1):78–93, 137. Medline:18271320

12. Ghemawat P. *Commitment.* 1st ed. New York: Free Press; 1991.

13. Williamson O. *The economic institutions of capitalism.* 1st ed. New York: Free Press; 1985.

14. Murray A. Top management group heterogeneity and firm performance. Strateg Manage J. 1989;10(S1):125–41. http://dx.doi.org/10.1002/smj.4250100710.

15. Daft R, Lengel R. Organizational information requirements, media richness and structural design. Manage Sci. 1986;32(5):554–71. http://dx.doi.org/10.1287/mnsc.32.5.554.

16. Galbraith J. Organizing modes: An information processing model. In: Galbraith J, editor. *Organization Design.* 1st ed., 1977. p. 33–57.

17. Prahalad C, Hamel G. The core competence of the corporation. Boston (MA). Harv Bus Rev. 1990; May:235–56.

III. LEADERSHIP, MANAGEMENT, ENTREPRENEURSHIP AND PERSONAL EFFECTIVENESS

CHAPTER 9

Leadership and Management

Kevin W. Hall, *B.Sc.Pharm., PharmD, FCSHP; Clinical Associate Professor, Faculty of Pharmacy and Pharmaceutical Sciences, University of Alberta*

Ron McKerrow, *BSc (Pharm), MBA; Principal, Concilio Consulting*

Learning Objectives

- Understand the differences between leadership and management.
- Understand there are both formal and informal leaders in the workplace and how informal leaders can contribute to, or detract from, the success of the organization.
- Understand the trait, situational and behavioural theories that have been proposed to help understand the factors that play a role in an individual's success in a leadership role.
- Understand the types of leadership models used to provide leadership within organizations.
- Understand the role of organizational charts and position descriptions.
- Recognize the historical disparity in male and female representation in the leadership ranks of organizations and the future trend toward greater female representation.

Creating competent pharmacy practitioners who work directly with patients to help manage their drug therapy is the focus of today's pharmacy undergraduate professional programs. Most students are looking forward to their career as a clinical practitioner and many express their lack of interest in subjects that do not seem to be related to developing clinical-practice skills. The perception that many students have of pharmacy management is that it involves being the boss, managing other people and dealing with problems in the workplace, none of which are very appealing to most pharmacy students.

It is perhaps not surprising, therefore, that many students question the need for courses that are focused on leadership and management. They may understand the need for managers and they may even have an open mind about eventually becoming managers themselves, but not anytime in the near future. They question why training in pharmacy management cannot be left to those few students who have an interest in becoming a manager soon after they graduate.

Even students who have an open mind about the possibility of becoming a manager often wonder if it would not be better to receive their leadership and management training sometime later in their career, when they are ready to make the transition to a management position. In their minds, it is unreasonable to expect that they are going to remember what they were taught about leadership and management many years later if they have not been using it in their practice.

Although these concerns are understandable, the reality is that everyone manages and leads, even if the only person managed and led is the one in the mirror. Many pharmacy students will find themselves managing other people far sooner than they had anticipated. Pharmacists often work in settings in which they must assume responsibility for managing and directing other staff members, such as pharmacy technicians and other support personnel. There may be a pharmacy manager onsite at the community pharmacy or hospital for eight hours a day, five days a week, but most pharmacies are open longer hours than that. In the absence of a formal manager in the workplace, pharmacists have to manage other people and attend to other management responsibilities. In many cases, new graduates will find themselves carrying out some management responsibilities almost as soon as they start their careers.

LEADERSHIP AND MANAGEMENT DEFINED

"Accountants are in the past, managers are in the present and leaders are in the future." – Paul Orfalea, founder of Kinko's, which later became FedEx, one of the world's largest courier companies[1]

The terms *leadership* and *management* are quite often used as though they were synonymous. Although some individuals may possess both strong leadership skills and strong management skills, there are many who are good leaders or managers but are weak in the other domain. Although there are overlaps, leadership involves a different focus and requires a different set of competencies than management does.

In his book *On Becoming a Leader*, Warren Bennis provides the following examples of the differences between leaders and managers[2]:

- The manager administers; the leader innovates.
- The manager accepts the status quo; the leader challenges it.
- The manager has a short-range view; the leader has a long-range perspective.
- The manager does things right; the leader does the right thing.
- The manager maintains; the leader develops.
- The manager focuses on systems and structure; the leader focuses on people.
- The manager relies on control; the leader inspires trust.
- The manager asks how and when; the leader asks what and why.
- The manager has an eye on the bottom line; the leader's eye is on the horizon.
- The manager is a copy; the leader is an original.
- The manager is the classic good soldier; the leader is his or her own person.

A few others that could be added to the Bennis list include the following:

- The manager is focused on efficiency; the leader is focused on effectiveness.
- The manager values order and stability; the leader values adaptability and change.
- The manager is detail-oriented; the leader has a big-picture orientation.

Although the roles of management and leadership are different, both are equally important in an organization.

Leadership involves envisioning what the organization will look like in the future. It has a long-term focus on doing the right things to ensure the organization remains vibrant and successful. Ensuring the organization will be effective in what it is trying to achieve is a key objective of leadership. Leadership requires ongoing attention to the big picture, and leaders must constantly monitor the environment in which their organization operates. By doing so, leaders can identify threats and opportunities at an early stage when it is easiest to do so, or take advantage of new opportunities as the world around us changes.

Management has a focus that is more about doing things right and being efficient in executing the plans that leaders develop. The focus of managers is more short term in nature, focusing on the *how*, rather than the *what* that leaders focus on. Although the differentiation between leadership and management is important to understand, it is also important to appreciate that the two domains overlap and many individuals carry out both leadership and management activities on a day-to-day basis.

FORMAL AND INFORMAL LEADERS

Leaders fall into two categories. Formal leaders occupy a leadership position that is accompanied by the power to reward or discipline. Informal leaders are those who have the ability to influence others as a result of their charisma, visionary ideas, intelligence or the history and trust they have built up with others in the group. It is important to realize that informal leaders have the potential to assist formal leaders in achieving their objectives, or they can represent a significant obstacle to the formal leader's efforts. Informal leaders may be supporting organizational efforts, or they may be leading the resistance to changes that are occurring within the organization. Astute formal leaders identify the informal leaders among their subordinates and determine if the leadership abilities of those individuals can be harnessed to help achieve the leader's goals. In other situations, informal leaders can be a negative influence in the workplace. In that case, efforts are needed to determine if the negative informal leader can be brought onside to support the formal leader or if other actions need to be taken to prevent the individual from having an ongoing negative influence on the organization.

APPROACHES TO LEADERSHIP AND MANAGEMENT OVER THE YEARS

It is useful to briefly review how the theories and approaches to leadership and management have evolved. In the early 1900s, large-scale manufacturing was developing. One of the best examples is the assembly-line production of automobiles by Henry Ford's Detroit-based company. Workers were usually assigned to a single task they repeated over and over again.

The job of managers in Ford's plants was to maximize the output of workers by closely monitoring their work. The belief was that such specialization would ensure that workers knew how to do their jobs correctly and could maintain a high pace of work output. However, the monotony of the work and the isolation of each worker's contributions from the end product (a finished automobile) created a work environment that was not very meaningful for workers. The quality of many products produced in assembly lines was less than ideal, and productivity was often a problem. Unions gained a bigger influence under those types of working conditions.

Following World War II, countries such as Japan began to produce products that were superior in quality to those manufactured in the traditional North American assembly-line plants. The focus on quality was accompanied by changes in the way workers were managed. Workplace models began to change to ones in which workers were given more variety in their work and were encouraged to focus on quality, rather than quantity or speed.[3]

Studies of these models showed that investing in quality was "free,"[4] meaning that the money spent on improving quality yielded greater savings than the cost of implementing the actual quality improvements. Just as important, workers were more motivated by an environment that encouraged their input and gave meaning to their work. The nature of leading and managing also changed. The concept of command and control, in which a manager's authority was used to coerce workers to produce a greater output, was slowly replaced by one in which motivation and persuasion were recognized as more effective ways to lead and manage.

In the latter part of the 20th century, the information age emerged, in which many of the outputs of organizations were information and communication products. The creation of those products required a very different approach to leadership and management. Effective leaders created a vision of where the organization wanted to go, encouraged creativity and "out-of-the-box thinking" and then largely stayed out of the way of the managers and workers who would achieve that vision. Leadership was about initiating and maintaining groups or organizations to accomplish shared goals.[5] Managers focused on providing needed resources and removing any obstacles that workers might face in achieving the organization's vision.

LEADERSHIP THEORIES

There are several publications that discuss the various theories of leadership and management, as well as the results of research that has been done to examine the validity of those theories. Several, such as *Leadership Theory and Practice* by Northouse[6] and *Organizational Behaviour: Understanding and Managing Life at Work* by Johns and Saks,[7] provide a detailed discussion of the theories and research results. A brief summary of leadership and management theories is provided here, and the textbooks mentioned can be consulted for more in-depth information.

TRAIT-BASED THEORIES

Johns and Saks report that interest in leadership traits first began in earnest during the WWI, when ways were being sought to identify individuals who were likely to be effective leaders (i.e., officers) during the war effort.[7] Many people believe that individuals are born with certain traits that predispose them to do well in different types of work, including leadership positions. Systematic attempts have been made to identify the traits of effective leaders and the role that those traits play in becoming an effective leader. Some traits that have been associated with success include need for achievement, motivation, energy, intelligence, self-confidence, emotional stability, sociability, honesty and integrity.[6,7] The trait theory was challenged in the mid-20th century when evidence accumulated indicating that good leaders in one situation might not be good leaders in a different situation.[6,7] Findings showed that leadership was not a passive state but resulted from working relationships between leaders and other group members. Despite those limitations, there has been renewed interest in the trait theory of leadership since the 1990s when research was being pursued in the areas of visionary leadership, as exemplified by individuals such as Steve Jobs of Apple fame and charismatic leadership as exemplified by Nelson Mandela.

The trait approach focuses almost exclusively on the leader, not on the followers or the situation. Essentially, it is a list of traits that leaders possess and that are thought to contribute to effective leadership. The assumption is that selecting people with the right traits for leadership positions will improve organizational effectiveness. Organizations that hold this belief often require job applicants to complete a personality trait test, such as the Myers-Briggs,[8,9] as part of the interview process.

Central to the trait approach is the question, *"Are leaders born or can an individual develop leadership traits over the course of a career?"* By studying leaders, several qualities have emerged that seem to help predict success. However, whether those traits are innate or learned remains uncertain.

SITUATIONAL-BASED THEORIES[6,7]

Leadership and management are complex processes that exist within different situational/environmental contexts. For example, there are still situations in which repetitive, assembly-line work is required. A pharmacy example might be the unit dose repackaging operations that exist in many hospital pharmacies. Management of that type of work will be different than other types of pharmacy activities, such as managing a group of specialized clinical pharmacy practitioners who work quite independently with minimal day-to-day supervision. Situational theories of leadership are based on the belief that the effectiveness of different styles of leadership depends on the setting or situation within which that leadership style is being used. Several situational leadership theories have been proposed.

The *Contingency Theory* of situational leadership was first proposed by Fiedler in the 1960s.[10] It is based on the premise that leadership effectiveness depends on three variables: leader/subordinate relationships, the nature of the tasks being performed and the power the leader has to direct, reward and discipline. Fiedler's theory is based on the belief that leadership style is fixed. He proposed a tool for measuring an individual's leadership style called the least-preferred co-worker scale.[10] However, that scale has been the subject of considerable criticism by other researchers.[7]

Cognitive Resource Theory is a later theory developed by Fiedler[11] in the 1980s, in which he proposed that whether or not a leader's intelligence or experience (cognitive resources) will be effective in a given situation depends on three conditions: the stressfulness of the situation, the level of support the leader receives from subordinates and how directive the leader is. For example, when stress is high, an individual's ability to reason effectively may become impaired. In such situations, an individual's ability to draw upon past experience of what worked and did not work in similar situations may be a more important determinant of leadership effectiveness.

The *Path-Goal Theory* was proposed by Robert House in the early 1970s.[12] This theory proposes that employees will be motivated and productive if they perceive they are capable of performing the work, their efforts will result in a desired outcome and the payoffs for doing the work are worthwhile. Effective leaders select the style that best meets subordinates' motivational needs. Leaders will be effective in motivating employees when the goals are well defined, the path to a goal is clear, obstacles are removed and the work itself is satisfying. In other words, this theory explains how leaders can help subordinates along the path to their goals by selecting specific behaviours that are best suited to their subordinates' needs and the situation in which staff are working.

MODELS FOR DELIVERING ORGANIZATIONAL LEADERSHIP

AUTOCRATIC LEADERSHIP

Autocratic leadership, in its extreme form, is one in which the leader makes virtually all the decisions with little or no input from others. The leader dictates what is done and how it is done. Group members are not entrusted with making decisions, even when the leader has little or no understanding of the work and the processes that are used to accomplish that work. Autocratic leadership can be an appropriate management model when immediate decisions may need to be made. The military is an example of an organization where autocratic leadership is an appropriate management model in some situations where immediate and cooperative action is required. In organizations that usually use a more participative model, the need may arise to adopt an autocratic style when a contingency occurs. For example, if a dramatic power failure occurred in a large hospital, someone needs to have the authority to mobilize and direct the available staff to deal with issues in a timely manner. In such situations, staff usually want and expect that the leader will take charge of the situation and provide clear direction to others.

Participative leadership[6,7] is a form of leadership in which employees participate in making work-related decisions. This can range from providing input and opinions to superiors, who will ultimately make the decision, to self-directed groups that make most of the decisions concerning how their work is carried out. In order for participative leadership to work, employees must have a clear understanding of the limits of their decision-making abilities. Potential advantages of participative leadership include increased employee motivation, higher levels of job satisfaction and improved quality of work.[6,7]

Team-based leadership[6,7] models are now commonly used to lead and manage in the workplace. They are composed of members who share common goals and coordinate their activities to accomplish their goals. Teams can be created purposefully or spontaneously to address several needs. They may take the form of projects, task forces, work unit initiatives, standing committees, quality teams, etc. Teams can be transient, coming together until a goal is completed, or can be longer-term in nature. Leadership in this context involves helping the group(s) to accomplish their goals. The strength of this approach is that it aligns well with real-life work situations, where teams are used extensively to get work done.

Servant leadership[6,7] is a paradoxical approach that challenges our traditional beliefs of what leadership is all about: the notion that leaders lead and followers follow. In essence, the leader's role in this model is to provide what the employees need in order for employees to achieve their full potential. This approach to leadership emphasizes the importance of listening to followers, being attentive to their needs, empowering them and helping them develop to their full potential. Leadership in this model involves listening to employees, empathizing with employees as they deal with challenges, providing support and guidance, assisting the personal growth of employees and building a sense of community with others.

Transformational leadership,[6,7] as the name suggests, is a form of leadership in which the leader exerts an exceptional form of influence over others in the organization. The leader creates a compelling vision of the future and engages others in achieving that vision. It moves followers to accomplish more than is usually expected of them. Transformational leaders are usually charismatic individuals who are able to articulate a clear vision and empower followers to pursue that vision.

Ethical leadership and authentic leadership[6,7] are two of the newer models of leadership delivery. Their origins can be traced to the recent rash of moral, ethical and criminal failures by individuals in leadership positions in both the public and private sector. Ethical and authentic leadership are a response to demands for trustworthy and effective leadership. These models are characterized as being morally grounded, value driven and responsive to the needs of their stakeholders. Leaders in these types of models understand the social purpose of their organization, have strong moral and ethical values and demonstrate self-discipline.

Discussion of the various leadership theories and models for delivering organizational leadership suggests that there is not just one standard approach. Understanding the characteristics of the different models will help in building an understanding of why a particular approach to leadership is successful, or not. In addition, the context of the organizational setting or situation in which the model is being applied is also an important consideration. Organizational leaders choose the leadership model they believe will achieve their goals.

THE ROLE OF ORGANIZATIONAL CHARTS AND POSITION DESCRIPTIONS

An organizational structure is needed in most business enterprises to ensure that work is arranged in a way that enables the goals of the organization to be achieved in a manner that is effective and efficient. In very small organizations, where there is one single boss, there may be little need for a formal organizational chart. However, as organizations grow and become more complex, there will be a need to define and document the work individuals carry out and to describe the relationships between the people doing the work. Job descriptions, also known as position descriptions or position profiles, are used to describe and document the work individuals are responsible for (see Chapter 32: Effective Management of Human Resources). Organizational charts are used to illustrate the relationships between the people who work in the organization (see Figure 9.1 and Figure 9.2).

An organizational chart provides the following information: the positions that exist in the organization, the reporting relationships that exist between the positions, the number of levels of management that exist, the span of control of managers and supervisors (i.e., the number of individuals who report to a given manager) and how individuals are grouped into departments or other organizational units.

Figure 9.1

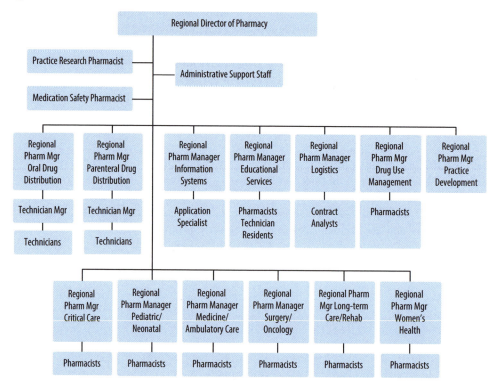

A Complex Organizational Model for a Large Multi-site Hospital Pharmacy Department

Figure 9.2

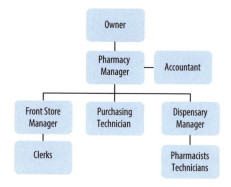

Organizational Chart for an Independent
Retail Pharmacy

Although there are several different types of organizational models, community and hospital pharmacy departments usually have a relatively simple, hierarchical organizational structure. Hierarchical organizational structures are pyramidal with the most senior position, such as the owner, president or chief executive officer (CEO), at the top. Below the top level in the pyramid are one or more layers of managers. The largest number of employees, termed the frontline staff, form the lowest level of the organizational chart. Figure 9.1 shows a typical organizational chart for a hospital pharmacy and Figure 9.2 shows one for an independent community pharmacy.

WOMEN AND LEADERSHIP

"We still think of a powerful man as a born leader and a powerful woman as an anomaly."
– Margaret Atwood, award-winning Canadian author[13]

According to 2011 data from the Canadian Institute for Health Information (CIHI), female pharmacists now represent approximately 60% of the pharmacist workforce in Canada.[14] In 2009, 68.3% of the graduates from all of the pharmacy faculties in Canada were female.[15] It appears that pharmacy is becoming a profession with increasing numbers of women both in the workforce and pharmacy schools. However, when the data has been examined to determine the female representation in the ranks of pharmacy managers and owners, a different picture emerges with only 39.1% of those leadership and management positions being occupied by females.[15] In the halls of academia in 2008/2009, females occupied only 30% of the Dean of Pharmacy positions in the United States and 20% of the Dean of Pharmacy positions in Canada.[15]

Over the past 30 or 40 years, there has been a heightened interest in gender and leadership. Prior to the 1990s, the widely held consensus, whether explicitly stated or demonstrated by a reluctance to hire or promote women into leadership positions, was that women were inferior to men in leadership roles. Since that time, however, the number of women in leadership roles has grown rapidly, particularly in high-profile areas such as elected office, academia, business, medicine and law. These changes have been accompanied by a considerable amount of research looking at the characteristics and leadership styles of male and female leaders. The only significant gender differences in leadership style that have been shown to date are that women tend to be more democratic and participative than men.[6]

Studies suggest that male and female leaders are equally effective overall but with some differences. There is some evidence that women are more effective in "female roles" (e.g., education, government, social services and middle-management positions), while men are more effective in "masculine roles" (e.g., the military and organizations with a large male workforce).[6] It should be noted again that these differences are small, both with respect to leadership style and effectiveness.

"Some leaders are born women." – Geraldine Ferraro, former candidate for vice-president of the United States[16]

Women make up half of the workforce in the United States and earn 57% of all bachelor's degrees awarded, 60% of master's degrees and slightly more than half of the doctoral degrees.

Despite those impressive statistics, women occupy only 3% of CEO positions and 14% of executive positions in Fortune 500 companies.[17] Politically, women hold 18.7% (80) of seats in the US House of Representatives,[18] while in Canada, 25% (76) of the members of the House of Commons are women.[19] Internationally, the average percentage of female parliamentarians is 22%.[20]

Although women have less work experience and more work interruptions than men, there is no evidence to suggest that women quit their jobs more often, are less committed to their jobs or are more likely to opt out of leadership-track opportunities than men.[5] Although women have had less opportunity for promotion and are given fewer responsibilities than men in the same jobs,[5,] the number of women who have successfully risen through the leadership maze continues to rise.[5,15] Changes in organizational culture, development opportunities and mentoring appear to have contributed to this slow but positive change for women in executive positions.

"In the future, there will be no female leaders. There will just be leaders." – Sheryl Sandberg, Chief Operating Officer of Facebook and author of *Lean In: Women, Work and the Will to Lead*[21]

REFERENCES

1. Paul Orfalea quote. Good Reads. Available: www.goodreads.com/author/quotes/461833.Paul_Orfalea (accessed Oct. 19, 2014).
2. Bennis W. *On becoming a leader*. New York: Addison Wesley; 1989.
3. Ouchi WG. *Theory Z: how American business can meet the Japanese challenge*. Reading, Massachusetts: Addison-Wesley Publishing Company; 1981.
4. Crosby PB. *Quality is free: the art of making quality certain*. New York: McGraw-Hill Companies; 1979.
5. Burns JM. *Leadership*. New York: Harper and Row; 1978.
6. Northouse PG. *Leadership theory and practice*. 6th ed. California: Sage Publications; 2013.
7. Johns G, Saks AM. *Organizational behaviour: understanding and managing life at work*. Toronto: Pearson Prentice Hall; 2011.
8. Quenk NL. *Essentials of Myers-Briggs type indicator assessment*. Hoboken, New Jersey: John Wiley and Sons; 2009.
9. Kroeger O, Thuesen JM, Rutledge H. *Type talk at work: how the 16 personality types determine your success on the job*. New York: Dell Publishing Random House; 2002.
10. Fiedler FE. *A theory of leadership effectiveness*. New York: McGraw-Hill; 1967.
11. Fiedler FE. The effective utilization of intellectual abilities and job-related knowledge in group performance: Cognitive resource theory and an agenda for the future. Appl Psychol. 1989;38(3):289–304. http://dx.doi.org/10.1111/j.1464-0597.1989.tb01259.x.
12. House RJ. A path goal theory of leader effectiveness. Adm Sci Q. 1971;16(3):321–39. http://dx.doi.org/10.2307/2391905.
13. Margaret Atwood quote. Quotes. Available: www.quotes.net/quote/10252 (accessed Jan. 31, 2015).
14. Canadian Institute for Health Information. Pharmacists in Canada, 2011. Available: www.cihi.ca/CIHI-ext-portal/pdf/internet/PHARM2011_INFOSHEET_EN (accessed Nov. 16, 2014).
15. Donica J, Fitzpatrick K, Jensen K, Suveges L. Women in pharmacy: a preliminary study of the attitudes and beliefs of pharmacy students. Can Pharm J. 2013;146(2):109–16.
16. Geraldine Ferraro quote. Good Reads. Available: www.goodreads.com/author/show/431087.Geraldine_Ferraro (accessed Jan. 31, 2015).
17. Catalyst. A statistical overview of women in the workplace. March 3, 2014. Available: www.catalyst.org/knowledge/statistical-overview-women-workplace (accessed Nov. 16, 2014).
18. USA. Center for American Women and Politics. Eagleton Institute of Politics Rutgers University, October 26, 2014. Available: www.cawp.rutgers.edu/fast_facts/levels_of_office/congress.php (accessed Nov. 23, 2014).
19. Canada. Women in Parliament: Library of Parliament. 41st parliament. Available: www.parl.gc.ca/parliamentarians/en/members (accessed Oct 26, 2014).
20. Inter-Parliamentary Union. Women in national parliaments June 2014. Available: www.ipu.org/wmn-e/classif.htm (accessed Oct 26, 2014).
21. Kaddouri O. Women mean business. Rotana Times. Available: www.rotanatimes.com/news/5761 (accessed Jan. 31, 2015).

CHAPTER 10

Change Management

Meagen Rosenthal, *PhD, MA, BA, University of Alberta*

Kevin W. Hall, *B.Sc.Pharm., PharmD, FCSHP; Clinical Associate Professor, Faculty of Pharmacy and Pharmaceutical Sciences, University of Alberta*

Ross T. Tsuyuki, *BSc(Pharm), PharmD, MSc, FCSHP, FACC; Professor of Medicine and Director, EPICORE Centre/COMPRIS, Faculty of Medicine and Dentistry, University of Alberta*

Learning Objectives

- Develop an understanding of the risks associated with failing to recognize and adapt to changes in the environment within which a profession or organization exists.

- Develop an appreciation of some of the major challenges that face pharmacy practitioners and how those are driving change in the profession.

- Become familiar with Kotter's eight-step model of change.

- Develop an appreciation of how Kotter's change model can be used to guide change initiatives to a successful conclusion.

There are many reasons why pharmacy managers and practitioners should understand managing change. Looking to the business world, there are numerous examples of once-successful companies that ultimately failed when they did not adapt to their changing environment.[1] For example, Kodak, a dominant player in the consumer photography sector for more than a century, was actually the first company to develop, and patent, many aspects of digital camera technology as it is known today.[2] However, leaders in the company feared that the new technology might adversely affect its traditional film photography business model and sat on their patents, while others exploited the potential.[2] By the time Kodak realized its mistake, it was too late.[2] After more than a century as a successful iconic business, Kodak declared bankruptcy in 2012.[2]

There are also numerous examples of companies weathering change. For instance, consider that 42 of the top 220 privately held companies are more than 100 years old.[3] Hallmark, one such company, has diversified over time and expanded its reach into non-English-language greeting cards, embraced the Internet with e-cards and recently developed products allowing customers to record video greetings.[3] Companies such as Hallmark embody the essence of the learning

Table 1. Kotter's Eight Steps[19]

1.	Establish a sense of urgency
2.	Form a powerful guiding coalition
3.	Create a vision
4.	Communicate the vision
5.	Empower others to act on the vision
6.	Plan for and create short-term wins
7.	Consolidate improvements and produce still more change
8.	Institutionalize new approaches

organization. These are companies that purposively take lessons from day-to-day experiences and translate them into new, and better, ways of achieving their vision.[4]

What does the story of Hallmark have to do with the profession of pharmacy? Since the 1960s, pharmacy leaders have argued that the long-term sustainability of the profession rests on its ability, and willingness, to assume responsibility for drug therapy management and outcomes.[5] In 1971, the Commission on Pharmaceutical Services in Canada published its final report that stated the following:

> Over the long term, the big question for pharmacy is whether the profession will be able to develop a role in which its specialized knowledge can be brought to bear where it is most needed—at the point where decisions about drug usage are made... [6]

How did pharmacy respond to these calls for change in the fundamental focus of the profession? More than 40 years after the Commission's 1971 report, evidence suggests that pharmacy practice is still largely drug distribution-centred, as the majority of its practitioners view drug distribution as their primary responsibility.[7,8] This is despite well-established evidence of pharmacists' benefit in patient care[9-16] and a recognition that the time for change is now.[17,18]

While convention dictates that change is inevitable, it is difficult, both for those who are leading change and for those affected by change. Fortunately, there are several popular change-management theories, including John Kotter's Eight Steps (Table 1),[19] Bridge's Transition Model,[20] Rogers' Diffusion of Innovations[21] and Lewin's Change Management Model,[22] to assist with the change process and the development of a learning organization. While each of these models has advantages and disadvantages, the model chosen for this chapter was put forward by John Kotter in 1995[19] and has been previously used by an author of this chapter (R.T. Tsuyuki) for investigating change in the profession of pharmacy.[23]

STEP 1: ESTABLISH A SENSE OF URGENCY

Kotter's first step in managing change is the creation of a sense of urgency within the group such that the status quo is no longer comfortable.[19] As discussed by Tsuyuki and Schindel, individuals and groups rarely engage in a change process without a compelling reason.[23] However, an examination of the current context of the pharmacy profession demonstrates that there is little immediate reason to change. First, members of the public already hold pharmacists in high esteem.[24] In fact, a recent Ipsos Reid poll ranked pharmacists as the fourth-most trusted out of 22 professions.[25] Second, market demands for pharmacists across Canada have exceeded supply for much of the past 10 to 15 years, resulting in rising salaries and many employment opportunities. Finally, and perhaps more importantly, a recent Government of Canada review of the profitability of pharmacies and drug stores found that more than 80% were profitable.[26]

However, pressures have been building within the health care system in Canada to force the profession's hand. For many years, community pharmacies generated considerable revenue from professional allowances and other forms of rebates received from generic pharmaceutical manufacturers. These professional allowances were paid to the pharmacies by generic drug companies for stocking their product and could be used by pharmacies to provide additional patient services or to offset waning dispensing fees.[27] Access to these funds changed dramatically in 2006 when the Ministry of Health and Long-Term Care in Ontario passed the Transparent Drug System Act for Patients, which reduced the price paid by the government for generic medications in an effort to curb rising costs.[28] This Act was followed in 2010 by Bill 16, which altered the definition of a rebate such that professional allowances were no longer permissible.[29] Seeing the potential cost savings for their own health care systems, provinces/territories across the country soon followed Ontario's lead by lowering the price governments would pay for generic drugs and reducing the rebates pharmacies are permitted to receive.[30]

In 2004, Ontario led the way in reforming pharmacy practice in Canada when the regulatory body for pharmacists in the province banned the use of customer loyalty programs.[31] These customer loyalty programs generally involved providing patients with inducements, such as points for filling their prescriptions in the pharmacy that could be exchanged for free merchandise. These inducements were deemed to be incongruent with the professional image of pharmacists as health care professionals. Following this example, the regulatory bodies in both Alberta and British Columbia attempted to ban customer loyalty programs.[32,33] While the ban in British Columbia has already been overturned by the Supreme Court,[34] it is clear that expectations of pharmacists by regulatory bodies and governments are changing.

Changes are also taking place in other professions. For example, expanding scopes of practice for other health care professionals, including nurses[35] and pharmacy technicians,[36] may place pressure on both pharmacists' traditional, and new, areas of expertise. For example, nurse practitioners in many Canadian jurisdictions can prescribe medications,[37] and pharmacy technicians in most provincial and territorial jurisdictions are, or soon will be, regulated. This is particularly important given that technicians will have responsibility and accountability for the accuracy and quality of drug product preparation and release, a role previously reserved for pharmacists. As such, it appears now, perhaps more than at any other time in the past, that there is an urgent need for pharmacists to transition their practices.

STEP 2: FORM A POWERFUL GUIDING COALITION

The second of Kotter's eight steps is to form a powerful coalition.[19] As described by Tsuyuki and Schindel, ". . . planned change, intended to achieve a desired outcome, is most likely to occur when a group of influential individuals come together to lead the change effort."[23] The profession of pharmacy in Canada began this process, which culminated in the Blueprint for Pharmacy[38] initiative, in the mid-2000s.

The Canadian Pharmacists Association (CPhA) originally spearheaded the development of a guiding coalition that included representation from all sectors of the profession on a steering committee for an initiative called Moving Forward: Pharmacy Human Resources for the Future.[38] The overriding vision of this coalition was that both the work and rewards of the initiative would be shared among members—a critically important factor in change management initiatives. This initiative was successful in obtaining $1.5 million in funding from the Government of Canada in 2005 to support a major study of human resources in the pharmacy profession.[38] A final report was released in 2008 containing 36 recommendations grouped around themes such as: managing the pharmacy workforce, educating and training the pharmacy workforce, regulating the pharmacy workforce and integrating internationally trained pharmacy graduates. An important outcome of the Blueprint for Pharmacy also concerned Kotter's third step: create a vision.

STEP 3: CREATE A VISION

According to Kotter, without a clearly articulated vision, change efforts can become unfocused, unhelpful or even counterproductive in achieving the intended change.[19] In April 2009, the Blueprint coalition released its final version of *The Vision for Pharmacy: Optimal Drug Therapy Outcomes for Canadians Through Patient-Centred Care*.[39] This strategic statement outlined, in broad terms, the profession's overall goals and objectives.[40]

STEP 4: COMMUNICATE THE VISION

Once the vision has been developed, Kotter's next step involves communicating that vision to the larger group.[19] This involves the commitment of substantial resources and effort to ensuring the vision is being effectively communicated to those who will be involved in implementing the change, as well as those who will be impacted by the change.[23] One of the key previous barriers to practice change within the profession of pharmacy, identified by Tsuyuki and Schindel, is inadequate communication of the vision.[23]

To the credit of the Blueprint for Pharmacy implementation plan, it has used numerous communication strategies in an effort to effectively communicate the vision to all stakeholders.[19] Those strategies include the development of a website of Blueprint-related material and resources, newsletters outlining the progress of Blueprint-related initiatives, as well as an opportunity for individual pharmacists, pharmacy businesses and pharmacy organizations to express their support of the Blueprint Vision through a Commitment to Act declaration.[41] The Commitment to Act was intended to be a catalyst in the change process. Signatories pledged their support for the Blueprint's vision and a commitment, "to work collaboratively with the Blueprint Task Force, and working groups," to further develop the implementation plan.[42]

However, a recent examination of the online mentions of the Blueprint for Pharmacy or the Vision for Pharmacy by the organizations signing the Commitment to Act found that only 35 of the more than 900 mentions provided detail about implementation activities.[42] Recipients of the other 865 messages were getting very little information about how the Blueprint for Pharmacy vision was being implemented or communicated.[42]

Turning to hospital pharmacists, in particular, there is also evidence to suggest that frontline pharmacists are not aware of these changes. In the early 2000s, the Canadian Society of Hospital

Pharmacists (CSHP) created a change initiative known as CSHP 2015 that set specific, measurable targets for improvements in hospital pharmacy practice.[43] Interestingly, a recent survey of more than 650 hospital pharmacists in Canada found that 35% of respondents were not aware of the CSHP 2015 initiative, 43% indicated they were aware of the initiative but did not know much about it, and only 6% indicated they were very familiar with it.[44]

To improve these statistics, pharmacists need more specific operational plans about what new pharmacy practice models might look like, what impact the changes would have on individual practitioners and how pharmacy team members could deal with those impacts.[40] One specific approach might be to develop a repository of pharmacy practice change stories. Stories are powerful because they allow individuals to make sense of their experiences and provide insight to others who can use those vicarious experiences to make sense of their own situations.[42]

STEP 5: EMPOWER OTHERS TO ACT ON THE VISION

Step five involves removing obstacles to change and encouraging risk-taking.[23] This is a particularly important step for the management team, as resistance to change may in fact be a symptom of systemic barriers not being removed, rather than individual resistance.[19] Furthermore, this step also demands *full* engagement in the change process by change leaders. According to Kotter, many change efforts will fail at this step if employees see leaders merely paying lip service to the new vision.[19]

Barriers to practice change within pharmacy have been well documented and include lack of time, payment for clinical services and support from employers and other practitioners.[45–48] Some of these barriers are being removed with development of payment schemes for clinical services[49,50] and the regulation of pharmacy technicians.[36] While overcoming these previously identified barriers is key, it is also not sufficient. The knowledge translation literature promotes the idea that an adequate understanding of the practice context, including the professional culture, is also necessary.[51] Work in the area of the professional culture of pharmacy is preliminary.[7,8,52] Future work should include an in-depth examination of how pharmacists understand and internalize new practice opportunities, as well as how these opportunities are understood by organizations employing pharmacists.

STEP 6: PLAN FOR AND CREATE SHORT-TERM WINS

The creation of short-term wins allows group members to observe improvements and be encouraged to continue the change process.[23] People need to receive regular positive messages reinforcing the vision and the change. These wins are success stories, which support and validate the change process. As pointed out by Kotter, planning for short-term wins is different than hoping for short-term wins.[19] An operational plan needs to be in place to deliver regular, positive news to keep individuals motivated. Examples of this include the addition of new professional services, such as comprehensive medication reviews, for which a pharmacist can receive reimbursement from patients, governments or other third-party payers. As new services become eligible for reimbursement, pharmacists can better appreciate that the new payment models for pharmacy services are creating an environment that will lead to profitable and satisfying careers that mirror the Blueprint's Vision for Pharmacy.

STEP 7: CONSOLIDATE IMPROVEMENTS AND PRODUCE STILL MORE CHANGE

In this step, short-term wins are placed into the overall context of the change process so that members can see how the larger vision is being achieved through these successive small wins.[23] This encourages individuals to continue with the change process.[19] For example, providing updates on expanding scopes of practice for both pharmacists and pharmacy technicians, the regulation of pharmacy technicians, new remuneration opportunities and the success of pharmacist-administered vaccination programs help individuals to see that progress is being made and should be more widely publicized and celebrated.[36,53]

STEP 8: INSTITUTIONALIZE NEW APPROACHES

Kotter's final step assumes that the changes are fully integrated into the day-to-day operations of the group.[23] The emphasis now transitions from trying new approaches to embedding those changes as components of the group's culture. An example of this is the role that pharmacy technicians now play in the drug distribution system in most hospitals and in some community pharmacies. In these practice model examples, after a pharmacist has verified that a prescription is appropriate for the patient, pharmacy technicians assume responsibility for the preparation and distribution of medications, working under a supervisor who, in many pharmacies, is a pharmacy technician, not a pharmacist. That change completes the transition from drug distribution-centred pharmacists to drug distribution-centred technicians. This has enabled pharmacists to more fully enact their role as clinical practitioners.

Implementing change is indeed a challenge, but change cannot be avoided. In fact, change can be a planned, proactive initiative that maximizes positive outcomes and minimizes negative ones. Those who decide to take charge of their own destinies can use a structured and proven approach to change, such as the Kotter model, to *manage* the change process. Even small changes in small organizations, such as a community pharmacy or a pharmacy department in a small hospital, are more likely to be successful if they use such an approach. While change can be intimidating, successful change will allow the pharmacy profession to achieve its ultimate goal of providing better patient care.

REFERENCES

1. Newman R. 10 great companies that lost their edge; how to avoid three traps that ensnare even breakthrough companies: US News and World Report; 2010. Available: http://money.usnews.com/money/blogs/flowchart/2010/08/19/10-great-companies-that-lost-their-edge (accessed July 7, 2014).

2. Mui C. How Kodak failed. Forbes.ca 2012. Available: http://www.forbes.com/sites/chunkamui/2012/01/18/how-kodak-failed/ (accessed July 5, 2014).

3. Upbin B. The six habits of successful private companies 2013. Available: www.forbes.com/sites/bruceupbin/2013/06/30/the-six-habits-of-successful-private-companies/ (accessed July 5, 2014).

4. Argote L, Miron-Spektor E. Organizational learning: from experience to knowledge. Organ Sci. 2011;22(5):1123–37. http://dx.doi.org/10.1287/orsc.1100.0621.

5. Francke DE. Prescription for pharmacy practice 1984. Drug Intell Clin Pharm. 1976;10(2):111–2. Medline:10236227

6. Canadian Pharmaceutical Association. *Pharmacy in a new age: report of commission of pharmaceutical services*. Toronto: Canadian Pharmaceutical Association; 1971.

7. Rosenthal MM, Breault RR, Austin Z, et al. Pharmacists' self-perception of their professional role: insights into community pharmacy culture. J Am Pharm Assoc (2003). 2011;51(3):363–7. http://dx.doi.org/10.1331/JAPhA.2011.10034. Medline:21555287

8. Al Hamarneh YN, Rosenthal M, McElnay JC, et al. Pharmacists' perceptions of their professional role: insights into hospital pharmacy culture. Can J Hosp Pharm. 2011;64(1):31–5. Medline:22479026

9. Charrois TL, Zolezzi M, Koshman SL, et al. A systematic review of the evidence for pharmacist care of patients with dyslipidemia. Pharmacotherapy. 2012;32(3):222–33. http://dx.doi.org/10.1002/j.1875-9114.2012.01022.x. Medline:22392455

10. Koshman SL, Charrois TL, Simpson SH, et al. Pharmacist care of patients with heart failure: a systematic review of randomized trials. Arch Intern Med. 2008;168(7):687–94. http://dx.doi.org/10.1001/archinte.168.7.687. Medline:18413550

11. Machado M, Bajcar J, Guzzo GC, et al. Sensitivity of patient outcomes to pharmacist interventions. Part I: systematic review and meta-analysis in diabetes management. Ann Pharmacother. 2007;41(10):1569–82. http://dx.doi.org/10.1345/aph.1K151. Medline:17712043

12. Machado M, Nassor N, Bajcar JM, et al. Sensitivity of patient outcomes to pharmacist interventions. Part III: systematic review and meta-analysis in hyperlipidemia management. Ann Pharmacother. 2008;42(9):1195–207. http://dx.doi.org/10.1345/aph.1K618. Medline:18682540

13. Elias MN, Burden AM, Cadarette SM. The impact of pharmacist interventions on osteoporosis management: a systematic review. Osteoporos Int. 2011;22(10):2587–96. http://dx.doi.org/10.1007/s00198-011-1661-7. Medline:21720894

14. Chisholm-Burns MA, Kim Lee J, Spivey CA, et al. US pharmacists' effect as team members on patient care: systematic review and meta-analyses. Med Care. 2010;48(10):923–33. http://dx.doi.org/10.1097/MLR.0b013e3181e57962. Medline:20720510

15. Wubben DP, Viven EM. Effects of pharmacist outpatient interventions on adults with diabetes mellitus: a systematic review. Pharmacotherapy. 2008;28(4):421–36. http://dx.doi.org/10.1592/phco.28.4.421. Medline:18363526

16. Santschi V, Chiolero A, Paradis G, et al. Pharmacist interventions to improve cardiovascular disease risk factors in diabetes: a systematic review and meta-analysis of randomized controlled trials. Diabetes Care. 2012;35(12):2706–17. http://dx.doi.org/10.2337/dc12-0369. Medline:23173140

17. Zardain E, Od VM, Loza MI, Garcia E, Lana A. Psychosocial and behavioural determinants of the implementation of pharmaceutical care in Spain. Int J Pharm Pract. 2009;31(2):174–82.

18. Jorgenson D, Lamb D, McKinnon NJ. Practice change challenges and priorities: a national survey of practicing pharmacists. Can Pharm J. 2011;144(3):125–31. http://dx.doi.org/10.3821/1913-701X-144.3.125.

19. Kotter JP. Leading change: why transformation efforts fail. Harv Bus Rev. 1995;(March–April):59–67.

20. Bridges W, Bridges S. *Managing transitions*. 3rd ed. USA: Da Capo Press; 2009.

21. Rogers E. *Diffusion of innovations*. 5th ed. New York: Free Press; 2003.

22. Levasseur RE. People skills: change management tools – Lewin's change model. Interfaces. 2001;31(4)71–3.

23. Tsuyuki RT, Schindel TJ. Changing pharmacy practice: the leadership challenge. Can Pharm J. 2008;141(3):174-80. . http://dx.doi.org/10.3821/1913-701X(2008)141[174:CPPTLC]2.0.CO;2.

24. Perepelkin J. Public opinion of pharmacists and pharmacist prescribing. Can Pharm J. 2011;144(2):86–93. http://dx.doi.org/10.3821/1913-701X-144.2.86

25. Ipsos R. Life-savers, medical professionals top the list of most trusted professionals 2012. Available: www.ipsos-na.com/news-polls/pressrelease.aspx?id=5663 (accessed April 23, 2014).

26. Pharmacies and Drug Stores. (NAICS 44611): Financial performance data 2014. Available: www.ic.gc.ca/app/scr/sbms/sbb/cis/benchmarking.html?code=44611&lang=eng - bec3 (accessed Sept. 30, 2014).

27. Stastna K. Top court backs Ontario's ban on pharmacy-brand generic drugs 2013. Available: www.cbc.ca/news/canada/top-court-backs-ontario-s-ban-on-pharmacy-brand-generic-drugs-1.2436368 (accessed Oct. 2, 2014).

28. Transparent drug system for patients act, 2006 2012. Available: www.health.gov.on.ca/en/common/legislation/bill102/ovr_drugsact.aspx (accessed Sept. 30, 2014).

29. Rosenthal MA, Austin Z, Tsuyuki RT. Ontario pharmacists crisis over Bill 16: a missed opportunity? Can Pharm J. 2012;145(1):35–9. http://dx.doi.org/10.3821/1913-701X-145.1.35.

30. Generic prices to fall in BC. CBC News. 2012.

31. Loyalty points program 2004. Available: www.ocpinfo.com/regulations-standards/policies-guidelines/loyalty-points (accessed Oct. 9, 2014).

32. Prohibition on the provision of incentives 2013. Available: www.bcpharmacists.org/about_us/key_initiatives/index/articles/304.php (accessed April 23, 2014).

33. Hoang L. Alberta College of Pharmacists to eliminate rewards programs in pharmacies 2013. Available: http://edmonton.ctvnews.ca/alberta-college-of-pharmacists-to-eliminate-rewards-programs-in-pharmacies-1.1243716 (accessed April 23, 2014).

34. Prescription rewards points ban struck down by BC Supreme Court 2014. Available: www.cbc.ca/news/canada/british-columbia/prescription-rewards-points-ban-struck-down-by-b-c-supreme-court-1.2720857 (accessed Oct. 9, 2014).

35. Position statement: the nurse practitioner: Canadian Nurses Association; 2008. Available: www.cna-aiic.ca/sitecore modules/web/~/media/cna/page-content/pdf-fr/ps_nurse_practitioner_e.pdf - search=%22nurse%20practitioner%20position%20statement%22 (accessed July 10, 2014).

36. *Professional competencies for Canadian pharmacy technicians at entry to practice*. Ottawa: National Association of Pharmacy Regulatory Authorities; 2007. p. 1–29.

37. Worster A, Sardo A, Thrasher C, et al. Understanding the role of nurse practitioners in Canada. Can J Rural Med. 2005;10(2):89–94. Medline:15842791

38. Blueprint for Pharmacy: the vision for pharmacy. 2008.

39. Blueprint for Pharmacy: implementation plan. Ottawa 2009.

40. Brown G. Differences between a strategic plan and an operations plan. Available: http://smallbusiness.chron.com/differences-between-strategic-plan-operations-plan-10634.html (accessed Oct. 1, 2014).

41. Commitment to Act Ottawa 2014. Available: http://blueprintforpharmacy.ca/about/commitment-to-act (accessed July 9, 2014).

42. Rosenthal M, Chen CB, Hall K, et al. Mixed messages: The Blueprint for Pharmacy and a communication gap. Can Pharm J (Ott). 2014;147(2):118–23. http://dx.doi.org/10.1177/1715163514520948. Medline:24660012

43. CSHP. 2015 - Targeting excellence in pharmacy practice 2014. Available: www.cshp.ca/programs/cshp2015/ (accessed Feb. 5, 2014).

44. Hall K, Bussieres J-F. Staff pharmacists perspectives on contemporary pharmacy practice issues. 40th CSHP Banff Seminar; Banff, Alberta, Canada2014.

45. Shoemaker SJ, Staub-DeLong L, Wasserman M, et al. Factors affecting adoption and implementation of AHRQ health literacy tools in pharmacies. Res Social Adm Pharm. 2013;9(5):553–63. http://dx.doi.org/10.1016/j.sapharm.2013.05.003. Medline:23759672

46. Hughes CA, Guirguis LM, Wong T, et al. Influence of pharmacy practice on community pharmacists' integration of medication and lab value information from electronic health records. J Am Pharm Assoc (2003). 2011;51(5):591–8. http://dx.doi.org/10.1331/JAPhA.2011.10085. Medline:21896456

47. Mak VS, Clark A, Poulsen JH, et al. Pharmacists' awareness of Australia's health care reforms and their beliefs and attitudes about their current and future roles. Int J Pharm Pract. 2012;20(1):33–40. http://dx.doi.org/10.1111/j.2042-7174.2011.00160.x. Medline:22236178

48. McCaig D, Fitzgerald N, Stewart D. Provision of advice on alcohol use in community pharmacy: a cross-sectional survey of pharmacists' practice, knowledge, views and confidence. Int J Pharm Pract. 2011;19(3):171–8. http://dx.doi.org/10.1111/j.2042-7174.2011.00111.x. Medline:21554442

49. Pharmacy services and prescription drugs Alberta: Government of Alberta; 2014. Available: www.health.alberta.ca/services/pharmacy-services.html (accessed April 23, 2014).

50. Pharmacy services agreement. British Columbia: Health Services Department; 2010.

51. Kitson A, Harvey G, McCormack B. Enabling the implementation of evidence based practice: a conceptual framework. Qual Health Care. 1998;7(3):149–58. http://dx.doi.org/10.1136/qshc.7.3.149. Medline:10185141

52. Rosenthal M, Austin Z, Tsuyuki RT. Are pharmacists the ultimate barrier to pharmacy practice change? Can Pharm J. 2010;143(1):37–42. http://dx.doi.org/10.3821/1913-701X-143.1.37.

53. Fletcher A, Marra F, Kaczorowski J. Pharmacists as vaccination providers: Friend or foe? Can Pharm J (Ott). 2014;147(3):141–2. http://dx.doi.org/10.1177/1715163514529725. Medline:24847364

CHAPTER 11

Personal Effectiveness

Kevin W. Hall, *B.Sc.Pharm., PharmD, FCSHP; Clinical Associate Professor, Faculty of Pharmacy and Pharmaceutical Sciences, University of Alberta*

Ron McKerrow, *BSc (Pharm), MBA; Principal, Concilio Consulting*

Learning Objectives

- Understand that achieving personal effectiveness can best be achieved through a conscious and structured approach, developed early in life.
- Understand the concept of personal branding.
- Become familiar with strategies for enhancing the quality of one's personal brand.
- Become familiar with Stephen Covey's *7 Habits* of personal effectiveness.
- Understand the concept of emotional intelligence and its importance in personal and workplace interactions.
- Understand the concept of cultural competency and its importance in pharmacy practice.
- Understand the benefits of delegation in the workplace.
- Understand the benefits of managing up in the workplace.

Over the course of people's careers and personal lives, they will interact with many others on a regular basis. People's personal effectiveness in dealing with others will depend, to a large extent, on the interpersonal skills and competencies they possess, as well as how they apply those in their day-to-day interactions with others. Almost everyone can recall interactions with others that might have been handled differently and resulted in a better outcome. Unfortunately, there are consequences associated with personal errors in judgment and actions that can ultimately diminish our personal effectiveness.

Fortunately, how people perceive others is rarely the result of a single interaction between individuals. It is usually a cumulative effect based on a series of interactions. Trust, or lack of trust, is the cumulative result of the past interactions that one person has had with another. If those past interactions have been positive and productive, the individuals involved are likely to expect that their future interactions will be worthwhile and beneficial as well. On the other hand, individuals with poor interpersonal skills will find that they have fewer and fewer opportunities for career advancement, and their personal relationships with colleagues, friends and family will fail to reach their full potential. How might someone get started on the journey to personal effectiveness?

WHY PERSONAL BRANDS ARE IMPORTANT

One approach to thinking about personal effectiveness is the concept of personal branding. The American Marketing Association defines the term *brand* as, "the name, term, design, symbol, or any other feature that identifies one seller's good or service as distinct from those of other sellers."[1]

For example, a major proportion of the population would almost instantly recognize the Apple® or Nike® logos. However, simple recognition of a logo is not what a company is aiming for with its branding strategy. A brand is effective when it has a positive psychological effect that results in the consumer favouring that company's products over similar products offered by other companies. In order for that to occur, the company's brand must be perceived as providing better quality and/or value than similar products provided by alternative companies.

To better acknowledge the psychological impact of a brand, other definitions of the term have been created such as, "A brand is the set of expectations, memories, stories and relationships that, taken together, account for a consumer's decision to choose one product or service over another."[2] Apple® and Nike® are examples of brands that a large proportion of the public would view favourably when making a purchasing decision. In contrast, the brand name Lada® (Russian-built cars that have poor reliability[3]), is a brand name that generally has a negative psychological effect on consumers.

Why does this matter? Individuals who wish to be hired, promoted or offered other opportunities need to sell themselves to those making the decision about who to choose for those opportunities. There are usually lots of other individuals who are being considered for those same opportunities. What identifies someone as a superior brand? Just like a successful brand, individuals who offer superior value are the ones who are likely to be favoured when those decisions are made.

In his 1999 book *The BrandYou50: Fifty Ways to Transform Yourself from an 'Employee' into a Brand That Shouts Distinction, Commitment and Passion,*[4] Tom Peters suggests that each individual has a personal brand that generates perceptions in the minds of others that range from highly favourable to highly unfavourable. In other words, a person's brand influences employers' willingness to buy into the brand by hiring and promoting.

Similarly, one's brand will play a role in determining if one will be offered other types of opportunities that are highly sought after, such as admission to certain university programs (e.g., graduate programs, professional programs such as pharmacy, medicine and nursing etc.), and being selected to serve as a board member of a professional licensing body.

Personal branding is the process through which a brand is established, either through conscious design or by default. There are two components to brand: how people are perceived by others (external brand) and how people perceive themselves (internal brand). Sometimes, there can be a significant disconnect between a person's own perception and others' perceptions.

Those who are interested in knowing if there is a difference between their internal and external brands might want to start by completing an exercise in which they ask friends and colleagues

Table 1. Examples of Personal Attributes and Skills That Contribute to a Personal Brand

Personal Attributes	Personal Skills
Reliable	Coaching
Trustworthy	Team-building
Honest	Communication
Dedicated	Conflict resolution
Passionate	Data analysis
Compassionate	Problem solving
Objective	Information technology
Innovative	Second-language fluency
Loyal	Cultural competency
Flexible	Emotional intelligence

to anonymously complete a survey. Several survey tools are available for this process.[5,6] Table 1 contains a few personal attributes and skills that many people would like to have recognized as part of their personal brand.

Before looking at the results of the surveys from friends and colleagues (external brand), complete the survey to establish the internal brand. Compare the external and internal results and consider areas that need work, what strategies might be helpful and overall alignment between the two perceptions.

STRATEGIES FOR ENHANCING PERCEPTIONS OF A PERSONAL BRAND

PRESENTATION AND APPEARANCE

Expectations about personal appearance vary from workplace to workplace, but people taking the time to show they care about their personal appearance will strengthen their brand in almost any work environment. In workplace situations where there is a lot of interaction with the public, a person's appearance can be an extremely important component of a personal brand.

In the health care setting, where most pharmacists and pharmacy technicians work, there is an expectation that individuals will dress professionally and maintain a high level of personal grooming. Failing to do so will have a negative impact on a personal brand in the eyes of an employer, colleagues and patients. The appearance of the work area also reflects on brand. Individuals with a disorganized, cluttered workspace will often be perceived as being personally disorganized. Dirty coffee mugs and the remains of yesterday's lunch also convey a message.

THE COMPANY YOU KEEP

Consider the old saying, "you are known by the company that you keep." If one's friends are complainers, disruptive in the workplace, dishonest, rude, unkind to others or demonstrate other negative personal characteristics, their association and effect on brand must be considered. Sometimes a discussion with such individuals can change their behaviour. In other cases, a decision may be needed about associating with individuals whose personal brand is contrary to the one desired. One of George Washington's "rules of civility and decent behavior" states, "Associate yourself with men of good quality if you esteem (value) your own reputation; for 'tis better to be alone than in bad Company."[7]

PERSONAL VALUES AND BEHAVIOUR

Table 1 lists some positive personal attributes and skills. Making a list of one's own personal attributes and values and reviewing them regularly in relation to one's actual behaviour in the workplace can help in developing and maintaining a desired brand. Questions to consider include the following: When you make mistakes, do you admit them and accept responsibility for your actions? Do you place your patient's well-being ahead of your own financial interests? Have you been careful not to over-promise and under-deliver, or do you make realistic commitments and strive to exceed them?

DIGITAL FOOTPRINT

The Internet is a well-established part of modern life, enabling large amounts of personal information to be broadly shared with others. The Internet has provided everyone with a platform for developing and promoting their personal brand through social and professional networking websites such as Facebook, Twitter, LinkedIn and other services. Unfortunately, many individuals have shared information about themselves that can later come back to negatively impact them. As health care professionals, pharmacists need to understand that patients may access information about them on the Internet. It is very important to focus on aligning one's digital footprint with the personal brand one is trying to build.

Establishing a positive personal brand takes time and effort, but the earlier people understand the concept of personal branding and start the journey to build a powerful personal brand, the sooner they will reap the rewards of having done so. It is important to remember that brands require ongoing maintenance—it takes time to establish a brand but only moments to destroy it. Many product brands, such as BlackBerry®, have fallen out of favour because they failed to maintain the perception that they represented superior value over other brands. The same holds true for personal brands where failure in personal conduct or failure to maintain skills can substantially weaken or even destroy an individual's personal brand.

BRAND DELIVERY

A good brand is a promise of quality. Once people have decided what they want their personal brand to be, they have to begin developing habits that will deliver on the promise of their brand. If Apple® or Nike® failed to deliver high-quality products, their brand credibility would diminish, and eventually the value of the brand would be worth nothing. The same is true of a personal brand; it needs to be translated into action. How does an individual begin to bring a brand to life?

Although there are many resources that can be used to help build interpersonal competency, one book about personal effectiveness stands out on the basis of its enduring sales and popularity, more than 25 years after its first publication in 1989. Stephen Covey spent many years studying leadership, management and organizational behaviour and wrote several books on the subject of personal effectiveness. His best-known book, *The 7 Habits of Highly Effective People*,[8] has sold more than 25 million copies in 40 languages.[9] In this book, Covey identifies seven habits that are common to many of the highly effective people he studied and worked with over the years. A brief summary of those habits is presented here.

HABIT 1: BE PROACTIVE

Covey describes this habit as taking responsibility for one's own words and actions rather than blaming others. Everyone has to deal with a wide range of external stimuli, such as the words and actions of others that individuals have little control over. However, people do have control over how they respond. They can react, or they can deal with the situation in a more thoughtful and effective manner.

HABIT 2: BEGIN WITH THE END IN MIND

This habit is about having a clear vision of what one wants to accomplish in both career and personal life, and the legacy that one wishes to leave. The story of Alfred Nobel is a powerful reminder of the importance of this.

Alfred Nobel was the inventor of dynamite and became extremely wealthy as a result of his invention. However, when Alfred's younger brother Ludwig died in 1888, a French newspaper incorrectly thought Alfred Nobel had died.[10] The newspaper printed an obituary for Alfred Nobel with the headline, "The merchant of death is dead." It went on to state, "Dr. Alfred Nobel, who became rich by finding ways to kill more people faster than ever before, died yesterday."[11] It is generally thought that his decision to leave his vast fortune for the creation of the Nobel prizes was driven by a desire to leave behind a better legacy than being remembered as the "Merchant of Death."

HABIT 3: PUT FIRST THINGS FIRST

Covey's third habit is about organizing your time and resources to achieve your personal vision. Unfortunately, many people spend much of their time doing things that do not contribute to achieving their personal vision. Covey argues that if we truly want to be effective, we need to "put first things first," spending more of our time and effort on things that are truly important to our interpersonal effectiveness, as opposed to spending large amounts of time watching television, surfing the web and other low-value activities.

HABIT 4: THINK WIN/WIN

Covey identified six paradigms of human interaction: win, win/win, win/lose, lose/win, lose/lose or no deal. In his book, he works through the advantages and disadvantages of each paradigm, making the case that in most of their interactions with others, highly effective people aim for win/win outcomes.

HABIT 5: SEEK FIRST TO UNDERSTAND, THEN TO BE UNDERSTOOD

Covey noted that in many interactions with others, people start out by trying to make sure their position or point of view is understood. Covey argues that effective people do the opposite; they seek to first listen to others with the intent of gaining a full understanding of the other's point of view.

HABIT 6: SYNERGIZE

Covey points out that successful interactions with others are based on trust and cooperation. By constantly working to improve the levels of trust and cooperation in our relationships with others, the result is not simply additive, but a synergistic one that greatly enhances the outcomes of our interactions with others.

HABIT 7: SHARPEN THE SAW

Covey's final habit is focused on self-renewal. If people do not maintain and sharpen themselves in four key areas (physical, mental, spiritual and social), their personal effectiveness will decline.

Covey's seven habits represent a powerful framework for maintaining personal effectiveness that is as current today as it was when it was first published. Habits are, by definition, practices that are repeated routinely and predictably. If these habits are developed early, and maintained over the course of a career, an individual's personal effectiveness will undoubtedly be enhanced.

OTHER TOOLS FOR ENHANCING PERSONAL EFFECTIVENESS IN THE WORKPLACE

EMOTIONAL INTELLIGENCE

An important leadership and management skill is the ability to work effectively with people. The workplace can be a stressful environment where managers have to deal effectively with people who are displaying a wide range of emotions. Over the past 20 years, the concept of emotional intelligence has received considerable attention.

Emotional intelligence has been defined as, "the ability to identify and manage your own emotions and the emotions of others."[12] Salovey and Mayer further define it as, "the subset of social intelligence that involves the ability to monitor one's own and others' feelings and emotions, to discriminate among them, and to use this information to guide one's thinking and actions.[13] They identify four components of emotional intelligence:
- accurately perceiving emotions, including non-verbal components of body language, facial expressions, etc.
- reasoning with emotions, which involves thinking about and analyzing the emotions that were observed, before responding
- understanding emotions by assessing a range of possibilities concerning what those emotions might mean
- managing emotions by responding appropriately and responding to the emotions of others

This concept is an important competency for managers to possess. Although some evidence suggests that emotional intelligence is largely determined in early life, there is evidence that with appropriate guidance, coaching and persistence, it can be improved.[14] Several tools and resources have been developed to assess an individual's emotional intelligence and to assist individuals in improving their emotional intelligence.[14]

CULTURAL COMPETENCY

Cultural competence refers to an ability to interact effectively with people of different cultures. Cross et al., indicate that the word *culture* is used because, "it implies the integrated pattern of human behaviour that includes thoughts, communications, actions, customs, beliefs, values and institutions of a racial, ethnic, religious or social group."[15] The word *competence* is used because, "it implies having the capacity to function effectively"[15] (see Chapter 44: Communicating with Your Patients and Across Cultures).

At the individual level, cultural competency encompasses five main components:[15]

- awareness of one's own cultural worldview
- attitudes toward cultural differences
- knowledge of different cultural practices
- awareness of the ways that different cultures view the world
- level of development of the individual's cross-cultural skills

At the organizational level, five characteristics are essential to the development and maintenance of cultural competence:[15]

- The organization values diversity.
- It has the capacity for cultural self-assessment.
- Staff are conscious of the dynamics inherent when cultures interact.
- They have institutionalized awareness and knowledge of cultural differences.
- They have developed adaptations to service delivery that reflect an understanding of cultural diversity.

Several provinces/territories and health care organizations in Canada have developed websites that provide information to assist their staff in developing cultural competency.[16–18]

DELEGATION: A STRATEGY FOR MANAGERS AND THEIR SUBORDINATES

The act of delegation frees up an experienced individual to take on higher-level responsibilities and spreads knowledge and skills to others in the organization. Those who delegate to others are making the transition from producers to managers since they become responsible for managing those to whom they have delegated their responsibilities. It builds reserve capacity within the organization to deal with staff departures and absences. Perhaps most importantly of all, it motivates staff by providing opportunities for growth and development.

Although delegation can be a powerful tool for enhancing personal effectiveness and productivity, there are potential pitfalls.[8] If individuals are assigned responsibility for certain tasks, without being delegated the authority and resources needed to accomplish the task, there is little chance they will be able to successfully accomplish the task they were given. Likewise, delegation is likely to fail if clear guidance regarding expectations and accountabilities is not provided. Delegation is most effective when it is results-focused and subordinates are given considerable latitude in how they achieve the desired results.

MANAGING UP: A STRATEGY FOR EMPLOYEES AND THEIR BOSSES

Managing up has been defined as, "the process of consciously working with your boss to achieve the best possible results for you, your boss and your organization."[19] In essence, the employee does not wait to be delegated responsibilities, but instead looks for opportunities to assist the manager by carrying out tasks that support the boss in carrying out his or her responsibilities. Managing up is most effective when there is a high degree of trust and cooperation between the two parties, combined with an understanding of the wants and needs of the boss. Managers stand to benefit by being able to offload some of their responsibilities and the employees benefit by gaining experience, proving their value and establishing themselves as having good potential for advancement within the organization. An employee going above and beyond what the boss had initially expected benefits both parties.

Employees should start out by learning as much as possible about the manager's personality and management style. Employees should attempt to develop a good understanding of how the manager sees the world and look for opportunities to help out when the manager is struggling with urgent or emergent issues. However, the work the employee does on behalf of the manager needs to fit with the manager's expectations of how things should be done. For example, some managers will, at least initially, want to review and approve everything the employee does. Other managers will be much more hands-off. The key is to understand the manager's style and expectations. Employees should touch base regularly with the manager, particularly in the early stages of developing a relationship with the boss.

Over time, the trust level should improve to the point where the employee is given a great deal of independence. However, in the early stages the employee should communicate regularly with the manager to make sure that the boss fully supports both the responsibilities the employee is taking on and the style or manner in which the employee carries out those responsibilities. Employees should keep managers informed of any matters that might develop into issues that the managers might have to deal with. Employees who are managing up should build networks with other employees so they are aware of issues that may be important considerations for the boss.

Employees who wish to establish a mutually beneficial relationship with their boss should be aware of some of the pitfalls that can damage or destroy that relationship. The employee may be aware of, but should avoid becoming involved in, office politics and should never share confidential information that they become aware of as a result of the managing-up activities.

Although an employee may have done work on behalf of the boss, and might like to be recognized for the contribution, it is best to let the boss decide how much credit to give. Although that might seem unfair, a good strategy is to allow the boss to decide when and how to recognize the contributions made. Others in the organization tend to learn about the work employees do on behalf of their boss without the employee making any direct efforts to be recognized for their contribution. In almost all cases, the employee will eventually benefit from managing-up efforts, but if the employee expects immediate payback and gratification, the relationship is likely to become strained. A longer-term perspective on the benefits that will accrue from managing up will serve the employee well. In addition, the employee should make sure the managing-up efforts provide real benefits and are, to the extent possible, viewed positively by other staff. Efforts should be made to avoid being perceived as "sucking up" to the boss. Finally, employees in a managing-up relationship with their boss should be very careful concerning information they share with others. In successful managing-up relationships, the boss places a significant amount of trust in the employee. Inappropriately sharing information or speaking critically of the manager can quickly destroy the trust that has been created in the relationship.

Many individuals struggle to achieve their goals without understanding how to improve their personal effectiveness. The earlier individuals begin to develop habits that improve their personal effectiveness, the more likely it is that that they will achieve their goals.

REFERENCES

1. American Marketing Association dictionary. Available: www.ama.org/resources/Pages/Dictionary.aspx?dLetter=B (accessed Aug. 15, 2014).

2. Godin S. Define: brand. Available: http://sethgodin.typepad.com/seths_blog/2009/12/define-brand.html (accessed Aug. 15, 2014).

3. Top ten Lada jokes. *The Telegraph.* Available: www.telegraph.co.uk/motoring/picturegalleries/9211301/Top-10-Lada-jokes.html?frame=2196460 (accessed Nov. 9, 2014).

4. Peters TJ. *The brandyou50: Fifty ways to transform yourself from an employee into a brand that shouts distinction, commitment and passion.* New York: Alfred A Knopf Inc; 1999.

5. PwC. Your Personal Brand Survey. Available: www.pwc.com/us/en/careers/campus/programs-events/personal-brand/assets/pb14-survey-gizmo-instructions-bw_4.pdf (accessed Nov. 14, 2014).

6. Cooly P. 33 questions to propel your personal brand forward this year. SteamFeed. Available: www.steamfeed.com/32-questions-propel-personal-brand-forward-year/ (accessed Aug. 15, 2014).

7. Foundations. George Washington's Rules of Civility & Decent Behavior in Company and Conversation. Available: www.foundationsmag.com/civility.html (accessed Nov. 9, 2014).

8. Covey SR. *The 7 habits of highly effective people.* New York: Franklin Covey Co.; 1989.

9. About Stephen Covey. Available: www.stephencovey.com/about/about.php (accessed Aug. 5, 2014).

10. Alfred Bernhard Nobel. Encyclopedia Britannica. Available: www.britannica.com/EBchecked/topic/416842/Alfred-Bernhard-Nobel (accessed Nov. 30, 2014).

11. Alfred Nobel was also known as "The merchant of death." Today I Found Out. Available: www.todayifoundout.com/index.php/2011/01/alfred-nobel-was-also-known-as-the-merchant-of-death/ (accessed Nov. 30, 2014).

12. Coleman A. *A dictionary of psychology.* 3rd ed., Oxford University Press; 2008.

13. Salovey P, Mayer JD. Emotional intelligence concepts, Journal Imagination, Cognition, and Personality. Available: www.unh.edu/emotional_intelligence/EI%20Assets/Reprints...EI%20Proper/EI1990%20Emotional%20Intelligence.pdf (accessed July 21, 2014).

14. Bradberry T, Greaves J. *Emotional intelligence 2.0.* California: TalentSmart; 2009.

15. Cross T, Bazron B, Dennis K, et al. Towards a culturally competent system of care, volume I. Washington, DC: Georgetown University Child Development Center, CASSP Technical Assistance Center. Available: http://files.eric.ed.gov/fulltext/ED330171.pdf (accessed Nov. 14, 2014).

16. British Columbia website for indigenous cultural competency, developed for the Provincial Health Services and their Ministry of Health. Available: www.culturalcompetency.ca/ (accessed Nov. 4, 2014).

17. Hospital for Sick Kids (Toronto) website for cultural competency. Available: www.sickkids.ca/culturalcompetence/ (accessed Nov. 4, 2014).

18. Winnipeg Regional Health Authority website for cultural competency. Available: www.wrha.mb.ca/community/commdev/files/Diversity-FrameworkForAction.pdf (accessed Nov. 4, 2014).

19. Zuber J, James E. Managing your Boss. Family Practice Medicine June 2001. Available: www.aafp.org/fpm/2001/0600/p33.pdf (accessed Nov. 30, 2014).

CHAPTER 12

Professional Competence and Ethics

Rene Breault, *BScPharm, PharmD; Clinical Assistant Professor, Faculty of Pharmacy and Pharmaceutical Sciences, University of Alberta*

Jill Hall, *BScPharm, ACPR, PharmD; Clinical Assistant Professor, Faculty of Pharmacy and Pharmaceutical Sciences, University of Alberta*

Learning Objectives

- Describe the role professional competence and bioethics play in improving the quality and acceptability of health care systems.

- Understand the five high-level, health-system competencies that have been recognized as key to close the quality gap that has been identified in recent reports.

- Describe strategies that pharmacists, pharmacy technicians and employers can use to maintain their professional competence.

- Describe the responsibility employers have for dealing with employees whose competence is in question.

- Understand the bioethical principles of beneficence, nonmaleficence, autonomy, justice, veracity, fidelity and confidentiality and be able to give examples of their link to pharmacy practice.

THE HEALTH CARE CONTEXT

There are many challenges facing the health care system in Canada, not the least of which is the public's concern with its quality. Reports of patient harm resulting from seemingly preventable failures in the delivery of care appear all too frequently in the media. In the late 1990s, the Institute of Medicine (IOM) published a report on medical errors titled *To Err is Human: Building a Safer Health System,* in which the magnitude of the medical error problem in the United States was quantified.[1] Based on the results from several studies, it was estimated that somewhere between 44,000 and 98,000 people were dying in hospitals each year as a result of preventable medical errors. A subsequent Canadian study indicated that medical errors were of a similar magnitude in the Canadian setting.[2] Medical errors outside the hospital setting have not been quantified reliably, but their inclusion would undoubtedly increase the estimated number substantially. The IOM report did emphasize that most medical errors are the result of failures in the design and operation of the health care system rather than the incompetence or negligence of individual practitioners. However, that is not always the case and there have been many situations in which health care professionals have been called before their profession's disciplinary committee to account for errors of commission or omission that led to patient harm. In a study of the medical profession in Canada, a total of 606 individual physicians were identified as having been disciplined by their licensing bodies over the period between 2000 and 2009.[3] Health care professionals have a covenantal responsibility to their patients to "first, do no harm" and are held to high expectations of competence and vigilance in the performance of their duties.

PROFESSIONAL COMPETENCE

When the word *competence* is used in the context of health care, what exactly is it referring to? A simple dictionary definition of competence is, "the ability to do something well," and that is actually a good starting point.[4] A more specific definition of competence, which is applicable to all health care professions, including pharmacy, is, "the habitual and judicious use of communication, knowledge, technical skills, clinical reasoning, emotions, values, and reflection in daily practice for the benefit of the individual and community being served."[5]

The IOM followed up its *To Err is Human* report with a second report titled *Crossing the Quality Chasm: A New Health System for the 21st Century*, in which they proposed five core competencies that all health care disciplines should possess, including the ability to do the following: provide patient-centred care, use an evidence-based approach to care, work effectively in interdisciplinary teams, apply continuing quality improvement strategies to their practice and use informatics effectively in the care delivery process.[6] At the individual discipline level, the IOM report acknowledged the role that professional associations had in setting performance standards, collaborating across disciplines with respect to standards and communicating with their members concerning practice expectations. At the individual pharmacy practitioner level, specific pharmacy competencies provide an overview of what pharmacists or pharmacy technicians should be able to do well, rather than how they are expected to perform the task.[7]

COMPETENCY AT ENTRY TO PRACTICE

In Canada, several organizations play a role in the establishment and assessment of competencies. For pharmacists and pharmacy technicians to meet the requirements for entry into practice, they must have graduated from an educational program that has met the standards and criteria set out by the Canadian Council for Accreditation of Pharmacy Programs (CCAPP).[8] Further, they must have met the entry-to-practice competencies as outlined by the National Association of Pharmacy Regulatory Authorities (NAPRA) and assessed by the Pharmacy Examining Board of Canada (PEBC). For entry-to-practice registration or licensure, each province/territory may also have other requirements for prospective pharmacists or pharmacy technicians (e.g., language proficiency, internship period, criminal record check, jurisprudence exam, fees).

The NAPRA professional competencies (Table 1) serve to guide the development of educational outcomes, educational program accreditation standards and national competency assessment

Table 1. Entry-to-Practice Competencies for Pharmacists and Pharmacy Technicians[7,9]

NAPRA Professional Competencies
Ethical, legal and professional responsibilities
Patient care
Product distribution
Practice setting
Health promotion
Knowledge and research application
Communication and education
Intra- and interprofessional collaboration
Quality and safety

examinations.[7,9] Educational outcomes have been developed for both pharmacist and pharmacy technician programs that align with the competencies established for each profession.[10,11]

The role of PEBC is to assess the qualifications of pharmacists and pharmacy technicians on behalf of provincial/territorial pharmacy regulatory authorities and to ensure entry-level pharmacists and pharmacy technicians have the necessary professional knowledge, skills and abilities to practise pharmacy within their scope of practice, in a safe and effective manner.[12] Successful completion of the qualifying examination indicates that candidates have met the required standard of competence at entry to practice.[12] PEBC also sets an evaluating examination for International Pharmacy Graduates (IPGs) to ensure graduates have completed a program of study comparable to that accredited by CCAPP.

CONTINUING COMPETENCE

Continuing competence has been described as, "the lifelong process of maintaining and documenting competence through ongoing self-assessment, personal development and implementation of a personal learning plan, and subsequent re-assessment."[13] While ensuring competence at entry to practice is essential, pharmacy regulatory bodies have the added task of ensuring continued competence, or fitness-to-practise. In contrast to measures used to assess competence at entry to practice, the focus of continuing competency assessment is *performance* as a health care professional.[14] Continuing competence evolved out of the demand from the public, provincial/territorial governments and third-party payers that health care professionals must be accountable to deliver high-quality services.[15] In some jurisdictions, competency assessment or continuing professional development programs are required by legislation.[16]

Provincial/Territorial pharmacy regulatory authorities, under a broader mandate of public safety, seek to ensure that all pharmacists and pharmacy technicians maintain their knowledge and skills at the highest possible level. Currently, all provinces/territories usually require that mandatory annual continuing education (CE) be completed to maintain pharmacist licensure. Similar requirements are in place for those provinces/territories that regulate pharmacy technicians.

Provincial/Territorial regulatory authorities employ several strategies to assess professional competency beyond traditional CE.[17] Knowledge-based exams, as the name suggests, are best at evaluating clinical knowledge, but are less useful as a measure of one's individual clinical practice.[18] Peer and patient assessments, along with objective structured clinical exams (OSCE) are variations of performance-based assessments with a focus on communication skills, demeanour and ethical and legal responsibilities.[17] These third-party assessments are challenging from a cost and implementation perspective and can be met with resistance from practising professionals.[14]

An ideal competency program would be structured to measure actual clinician performance, assess outcomes of care and be incorporated into a model of continuing professional development.[14,19]

STRATEGIES FOR MAINTENANCE OF COMPETENCE

While pharmacists and pharmacy technicians have traditionally only completed required CE hours, it is now widely recognized that reliance on traditional CE is a flawed approach, which is likely inadequate for maintaining the competence of professionals over the course of their careers.[20,21] There is little evidence that a relationship exists between CE hours and maintenance of practitioner competency or practitioner adoption of practice changes that lead to better patient outcomes.[15,22] Mandatory CE focuses on meeting regulatory requirements versus identifying gaps in knowledge and skills and finding strategies to address them.[21] An alternative method professionals can incorporate to maintain competence is continuing professional development (CPD). CPD is a systematic, self-directed, ongoing and cyclical process where a practitioner 1) reflects on learning needs and goals; 2) plans learning activities to meet needs and goals; 3) implements the learning plan; 4) evaluates success of the plan; and 5) documents learning activities in a professional portfolio.[23] The CPD concept aligns with the idea of continuing competency across a lifespan of one's career and is different in many aspects from traditional CE (Table 2).[24]

Unfortunately, pharmacy professionals frequently find the CPD steps of self-assessment and developing learning plans to address their learning needs to be a challenge.[14] Individuals generally have limited ability to accurately self-identify and correct practice deficiencies.[25] Further, there is conflicting evidence as to whether the CPD process itself is effective at ensuring competence or a high quality of practice.[26,27]

The specific learning activities pharmacists and pharmacy technicians participate in as part of the CPD process can vary depending on their identified needs and goals and may include

Table 2. Comparison of Continuing Education (CE) and Continuing Professional Development (CPD)[24]

Parameter	Traditional CE Model	CPD
Educational needs	Predetermined by program speaker	Self-identified through personal reflection
Motivation to participate	External	Internal
Relevance to practice	May be absent; no requirement to link to practice	High
Outcomes	May be absent, poorly defined and may not be assessed	Process dependent
Duration	Isolated event	Ongoing, cyclical
Process	Passive	Active

CE hours, workshops, practice-based activities or credentialling/certification.[14] Many of these learning endeavours are accredited through various organizations such as the Canadian Council on Continuing Education in Pharmacy (CCCEP),[28] the Accreditation Council for Pharmacy Education (ACPE)[29] and the American-based Board of Pharmacy Specialties (BPS).[30] Pharmacy professionals can also incorporate informal learning to keep up to date within their practice, using resources such as subscriptions to relevant journal electronic table of contents, web-based forums and newsletters.

Employers have an important role in supporting pharmacists and pharmacy technicians to maintain professional competence. Strategies may include supporting professional development with educational funding and paid days off to attend courses, as well as internal training programs (e.g., for new standards of practice, such as provision of injections) and informal workplace learning (e.g., lunchtime journal club, case discussions).[31] Employers can also assist in creating environments that are favourable to informal workplace learning and provide feedback to help focus pharmacists and pharmacy technicians on their educational and professional goals.[32]

MANAGING COMPETENCE ISSUES

All pharmacists are responsible for ensuring their competence. Regulatory authorities set standards of practice and administer competence programs to ensure fitness-to-practise and to protect the public. However, employers also have the responsibility to ensure their staff practise at accepted standards.[7] In the context of provision of professional services, employers should establish policies and procedures for patient care, which are focused on clinical performance, *not* business targets, and have a structure in place for performance appraisal and remediation, if necessary.[33] There must also be systems in place to identify performance concerns in the workplace that require the employer to address an individual practitioner's performance concerns.[34] Challenges to managing pharmacists with performance concerns include difficulty in effective self-appraisal, lack of clear performance standards and professional isolation (e.g., locum and solo-practice pharmacists).[34] Error reporting systems, such as "good catch" systems where errors are detected and corrected before reaching the patient, peer reporting systems and routine audits, can all help to identify issues.[34] When identified, performance concerns should be dealt with internally, ideally in a non-punitive fashion and with support for any well-being issues and remediation using a directive corrective action pathway, such as Studer's D.E.S.K. approach,[34,35] which involves a conversational approach to providing feedback to low performers with the objective of improving their behaviour. The specific steps involve *describing* to the employee the behaviour of concern that has been observed, the *evaluation* of the behaviour, *showing* what needs to be done to address the problematic behaviour, and ensuring the employee *knows* what the consequences will be if the behaviour is not corrected. Disciplinary action may be necessary, as may referral to the regulatory body for ongoing competence concerns.[34]

ETHICS IN PHARMACY PRACTICE

Pharmacists are bound by a collective set of professional ethics that supersede their personal values.[36] Although an individual's personal values may have some impact on how he or she conducts patient care assessments and makes decisions, normative bioethical principles (Table 3) must guide

Table 3. Bioethical Principles and Their Link to Pharmaceutical Care[37,39,40]

Bioethical Principle	Brief Definition	Link to Pharmacy Practice
Beneficence	Do what benefits others	Moral obligation to do the best you can for every patient, considering your professional knowledge as well as patient preferences with respect to guiding therapy decisions. Moreover, always consider the fact that it may be better not to subject patients to more treatment, so as not to risk causing more harm than good.
Nonmaleficence	Do no harm, prevent harm, or remove harm	
Autonomy	Respect each individual's right and ability to make decisions and to determine their own actions	While advocating for patients' well-being, respect their preference(s) and right to provide consent to accept or refuse treatment, enabling informed patients to make their own (guided) decisions.
Justice	Treat all people fairly	Provide fair, equitable and appropriate treatment in light of what is due to an individual patient and society (through resource allocation: time, effort, money), aiming to improve health and quality of health care.
Veracity	Tell the truth	Be honest and forthcoming in the provision of care and conduct of research, aiming to serve patients' best interests.
Fidelity	Honour the professional promise of care	Uphold responsibility to patients, employers and society granted by licensing bodies (Code of Ethics, Standards of Practice), putting these interests ahead of self-interest.
Confidentiality	Keep private information entrusted	Protect patient privacy and right to information access to maintain patient trust in an established patient-care relationship.

the pharmacist's duty of care and professional responsibilities[37] as set forth by each provincial/territorial regulatory body in a code of ethics (or conduct). As society grants professional autonomy to pharmacists based on their unique knowledge and skill set, this code ensures that pharmacists uphold high ethical standards while acting in the best interests of their patients and society.[38]

Although pharmacists are generally aware of these normative bioethical principles, they may prefer to rely more on their personal or religious values, past experiences and legislation to guide decision making.[39,41] Without formal training, it is difficult to recognize ethical dilemmas and make appropriate decisions in today's complicated health care environment. Several tools are available to support pharmacists in ethical decision making,[42,43] many based on Rest's four-stage model, where one must be able to do the following: 1) recognize an ethical problem, 2) reason through it with the 3) intention of acting in the best interests of the patient rather than one's own interest and finally, 4) enact what one has deemed to be the ethically most sound decision.[44,45]

Having a decision-making framework is essential, as ethical dilemmas are encountered daily in contemporary pharmacy practice. This can be defined as any situation wherein ethical principles conflict and there is no clear right or wrong answer, often creating an "uneasy feeling" in practice.[46] Pharmacists need to weigh the best interests of their patients with all of the other factors involved. This internal conflict frequently causes stress or even moral distress that "occurs when one knows the right thing to do, but institutional or other constraints make it difficult to pursue the desired course of action."[47,48] Dilemmas can take many forms and can impact pharmacy practice at an individual, organizational or societal level.[49]

AT AN INDIVIDUAL LEVEL

As North American culture is generally focused on individualism, considering the bioethical principles at this level is somewhat straightforward as a health care provider:[49]

- ensuring patient autonomy in decision making
- confirming informed consent in the therapeutic relationship and in research
- acting with veracity and fidelity
- guarding confidentiality of health information

A conflict of interest, whether real or perceived, where professional judgment is influenced by another interest such as financial gain or personal recognition, may affect one's ability to act in the best interest of patients.[50,51] This may include receiving restricted or superfluous funding for a research project or simply attending an industry-funded educational event or receiving industry-labelled items. Asking oneself, "Would I feel comfortable if patients and other people found out about my . . . "[51] can help identify potential conflicts of interest. Disclosure is key, regardless of intentions, to ensure fidelity in patient-centred care.

Objections of conscience are another commonly cited example of ethical dilemmas in patient care, where one's personal beliefs or moral values conflict with a professional duty of care. Refusal to fill oral contraceptives or emergency contraception, based on religious or personal beliefs, has been argued to be a breach of a professional's duty to provide patient care and respect patient autonomy. In such situations, pharmacists are placing their own professional autonomy (paternalism) over their professional obligations, based on religious beliefs.[52]

Legislation concerning refusal to fill exists in many provinces/territories. The legislation usually recognizes the right of an individual professional to personally decline to participate in providing a service they are morally opposed to *provided* they inform the patient of alternative methods of accessing the product or service. That proviso is intended to ensure patients do not suffer harm as a result of a professional's personal beliefs.[36]

AT AN ORGANIZATIONAL LEVEL

However important ethical practice is between individuals (pharmacist-patient), trade-offs must sometimes be made to balance the needs of individuals with the needs at an organizational and societal level.[49] While pharmacists have an obligation to support organizational and societal interests, patient autonomy and well-being should always remain the primary concern.[53] Aiming to maximize profit in a business can be a challenge to this principle. With expanding scopes of practice, there are increasing opportunities for both improving patient care and improving profitability. The challenge for some community pharmacy owners is whether they are first and foremost a health care professional or a retailer of pharmacy goods and services.[54]

Patient counselling is a standard of practice that is key to positive patient outcomes. It ensures autonomy and guards the covenants of trust, fidelity, confidentiality and justice in patient-centred care.[40,55] However, several business practices put this at risk, including minimizing human resource utilization (pharmacists) and maximizing workload (prescriptions filled), along with policies supporting quantity rather than quality, putting profit ahead of professional duty.[53] Internet pharmacies (before a rigorous framework was established) and drive-through pharmacy outlets, where counselling may be entirely absent, direct-to-consumer advertising on over-the-counter products, discounted services and poaching patients from facilities already under pharmacy service contracts are clear examples of placing business practice over professional practice.[54]

Organizations may also act to protect patients and reduce potential conflicts of interest and ethical dilemmas through policies such as limiting staff interactions with the pharmaceutical industry. They can also act to ensure justice in resource allocation in an attempt to provide equitable access to effective and safe medications; for example, through formulary decisions.[40]

AT A SOCIETAL LEVEL

At a broad level, in publicly funded health care systems, policy makers need to balance conflicting needs of individuals, organizations and society. An example of an ethical dilemma here is distributive justice. Policy makers must not only ensure effectiveness, safety and fair pricing of all drugs, but balance equitable allocation of public resources in acute and chronic care, in primary prevention versus treatment/cure and in human resources allocation.[49]

Consider as an illustration cancer treatment, where several established, cost-effective therapies exist alongside novel, potentially more efficacious but also more expensive treatments. No drug guarantees a cure, but may extend survival or improve quality of life. At an individual level, one would treat each patient with the best available therapy, regardless of cost, to optimize that patient's outcome. At an organizational level, there may exist a formulary, limiting the type and use of both established and novel therapies. At a societal level, restrictions on the use of the novel therapies may be in place to limit treatment only to those who have failed all other options. This may create moral distress for pharmacists, who recognize the potential benefit of a novel therapy for an individual patient but cannot provide it due to organizational or societal policies restricting its use. However, there is broad agreement that to best treat all patients requires consideration of the common good, and often organizational and societal ethics need to be contemplated before one can truly succeed in benefiting an individual.[49]

This chapter provides an introduction to two topics that are relevant to both pharmacy managers and frontline pharmacy practitioners. Both individual pharmacists and their managers must recognize the need to optimize the quality of care in the health care system. That objective can only be achieved if individuals and their managers understand the need to develop and maintain professional competency. Similarly, both pharmacists and pharmacy managers must have a solid understanding of, and commitment to, a high standard of ethical behaviour. Additional reading and reflection on these topic areas will help individuals to achieve their full potential as competent and highly ethical health care professionals.

REFERENCES

1. Kohn LT, Corrigan JM, Donaldson MS, eds. To err is human: building a safer health system. [Internet]. Committee on Quality of Health Care in America, Institute of Medicine. Washington, D.C.: National Academy Press; 1999 [cited 2014 Oct 14]. 311 p. Available: http://books.nap.edu/openbook.php?record_id=9728.

2. Baker GR, Norton PG, Flintoft V, et al. The Canadian Adverse Events Study: the incidence of adverse events among hospital patients in Canada. CMAJ. 2004;170(11):1678–86. http://dx.doi.org/10.1503/cmaj.1040498. Medline:15159366

3. Alam A, Klemensberg J, Griesman J, et al. The characteristics of physicians disciplined by professional colleges in Canada. Open Med. 2011;5(4):e166–72. Medline:22567070

4. Competence [Internet]. Merriam-Webster 2014. Available: http://www.merriam-webster.com/dictionary/competence (accessed Oct. 14, 2014).

5. Epstein RM, Hundert EM. Defining and assessing professional competence. JAMA. 2002;287(2):226–35. http://dx.doi.org/10.1001/jama.287.2.226. Medline:11779266

6. Committee on Quality of Health Care in America. Crossing the quality chasm: A new health system for the 21st century [Internet]. Washington, D.C.: National Academies Press; 2001. Available: www.nap.edu/catalog/10027.html (accessed Oct. 5, 2014).

7. Professional competencies for Canadian pharmacy technicians at entry to practice [Internet]. Ottawa: National Association of Pharmacy Regulatory Authorities; 2014. Available: http://napra.ca/Content_Files/Files/Comp_for_Cdn_PHARMTECHS_at_EntrytoPractice_March2014_b.pdf (accessed Oct. 14, 2014).

8. Accreditation standards for first professional degree in pharmacy programs [Internet]. Toronto, ON: Canadian Council for Accreditation of Pharmacy Programs; 2013. Available: www.ccapp-accredit.ca/site/pdfs/university/CCAPP_accred_standards_degree_2012.pdf (accessed April 12, 2014).

9. Professional competencies for Canadian pharmacists at entry to practice. [Internet]. Ottawa: National Association of Pharmacy Regulatory Authorities; 2014. Available: https://scp.in1touch.org/document/1745/NAPRA_Comp_Cdn_PHARMACISTS_CURRENT.pdf (accessed Oct. 14, 2014).

10. Educational outcomes for first professional degree programs in pharmacy (entry to practice pharmacy programs) in Canada [Internet]. Vancouver: Association of Faculties of Pharmacy of Canada; 2010. Available: www.afpc.info/sites/default/files/AFPC%20Educational%20Outcomes.pdf (accessed Oct. 5, 2014).

11. Educational outcomes for pharmacy technician programs in Canada [Internet]. Canadian Pharmacy Technician Educators Association; 2007. Available: www.ccapp-accredit.ca/site/pdfs/technician/CPTEA_Educational_Outcomes_for_Pharmacy_Technician_Programs_in_Canada_(Mar_2007).pdf (accessed April 21, 2014).

12. Pharmacist qualifying examination [Internet]. Toronto, ON: Pharmacy Examining Board of Canada. Available: www.pebc.ca/index.php/ci_id/3147/la_id/1.htm (accessed April 2, 2014).

13. Continuing competence in physical therapy: An ongoing discussion [Internet]. American Physical Therapy Association and the Federated State Boards of Physical Therapy; 2009. Available: www.fsbpt.org/download/CCDiscussionPaper.pdf (accessed April 12, 2014).

14. Winslade NE, Tamblyn RM, Taylor LK, et al. Integrating performance assessment, maintenance of competence, and continuing professional development of community pharmacists. Am J Pharm Educ. 2007;71(1):15. http://dx.doi.org/10.5688/aj710115. Medline:17429515

15. Shord SS, Schwinghammer TL, Badowski M, et al. Desired professional development pathways for clinical pharmacists American college of clinical pharmacy. Pharmacother. 2013;33(4):e34–42. http://dx.doi.org/10.1002/phar.1251.

16. Government of Alberta Health professions act: Pharmacists and pharmacy technicians profession regulation [Internet]. Alberta: Queen's Printer; 2011. Available: http://142.229.230.30/1266.cfm?page=2006_129.cfm&leg_type=Regs&isbncln=9780779758197&display=html (accessed April 12, 2014).

17. National model continuing competence program for pharmacists [Internet]. Ottawa: National Association of Pharmacy Regulatory Authorities; 2002. Available: http://napra.ca/pages/Practice_Resources/contiuning_competence.aspx?id=2091 (accessed April 12, 2014).

18. Leigh IW, Smith LI, Bebeau MJ, et al. Competency assessment models. Prof Psychol Res Pr. 2007;38(5):463–73. http://dx.doi.org/10.1037/0735-7028.38.5.463.

19. Head K. Improving the practice of continuing competency: An exploration of continuing competency programs amongst regulated health care professionals in Canada. A consulting project for Physiotherapy Alberta. Unpublished document/personal communication with author.

20. Austin Z. CPD and revalidation: our future is happening now. Res Social Adm Pharm. 2013;9(2):138–41. http://dx.doi.org/10.1016/j.sapharm.2012.09.002. Medline:23062784

21. Institute of Medicine. Redesigning continuing education in the health professions. [Internet]. Washington, D.C.: National Academies; 2009. Available: www.iom.edu/~/media/Files/Report%20Files/2009/Redesigning-Continuing-Education-in-the-Health-Professions/RedesigningCEreportbrief.pdf (accessed April 19, 2014).

22. Albanese NP, Rouse MJ, and the Council on Credentialing in Pharmacy. Scope of contemporary pharmacy practice: roles, responsibilities, and functions of pharmacists and pharmacy technicians. J Am Pharm Assoc (2003). 2010;50(2):e35–69. http://dx.doi.org/10.1331/JAPhA.2010.10510. Medline:20199947

23. The council on credentialing in pharmacy resource document: Continuing professional development in pharmacy. [Internet]. Washington, D.C. Council on Credentialing in Pharmacy; 2004. Available: www.pharmacycredentialing.org/Files/cpdprimer.pdf (accessed Oct. 14, 2014).

24. Schindel T, Moulton J, Stasyk R, et al. Continuing professional development for the CE provider. implementing CPD: Our stories. Paper presented at: 11th annual accreditation council for pharmacy education conference; 2005 Sep 29-Oct 2; Chicago, IL.

25. Eva KW, Regehr G. Self-assessment in the health professions: a reformulation and research agenda. Acad Med. 2005;80(10 Suppl):S46–54. http://dx.doi.org/10.1097/00001888-200510001-00015. Medline:16199457

26. Goulet F, Hudon E, Gagnon R, et al. Effects of continuing professional development on clinical performance: results of a study involving family practitioners in Quebec. Can Fam Physician. 2013;59(5):518–25. Medline:23673591

27. Norman GR. The adult learner: a mythical species. Acad Med. 1999;74(8):886–9. http://dx.doi.org/10.1097/00001888-199908000-00011. Medline:10495727

28. Canadian council on continuing education in pharmacy [Internet]. Saskatoon, SK; c2008. Available: www.cccep.org (accessed April 17, 2014).

29. Accreditation council for pharmacy education [Internet]. Chicago, IL; 2014. Available: www.acpe-accredit.org (accessed April 17, 2014).

30. Board of pharmacy specialties [Internet]. Washington, D.C.: American Pharmacists Association; c2014. Available from: http://bpsweb.org (accessed April 17, 2014).

31. Hassell K. Good management is critical to professional development and employee well-being. Int J Pharm Pract. 2012;20(6):347–8. http://dx.doi.org/10.1111/j.2042-7174.2012.00251.x. Medline:23134092

32. Noble C, Hassell K. Informal learning in the workplace: What are the environmental barriers for junior hospital pharmacists? Int J Pharm Pract. 2008;16(4):257–63. http://dx.doi.org/10.1211/ijpp.16.4.0008.

33. Poppe LB, Granko RP. Managing underperformers. Am J Health Syst Pharm. 2011;68(22):2123–5. http://dx.doi.org/10.2146/ajhp110074. Medline:22058097

34. Jacobs S, Hassell K, Seston E, et al. Identifying and managing performance concerns in community pharmacists in the UK. J Health Serv Res Policy. 2013;18(3):144–50. http://dx.doi.org/10.1177/1355819613476277. Medline:23620581

35. Studer Q. Hardwiring excellence. Gulf Breeze, FL: Fire Starting Publishing; 2003.

36. Altilio JV. The pharmacist's obligations to patients: dependent or independent of the physician's obligations? J Law Med Ethics. 2009;37(2):358–68. http://dx.doi.org/10.1111/j.1748-720X.2009.00379.x. Medline:19493080

37. Cipolle R, Strand L, Morley P, editors. Pharmaceutical care practice: Patient centered approach to medication management. 3rd ed. New York, NY: McGraw Hill; 2012.

38. Fassett WE. Ethics, law, and the emergence of pharmacists' responsibility for patient care. Ann Pharmacother. 2007;41(7):1264–7. http://dx.doi.org/10.1345/aph.1K267. Medline:17595303

39. Chaar B, Brien J, Krass I. Professional ethics in pharmacy: Australian experience. Int J Pharm Pract. 2005;13(3):195–204. http://dx.doi.org/10.1211/ijpp.13.3.0005.

40. Salari P, Namazi H, Abdollahi M, et al. Code of ethics for the national pharmaceutical system: Codifying and compilation. J Res Med Sci. 2013;18(5):442–8. Medline:24174954

41. Cooper RJ, Bissell P, Wingfield J. Ethical decision-making, passivity and pharmacy. J Med Ethics. 2008;34(6):441–5. http://dx.doi.org/10.1136/jme.2007.022624. Medline:18511616

42. IDEA. Ethical decision-making framework - Guide & worksheets [Internet]. Toronto, ON: Trillium Health Centre. Available: www.trilliumhealthcentre.org/about/documents/TrilliumIDEA_EthicalDecisionMakingFramework.pdf (accessed April 18, 2014).

43. Model for ethical decision making [Internet]. Vancouver, B.C.: College of Pharmacists of British Columbia; 2011. Available: http://library.bcpharmacists.org/D-Legislation_Standards/D-2_Provincial_Legislation/5112-Code_of_Ethics_Model_for_Ethical_Decision_Making.pdf (accessed April 18, 2014).

44. Cooper RJ, Bissell P, Wingfield J. A new prescription for empirical ethics research in pharmacy: a critical review of the literature. J Med Ethics. 2007;33(2):82–6. http://dx.doi.org/10.1136/jme.2005.015297. Medline:17264193

45. Rest J. Moral development: Advances in research and theory. New York: Praeger Publishers; 1986.

46. Roche C, Kelliher F. Exploring the patient consent process in community pharmacy practice. J Bus Ethics. 2009;86(1):91–9. http://dx.doi.org/10.1007/s10551-008-9836-7.

47. Raines ML. Ethical decision making in nurses. Relationships among moral reasoning, coping style, and ethics stress. JONAS Healthc Law Ethics Regul. 2000;2(1):29–41. http://dx.doi.org/10.1097/00128488-200002010-00006. Medline:10824015

48. Kälvemark S, Höglund AT, Hansson MG, et al. Living with conflicts-ethical dilemmas and moral distress in the health care system. Soc Sci Med. 2004;58(6):1075–84. http://dx.doi.org/10.1016/S0277-9536(03)00279-X. Medline:14723903

49. Glaser J. Three realms of ethics. 1st ed. Kansas City, MO: Sheed & Ward; 1994.

50. Hatton RC, Chavez ML, Jackson E, et al, and the American College of Clinical Pharmacy. Pharmacists and industry: guidelines for ethical interactions. Pharmacotherapy. 2008;28(3):410–20. http://dx.doi.org/10.1592/phco.28.3.410. Medline:18294122

51. Lemmens T, Singer PA. Bioethics for clinicians: 17. Conflict of interest in research, education and patient care. CMAJ. 1998;159(8):960–5. Medline:9834723

52. Cantor J, Baum K. The limits of conscientious objection--may pharmacists refuse to fill prescriptions for emergency contraception? N Engl J Med. 2004;351(19):2008–12. http://dx.doi.org/10.1056/NEJMsb042263. Medline:15525728

53. Schafer A. Canadian internet pharmacies: Some ethical and economic issues. Can Pharm J. 2008;141(3):191–7. http://dx.doi.org/10.3821/1913-701X(2008)141[191:CIPSEA]2.0.CO;2.

54. Wingfield J, Bissell P, Anderson C. The Scope of pharmacy ethics: an evaluation of the international research literature, 1990-2002. Soc Sci Med. 2004;58(12):2383–96. http://dx.doi.org/10.1016/j.socscimed.2003.09.003. Medline:15081191

55. Resnik DB, Ranelli PL, Resnik SP. The conflict between ethics and business in community pharmacy: what about patient counseling? J Bus Ethics. 2000;28(2):179–86. http://dx.doi.org/10.1023/A:1006280300427. Medline:12530432

CHAPTER 13

Personal Finance

Mike Sullivan, RPh, BSP, MBA; President, Cubic Health Inc.

Learning Objectives

- Understand the fundamentals of personal financial management to develop the confidence and ability to achieve goals, and the ability to understand where to go to find needed assistance in managing financial affairs.

- Understand how to create a personal financial plan and how to update that plan each year and with each new life milestone that arrives.

- Dispel the myth that the topic of personal financial management is complicated and beyond the understanding of the average pharmacy student/graduate.

Pharmacists are privileged to be members of a highly regarded profession that can have a meaningful impact in people's lives. With a typical starting income of $80,000 or more, one would tend to put pharmacists at the top end of the income spectrum in Canada. Given that the median household income in 2011 was $74,540, according to Statistics Canada, pharmacists are certainly doing better than the average Canadian in terms of income.[1]

The offsetting reality, however, is that most pharmacists will not see significant annual increases in compensation over the course of their career—to the extent that steady climbs in the costs of living can become a challenge over time. In addition, unless pharmacists work for public employers such as hospitals, governments or universities, their odds of having a pension plan are slim. The onus is on most pharmacists to provide for themselves and their families in retirement.

A working knowledge of the fundamentals of personal financial management is, therefore, vital for today's pharmacist. Having one's personal finances in order enables the following:

- career flexibility and the opportunity to pursue a dream job or independent business, rather than having to work at a job that pays the bills but is not fulfilling
- the achievement of short- and long-term financial goals
- retirement with a lifestyle comparable to the lifestyle before retirement
- financial support for aging parents and/or a family
- healthier relationships (Family and marital conflicts often arise from poor decisions about personal finance and the management of family assets.)

INCOME VERSUS COST OF LIVING

Regardless of when they graduated, all pharmacists face similar financial challenges when it comes to having an income that does not keep pace with the cost of living. Consider the case of a pharmacist who graduated 15 years ago and started with a salary of $90 000 (higher than today's average starting salary because, at the time, pharmacists were in short supply). What would that annual salary need to look like today to have kept up with an average, reasonable inflation rate of 3% per year?

The answer is $140,000, or nearly $72.00 per hour. Yet how many pharmacists working in community or hospital practice earn $72.00 per hour? Five years from now, the wage would have to increase to $83.50 per hour to match inflation. That is clearly not realistic for most pharmacists.

The bottom line: pharmacists can enjoy a very comfortable middle-class lifestyle, but by no means will most have the earning potential to live a lifestyle where they can be ignorant of how to manage their financial affairs. The key steps to pharmacists being smart with money are to make the right decisions and avoid common mistakes (especially early in their career) that can set them back years in terms of achieving financial goals, or even prevent them from achieving their personal dreams.

WHY CANADIANS DO NOT MEET THEIR FINANCIAL GOALS

The following are primary reasons why Canadians do not meet their financial goals:
- procrastination: People procrastinate in setting financial goals, developing a plan, budgeting and saving. The longer they procrastinate, the less they benefit from the power of compound growth (see Table 1)—and they stand to miss out on tens if not hundreds of thousands of dollars in potential investment earnings.
- unrealistic expectations: Nothing is wrong with having a second home on the lake, travelling the world or putting three kids through university. What is not so good, and what can be very demoralizing financially, is setting unrealistic expectations based on the current financial position, risk tolerance and future earnings prospects.
- ignorance of the resources required: Most pharmacy students are used to making very little money and living with debt. Earning a salary that exceeds the median Canadian household income seems like a guaranteed way to financial success after years of scrimping, but ignorance of the fundamentals of financial planning—such as the types of savings required, expected returns and how to minimize taxes—can put such success forever beyond reach.

Last but not least, people often struggle to meet their financial goals because they believe financial planning is beyond their capability and understanding. Yet the fundamental concepts of personal finance are not particularly challenging. In fact, any pharmacy graduate who has learned organic chemistry, pharmacology, physiology and therapeutics has grasped far more complicated and challenging concepts.

TIME VALUE OF MONEY AND INFLATION

The most fundamental concept in personal financial management is the time value of money (TVM), which essentially means knowing the value of a sum of money at different points in time. This enables the comparison of the value of a sum of money today with its value in the future, or conversely, the determination of what an amount of money in the future is really worth today.

TVM states that a dollar today is worth more than a dollar tomorrow because purchasing power diminishes over time due to inflation. Inflation is defined as an increase in the prices of goods and services in an economy over time. Fifty years ago, for example, a cup of Tim Horton's coffee sold for 10 cents. In a developed economy, inflation is a fact of life, and ignoring its impact is an enormous oversight when it comes to personal financial management. Particularly when the costs of living increase at a faster rate than earnings—as is the case for most pharmacists—how does one stay ahead?

TVM is expressed as an equation comprised of present value (PV), future value (FV) and the rate of return (or the discount rate) of (k) over a period of years (t) where:

$$PV = FV/(1 + k)^t$$

An investor uses TVM to assess investment opportunities and compare the value of different amounts at different periods. For example:

Bridget is looking at a real estate investment. She feels an investment of $400,000 that she and a couple of business partners are looking to make will be worth $700,000 in six years. What rate of return would that provide?

If one solves for k in the equation, where PV = $400,000, FV = $700,000 and t = 6, Bridget would earn a 9.75% return compounded annually. In other words, $700,000 in six years is the same as earning a 9.75% return on an investment of $400,000 over a six-year period.

With this information, Bridget would then have to answer the following questions:

- Is an average annual return of 9.75% acceptable for the risk of the investment? Is she happy with that?
- How confident is she of that return?
- Are there other investments with less risk that could earn a similar return?

Here is another example, related to inflation. Logan works hard to save money but is afraid of losing it in the stock market or with risky investments. As a result, Logan keeps his money in a savings account that pays virtually no interest. If Logan has $10,000 in savings that he does not invest and inflation averages 3% per year, what will his $10,000 be worth in 15 years?

If one solves for FV, where PV = $10,000, k = −0.03 (i.e., −3% because inflation eats away at money) and t = 15, Logan's savings would be worth $6,333 in 15 years. In other words, the purchasing power of $10,000 in today's money, earning no interest, would be only $6,333 in 15 years.

It is safe to assume that inflation averages around 3% per year. Therefore, any returns less than 3% per year means money is being lost, and hard-earned savings will have less purchasing power. People often overlook this critical fact, however, because no one can see inflation—it is intangible. When Logan checks his bank account balance in 15 years, for example, it will still contain $10,000.

In another example, if a pharmacist in Ontario earns $85,000 per year, the take-home income after taxes would be $5,145 per month in 2014.[2] The pharmacist's monthly expenses include rent ($1,200), student debt payment ($800), car loan payment ($350) and phone/Internet/cable

($150). That equals $2,500 in monthly expenses plus food, clothing, auto expenses, utilities, personal care, entertainment, travel, gifts, gym membership, charitable donations, furniture, etc. Through careful planning and budgeting, let's assume total costs of $4,300, which leaves $845 per month to save and invest.

What happens if the pharmacist's salary is frozen for the next three years (as is the case for many pharmacists in today's market), yet expenses escalate with inflation? Monthly costs would grow from $4,300 to $4,700 after three years. Potential monthly savings will decline from $845 to $445 in three years. Thanks to inflation, the pharmacist is effectively taking home nearly $5,000 less per year after three years.

Inflation is the single greatest threat to pharmacists who do not have a properly constructed financial plan and do not take the time to update and track their financial progress.

THE POWER OF COMPOUND GROWTH

Inflation can be a depressing topic. There is good news: the weapon to fight inflation, and the tool that will allow pharmacists to realize their financial dreams, is the power of compound growth (see Table 1).

Compounding growth means that savings/investments and the returns earned on those savings compound progressively year after year. For example, if an investment of $100 earns an average return of 7%, it is worth $107 at the end of year one. In year two, that $107 would grow by 7% to $114.49. The gains may not seem like much at first, but over time they become significant. The power of compounding is subtle but very substantial.

Table 1 speaks for itself:

- If a 25-year-old pharmacist invested $5,500 every year in a Tax-Free Savings Account (TFSA), with an average return of 7% every year, by age 65 the account would contain almost $1.1 million. Think about that for a moment: a total of $220,000 invested over 40 years (or $15 per day) would result in an investment portfolio of more than $1 million.

- If a pharmacist waited until age 35 to start investing $5,500 per year, that portfolio would be $519,534 at age 65. In other words, the pharmacist would have left nearly $600,000 on the table from procrastinating for 10 years before starting to invest. Sure, this pharmacist ended up investing $55,000 less than the eager classmate, but that $55,000 of investment between the ages 25 and 35 translated into nearly $600,000 more in a tax-free account at retirement.

- Now consider the situation in which another pharmacist starts saving diligently at age 25, again investing $5,500 per year to age 65. If the investment earned 9% on average due to shrewd investing and discipline, the portfolio would be worth $1.86 million at age 65. Conversely, if the pharmacist was very conservative and put his money in low-risk investments that earned only 3%, the portfolio would not even be worth $415,000 by age 65.

The secret to beating inflation is starting the power of compound growth early and learning enough as an investor to earn solid returns on a portfolio—or finding the right financial advisor who can do it on behalf of their clients.

Table 1. The Power of Compound Growth

Annual Investment in TFSA	Average Annual Return	Age When Saving Begins	Value at Age 35	Value at Age 55	Value at Age 65	Value at Age 66
$5,500	7%	25	$75,990	$519,534	$1,098,000	$1,180,350
$5,500	7%	35	-	$225,475	$519,534	$561,400
$7,500	7%	25	$103,623	$708,456	$1,497,265	$1,609,570
$7,500	7%	35	-	$307,466	$708,456	$765,550
$5,500	9%	25	$83,561	$749,692	$1,858,350	$2,031,105
$5,500	3%	25	$63,051	$261,665	$414,707	$432,650

THE BIG THREE PERSONAL FINANCIAL CONSIDERATIONS: CASH, DEBT AND RISK MANAGEMENT

Personal finance is straightforward but, like losing weight, it is easier said than done. To help develop the right financial habits, focus on just three main areas: cash management, debt management and risk management.

CASH MANAGEMENT

Cash management is just a fancy term for budgeting. Pharmacists must ensure what they spend does not exceed what they take home after taxes. It may seem basic, but many people come to live well beyond their means with relative ease. Cash management becomes even more challenging when incomes do not grow as fast as inflation.

Many expenditures eat into every paycheque and can leave little (or nothing) behind for savings and investment, especially as inflation drives higher prices for food, gas and other costs of living (including discretionary items such as clothing, entertainment and travel). Yet many working-age Canadians are completely unaware of two key pieces of information:

- where they spend their money
- how their expenses are tracking year-over-year compared to their earnings

Without a proper financial plan that sets limits for monthly and annual spending, and incorporates a plan for investing any savings in the most tax-efficient and effective way possible, it is very easy to lose control of something as basic as cash management.

DEBT MANAGEMENT

Debt is a fact of life for most Canadians, and by no means is all debt bad. A student loan is good debt if it leads to a sustainable and fulfilling career. A mortgage is debt, but since most people cannot pay for a home in cash, a mortgage is a necessity to eventually become a homeowner.

Some experienced investors will take out investment loans to help bulk up investment portfolios if they are confident the returns will far exceed what they will pay in interest. This can be a good form of debt. Debt incurred to invest in a business, such as a pharmacy, is also generally good debt.

However, for every piece of good debt, there are many examples of bad debt:

- Any balance outstanding on a credit card is bad debt and an immediate signal that people may be living beyond their means.

- A mortgage payment that consumes the bulk of disposal income is not good debt—the household is living beyond its means. Most banks and financial advisors suggest that home-related expenses should not exceed 30% to 35% of gross monthly income.
- An investment loan taken out on poorly researched speculative investments (or without proper diversification) that lose money is clearly bad debt.
- A car payment that is difficult to pay is bad debt.
- A line of credit for discretionary lifestyle expenses (e.g., vacations) is clearly bad debt.

DEBT CONSIDERATIONS FOR PHARMACY STUDENTS

Paying back student loans

Pharmacy students can incur remarkable levels of debt through student loans. It is not unusual to graduate with debts of $80,000 to $90,000 or, when two or more degrees are earned, debts of more than $100,000. That is a big financial weight to carry at the start of a career.

Here are a few tips to speed repayment of Canada Student Loans:

- The government gives a six-month grace period before repayment must begin. Pharmacists should *not* take advantage of it because the interest compounds during that time.
- The default repayment period is 10 years, which can be shortened to reduce the total amount of interest paid.
- Make lump sum payments against the outstanding principal whenever possible.
- Debtors can choose between a floating interest rate of prime plus 2.5% or a fixed interest rate of prime plus 5%. In today's economic climate (at time of writing), most choose the floating rate. Even better, if feasible, consolidate a student loan debt into a line of credit that has an interest rate of less than prime plus 2.5%.
- Debtors can receive a 15% federal tax credit for interest paid on qualifying student loans and, possibly, an additional provincial/territorial tax credit, depending on the province/territory.

Paying back student debt versus investing

The first major financial dilemma for most graduates is how to save money with tens of thousands of dollars of student debt hanging over their heads. Many decide to put debt repayment ahead of investing. But if they wait 10 years to start investing, they lose a decade's worth of compound growth, which could mean hundreds of thousands of dollars in lost returns. At the very least, inflation will eat away at the purchasing power of annual income.

Debt is a fact of life for many Canadians, which means that paying off debt cannot come at the expense of future financial security. Pharmacists need to consider the big picture, with a financial plan that encompasses both short- and long-term financial goals.

Every year, pharmacists must consider their budgets, obligations and financial plans to determine how best to allocate resources toward investment and debt repayment. There is no one right answer because circumstances change, but one must avoid the trap of tunnel vision that focuses on paying off debt only.

Mortgages: A brief overview

Buying a house is a major step for any young professional. Mortgage lenders, mortgage brokers, real estate brokers and others associated with real estate continue to perpetuate the belief that home ownership is a rite of passage into adulthood. Before taking this big step and assuming a mortgage, consider the following:

> A $400,000 mortgage with an initial interest rate of 4% and repayment period of 25 years will result in weekly mortgage payments of $485, or $25,200 per year in after-tax income. After five years, one will have paid $126,000—of which $75,000 is for interest—which goes directly to the bank.

If it takes 25 years to pay off a $400,000 mortgage with an average interest rate of 5%, the bank receives a total of $293,500 in interest, which is nearly 75% of the value of the original mortgage. While those who work in the banking and real estate industries will run the numbers and make it seem easy to "afford" a home, one needs to carefully consider the long-term impact on financial health.

RISK MANAGEMENT

Risk management is an area that is not well understood and often overlooked. The flood of new insurance products in recent years raises questions about being over-insured. People tend to insure their cars and houses. Pharmacists have professional insurance. How much additional insurance is really necessary?

Long-term disability insurance

Personal long-term disability (LTD) insurance is a must. Pharmacists' biggest financial asset is their ability to earn an income, yet over the course of a career, a person stands about a 50% chance of being disabled and off work for 90 days or more. If this occurs, LTD insurance provides tax-free monthly payments to replace lost income.

Some pharmacists incorrectly assume that they do not need to purchase their own LTD insurance if they already have one through their employer's benefit plan. However, company policies may have significant limitations on coverage, and they are available to current employees only. It is essential to purchase a personal policy that travels from job to job, and/or from career to career.

It is important to purchase an individual policy early in one's career, when health is likely at its peak and premiums will be lower. Otherwise, certain pre-existing medical conditions will increase the cost of premiums and may even disqualify a person from coverage.

When shopping for an LTD plan, look for the following features:

- A minimum monthly payment equal to two-thirds of salary before tax. For example, a person with an annual income of $100,000 should purchase a policy that pays $67,000 tax free each year, or about $5,583 per month.
- The option to purchase additional coverage as income increases, without the need for a medical. This is sometimes referred to as a "future earnings protector option."
- A cost of living allowance (COLA) that increases coverage annually to keep up with inflation.
- An "own-occupation" clause that prevents the insurance company from cutting off coverage after deeming that a beneficiary is competent for other employment.
- A "washout period" of 90 days, which means that coverage begins 90 days after the incident that caused the disability. Premiums are substantially higher for policies that start coverage before 90 days.

Life insurance

Pharmacists who have dependents and/or a family need to consider life insurance. The level of insurance is determined in one of two ways:

- income approach: Determine the amount of lost future income (e.g., $4 million over the next 30 years) and purchase a policy to replace 75% (or $3 million) of that amount (keeping in mind 100% is not necessary because there is one less person to cover).
- expense approach: Calculate the expenses that need to be paid on behalf of dependents (e.g., mortgage, other debts, funeral expenses) and purchase a policy for that amount.

Pharmacists can choose from two major types of life insurance:

- Term life policies have a fixed annual premium for a specific period (e.g., 10 or 20 years). After the term is up (or during the term of an existing policy), one can apply to purchase additional insurance. Alternatively, the insurance policy does not need to be renewed if life insurance is no longer needed. The advantage of term life is the flexibility it provides; the major disadvantage is higher premiums over time.
- Whole life plans are life insurance contracts that feature fixed premiums over time. Whole life policies contain both a savings and an investment component. If they are purchased earlier in life by adolescents or young adults, they can have lower annual premiums than term policies over time. As a result, whole life policies are generally best suited for younger buyers. The disadvantage of whole life plans is that they lack the flexibility of term life policies if insurance needs change.

Life insurance premiums depend primarily on age, gender, smoking status, health status and family health history. Medicals are required to determine eligibility and, in some cases, pre-existing medical conditions can be exclusions within a policy (i.e., coverage is not provided if the cause of death is related to a pre-existing medical condition).

TAX-SHELTERED SAVINGS VEHICLES IN CANADA

Canadians can use two tax-sheltered savings vehicles to prepare for retirement: Registered Retirement Savings Plans (RRSPs) and Tax-Free Savings Accounts (TFSAs). Other vehicles, such as Registered Education Savings Plans (RESPs) and non-registered investment accounts also exist, but given the popularity and relevance of RRSPs and TFSAs for all pharmacists, this section will focus on these two offerings.

RRSPS

An RRSP is a registered account for savings that can be invested in eligible investment options such as stocks, bonds, mutual funds, real estate income trusts and more. Each year, a person can contribute up to 18% of income from the previous year, up to a maximum amount determined by the federal government. If one does not contribute the full allowable amount, the difference is carried forward to future years' contributions.

The biggest benefit of RRSPs is the government gives a tax refund based on the amount of the contribution and a person's marginal tax rate (for more on taxes, see the next section). For someone living in Ontario who made $100,000 and contributed $10,000 to an RRSP, for example, the tax refund would be $4,340 (based on tax rates at the time of publication).

RRSPs also grow tax free until withdrawals begin. This allows compounded returns without the worry about taxes—hence the power of compound growth is accelerated in tax-sheltered vehicles such as RRSPs.

However, RRSPs come with potential downsides that underscore the need for continuous financial planning throughout a career:

- A person must start withdrawing a minimum percentage of RRSP savings by age 72, and every year thereafter, whether or not the money is needed.
- All RRSP withdrawals are taxed at a person's highest marginal tax rate, raising the risk of having an RRSP that is too big because of the taxes that eventually would be paid.
- RRSPs have no provisions for capital losses. If money is lost on investments in an RRSP, one cannot claim these losses against other capital gains or receive any tax relief.
- An RRSP is a government-controlled tool, which means government can change the rules at any time.

TFSAS

TFSAs were introduced in 2009 and, like RRSPs, enable Canadians to invest their savings in investments that can grow tax free. Unlike RRSPs, TFSAs do not require the payment of taxes upon withdrawals. On the other hand, TFSAs do not generate tax refunds when contributions are made.

In 2013, the government increased the maximum annual contribution to TFSAs to $5,500 from $5,000. Like RRSPs, if people do not contribute the maximum amount in a given year, they can carry forward the difference to future years. If withdrawals are made, those amounts are also added to amounts carried forward for future contributions.

TFSA OR RRSP: WHICH IS BETTER?

The decision to invest in a TFSA or an RRSP depends on several personal factors, guided by the following golden rule: if a person's marginal tax rate is lower today than it will be down the road when he or she cashes in his or her investments (as is the case with most new graduates), then it often makes more sense to invest in a TFSA first and save the RRSP contributions for later. Conversely, if the tax rate is higher today than it will be down the road, it may make more sense to invest initially in an RRSP.

FORMS OF INCOME AND TAXES—CONSIDERATIONS FOR PHARMACISTS

Tax planning and tax reduction are useful practices to help improve personal finances. To do so, it is important to have a basic understanding of income taxes.

There are three major types of income, and all are taxed differently in Canada:

- salary income and interest income
- dividend income
- capital gains income

SALARY INCOME

Canada uses a marginal system of tax, which simply means that the more someone makes, the higher the tax rate. However, this does not mean that all income is taxed at the marginal tax rate. It means that the next dollar of income is taxed at that rate.

Using Ontario as an example, Table 2 illustrates the various tax rates in the province in 2015. Based on an income of $100,000, the marginal tax rate (i.e., the amount of tax paid on the next dollar of salary earned) would be 43.4%. However, that rate applies only on the amount between $87,907 and $100,000. As for all Ontarians, the tax rate is 20% on the first $40,120 of salary earned, over and above the tax-free basic personal amount of $9,670. Therefore, someone earning an income of $100,000 in Ontario, without any tax deductions for RRSP contributions or any other tax credits, would pay $29,596 for federal and provincial taxes, the Canada Pension Plan (CPP) and Employment Insurance (EI). This translates into an average tax rate of 29.6% on every dollar earned, and a marginal tax rate of 43.4%.

DIVIDEND INCOME

Dividends are payments received from the profits of a company (public or private) in which people have invested and that distributes some (or all) of its profits to shareholders. Tax rates on dividends are lower than for salaries or interest income because dividends are paid with after-tax corporate profits. To avoid double taxation, the tax rates on dividends are much lower (see Table 3). (Eligible and non-eligible refer to whether or not a dividend qualifies for the enhanced dividend tax credit.[3])

CAPITAL GAINS

Capital gains represent the profit made after buying an asset at X dollars and selling it at a higher price of Y dollars. The difference between Y and X is the capital gain. Tax rates on capital gains are lower than for other forms of income to encourage investment in the economy and the buying and selling of assets (see Table 4).

Table 2. 2015 Combined Federal and Ontario Tax Rates[2]

Taxable Income*	Marginal Tax Rates
First $40,922	20.05%
Over $40,922 up to $44,701	24.15%
Over $44,701 up to $72,064	31.15%
Over $72,064 up to $81,847	32.98%
Over $81,847 up to $84,902	35.39%
Over $84,902 up to $89,401	39.41%
Over $89,401 up to $138,586	43.41%
Over $138,586 up to $150,000	46.41%
Over $150,000 up to $220,000	47.97%
Over $220,000	49.53%

*This income does not include dividends or capital gains.

Table 3. 2015 Combined Federal and Ontario Tax Rates for Dividends[2]

Taxable Income*	Eligible Dividends	Non-Eligible Dividends
First $40,922	−6.86%	5.35%
Over $40,922 up to $44,701	−1.20%	10.19%
Over $44,701 up to $72,064	8.46%	18.45%
Over $72,064 up to $81,847	10.99%	20.61%
Over $81,847 up to $84,902	14.31%	23.45%
Over $84,902 up to $89,401	19.86%	28.19%
Over $89,401 up to $138,586	25.38%	32.91%
Over $138,586 up to $150,000	29.52%	36.45%
Over $150,000 up to $220,000	31.67%	38.29%
Over $220,000	33.82%	40.13%

*This income does not include dividends or capital gains.

Table 4. 2015 Combined Federal and Ontario Tax Rates for Capital Gains[2]

Taxable Income*	Capital Gains
First $40,922	10.03%
Over $40,922 up to $44,701	12.08%
Over $44,701 up to $72,064	15.58%
Over $72,064 up to $81,847	16.49%
Over $81,847 up to $84,902	17.70%
Over $84,902 up to $89,401	19.70%
Over $89,401 up to $138,586	21.70%
Over $138,586 up to $150,000	23.20%
Over $150,000 up to $220,000	23.98%
Over $220,000	24.76%

*This income does not include dividends or capital gains.

Here is a summary of the differences in taxes paid based on forms of income (using 2015 tax rates in Ontario for the following examples[2]):

- A salary of $100,000 would pay $29,596 for taxes, CPP and EI.
- Dividend income of $100,000 after taxes, with no other sources of income, would pay $16,700 in total taxes. That is nearly $12,000 less than taxes paid on a salary.
- A $100,000 capital gain from an investment that is outside of an RRSP or TFSA, and barring other sources of income, would pay only $9,294 in total taxes. That is $20,000 less in taxes than earning income as salary.

FINANCIAL ADVISORS

While most pharmacists hire a financial planner to manage their financial affairs since they feel they do not have the time, competence and/or inclination to do so themselves, it is vital that pharmacists understand the basics of personal finance so they can be sure their financial advisor has their best interests at heart and is providing good information that ultimately delivers optimal returns on investments—and not just commissions in the advisor's pocket.

Finding a trustworthy financial advisor is one of the most important financial decisions a pharmacist will ever make. Several types of advisors are available:

- fee for service: independent advisors who have the freedom and flexibility to invest money where they feel it is a best fit for their clients' goals and risk tolerance. They are paid fees for services much like an accountant or a lawyer.
- salaried advisors: advisors who typically work for a bank, which usually requires them to sell their own company's products or portfolio of products. While clients may not pay them directly, they will likely pay fees related to the investments purchased on their behalf.
- commission-based advisors: mutual-fund and insurance salespeople who sell a wide range of financial and insurance products. However, they may steer clients toward products with the highest commissions because that is how they are paid—whether or not these investments are in clients' best interests.

Pharmacists must take the time to interview and get to know prospective financial advisors. The best financial advisors will listen to and understand their clients' goals, build a suitable financial plan that can evolve over time and disclose all fees and commissions along the way so there are no surprises.

COMPONENTS OF A FINANCIAL PLAN

The only path to success in personal finance is to have a plan, one that can easily be modified over time. The key components of a financial plan include the following:

- personal and financial goals, both short and long term
- career aspirations and other personal needs and priorities
- analysis of current financial position (cash flows, personal balance sheet, etc.)
- consideration of risk tolerance and an analysis of the investment returns required to achieve goals (For example, if 12% annual returns are needed but the person is conservative in nature, then goals and/or risk tolerance need to be revisited.)
- cash flow projections from year to year to understand how life events (birth of a child, change in career, purchase of a house, etc.) will affect finances
- retirement plans and aspirations

RESOURCES AND SUGGESTED READINGS

Canadian Moneysaver independent personal finance magazine: www.canadianmoneysaver.ca

Financial calculator for PV, FV calculations: Texas Instruments BA II Plus Calculator App at the Apple App Store or on Android platform.

Ho K, Robinson C. *Personal financial management basics: personal financial planning*. 5th ed. Concord, ON: Captus Press; 2012.

Income tax calculator. www.taxtips.ca/calculators/taxcalculator.htm

Mortgage payment calculator. www.rbcroyalbank.com under Personal Banking, Mortgages.

Student loan repayment calculator. tools.canlearn.ca under Loan Repayment Estimator.

REFERENCES

1. Statistics Canada. Median total income by family type, by province and territory. Available: www.statcan.gc.ca/tables-tableaux/ sum-som/l01/cst01/famil108a-eng.htm (accessed Nov. 13, 2014).

2. TaxTips.ca. Detailed Canadian income tax and RRSP savings calculators for 2015, 2014 and earlier years. Available: www. taxtips.ca/calculator/cdncalculator.htm (accessed Nov. 30, 2014).

3. GE Solutions. Eligible vs ineligible dividends. Available: www.ge-solutions.ca/what-are-eligible-and-ineligible-dividends.html (accessed Dec. 1, 2014).

TEVA

Learn how to interpret your financials — and improve your profitability

Sample pharmacy balance sheet and income statement

BALANCE SHEET		($, 000)	
		2015	2016
ASSETS			
Current			
Cash	$	150	$ 100
Accounts receivable		600	550
Inventory			
Rx		400	375
FS		300	375
Prepaid expenses		10	10
Total current assets		1,460	1,410
Capital assets (equipment)		120	140
Total assets		**$ 1,580**	**$ 1,550**
LIABILITIES & SHAREHOLDERS' EQUITY			
Current liabilities			
Accounts payable & accruals	$	800	$ 850
Income taxes payable		50	30
Current portion of loans payable		20	20
Total current liabilities		870	900
Long-term debt			
Loans payable		25	40
Due to shareholder		200	200
Total long-term debt		225	240
Total liabilities		1,095	1,140
Shareholders' equity			
Share capital		1	1
Retained earnings		484	409
Total shareholders' equity		485	410
Total liabilities & shareholders' equity		**$ 1,580**	**$ 1,550**

INCOME STATEMENT	($, 000)	
	2015	2016
Sales		
Rx	$ 7,600	$ 7,400
FS	700	600
Total sales	8,300	8,000
Cost of goods sold		
Rx	5,800	5,700
FS	500	400
Total cost of goods sold	6,300	6,100
Gross profit		
Rx	1,800	1,700
FS	200	200
Total gross profit	**$ 2,000**	**$ 1,900**
Expenses		
Wages	$ 1,200	$ 1,100
Occupancy	50	50
General & administrative		
Advertising & promotion	150	175
Delivery	70	65
Store supplies	50	48
Bad debts	40	45
Credit card charges	25	23
Computer	20	25
Other general & administrative	120	119
Total expenses	1,725	1,650
Net income before income taxes	**$ 275**	**$ 250**

OTHER	(000)	
	2015	2016
Number of prescriptions	110	107

CHAPTER 14

Financial Statements and Forms of Business Ownership

Rubin Cohen, *CA, CPA*

Please see the example financial statements included at the beginning of this section. *They have been adapted with permission from the course, "Learn how to interpret your financials and improve profitability," sponsored by Teva Canada Limited.*

Most will agree that the language of business is accounting. The story of any pharmacy business, regardless of size, the market and patients it serves or the community it operates within, is told through its financial records. Income, debt, revenue versus expenses, compensation and cost of retaining customers can all be found in financial statements.

This chapter introduces readers to financial literacy so they can begin to engage in numbers-based discussions by being aware of the best questions to ask of the most appropriate people.

Learning Objectives

- Identify the primary users of financial statements.
- Understand the purpose of financial statements.
- Specify what "prepared in accordance with generally accepted accounting principles" refers to, with respect to objectivity, conservatism, consistency, matching, materiality and going concern.
- Compare and contrast the concept of cash versus accrual basis of accounting.
- Distinguish between three different types of accountants' letters: auditor's report, review engagement report, notice to reader.
- Define three forms of ownership: sole proprietorship, partnership, incorporation.

WHAT ARE FINANCIAL STATEMENTS?

When operating a pharmacy, there will come a point where you will need to determine how the business is doing financially. Is it generating a profit or a loss? Is payroll expense too high? Are there improvements that can be made operationally that can lead to improved profitability?

Financial statements are prepared to answer these types of questions. These documents are typically prepared by an accountant and quantitatively describe the financial well-being of a company. By summarizing all the transactions that took place during a specific period, the accountant can provide the reader of the financial statements with a financial report card that assesses the financial health of a company.

The following are examples of those most interested in financial statements and what information they would expect to extract from these documents:

Managers will review the financial statements to assess whether sales projected at the beginning of a fiscal period match actual sales, if there are any expenses that are unexpectedly high or whether the store is carrying too much inventory.

Shareholders and potential investors will assess whether the business is running profitably and whether they should maintain their investment in the company. A shareholder (or someone contemplating becoming a shareholder) will review the financial statements looking to assess the company's earnings potential, internal efficiencies and management effectiveness, market share in the industry and profitability.

Lenders who have advanced money to a business will review the financial statements to determine if their loan is secure. If the financial statements reflect a large operating loss and dwindling cash reserves, then the lenders aim to minimize their exposure to non-payment by requiring an immediate loan repayment.

Canada Revenue Agency will use the financial statements to determine how much income tax will be owing to government.

HOW ARE FINANCIAL STATEMENTS PREPARED?

Financial statements are generally prepared by accountants who adhere to a series of principles called generally accepted accounting principles (GAAP). These principles help to ensure that financial statements, regardless of the preparer, are organized in a way that is universally understood.

GAAP include the following:

- objectivity: Transactions should be recorded on the basis of objective evidence. For example, if the financial statements indicate the business has purchased a car for $40,000, they must be supported by an invoice from the car dealer in that same amount.
- conservatism: In addition to reflecting transactions objectively, the accountant must reflect them in a conservative manner. To illustrate, a pharmacist purchases a large supply of a particular drug in April, but the value of the drug is now significantly higher in the open market due to a production shortage. While the pharmacist may want to reflect the increased value of the drug in the pharmacy's financial statements, the accountant— following the principle of conservatism—will state the inventory at its original cost, given that there is no guarantee the current market price will be in effect when that drug is ultimately sold.
- consistency: Businesses should use the same accounting methods and procedures from one time period to another because financial statements typically include comparative

data. For example, a statement will have one column for the current year and another for the year prior. To ensure the reader is comparing "apples to apples," the accountant must use the same procedures of tabulation for both years.

- matching: It is critical that expenses be recorded in the same fiscal period as the revenues they triggered. For example, a pharmacy that has a December 31 fiscal year-end places an order to a supplier and receives the goods on December 27, 2013. However, because most of the accounting staff on the supplier's end are on Christmas break, the invoice for the goods arrives to the pharmacy on January 8, 2014. Were the accountant to prepare the financial statements strictly based on the underlying date of the transaction, the 2013 statements would look unrealistically good because they would include the goods but not the corresponding costs associated with the purchase.

- materiality: In preparing the financial statement, the accountant must pre-assess the dollar amount of a transaction that should be reported in the statement. Disclosing each and every transaction would make the financial statements too lengthy, so the accountant has to determine what transactions are material or significant enough to warrant separate disclosure.

- going concern: A critical assumption used by an accountant in preparing financial statements is that the business will continue to operate into the future, thereby reflecting assets at their original cost. This is in contrast to the preparation of financial statements of a business that is seriously struggling and likely to shut down operations. In the latter case, the accountant has to reflect the assets at liquidation.

CASH VERSUS ACCRUAL BASIS OF ACCOUNTING

Earlier in this chapter, the importance of matching revenues and expenses was discussed. Before GAAP was established, many financial statements were prepared on what is referred to as the cash basis of accounting. This means only transactions involving either cash going in or out of the bank account in that fiscal period (i.e., payments received from customers or supplier invoices paid) were reflected in that year's financial statement. As a result, financial statements prepared in this way often contained inaccuracies. Imagine that a business needs to show its financial statements to the bank to qualify for a loan. Knowing that the bank will lend money only if the business shows a healthy profit, the business purposely does not pay its supplier invoices before the end of the year. Therefore, the financial statements look healthy because all revenues have been incorporated into the statements whereas the expenses have not. For this reason, a statement prepared using the cash basis of accounting is deemed non-compliant with GAAP.

Alternatively, the accrual basis of accounting is in compliance with GAAP where transactions are recorded regardless of whether cash is received or paid. Sales are recorded when customers pick up their prescription regardless of whether or not they pay for it. An expense is recorded when the service is rendered by the supplier regardless of whether or not it is paid for by the business in that period. Effectively, the key point for the accrual basis of accounting is the time in which the transaction took place, as opposed to when the payment is made or received.

In Canada, as of the last few years, financial statements are now prepared by accountants who are guided by accounting principles based on International Financial Reporting Standards

(IFRS) and Accounting Standards for Private Enterprises (ASPE).

ACCOUNTANTS' LETTERS

When looking at financial statements in which an accountant was involved, a letter from that accountant often appears, attesting to the nature of his or her role in the preparation of the documents. There are three types of accountants' letters.

AUDITOR'S REPORT

A certified public accountant performs, by way of various methods of investigation and corroboration, a detailed examination and verification of a company's books and records to determine the accuracy of the financial statements. Generally, when financial statements are audited, it should provide the reader with the highest degree of assurance as to the accountants' verification of the contents. Most public corporations and charitable organizations have their financial statements audited to satisfy the readers of the financial statements, who generally require that an independent, objective accountant provide them with the assurance of accuracy.

A company's directors will determine whether IFRS or ASPE is more appropriate. Given the complexity in the preparation of financial statements under IFRS (used mainly for public companies), most pharmacy financial statements will be prepared under ASPE. Therefore, regardless of where you are in Canada, the presentation of the financial statements should be comparable. Note: These reporting standards apply to audits and reviews but not to compilations (notice to reader). Although the balance sheet and income statement will appear the same in a compilation vis-à-vis audit and review, the compilation does not have a statement of cash flows and, typically, has no notes to the financial statements. Furthermore, there are required procedures when an accountant performs an audit or review that are not required when preparing a compilation. The notice to reader signed by the accountant clearly states, "Readers are cautioned that these statements may not be appropriate for their purposes." The word *caution* does appear ominous. However, the reader should be comforted by the fact that accountants do use GAAP when preparing compilation financial statements and are forbidden to disclose information that is false and/or misleading.

REVIEW ENGAGEMENT REPORT

This report's first objective is to stress that the accountant has *not* performed an audit and that readers should not, therefore, rely on the figures as they would if the statements had been audited. It also explains why each page in a financial statement that includes the accountant's review engagement report is clearly marked "unaudited." In this report, the accountant confirms that the statements conform to GAAP and he or she has performed an "on-the-surface" verification of the plausibility of the figures.

NOTICE TO READER

When the financial statements include a Notice to Reader letter, the readers are alerted that the accountant has only compiled the financial statement and has not assessed GAAP compliance or verified the accuracy of the figures within the financial statement. Most smaller, private businesses prepare statements in this way.

The cost of retaining an accountant varies depending on the type of letter to be attached to a company's financial statement. An auditor's report is generally the most costly because it is the most labour intensive.

FORMS OF OWNERSHIP

There are options of setting up a pharmacy as a sole proprietorship, partnership or incorporated business. The key determinants in making that decision are exposure to liability and taxation (see Chapter 53: Business Planning to Business Plan for a comparison chart).

SOLE PROPRIETORSHIP

A sole proprietor owns 100% of the business and is personally responsible (liable) for its debts and obligations. It is the simplest form of operating a business; however, a major drawback is the inability for the owner to protect personal assets if anyone were to sue the business. To illustrate, Mr. Smith runs a construction business as a sole proprietor. He forgets to hammer a nail on the wall, which eventually collapses and extensive damage occurs. The homeowner successfully sues Mr. Smith's sole proprietorship business and the judge awards the homeowner a $2 million settlement. Unfortunately, because the business is a sole proprietorship, Mr. Smith will have to pay this settlement personally, which will probably require him to sell his home and other personal assets. Under current law, a sole proprietorship and the owner are the same legal entity.

Given that the sole proprietorship is indistinguishable from the owner, whatever the company earns in the year is deemed to be the income of the owner and, therefore, reported on the owner's personal income tax return. Since personal tax rates are generally higher than corporate tax rates, a high amount of income earned in a sole proprietorship will lead to a high personal tax bill as well.

PARTNERSHIP

A partnership only differs from a sole proprietorship in that there is more than one owner. The partners are also personally liable and report their share of the partnership income on their personal tax returns. Creditors will often insist that the partners be joint and severally liable as this allows creditors to collect all their debts from one partner as opposed to claiming from each based on their percentage ownership. The "easier" partner would then pay the creditor in full and have to sue the partner for their share of the liability. Simply put, this allows the creditor to do less work in collecting debts.

CORPORATION

Incorporating a business is more expensive to set up in that it requires registering the corporation with the government. (One can identify if a business is incorporated if "Limited," "Ltd.," "Incorporated" or "Inc.," is included at the end of the business name.) As a legal entity, a corporation is separate from its owner(s). As such, any debts and obligations become the responsibility of the corporation, and the owner's personal assets are not exposed to creditors as they would be under a sole proprietorship. (There are exceptions to this where a creditor, such as a bank or landlord, will insist that the shareholder[s] of the corporation personally guarantee the obligation as a means of ensuring that the commitment is paid.) A corporation issues shares and each owner's percentage of ownership is based on the number of shares owned over the total number of shares issued by the corporation.

From a taxation point of view, because the business is a separate legal entity, it must file a separate corporation income tax return. There are various tax advantages that can accrue under a corporate ownership structure because the tax liability on income earned by the corporation can be split between the corporation and its owners by way of salaries and dividends.

In conclusion, it is essential to understand that the primary purpose of a financial statement is for external reporting. It is prepared using a set of accounting rules that can be applied in different ways by different people.

CHAPTER 15

Statements Included Within Financial Statements

Michael S. Jaczko, *BSc. Phm., RPh, CIM® (Chartered Investment Manager); Partner and Portfolio Manager, K J Harrison & Partners Inc., Toronto, ON*

Please see the example financial statements included at the beginning of this section. *They have been adapted with permission from the course, "Learn how to interpret your financials and improve profitability," sponsored by Teva Canada Limited.*

Learning Objectives

- Describe, in general terms, how to interpret an income statement.
- Describe the importance of and difference between gross margin and gross profit.
- Describe the various elements of the balance sheet.
- Define and provide examples of assets and liabilities.
- Recall and use the equation Assets = Liabilities + Owner/Shareholder Equity.
- Recognize the importance of the statement of retained earnings and explain the role of retained earnings.
- Explain the purpose of dividends and their financial effects.
- Explain the concept of "goodwill" with regard to a pharmacy business.
- Discuss the value and importance of the cash flow statement.
- Discuss the importance of the notes to the financial statements.

KEY CONCEPTS

Financial statements provide quantitative information about the economic realities of a pharmacy business. In addition, financial statements communicate information that is useful to a variety of stakeholders: investors, creditors and pharmacy owners/operators. This information helps assess management's stewardship and the overall financial health of a pharmacy business.

The next two chapters look to accounting for answers to questions relevant to the above-mentioned stakeholders such as the following:

- What debts does the pharmacy owe to debt holders such as lenders, bankers? (Important to creditors and investors)
- Does the pharmacy have earnings? (Important to investors and owners)
- Are expenses too large in relation to sales? (Important to owners and managers)
- Are appropriate levels of inventory being kept on the shelves? (Important to owners and managers)
- Are amounts owed to the pharmacy by its customers being collected regularly and rapidly? (Important to investors and owners)
- Will the business be able to pay its debts as they mature and come due? (Important to investors/owners and lenders such as banks)

THE INCOME STATEMENT

Often called the profit and loss statement (P&L), the income statement describes the performance of a pharmacy business over a period of time.[1] The examples in this chapter use a one-year timeframe as illustrated in the sample pharmacy income statement provided at the beginning of this section.

The income statement measures the pharmacy's revenue and the expenses incurred to produce a profit or loss. It is summarized as follows:

$$Revenue - Expenses = Profit$$

The difference between revenues earned and the respective expenses incurred is called the profit (loss) or net income (see Chapter 16: Financial Ratios: Putting the Numbers to Work). The heading of an income statement indicates the name of the pharmacy business for which it is prepared and the time period covered by the statement.

Revenue is the dollar amount of products (including prescriptions) and professional services the pharmacy provided to its patients and customers during the year. The customer, patient or third-party payer pays cash or promises to pay in the future, in the latter case, for products and services; the amounts are recorded as accounts receivable. In this example, revenue is recorded as $8,000,000 and $8,300,000 for the financial years 2015 and 2016 respectively.

COST OF GOODS SOLD

Cost of goods sold (COGS) is the cost of purchasing the goods that are subsequently sold to customers and patients of the pharmacy. This amount is subtracted from revenue to determine the gross profit and gross margin. COGS is an expense to the business. In the example, cost of goods sold is recorded as $6,100,000 and $6,300,000 for the financial years 2015 and 2016, respectively.

GROSS PROFIT/MARGIN

Gross profit measures the profitability achieved as a result of selling products and professional services. Two terms that are often used interchangeably but have different meanings are *gross profit* and *gross margin*. Gross profit is expressed as a number (stores sales less cost of goods sold). Gross margin is expressed as a percentage (gross profit divided by sales x 100). Gross profit and gross margin calculations are ideally broken out by dispensary and front store (see Chapter 16: Financial Ratios: Putting the Numbers to Work). In the example, gross profit was recorded as $1,900,000 and $2,000,000 for the financial years 2015 and 2016, respectively.

EXPENSES

Expenses represent the dollar amount of resources the pharmacy business used or consumed, to earn revenues during a specific period (e.g., one year).[2] Expenses can be formatted and listed in several ways. The largest expenses after COGS are the salaries and wages paid to employees such as pharmacists, pharmacy technicians, front store personnel and clerical staff. In the example, wages were recorded as $1,100,000 and $1,200,000 for the financial years 2015 and 2016, respectively. Occupancy expenses represent the costs associated with having a store location. Items included in this expense item are rent, common area expenses, municipal taxes and building maintenance.

General and administrative expenses include several expense items such as advertising and promotion, delivery, store supplies, bad debts and expenses associated with technology (computer). The list of expense items included can vary from accountant to accountant. In the example, general and administrative expenses were recorded at $1,650,000 and $1,725,000 for the financial years 2015 and 2016, respectively.

> One line item worthy of note but not included in the example is interest expense; an expense reflects the cost of using borrowed funds to finance the operations of a pharmacy business and is not deemed part of an operational analysis.

ACCRUALS

Expenses may require the immediate payment of cash, a payment of cash at a future date or the use of some other resource such as an inventory item that may have been paid for in a previous period. For accounting purposes, the expense reported in one accounting period may actually be paid for in another accounting period. As mentioned in the previous chapter, under generally accepted accounting principles (GAAP), the pharmacy business recognizes all expenses (cash and credit) incurred during a specific accounting period regardless of the timing of the cash payment. Prepaid expenses (an asset) (e.g., registrations to conferences occurring in the next year) would be an example, and it appears as $10,000 on the balance sheet in years 2015 and 2016.

NET INCOME BEFORE INCOME TAXES

As a corporation, the pharmacy must pay income tax to the government. In the example, income tax expense is not identified but is always itemized as a general rule. Therefore, note that "Net income before income taxes" is an important line item typically listed in Canadian retail pharmacy income statements. It is the difference in dollars obtained by subtracting expenses from total gross profit; the amount does not reflect income tax expenses.

Net income or net earnings is the excess of total revenues over total expenses. If total expenses exceed total revenues, a net loss is reported on the income statement. By way of convention, net losses are normally identified by parentheses around the income figure. The term *break-even* is used when revenues and expenses are equal for the accounting period. Whether it is a net income, net loss or break-even, the number is also referred to as the bottom line.

THE BALANCE SHEET

The purpose of the balance sheet is to report the financial position (amount of assets, liabilities and shareholders' equity) of a pharmacy business at a particular point in time. The heading of the balance sheet identifies four significant items related to the statement:[3]

- name of the entity (e.g., Anytown Pharmacy Inc.)
- title of the statement – Balance Sheet
- specific date of the statement (e.g., at December 31, 2015. Note: a reminder that in contrast, the income statement measures activity over a period, usually one year)
- unit of measure – typically stated in thousands of dollars

The example balance sheet begins by listing the pharmacy business's assets. Assets are economic resources legally owned by the pharmacy business as a result of past transactions and from which future economic benefit can be obtained.

ASSETS – CURRENT ASSETS VERSUS LONG-TERM ASSETS VERSUS CAPITAL ASSETS

Assets in the sample balance sheet include cash (money in the pharmacy business bank account), accounts receivable (representing monies owed to the pharmacy business; e.g., by a government third-party payer), inventory and prepaid paid expenses. Because the pharmacy business expects to convert these assets into cash, sell or consume these assets in one year, they are categorized as current assets and are presented on the balance sheet in order of their ability to be converted to cash or their liquidity.[4]

Conversely, long-term assets are assets the pharmacy business will not convert into cash or use to pay a debt within one year; these assets are often referred to as non-current assets. Capital assets, such as store fixtures, land and a building, are the most common examples of capital assets found on a Canadian pharmacy business's balance sheet.[5] In the example, capital assets are recorded as $140,000 and $120,000 for the financial years 2015 and 2016, respectively.

Capital assets represent physical property and, with the exception of land, are depreciated on the pharmacy business's income statement. When tangible assets are purchased and recorded on the balance sheet as long-term or fixed assets, their value must be allocated over the course of their useful life expectancy in the form of a non-cash expense on the income statement called depreciation. For simplicity, our sample pharmacy does not reflect the concept of depreciation.[6]

GOODWILL

Many types of assets can be readily seen, understood and referred to as tangible assets. Examples of readily recognizable tangible assets would be cash, inventory and the building in which a pharmacy operates. Conversely, intangible assets have no physical substance but they have a long life. Intangible assets include items such as patents, trademarks, copyrights and goodwill. Their values arise from the legal rights and privileges of ownership.[7] Goodwill is a special type of intangible asset related to the purchase of a pharmacy business in the past.

Alternatively, in a "non-accounting" sense, goodwill is commonly inferred to mean a favourable reputation a pharmacy business has with its patients and customers. Goodwill comes from business factors such as customer shopping habits, patient confidence in staff pharmacist relationships, a positive reputation for excellent service and quality patient care. Reinforcement of these attributes daily over time invariably builds goodwill associated with a pharmacy business and results in increased sales and profits. This ultimately creates value when it comes time to sell the pharmacy business. As a result, goodwill is said to be internally created and is not reported as an asset on the balance sheet.[8]

Practically speaking, goodwill is the amount of money a pharmacy business can garner above and beyond the value of its tangible assets. It becomes a very important element when placing a value on a pharmacy business at the time of sale.

LIABILITIES

Assets are followed by liabilities and shareholders' equity on the balance sheet. Both are sources of financing and represent claims against the pharmacy business. Liabilities represent financing provided by creditors (through debt owed by the pharmacy), while financing provided by the owner is presented by owner's equity. Therefore, it logically follows that since each asset must have a source of financing, a pharmacy business's assets must equal the sum of its liabilities and shareholders' equity.

The basic accounting equation, referred to as the balance sheet equation, is expressed as follows:

Assets	=	Liabilities + Owner's Equity
Business resources:		Sources of financing for the pharmacy business:
e.g., cash, inventory, prepaid expenses and capital assets such as equipment		liabilities (debts incurred by creditors) and shareholders' equity (or owner's equity) is received from shareholders

Financial position is a term often illustrated by the basic accounting equation relating the economic resources the pharmacy business owns to the sources of financing received by the pharmacy business to purchase those resources in the first place.

LIABILITIES—CURRENT VERSUS LONG TERM

Similar to assets, pharmacy businesses classify liabilities as either current or long term. Current liabilities represent the obligations a pharmacy business reasonably expects to settle through the use of current assets such as cash. In the example, current liabilities are recorded as $900,000 and $870,000 for the financial years 2015 and 2016, respectively. Current liabilities include such items as accounts payable (who the pharmacy owes money to), income taxes payable and the portion of long-term debt such as a mortgage that is coming due within the following fiscal year. Note how these items are recorded in the sample balance sheet.

The excess of total current assets over total current liabilities is referred to as working capital (or net working capital) and represents the amount of a pharmacy business's assets that can be relatively quickly converted to cash (liquid resources). Think of this net amount as the liquidity buffer—the amount of cash available to meet the short-term financial demands of the pharmacy's business.[9] Bankers and other creditors calculate and consider this as an indicator of the short-term financial health of a pharmacy business (see Chapter 16: Financial Ratios: Putting the Numbers to Work for more on this important concept).

Long-term liabilities are obligations a pharmacy business expects to have to pay beyond the current fiscal year. Therefore, it does not reasonably expect to settle long-term liabilities over the short term. On the sample balance sheet, loans payable represents monies owed to a creditor (likely associated with a mortgage) as well as a loan made by a shareholder to the pharmacy business. Note that these amounts rise and decline based on the business activity of the pharmacy business. As the business pays off its loans, these amounts are generally referred to as debt-servicing. In the example, long-term debts (or liabilities) are recorded as $240,000 and $225,000 for the financial years 2015 and 2016, respectively.

SHAREHOLDERS' EQUITY

The shareholders' equity or owner's equity section represents the cumulative amount of money the shareholders have invested and retained in the business. For the purposes of this discussion, this section can be divided into two parts:

- contributed capital, which primarily reflects contributions of capital from shareholders, referred to as capital stock disclosed at the par or stated value of the shares authorized and issued
- earned capital, referred to as retained earnings, which results when the owners of the pharmacy business leave the profits of the business in the business rather than taking the money out of the business in the form of dividends. The cumulative amount of this reinvestment is represented on the balance sheet by the retained earnings, which in the sample balance is $409,000 and $484,000 in 2015 and 2016, respectively.

Observers of financial statements are always interested in the share of a pharmacy business's assets furnished by creditors and the share furnished by its owner or owners.[10]

Note: Creditors recognize that if the pharmacy business must be liquidated and its assets sold, the shrinkage in converting assets into cash must exceed the equity of the owner or owners or the pharmacy's creditors will lose.

STATEMENT OF RETAINED EARNINGS

Like the income statement, the statement of retained earnings covers a specific period (the accounting period), which in the example is one year. The statement of retained earnings reports the way net income and the distribution of dividends affect the pharmacy business's financial position during the year. Net income

Note: Reinvesting earnings is an important source of financing, particularly in the early years of a startup pharmacy. Owner's behaviour on dividend payment to its shareholders affects the ability of the pharmacy to repay its debts. Every dollar a pharmacy business pays to shareholders as a dividend is not available to use in paying back its debt to creditors. This becomes particularly important when the pharmacy requires sufficient reinvestment of its surplus earnings to support future growth or expansion.

earned during the year increases the balance of retained earning, while the payment of dividends (declared) to the shareholders decreases retained earnings.[11]

The retained earnings equation that describes these relationships is shown:

Beginning Retained Earnings + Net Income – Dividends = Ending Retained Earnings

DIVIDENDS

Dividends are a distribution of economic value to the shareholders of a pharmacy business corporation. While distributions can take the form of property and/or company stock, the most common form of dividend payment is in the form of cash.[12] Dividends are declared by a formal resolution of the pharmacy business corporation's directors, typically at the end of the pharmacy's fiscal year. Strategies surrounding the payment of dividends are often suggested by income tax considerations and recommendations by the pharmacy business accountant and are beyond the scope of this textbook.

CASH FLOW STATEMENT

A brief note about the cash flow statement as a matter of simple introduction as the analysis of cash flow is beyond the scope of this introductory chapter. The pharmacy business cash flow statement details the cash inflows (sources of cash or receipts) and cash outflows (uses of or payments) into three primary categories:

- Cash flows from operations would include examples such as collections of accounts receivables from customers, cash paid to suppliers such as a wholesaler (e.g., McKesson), wages paid to employees and cash paid for interest and taxes.
- Cash flows from investing activities would include, for example, cash paid to purchase the building in which the pharmacy business operates.
- Cash flows from financing activities would include repayment of long-term debt such as a mortgage, or a source of cash (inflow) from an increase in bank indebtedness. Cash received from a shareholder from the issuance of new share capital would present a source of cash, while cash paid out for dividends would represent a use of cash.

The cash flow statement equation describes the causes of the change in cash reported on the balance sheet from the end of the last period to the end of the current period.

+/– Cash Flows from Operating Activities (related to earning income)
+/– Cash Flows from Investing Activities (related to the purchase or sale of fixed assets)
+/– Cash Flows from Financing Activities (related to the financing of the pharmacy business)
Net Change in Cash

In the example, the net change in cash as a net result of all operating, investing and financing activities of our pharmacy business from the year ended 2015 to 2016 is $50,000.

With the introduction of the four basic financial statements, the various elements associated with each and equations linking them, it can now be recognized how they are related to one

Table 1. Summary of Four Basic Financial Statements[2]

Financial Statement	Purpose	Structure/Equation	Examples
Income statement	Measures financial performance during the accounting period	Revenue – Expenses	Cash, accounts receivable, inventory, accounts payable, loans payable and shareholders' equity
Net income	Sales revenue, costs of goods sold, expenses including wage, occupancy, interest and taxes		
Balance sheet	Reports the financial position including economic resources and sources of financing at a point in time	Assets = Liabilities + Shareholders' (owner's) equity	
Statement of retained earnings	Reports how net income and dividend distribution affected the financial position of the pharmacy business during the year	Beginning retained earnings + Net income – Dividends = Ending retained earnings	Net incomes come from the income statement, while dividends are distributions to shareholders
Cash flow statement	Reports inflows (receipts) and outflows (payments) of cash during the year listed under the categories of operating, investing and financing	+/– Cash flows from operating activities +/– Cash flows from investing activities +/– Cash flows from financing activities = Change in cash	Cash collected from customers and third parties, cash paid to suppliers, cash paid to buy equipment, cash borrowed from banks

another to tell the complete story of what happened in the pharmacy business throughout the year. Table 1 summarizes the four basic financial statements as a brief overview.

NOTES TO THE FINANCIAL STATEMENTS

A very important element of all financial statements relates to the notes located at the bottom of financial statements. There are three basic types of notes:

- notes that provide descriptions of the accounting rules applied to construct the pharmacy business's financial statements
- notes that present supplemental information about what is behind statement item amounts that appear in the financial statements (A common example pertains to how inventory is allocated to cost of goods sold.)
- notes that present additional financial disclosures about items not listed on the statements themselves such as a description of the pharmacy business lease

In summary, notes provide supplemental information about the financial statements to allow the user to better understand the assumptions and accounting methods applied in their construction and to disclose important information not found directly in the financial statement.

Chapter 16 builds on the information presented in this chapter and Chapter 14 with a view to applying the concepts introduced, including the calculation and interpretation of financial ratios.

REFERENCES

1. Fields E. The income statement. In: *The essentials of finance and accounting for nonfinancial managers*. 2nd ed. New York: American Management Association; 2011. p. 55–63.
2. Libby R, Libby PA, Short DG, et al. Financial statements and business decisions. In: *Financial accounting*. 3rd Canadian ed. Toronto: McGraw-Hill Ryerson Limited; 2007. p. 10–1.
3. Libby R, Libby PA, Short DG, et al. Financial statements and business decisions. In: *Financial accounting*. 3rd Canadian ed. Toronto: McGraw-Hill Ryerson Limited; 2007. p. 5–8.
4. Kieso DE, Weygandt JJ, Warfield TD. Classifications in the Balance Sheet. In: *Intermediate Accounting*. 13th ed. New Jersey: John Wiley & Sons; 2010. p. 179–89.
5. Jaczko MS. *K J Harrison & Partners Inc*. Canadian retail pharmacy database; 2014.
6. Fields E. The income statement. In: *The essentials of finance and accounting for nonfinancial managers*. 2nd ed. New York: American Management Association; 2011. p. 30.
7. Libby R, Libby PA, Short DG, et al. Financial statements and business decisions. In: *Financial accounting*. 3rd Canadian ed. Toronto: McGraw-Hill Ryerson Limited; 2007. p. 51.
8. Libby R, Libby PA, Short DG, et al. Financial statements and business decisions. In: *Financial accounting*. 3rd Canadian ed. Toronto: McGraw-Hill Ryerson Limited; 2007. p. 488.
9. Kieso DE, Weygandt JJ, Warfield TD. Classifications in the balance sheet. In: *Intermediate accounting*. 13th ed. New Jersey: John Wiley & Sons; 2010. p. 186–7.
10. Libby R, Libby PA, Short DG, et al. Financial statements and business decisions. In: *Financial accounting*. 3rd Canadian ed. Toronto: McGraw-Hill Ryerson Limited; 2007. p. 12.
11. Libby R, Libby PA, Short DG, et al. Financial statements and business decisions. In: *Financial accounting*. 3rd Canadian ed. Toronto: McGraw-Hill Ryerson Limited; 2007. p. 12.
12. Pratt J. Shareholder's equity. In: *Financial accounting in an economic context*. 7th ed. New Jersey: John Wiley & Sons. Inc; 2009. p. 531.

CHAPTER 16

Financial Ratios: Putting the Numbers to Work

David Cunningham, *CPA, CA, LPA, CMA, BMath (Hons.)*

Please see the example financial statements included at the beginning of this section. *They have been adapted with permission from the course, "Learn how to interpret your financials and improve profitability," sponsored by Teva Canada Limited.*

Learning Objectives

- Define and differentiate between key financial ratios.
- Calculate the ratios from a pharmacy's income statement and balance sheet.
- Interpret key ratios by comparing their values to budgets, previous-year results and industry averages.
- Determine how to "put the numbers to work" once key ratios are calculated and analyzed/interpreted.

KEY FINANCIAL RATIOS

There are hundreds of ratios that can be calculated from financial statements and the details of the trial balance. A ratio simply relates one figure appearing in the financial statement to another figure appearing elsewhere in the financial statements.[1] The pharmacist entrepreneur has little time to calculate, let alone analyze, hundreds of ratios. Therefore, by identifying the key ratios, the process of problem identification and corrective action can happen more efficiently and effectively.

Think of financial ratios as statistics that tell a financial story about the pharmacy business. Mark Twain popularized the quote, "There are three types of liars in this world: liars, damn liars and statistics." It is not that statistics lie but, rather, they lend themselves to be subjectively interpreted. Therefore, it is important to review financial ratios in context. Evaluation of the results is critical, and common sense must always be applied.

To begin examining the key financial ratios, refer to the sample pharmacy balance sheet and income statement for Anytown Pharmacy found at the beginning of this section.

FINANCIAL RATIO CLASSIFICATIONS

Ratio analysis represents an important and necessary process for the development and monitoring of performance goals. Meeting these goals ensures the pharmacy remains on a solid financial and operational footing to withstand the economic challenges pharmacies face today, and to ultimately allow the business to grow and prosper.

These ratios can be categorized to help answer several important questions:[2]

- liquidity: Can the pharmacy pay its short-term commitments?
- financial efficiency: Are the pharmacy's assets being managed efficiently?
- solvency: Can the pharmacy pay its long-term commitments?
- profitability: Does the pharmacy earn adequate profits?
- operational productivity: Is the dispensary operationally productive?

It is important to compare the pharmacy's ratios to both internal benchmarks (referred to as historical trend analysis) as well as external benchmarks accepted within the Canadian pharmacy industry. This chapter examines the use of five categories of ratios from a practical application perspective.

Some of the ratios calculated from the pharmacy's balance sheet reflect a measure of risk to the pharmacy operation. Liquidity is the ability of a pharmacy to pay obligations expected to become due within the next year.[3] Therefore, it is essential to measure the liquidity of the operation. Liquidity ratios are current ratio, quick ratio and accounts payable days. The liquidity ratio can be affected by the financial efficiency of certain assets. The financial efficiency ratios are inventory turnover (both dispensary and front store) and accounts receivable days. The other aspect of risk on the balance sheet is debt. The debt to equity ratio (sometimes called debt to tangible net worth) measures solvency of the company.

Some of the ratios calculated from the pharmacy's income statement measure profitability. The key ratio is gross margin (usually distinguishing between dispensary and front store). Other ratios will focus on front store categories such as return on investment/assets. Still other ratios compare the relationship between wages and gross profit or sales; occupancy costs to gross profit or sales; other expenses to gross profit or sales; and normalized income before tax to gross profit or sales.

CURRENT RATIO

The current ratio provides an indication of the company's ability to meet short-term debt obligations (e.g., liquidity). This ratio is considered by many bankers and other creditors to be a good indicator of a company's ability to pay its bills and to repay outstanding loans.[4] It is calculated by dividing current assets by current liabilities in the sample financial statements ($1,460,000/$870,000 = 1.68). The higher the ratio, the less likely there will be cash flow problems. Typically, a ratio of 2.0 is good and a ratio of less than 1.0 means the pharmacy is technically insolvent. Is the objective to increase this ratio as much as possible? How does one avoid technical insolvency? There are pharmacies that discover a ratio of more than 2.0 as problematic. Further, there are pharmacies quite satisfied with a ratio of 1.0 or less.

Leverage refers to using borrowed funds to generate returns for the owners of a pharmacy business.[5] Leverage is a method to increase profitability. The more borrowed cash (e.g., bank loan) used in a pharmacy business, the higher the profitability to the pharmacy entrepreneur.

However, this could leave the pharmacy vulnerable in the event that one or more doctors in the area were to leave, as an example. The drop in prescription revenue could render the pharmacy unable to pay its expenses. On the other hand, too much cash left unused will reduce the return on assets. Pharmacy entrepreneurs should determine how much risk they are willing to take. Some leverage is a good thing; however, too much could be problematic.

The current ratio in the example provided is calculated at 1.68. This should be compared to the budget and the trend over five years (less if the business has not operated for five years). The Canadian industry average is 1.4–1.5.[6]

QUICK RATIO

The quick ratio is similar to the current ratio with the proviso that inventory and prepaid expenses are eliminated from the current asset total. Prepaid expenses are eliminated because there is no cash generated from this asset. (The cash has been paid and the expense is amortized over time.) The inventory is notionally eliminated because it first has to be converted into accounts receivable and then, subsequently, converted into cash. Simply, the ratio measures whether the cash and accounts receivable are sufficient to pay the accounts payable and other current liabilities. It is a more stringent test of a pharmacy's ability to pay its bills.[7]

In the example, cash ($150,000) plus accounts receivable ($600,000) is $750,000. When divided by the current liabilities of $870,000, the result is a ratio of 0.86. The standard rule of thumb is that the ratio should be at least 1:1.[6]

However, note that this ratio can be misleading in a retail pharmacy business, especially in a pharmacy with a large front store. In most businesses, when inventory is sold it is converted into accounts receivable and/or cash. In a pharmacy or other retail businesses, however, inventory is often converted directly into cash. For "quick" liquidity purposes, the business can rely on cash, accounts receivable and inventory to pay short-term liabilities. The extent to which this ratio should be relied on should be considered in concert with the results from the calculation of the number of days of accounts receivable, inventory and accounts payable.

NUMBER OF DAYS OF ACCOUNTS RECEIVABLE

The calculation is often referred to as the average collection period and reflects how well the pharmacy operator is collecting on payments owed to the pharmacy business. The number of days of accounts receivable is calculated by dividing accounts receivable ($600,000) by sales ($8,300,000) and multiplying the result by 365 days in one year. In this example, the result is 26.4 days.

Accounts receivable in a pharmacy operation typically consists of provincial/territorial plan billings, insurance companies (also known as third-party billings) and house accounts. House accounts consist of receivables from customers/patients and doctors. Each pharmacy has a different policy regarding house accounts. Some will decide on "none at all" or "only to doctors." Others may stipulate "only to doctors and customers who are waiting to get reimbursed by a plan." Some will open credit to just about anyone. This decision to offer credit is an important operational and philosophical choice left up to the pharmacy owner or manager.

A pharmacy's customer base and competition may impact policies as well. Keep in mind that there are costs associated with administering accounts. A pharmacy will need to entrust a staff member to maintain these accounts to ensure timely collection. If customers do not pay, it will require "writing off" such bad debts ($40,000). A key question to consider is what is more critical to the business: the cost of maintaining a larger list of receivables or the loss on income by not allowing house accounts? Typically, the cost of maintaining the list is higher, but each store should evaluate its own situation. Ideally, the average collection period is 30 days or less.[3]

If a store has government and insurance accounts receivable only, the average collection period should be 15 to 20 days.

INVENTORY MANAGEMENT

There is a delicate balance between having too little and too much inventory. Two ratios to help a pharmacy operator manage inventory levels are the inventory turnover and the number of days of inventory ratios.

The inventory turnover ratio measures the number of times, on average, that inventory is sold or "turned over" during a particular period.[7] It is calculated as the cost of goods sold ($6,300,000) divided by the average inventory (i.e., the average of beginning and ending inventory for the period being measured) ($700,000 + $750,000)/2. This example results in an 8.69 turnover ratio. It is recommended that pharmacy operators calculate turnover ratios for both prescription dispensary and front store inventories separately for further clarity and monitoring purposes. A complement to the inventory turnover ratio is the number of days of inventory ratio.

NUMBER OF DAYS OF INVENTORY

The number of days of inventory is calculated by dividing inventory ($700,000) by cost of goods sold ($6,300,000) times 365. This results in 40.6 days in the current example. It is advisable to calculate both the dispensary and front store amounts. This results in 25.2 days ($400,000/$5,800,000 × 365) for the dispensary and 219 days ($300,000/$500,000 × 365) inventory for the front store.

The industry norm for the number of days of inventory for a typical dispensary should be about 30 days. At 25 days, this example appears to be acceptable. Another indicator of the appropriate size of inventory is stock outs. If a store is continually experiencing stock outs to the point of "chasing customers away," increasing the inventory should be considered. Conversely, there is a cost associated with carrying every inventory item, especially expensive medications that are seldom dispensed. Depending on the product and customer needs, a store may be able to satisfy customer demand by bringing the product in as needed. Further, every dispensary requires a base stock. Those with low annual prescription volumes will find it difficult to maintain dispensary inventory of 30 days or less. In the example, this dispensary fills approximately 110,000 retail prescriptions per year. Therefore, it should be fairly straightforward to keep the inventory under 30 days.

The number of days of inventory for the front store can vary depending on the product mix and sales volume. For example, gift items typically turn over twice per year, while confectionary items will turn over much more frequently. In addition, profitability of the product will have an impact on the quantity (see information on gross profit return on inventory in the discussion of profitability ratios). It is fair to say that 219 days of inventory is excessive and, typically, the management of front store inventory represents one of the most difficult challenges for owners/managers of retail pharmacies in Canada. Practically speaking, it is difficult to balance the patient/customer need for products with space constraints and the costs associated with carrying inventory.

NUMBER OF DAYS OF ACCOUNTS PAYABLE

The number of days of accounts payable is calculated by accounts payable ($800,000) divided by cost of goods sold ($6,300,000) times 365. This results in 46.3 days.

Refer back to the receivable and days of inventory calculation and note that dispensary inventory is sold in 25 days. Of those that are not cash (e.g., accounts receivable), these will be collected in 26 days. This means the dispensary inventory should be converted into cash in 51 days. Since the accounts payable is paid in 46 days, there is a large portion of the accounts receivable that can be used for quick liquidity. Therefore, the quick ratio should not be relied upon in this pharmacy operation.

DEBT TO EQUITY RATIO

By comparing liabilities to shareholders' equity, an owner or manager can measure capital structure leverage in a pharmacy operation. This is also known as the debt to tangible net worth ratio or the leverage ratio. This is calculated as total liabilities ($1,095,000) divided by shareholders' equity ($485,000). This results in a ratio of 2.26.

The debt to equity ratio relates the proportion of the pharmacy operations financed by creditors compared to that financed by stockholders.[4] Typically, a low-risk operation will have a ratio of 1.0 or less. This means the shareholders are not relying on outsiders as much as the shareholders for financing the business. A high-risk operation is deemed to have a ratio of 2.0 or more. Which is better? This all depends on the risk tolerance of the pharmacy owner. Some will want to maximize return on equity. The less equity injected into the operation, the more of the creditor's cash is used. This will increase the return. Many startup or recently acquired pharmacy operators will have very high debt to equity ratios in their early years of operation reflecting the relative risks associated with debt borrowing. As the store continues to pay off debt, this ratio will decline over time to more acceptable levels.

Example: If a pharmacy owner invests $100,000 in a stock that pays 5%, the return will be $5,000. If the owner invests $100,000 of his or her own money and borrows another $100,000 with an interest rate of 3%, the total investment of $200,000 will earn $10,000. The owner pays $3,000 in interest and the resulting return is $7,000. This is an example of using the creditor's money to increase one's return. Note: The downside of this example occurs when the investment decreases in value. If the value decreases by 10%, the owner will lose $5,000 in the first year. (The loss on the investment is 10% of $100,000, mitigated by the $5,000 dividend.) In the second scenario, the owner will lose $13,000 (the $7,000 gain, less 10% of $200,000).

The pharmacy industry is full of examples of pharmacy owners who extended themselves with bloated debt to equity ratios. Some are success stories and others, unfortunately, end in bankruptcy.

On the sample balance sheet, note that there is a $200,000 amount in liabilities "due to shareholder." Should this be included as debt or equity? Conventional calculations suggest it should be included in debt. However, the point of the debt to equity ratio is to measure financing by third parties compared to shareholders. This would suggest that the due-to-shareholder balance should be included in equity. Regardless of the method chosen, the key is to be consistent.

The previous examples demonstrate why balance sheet ratios are considered risk ratios. While there are rules of thumb about acceptable values, the resulting calculations are more dependent on the individual pharmacist owner's tolerance for risk. In general, it is recommended that the pharmacy owner/manager produce monthly financial statements and budgets. For those accepting a higher degree of risk, this becomes critical. The timing of identification and correction of negative financial results may mean the survival of the business.

> Financial institutions will typically refer to this ratio as debt to tangible net worth. Shareholders' equity will typically be reduced by goodwill and due to related parties, but what about the due-to-shareholder balance? The financial institution will allow the amount to be included in equity if the shareholder signs a subrogation agreement. (Basically, the shareholder will not be paid until the bank loans are paid.) If there is no such agreement, the bank includes the due-to-shareholder in debt.

INCOME STATEMENT AND EVALUATION OF PROFITABILITY – PROFITABILITY RATIOS

As the various profitability ratios are calculated and presented, the pharmacist owner should always be looking at ways to make them better. Start with projections, monitor and evaluate results and take corrective action as required.

GROSS PROFIT/ GROSS MARGIN

Two terms that are often used interchangeably but have different meaning are *gross profit* and *gross margin*.

> Many pharmacist owners compare various ratios to the average or the upper quartile. One must ask if the financial goals set are average and if this is acceptable. In the book *Good to Great* by Jim Collins, he suggests that the great companies produce BHAGs (Big Hairy Audacious Goals). When presented with industry averages and upper quartile results, one pharmacist owner exclaimed, "I have no interest in the averages and middling interest in the upper quartile. What I want to know is whether mine are the best!"

Gross profit is expressed as a number (store sales less cost of goods sold). Gross margin is expressed as a percentage (gross profit divided by sales times 100). Gross profit and gross margin calculations are ideally broken out by dispensary and front store. Furthermore, depending on the requirements of the pharmacist owner and the ability of obtaining more granular information, gross profits and margins can further be calculated by product groups and individual products.

The use of industry averages for gross margin is often not a useful exercise. Consider that the average gross margin for a typical pharmacy is approximately 30%. The dispensary margin is in the high 20s and the front store margin in the low- to mid-30s. However, depending on the clientele of the pharmacy (case mix), a dispensary gross margin can range from 15% to 55%. With the advent of professional service fees (typically included in sales), the dispensary margin could grow even larger in the future. Front store gross margins can also vary widely from pharmacy to pharmacy. The reason is product and service mix.

If the pharmacy is a typical retail operation, the averages could be appropriate; however, pharmacy operations tend to be akin to snowflakes—each one is a little different. Does the store tend to have an older or younger client base? Stores with older patient clientele tend to experience higher margins as lower-cost government-subsidized prescriptions tend to dominate the patient case mix. These types of operations typically see more prescriptions that require medication reviews (which are reimbursed in some provinces/territories), as well as an increased use of blister packs and strip packaging. These compliance tools drive lower prescription prices and more frequent renewals of government-funded prescriptions. The end result could be more pharmacist/patient interaction leading to greater pharmacist patient affinity. Further specialization can also affect margins. For example, a practice with an active methadone patient population with frequent refill renewals will experience relatively higher margins than average. Conversely, pharmacies dispensing expensive specialty drugs (e.g., biologics) will experience markedly lower-margin percentages. Identifying and understanding your product mix is the key to monitoring and managing your financial results.

Similarly, the product mix in the front store may have an effect on the overall margin. Specifically, over-the-counter products may enjoy margins in the range of 30% to 40% (on average), while other product categories will have varying margins. Paper products and food items typically experience margins of less than 10% as they represent more competitive categories in the marketplace. Conversely, home health care products may enjoy margins greater than 50%. Some pharmacy owners identify specialized products for their customer base and realize margins well over the averages. Therefore, it is important for pharmacy owners and managers to identify and evaluate product mix, monitor the results and make changes if and when necessary in an ongoing and recurring process.

In the Anytown Pharmacy example, the gross profit of $2,000,000 and the sales of $8,300,000 result in a gross margin of 24.1%. Is this a good or bad result? If the expected margin was 20%, the result is good. However, given that the expected margin for this operation was 28%, there is a shortfall of 3.9%. When the pharmacist/owner determines differences, it is important to think in terms of dollar values rather than abstract percentages. After all, gross profit dollars pay the bills! In the example, a shortfall of 3.9% seems insignificant, but the gross profit dollars could have been increased by $323,700 (3.9% x $8,300,000)! A shortfall in planned gross profit may be a result of a shift in sales mix (from high-margin products to low-margin products), pricing errors or perhaps even theft or loss prevention issues.

The dispensary's gross profit is shown to be $1,800,000 on sales of $7,600,000, resulting in a gross margin calculation of 23.7%. Furthermore, the front store gross profit is shown to be $200,000 on sales of $700,000, which results in a gross margin of 28.6%. The use of retail point-of-sale (POS) systems allows for more detailed evaluation of both dispensary and front store margins. For example, margin calculations can be completed on a product-by-product basis.

Pricing products in the pharmacy will have a large impact on gross margins. However, applying a markup to product cost should be done with consideration. If a margin of 33.3% is required, the markup on cost should be 50%. For example, if a product cost is $1, the markup of 50% results in a sales price of $1.50. The margin would be calculated as 50 cents divided by $1.50, which is 33.3%.

FRONT STORE – GROSS PROFIT RETURN ON INVENTORY

Another measure of the efficiency of inventory control is the gross profit return on inventory (GPROI).[8] This ratio measures the number of dollars of gross profit earned for every dollar of inventory. The resulting number is expressed as a percentage by multiplying the total by 100. This ratio is used to evaluate the profitability of the front store and compares the profitability of individual product lines.

Example: If Product A has a gross margin of 33% and Product B has a gross margin of 10%, one might conclude that Product A is better. If Product A has four inventory turns per year (90 days' inventory) and Product B has 10 turns per year (36.5 days' inventory), one might conclude that Product B is better. If Product A has a margin of 33% and four turns per year and Product B has a 10% margin and 10 turns per year, which product is more profitable? To draw an appropriate conclusion, the inventory value for both products would be required.

Overall, the goal for a pharmacy is to earn $2 gross profit for every $1 of front store inventory. Based on industry averages, most pharmacies are fortunate if they earn $1.25 to $1.50.[6]

In the example provided, the front store gross profit is $200,000 and the front store inventory is $300,000. This results in a GPROI of 0.67 or 67%. The result is well below what is acceptable. In this case, front store inventory should be evaluated and corrective action should be taken immediately.

RETURN ON OPERATING ASSETS

Both the profit margin and inventory ratio calculation have some limitations. The profit margin ratios do not take into consideration the assets necessary to produce income, and the inventory turnover ratio does not take into account the amount of income produced.[4]

Assume there is a $1,000 budget to invest in inventory. The goal is to choose inventory that gives the maximum return on investment.

Product A has a 33% margin and the total proceeds from the sale would be $1,500. Given that the example states there are four turns, the sales would be $6,000 (4 x $1,500) and the cost of goods sold would be $4,000 (4 x $1,000). The gross profit would be $2,000 ($6,000 less $4,000). This means $2 has been earned for every $1 of inventory ($2,000 gross profit divided by $1,000 in inventory). The GPROI would be 200 (gross profit divided by inventory times 100).

Alternatively, Product B has a 10% margin and the total proceeds from the sale would be $1,111. With 10 turns, the sales would be $11,110, while the cost of goods sold would be $10,000, providing a gross profit of $1,110. This means $1.11 was earned for every $1 of inventory. The GPROI would be 111.

This example illustrates how to evaluate the relative profitability of two products with the same amount of inventory invested. It is understood that the inventory and gross profit will differ when evaluating the various products and product lines. However, calculating the GPROI can determine which product/line is more profitable. Note: Pricing decisions will affect inventory turnover (supply and demand). When expanding a product line without expanding prices, overall section turnover may be affected as well. Therefore, it is important to consider the overall profitability to the store and GPROI before making a pricing or product adjustment.

Specifically, return on operating assets combines profit margin and operating asset utilization into one ratio. The return on operating assets is calculated as normalized income before taxes divided by operating assets and shown as a percentage. The calculation of this ratio is akin to calculating the return on any investment (whether it is shares of stock, real estate, etc.). It answers the following question: How productive are your operating assets (accounts receivable, inventory and capital assets) at generating income? First, look at normalized income. Note that the components of income and expenses of the income statement may require some "normalization" to weed out elements included that are not part of a "normal" pharmacy operation. The non-pharmacy income and expenses must be eliminated from the calculation income before taxes to result in normalized or pharmacy operation income before taxes. The following items are examples that would have to be adjusted to calculate normalized income:

- investment income
- long-term interest expense
- owner manager salary/wages: Owner managers take remuneration based on what is needed, not what is normal for their contribution to the business. Sometimes, the owner manager takes dividends and no salary. The owner manager salary should be adjusted to fair market remuneration for the contribution the owner manager makes to the company.
- related party expenses: Sometimes related parties charge rent or other expenses to assist the pharmacy operation. Again, this should be adjusted to a "normal" amount.
- expenses paid to related parties at above market rates: Again, these should be reduced to "normal" amounts.

The number of example items to be normalized can be exhaustive. The key is to remove all components that are not related to the pharmacy operation and to increase those to normal rates. For the purposes of the attached income statement, the assumption is that the net income before taxes is normal.

In the example provided, the operating assets are accounts receivable ($600,000) plus inventory ($700,000) plus capital assets ($120,000) to total $1,420,000. Since the normalized income is $275,000, the return on operating assets is 19.4%. If the pharmacy had a goal of 20%, it would have just missed the mark.

EXPENSE ANALYSIS

It is important that a horizontal and vertical analysis of expenses be conducted. The horizontal analysis compares this year's results to last year's and is often referred to as a trend analysis or historical analysis. A vertical analysis compares a component (an expense) found in the financial statements to another component found on either the balance sheet or income statement of the same fiscal year. For the purpose of analyzing expenses, gross profit is often compared from one year to another. Stringing subsequent years begins to illustrate various trends. As discussed previously, gross margins can vary greatly between pharmacies, often as a result of varying product costs and as such, is beyond the control of the pharmacist owner. Once the cost of sales is subtracted from the sales, the gross profit is then available to pay wages, occupancy cost (e.g., rent and utilities) and general and administrative expenses. The ratio of these expenses, which are controlled by the decisions of the pharmacist owner, is either compared to store sales or alternatively to gross profit. Either comparison is expressed as a percentage as a general rule. To illustrate this concept, compare such costs to gross margin for relevancy. Note: When analyzing different base components, ensure consistency when comparing to avoid drawing inappropriate conclusions.

WAGES EXPENSES

Outside of inventory, which is a working capital item, wages are the second-largest investment a pharmacy owner or manager is required to control. Wages as a percentage of gross profit indicate wage efficiency and wage productivity. Typically, wages are 45% to 50% of gross profit[6] (or 12% to 14% of sales). If it is a high-sales-volume store (more than 100,000 prescriptions per year) or a clinic pharmacy, the wages can range from 30% to 40% (or 8% to 11%, respectively). The wage percentage should be assessed on an individual store basis.

Wages expenses typically include salaries, wages and benefits to all employees, amounts paid to part-time employees or locums and any other payroll remuneration. If the owner manager is not taking a real appropriate salary (as reflected in real market economic value), the wages should be adjusted so that an appropriate industry market comparison can be determined. Normalization is an important concept used in valuation analysis. Valuation is beyond the scope of this introductory chapter.

In the example provided, wages are $1,200,000, gross profit is $2,000,000 and sales are $8,300,000, resulting in a ratio of 60% (or 14.5%). The expected ratio for this store is 45% or 14%, respectively.

OCCUPANCY EXPENSES

Occupancy expenses typically include rent, utilities, repairs, maintenance, insurance and any other cost related to the store space occupied. This ratio tends to be about 10% of gross profit (1% to 3% of sales); however, urban areas tend to be higher than rural. Clinic-based pharmacy operations tend to experience higher occupancy expenses than stores located in stand-alone and front/plaza locations. Furthermore, normalization adjustments are often requirements in the event that the pharmacy owner owns the building but fails to charge back rent to the pharmacy operation. Failure to charge back rent results in overstated profitability and artificially low occupancy expenses.

In the example provided, the occupancy cost is $50,000, gross profit is $2,000,000 and sales are $8,300,000, resulting in a ratio of 2.5% of gross margin (0.6% of sales). Since this pharmacy enjoys a relatively high annual prescription volume, the resulting lower ratio is not unexpected yet well below industry averages.

OTHER EXPENSES

Other expenses (general and administrative) include advertising, supplies, delivery, credit card cost and other bank charges, computers, pharmacist memberships, professional fees and others. This can fluctuate from store to store but averages 20% of gross margin (6% to 9% of sales). A clinic-based pharmacy will experience lower relative ratios since some expenses (e.g., advertising) are not required to the same extent. Conversely, a high-volume store operation will benefit from economies of scale.

In the example provided, the other expenses are $475,000, gross profit is $2,000,000 and sales are $8,300,000, resulting in a ratio of 23.75% (5.7% of sales).

NET INCOME BEFORE INCOME TAXES

The general target is 25% of gross profit (5% to 10% of sales). The example illustrates that the net income is $275,000, the gross profit is $2,000,000 and sales are $8,300,000, resulting in a ratio of 13.75% (or 3.3% of sales).

Financial ratios are statistics that can assist in the evaluation of financial statements and ultimately how well a pharmacy operation is performing. They can be an optimal tool if correctly applied to timely financial information.

Pharmacy owners and managers are encouraged to have their bookkeepers do the following:

- Prepare a monthly balance sheet and income statement.
- Calculate the ratios and compare to budget/expectations.
- Identify the areas of concern.
- Develop a plan to investigate and resolve areas of concern.
- Repeat every few months.

REFERENCES

1. Atrill P. *Financial management for decision makers.* 5th ed. Pearson Education, Edinburgh Gate, Harlow Essex CM20 2JE, England; 2009. p. 68.
2. Jaczko MS, Adams P, Lockie P, et al. Essential business principles in preparation for expanded services in pharmacy practice; practice change solutions, a practical CE series for pharmacists seeking to sustain and build an expanded scope of practice, 2010.
3. Kimmel PD, Weygandt JJ, Kieso DE, et al. *Financial accounting tools for business decision making.* 5th ed. Mississauga, Ontario: John Wiley & Sons Inc; 2011..
4. Needles BE, Powers M. In: *Financial accounting special edition for the Association of Investment Management Research*, 6th ed. Boston, MA: Houghton Mifflin Publishing; 2000.
5. Pratt J. *Financial accounting in an economic context.* 7th ed. New Jersey: John Wiley & Sons, Inc; 2009. p. 180.
6. Cunningham LLP, chartered accountants.
7. Bachynsky JA, Segal HJ. *Pharmacy management in Canada.* 2nd ed. Toronto: Grosvenor House Press Inc; 1998.
8. Jaczko MS. K J Harrison & Partners Inc. Canadian retail pharmacy database; 2014.

CHAPTER 17

The Canadian Third-Party Payer Market

Mike Sullivan, *RPh, BSP, MBA; President, Cubic Health Inc.*

According to the Canadian Institute for Health Information (CIHI), spending on medications in Canada consumes approximately 16% of all health care expenditures.[1] This places pharmacists at the heart of a significant proportion of the resources invested in the health care of Canadians. However, one of the greatest weaknesses of the profession over the past 40 years has been a lack of understanding of who pays for drugs in this country, and the needs of these different stakeholders. As a result, pharmacy's relationships with key stakeholders in the administration of prescription drug plan benefits in Canada are not as developed as they should be.

There has been an intense focus on behalf of pharmacy advocacy groups in each province/territory in recent decades in lobbying the provincial/territorial governments who control the publicly funded programs in each province/territory, but private payers (i.e., non-government payers) have been completely ignored. For pharmacy to succeed, this needs to change dramatically, and it needs to change quickly.

Learning Objectives

- Understand who all of the stakeholders are in the third-party provision of drug plan benefits, their roles and their business models.
- Understand how drug benefit plans are structured in Canada for private payers.
- Understand why drug plan cost containment has become a consistent theme for plan sponsors (employers).
- Highlight trends in drug plan management within third-party payer plans in Canada.
- Outline threats and opportunities for pharmacists, and the profession of pharmacy, as they relate to third-party payers.

The third-party payer (TPP) market has been a topic of confusion ever since the 1940s when Tommy Douglas and the Co-operative Commonwealth Federation government of Saskatchewan passed the Saskatchewan Hospitalization Act, which evolved into the Federal Medical Care Act in the mid-1960s, and eventually into the Canada Health Act introduced in 1984. The Canada Health Act only required that the public budget cover drugs administered in a hospital. As a result, drug coverage outside of a hospital would become the responsibility of the provinces/territories and individual Canadians.

One of the challenges of the current health care system in Canada is that there is no standard for drug coverage for residents from one province/territory to the next. This is a significant issue when one considers that CIHI estimated in their *Drug Expenditure in Canada 1985 to 2012* publication that $27.7 billion was spent in 2012 on prescription drugs, with only 44.5% of the amount being paid for by government-funded plans.[1]

For example, the Ontario Drug Benefit (ODB) program was started in 1974 to cover seniors, residents on social assistance and Ontarians residing in care homes and long-term care facilities. Despite its 40-year history, ODB has never evolved into the type of coverage seen in provinces such as British Columbia and Saskatchewan where *all provincial residents* are covered by the public program once relevant out-of-pocket cost thresholds have been reached.

Perhaps it is the lack of consistency and uniformity in coverage across the country that has caused pharmacy to focus its lobbying efforts with respective provincial/territorial governments around compensation such as dispensing fees, markup allowances, capitation fees, etc. However, lost in this complex web of provincial/territorial differences and anomalies is the fact that if only 44.5% of the prescription drug spending in Canada is being paid for by government-funded plans, what about the biggest chunk of pharmacy's market—namely non-government payers? What is pharmacy doing to build relationships and positively impact TPPs?

This chapter highlights the structure of the TPP market in Canada. A TPP is defined as any payer of drug benefits that is a non-government payer or patients paying out of their own pocket for their medications because they lack drug benefit coverage (a common occurrence for self-employed individuals or unemployed Canadians who do not qualify for social assistance). The TPP market in Canada today is dominated by employer-sponsored health care benefit plans.

WHY DO TPPS OFFER A DRUG BENEFIT PLAN?

As the cost of providing drug benefits has grown dramatically over the last two decades, a common question asked by many TPPs is why are they are even bothering to offer a drug benefit plan in the first place? Given that the most prevalent TPP is an employer-sponsored plan, consider the question from the perspective of an employer.

There are many reasons why an employer offers a prescription drug benefit plan to its employees and their eligible dependents (i.e., spouse and dependent children):

- A comprehensive benefits package, including drug plan coverage, is a compensation tool that many employers need when recruiting or retaining top talent. If the warnings from statisticians are to be believed, employers are regularly reminded that there will be an ever-increasing competition for top talent in the years ahead as baby boomers move out of the workforce and the supply of specialized skill sets is strained. As a result, employers feel that employee benefits will continue to be an important component of the overall compensation plan.
- When employers hire an employee, they recognize they are hiring the whole person, not just the person who shows up for work. They are hiring the productive talents of the individual, but also the health liabilities of the employee and the employee's family. Employers recognize they stand to gain profoundly if they can help their employees and their families achieve and maintain optimal health. As a result, they want to minimize any barriers to accessing necessary health care benefits.

- Employers recognize that if members' drug plans were not heavily subsidized, and if members had to pay out of pocket for their medications, it is very likely they would be far less adherent to their medication regimens. Employers depend on healthy, engaged employees to ensure maximum productivity. Unhealthy, absent and/or unproductive workers are a liability.

However, the most important reason why employers offer a drug plan benefit is the fact that it is a tax-effective form of compensation. The health care benefit costs an employer bears is tax deductible to the employer and is a tax-free benefit for plan members. This tax efficiency is the key reason why many plans have not moved away from providing benefits. Employers look at total compensation for employees, which includes salary, bonuses, benefits and pension. The benefits portion of total compensation is a very tax-efficient way to compensate employees.

PRESCRIPTION DRUGS NOT THE ONLY BENEFIT TO CONSIDER

In many employer-sponsored benefit programs in Canada, prescription drugs commonly make up 60% or more of all health care benefit spending.[2] That figure used to be closer to 75% to 80% 5 to 10 years ago,[2] but the decrease in generic drug prices, the relative lack of new blockbuster drug products coming to market over the last few years and the growth in other health care benefits used within employee benefit plans have continued to shrink the drug benefit's share of total plan spending. However, the substantial growth in the use of and plan spending on expensive specialty (i.e., high cost) drugs since 2010 will likely start to focus more benefits-spending back on drug plan benefits.

As a result, prescription drug plan benefits are not likely to move off the radar screen of a vast majority of TPPs anytime in the near future. Although, while drugs will continue to command attention from TPPs, pharmacy often loses sight of the fact of two very important points as it relates to employer spending on prescription drug benefits:

- Prescription drug spending is not the only concern of an employer. Within the health care benefits portfolio, there is a growing significance of the spending on paramedical benefits such as chiropractic and massage therapy claims, acupuncture, vision care and physiotherapy. Pharmacy is only concerned about the drug plan benefit, but TPPs have an array of health care benefits to manage.
- There is a host of other employee benefits employers have to consider that are not related to the portfolio of health care benefits. Therefore, excessive spending in the area of drug plan benefits can impact an employer's ability to meet other benefit obligations. The other benefits that many employers offer include short-term disability (STD), long-term disability (LTD), life insurance and either defined benefit or defined contribution pensions. Often, cost-containment initiatives around drug benefits costs are undertaken to help relieve pressure elsewhere in the employee benefit portfolio.

INSURED VERSUS NON-INSURED DRUG BENEFITS

The common misperception of pharmacists is that drug plan benefits are paid for by a faceless insurance company or claims processor. This is the primary reason why many pharmacists do not appreciate why there continues to be substantial focus by TTPs on cost-containment strategies that impact the economics of pharmacy practice. The idea that drug benefits are the concern and responsibility of an insurance company could not be further from the truth.

The majority of the cost of a TPP drug plan is paid for by the employer. In a growing number of cases every year, there is also some cost-sharing with plan members.

It is very easy for pharmacists working in community practice to get the sense that benevolent insurance companies are generously picking up the cost of drug benefit plans when plan members arrive at the pharmacy counter with a drug benefit card that features the logo of an insurance company such as Manulife, Sun Life, Great-West Life, Green Shield, Medavie Blue Cross or Alberta Blue Cross. Pharmacists need to keep in mind that TPP plans are funded primarily by employers and that insurance companies act primarily as administrative third-party vendors. Every dollar spent on drug plan benefits within the TPP market in Canada is being paid for largely by an employer or the other entity sponsoring the plan. The insurance company is simply being asked to administer and manage the plan on behalf of the TPP.

Pharmacists in community practice will typically have much more interaction with the pharmacy benefits manager (PBM) who processes the claims than they will with the actual insurance company. The majority of Canada's largest insurance companies outsource drug claims processing to a PBM. For example, Sun Life Financial and Great-West Life use TELUS Health to process their drug claims, while Manulife Financial and Desjardins Financial Services use Express Scripts Canada.

While the typical practice in the past has been to outsource claims processing, there are some insurance companies that process their own claims (such as Green Shield Canada, Medavie Blue Cross, Alberta Blue Cross and Pacific Blue Cross).

There are two major types of drug benefit plans available in Canada:

- administrative service only (ASO) plans
- fully insured plans

ASO plans are typically reserved for groups of 100 plan members or more plus their dependent children and spouses. Typically, TPPs in Canada are defined by the number of primary lives under the plan (e.g., number of employees, whereby 150 employees in the company would constitute a 150 life plan), so many plans for greater than 100 people are often structured in an ASO format.

In an ASO plan structure, the insurance company is simply an administrator. It assumes no financial risk in providing a drug plan benefit. The insurance company pays claims on behalf of an employer and adds in an administrative charge on top to cover expenses and profit margin. Whenever a pharmacist receives a drug plan benefit card for a patient covered by a large employer plan, it is a certainty that the plan is structured in an ASO manner where the plan sponsor and its members have to pay the full costs of the claims incurred in a given year.

This responsibility for plan costs is why ASO plans have long been eager to control benefit costs, because every additional dollar spent on employee benefits is a dollar less on the company's bottom line. Most pharmacists are completely unaware that ASO plans even exist, and that they exist in such large numbers. There is even a trend in benefits to try to move ASO plan structures into smaller employers. However, that being said, the explosion of the use of expensive specialty drugs in Canada is causing premiums for catastrophic drug claims insurance within ASO plans to skyrocket. This is threatening the viability of an ASO model for smaller plans because most ASO plans want to protect themselves from catastrophic claims for drugs that could cost $50,000 or more per year.

The other type of plan structure is a fully insured plan. This is typically reserved for smaller plans that do not like uncertainty and volatility. Typically, any employer plan between 2 and 100 employees will be in a fully insured environment. In these cases, insurance companies will typically offer companies various health care benefit plan options with a fixed premium per month based on the demographic profile and past claims experience of a group. The premium will include the expected claims experience for the coming year, as well as a profit margin.

In cases of fully insured groups, if their drug claims exceed what they have paid in premium in a given year, that will be added to their premium the next year since these plans renew every year. So while a cynic might suggest that it is the insurance company that is actually responsible for drug plan costs, in reality, if the plan members claim more than the premium paid over the course of the year, the premium will increase in the next year. Insurance companies are not in the habit of losing money, so at the end of the day, if claims increase, the TPP will eventually be paying for the increase.

ASO plans have become popular in recent years because plan holders feel that the profit margins built into fully insured plan premiums are too high and that an ASO model will lead to lower costs. There are different schools of thought on the subject, but the move to ASO has been steady for many years.

Bottom line—it does not matter how a TPP drug benefit plan is structured; it is the plan sponsor and its members who will be picking up the costs, not an insurance company or claims processor.

STAKEHOLDERS IN THE PROVISION OF DRUG PLAN BENEFITS AND ECONOMIC MODELS

An awareness and understanding of the various stakeholders in the provision of drug plan benefits and insight into their business models is vital for understanding how to strategically influence TPPs. One of pharmacy's most significant shortcomings in this area over the years has been a lack of understanding of who the stakeholders are and what role they play.

The biggest oversight in this space is that insurance companies (referred to as "carriers") are the most important stakeholder. They are not the focal point—the most important stakeholder by far is the group subsidizing most drug plan spending: *the plan sponsor*. See Figure 17.1 for an overview of who the stakeholders are in the area and how they are interconnected.

PLAN SPONSOR

In most cases, the plan sponsor is the employer who is offering the benefit to the plan member. In a vast majority of cases, the employer assumes the majority of the financial responsibility for drug plan funding as discussed in the previous section related to plan structures. There are different types of plan sponsors, the most common including the following:

Figure 17.1

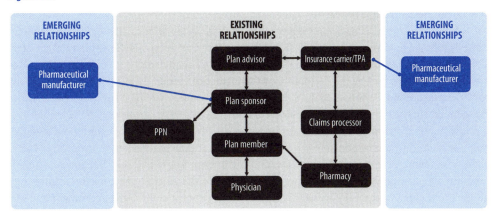

Stakeholders and Their Relationships

- single employer plan sponsor: where an individual employer offers a drug plan to its employees
- multi-employer plan sponsor: where more than one employer comes together under one plan (There are many cases, especially in the public sector, where more than one employer will come together under one plan. This is done to achieve better administration costs from the carrier as well as to access cheaper premiums on true insured benefits such as life insurance and disability insurance.)
- association plans: where members of a particular association can purchase a common drug benefit plan that the association offers and manages on its members' behalf
- trusteed plan sponsor: where a Board of Trustees oversee the plan (Some TPP drug plans are run not by an employer but a Board of Trustees who oversee the benefits plan on behalf of a collection of members. This is commonly seen in union-based environments where the unions are provided with a certain level of funding for benefits and must manage the plans themselves.)

As described earlier in the chapter, there are two common financial arrangements for plan sponsors: they can become ASO and self-insure their own drug benefit plan, or they can be an insured plan where they pay premiums to an insurance company who underwrites the plan and takes on more risk. However, in the end, how the plans are structured makes little difference to the plan sponsor in the big picture because even if a plan is fully insured, if what the insurance company took in as drug plan premiums is far lower than what it paid out in prescription drug claims for members, it stands to reason that the plan sponsor will see a significant increase in premiums the next year.

It is the plan sponsor who absorbs most of the cost of the drug plan and they have the authority to decide which drugs are covered, which drugs are not covered, how much cost plan members will have to bear, whether or not a preferred pharmacy network (PPN) program is considered and which cost-containment items are placed into plans. The person who pays the bill makes the decisions and, surprisingly, pharmacy to date has been very slow to understand that it is the plan sponsor at the centre, not the carrier.

It is important for pharmacists to realize that while the plan sponsor is funding the benefit, most do not get involved in making individual drug coverage decisions. Drug plan design decisions are usually outsourced to external consultants or plan advisors, and formulary decisions are usually taken care of by the PBM and/or the insurance carrier. As a result, pharmacy needs to communicate and demonstrate the value of its services not only to plan sponsors, but to other stakeholders in the provision of drug plan benefits.

While many pharmacists assume that plan sponsors are only concerned about cost management because they are responsible for paying for most of the costs related to drugs, that is not a fair assessment. Plan sponsors have an economic interest to get the most benefit out of their investments in employee health care benefits and obtain the greatest value for the money they allocate to these benefits. They are very receptive to the concept of investing in products and services that provide tangible returns, so there are great opportunities for pharmacists in this area.

PLAN MEMBER

The plan member is an eligible participant in a given plan sponsor's TPP plan. Often, the plan member is an employee of a specific plan sponsor, or a spouse or dependent child of an employee. It is the plan member who pharmacists deal with at the dispensary counter. Contrary to popular understanding, even though plan members are eligible for coverage under a given plan, they often have very little insight into what is covered and how the coverage is structured.

Plan members are provided with plan coverage documents, but they are often very vague and can be confusing. Coverage can also change from year to year, so it is very common to encounter members who have very little insight into what is covered and the level of coverage.

In most cases, plan members also have a financial stake in the plan as well through one of (or a combination of) the following:
- payroll deductions for a portion of the cost of their health care benefit plan
- a given level of co-insurance for a claim (Co-insurance is defined as the percentage of the amount of the claim for which the member is responsible to pay; a 20% co-insurance on a $100 claim means the member has to pay $20 of the claim cost.)
- an annual deductible
- a co-payment per prescription (Co-payment is defined as a flat cost per claim for which the member is responsible.)

The financial interest of the plan members is entirely dependent on their level of coverage and whether or not they have additional coverage through a secondary plan or spousal plan. Members who have very generous plans and/or secondary coverage with more than one plan tend to be far less concerned about cost than members who are responsible for a larger proportion of the cost.

INSURANCE CARRIER

Insurance carriers are the dominant plan administrators for drug benefit plans in Canada. For ASO plans, their primary focus is on all of the administrative functions, but they do not take on risk because, in the case of ASO plans, the plan sponsor is self-insuring their risk. ASO plans still rely on carriers for catastrophic stop-loss coverage to protect them in the event they experience very high cost claims, and they pay an insurance company an additional premium for the coverage.

For fully insured plan sponsors, carriers take on the role of underwriting the risks involved with a drug plan as well as administering the plans. For example, if a small plan pays $20,000 in drug plan premiums and incurs $30,000 worth of claims, the carrier is responsible for covering the additional $10,000 in claims over $20,000. However, in this case, the plan sponsor can expect a sizable premium increase next year.

The other advantage that carriers have in the market is that they can provide additional products and services to plan sponsors such as disability and life insurance, employee assistance programs, health and wellness offerings, as well as pension/group Registered Retirement Savings Plan (RRSP) management. Drug benefits are only one line of the health care benefit portfolio carriers offer, and just one of the products and services in the suite of offerings for plan sponsors.

Since benefit plans renew every 12 months, plan sponsors have the freedom to leave a carrier at any point after their first year, so there is competition to win new business between the carriers.

The economic interest of carriers may seem counterintuitive to some. If they have covered their risk exposure adequately, more claims and more money flowing through drug benefit plans is actually a positive thing for carriers because they stand to make more administration fees, and it helps justify ever-increasing premiums. Traditionally, carriers have not had to worry a great deal about cost containment. Many carriers make relatively modest returns administering health care benefit plans compared to the returns that can be made from insured benefits such as life and disability.

THIRD-PARTY ADMINISTRATORS

The alternative for a plan sponsor using an insurance carrier to administer their plan is to use a third-party administrator (TPA). A TPA provides all the administrative and claim payment functions a carrier would provide. The major difference from a plan sponsor's perspective is that a TPA does not take on any risk. They are simply plan administrators.

The main advantage a TPA offers a plan sponsor is the ability to use multiple carriers to serve the same plan, and to have all the billing and administration flow through one TPA system. This way, if a plan sponsor wants to use carrier A for its health benefits, carrier B for life insurance and carrier C for disability insurance, it can do so seamlessly. It also allows a plan sponsor to change carriers much more easily if they feel they are not being serviced properly.

Some multi-employer plans have formed their own TPAs to help minimize administrative costs and to gain greater control of their plan.

CLAIMS PROCESSORS

Claims processors are commonly referred to as PBMs. They are familiar entities to pharmacists because outside of the plan member, this is the stakeholder with whom pharmacists interact the most. Some carriers and TPAs have made the decision to outsource claims processing to external technology companies, and others have seen a strategic benefit in processing claims in-house. Examples:

- TELUS Health Solutions processes drug claims for Great-West Life and Sun Life Financial—two of the biggest carriers in Canada. They also process claims for smaller carriers and some TPAs.
- Express Scripts Canada (ESC) is a subsidiary of Express Scripts—the largest pharmacy benefit management company in the world. ESC processes claims for Manulife Financial and Desjardins Financial. ESC also processes claims for some TPAs.

By contrast, carriers such as Green Shield Canada, Medavie Blue Cross, Alberta Blue Cross and Pacific Blue Cross, and some TPAs such as Johnson Inc., have made the strategic decision to keep claims processing in house. While claims processors are commonly referred to in Canada as PBMs, that term is very misleading. In the United States, PBMs are involved in drug procurement, distribution, formulary management, medication access and claims processing. PBMs are full-service drug plan managers in the United States, but in Canada, they are effectively relegated to the role of claims processor, although a few groups are trying to break that mould by offering programs such as mail-order pharmacy and enhanced prior authorization programs.

In most cases, any carrier that uses an external PBM retains complete control over the PBM. Hence, for stand-alone claims processors, the economic model is the more claims processed, the better. They incur no risk whatsoever, and have no direct access to plan sponsors; therefore, they have little influence over plan design.

The carrier and PBM relationship is an important one for pharmacists to consider because until relatively recently, insurance carriers were still involved in processing a substantial proportion of drug claims. For many years, Canada had been very slow in embracing the electronic, real-time reimbursement of drug claims using pay-direct drug cards (PDD). Many plans were still on a paper reimbursement system whereby a member made a claim in the pharmacy, paid for their claim and then submitted the receipt to the insurance carrier manually for reimbursement.

There was a widespread belief in the insurance industry that if plans moved to a PDD card, they would see substantial increases in plan use and cost—partly because all claims would be paid immediately (and plans would lose out on the benefit of members forgetting to submit claims manually), and because there was an impression that increased convenience would lead to people making more claims. Thankfully, in recent years, that has all begun to change. Plans realize that without real-time adjudication, they cannot adopt more meaningful plan designs and cannot institute necessary controls. Evidence of the change in thinking is best demonstrated by the biggest plan in the country—the federal government's Public Service Heath Care Plan for all government workers and retirees, which moved to a PDD plan structure.

It is often the PBM/claims processor who is called upon by the insurance carrier or plan sponsor to conduct audits at the pharmacy level to ensure claims are being adjudicated properly. These audits have become a source of great frustration to many pharmacy stakeholders as pharmacists perceive the audits to be unfair at times (i.e., arbitrarily cutting back reimbursement on a given claim after the fact), and disruptive to the business. PBMs are contractually required by their insurance company partners to carry out a fixed number of audits on site per year, and to flag claims that meet certain criteria for same-day or next-day audits. This is a fact of life for pharmacy that is not likely to change dramatically moving forward unless a given pharmacy or pharmacy chain wished to stop accepting claims for a specific insurance carrier or PBMs.

BENEFITS CONSULTANTS AND INSURANCE BROKERS (PLAN ADVISORS)

A large number of plan sponsors engage external advisors to assist them in managing their benefits plans. Some larger firms may in-source that work by hiring on an internal plan advisor within the human resources function, but most plan sponsors retain external advisors. In many cases, this is because the majority of companies in the Canadian economy are small- to medium-size businesses that do not have the need for or the resources to engage a full-time internal advisor.

There are two major types of plan advisors:

- benefits consultants: focused primarily on large plan sponsors
- insurance brokers: focused primarily on small- and medium-sized plan sponsors

Benefits consultants typically work for large, international human resource consulting firms such as Mercer, Aon Hewitt, Towers Watson and Morneau Shepell. In most cases, these firms are engaged with large plans, and often those that have pension considerations and, therefore, require regular actuarial reviews of their pension plans. Given that the plans they assist on the investment/pension side also provide health benefits, the same advisory firm completing actuarial work or investment management services is often retained to help manage benefits. Many benefits consultants in Canada have an actuarial background, which underlines the close ties between pensions and benefits.

The typical business model for a benefits consultant is much like a lawyer—an hourly billable rate and clients are billed for hours spent on their file. The business is assisted by the fact that benefit plans renew annually. It is noteworthy that of all the benefits consultants working in Canada who have a stake in managing drug benefit plans, fewer than 1% are pharmacists.

Insurance brokers represent various insurance companies and typically build relationships with the owners of small- and medium-size businesses. Often, brokers are involved in selling business owners life and disability insurance, and from there assist in putting together benefits plans for the employees of the business. Insurance brokers come from a variety of backgrounds, but most started their career working for a carrier.

Insurance brokers typically make a commission based on the premiums paid by the employer for health benefits. The obvious challenge here is that from an economic standpoint, brokers typically have no interest in trying to contain plan costs because that can negatively impact their commissions. One of the complaints in the benefits industry centres around the lack of complete transparency in broker compensation. While the commission they are paid by the carrier for the business is typically disclosed to the plan sponsor, other forms of commissions, such as bonuses paid by carriers to brokers to drive given thresholds of business their way, are typically not disclosed.

Overall, given the billable hourly model of a benefits consultant and a commission-based model of a broker, there has not been a tremendous need for plan advisors to push the cost-containment mandate in the past. Plan advisors have been more active in that discussion these days in an effort to recruit and retain key clients given the financial pressures many benefit plans are under these days.

PHARMACEUTICAL MANUFACTURERS

For many years, pharmaceutical manufacturers were not active stakeholders in the provision and management of drug plan benefits, but that is beginning to change, precipitated by the following factors:

- The patent cliff that has seen many blockbuster brand-name drug products lose patent protection in recent years is forcing brand-name manufacturers to look for new ways to protect their market share.
- Brand-name manufacturers who feel their products provide substantial value that justifies higher prices are looking to build business cases that highlight to plan sponsors where investments in drug plan benefits have positive impacts on decreasing absence from the workplace, minimizing the number and average duration of short-term and long-term disability claims and increasing productivity.
- Decreasing generic drug prices, a declining generic pipeline and competition from brand products that have lost patent protection and are trying to keep market share from generic products post-patent expiration have forced generic manufacturers to engage plan sponsors more actively in an attempt to increase generic drug penetration rates.
- The rise in use of expensive specialty drugs products threatens to change how employers fund their drug benefit plans. Specialty manufacturers are looking to work more closely with plan sponsors so they do not lose access to a significant source of financial support.

The pharmaceutical industry's willingness to invest in building relationships with large, influential plan sponsors should serve as a role model for pharmacy, which to date has been very slow in doing so. The business models of both brand and generic manufacturers are greatly impacted by the degree to which they can influence plan sponsors.

PHARMACY

Since the emergence of TPP drug plans, pharmacy has been content to simply focus on the distribution of drugs to members and the simple act of filling prescriptions. Pharmacy has long been reimbursed primarily for distributing a product (i.e., a prescription) as opposed to rendering a service, so the economic model of pharmacy has been a barrier to proactive engagement of plan sponsors.

Pharmacy stakeholders have long complained that as the most accessible and trusted health care service provider, the pharmacist is an underused asset for plan sponsors and their members. While that may well be the case, pharmacy has done very little to build concrete business cases as to how their interventions can financially impact a plan sponsor.

Some of the landmark community practice research on the impact of pharmacists in helping to manage hypertension or Type 2 diabetes has focused on how pharmacists have affected health metrics such as blood pressure readings or HbA1c levels, but the research has not focused on the financial impact on plan sponsors of better health. If plan sponsors are the ones paying the bill, without the ability to quantify the impact of pharmacy services on benefits plan spending and productivity, pharmacy will continue to fail in their attempt to build relationships with TPP and plan a more central role in drug plan management.

ATTENTION PAID TO DRUG BENEFITS AND THE LACK OF PLAN SPONSOR REPORTING

In recent years, there has been an ever-increasing focus on containing costs within drug benefit plans among TPPs that mirrors the efforts governments have taken in reducing the cost burden of drug benefit plans. Pharmacy stakeholders are often frustrated at why the focus of many large health benefit plans seems to be consistently on containing drug plan costs. The following are the major factors why prescription drug costs are routinely targeted by plans looking to better manage their experience:

- As mentioned previously, prescription drugs continue to dominate health plan spending, so they will always be on a plan sponsor's agenda at plan-renewal time every year.
- The reporting that plans receive every year at renewal time is limited. Often, they only receive a listing of the top drugs by amount paid and the number of claims paid. This limited reporting makes it very difficult for plans to effectively manage their plans. It is also the reason why they look to very basic cost-containment solutions such as dispensing fee caps and markup caps because plans and their advisors lack deeper information to make more strategic changes.
- Catastrophic claims employers deal with, and need to insure against, are driven primarily by expensive specialty drugs. Therefore, even if a plan has seen strong performance within the drug plan benefit from a cost perspective in recent years, any time there are catastrophic drug claims incurred, this brings the topic of drug plan cost-containment back to the top of the agenda.
- There exists a substantial price discrepancy for the same quantity of the same drug at pharmacies within the same province/territory, as well as from one province/territory to another. These pricing discrepancies have led plan sponsors and their advisors to explore preferred provider networks (PPN) and markup limits on drug claims.
- There is a perception with the TPP community that the pharmacy business model is broken and that the financial interests of community pharmacy are in direct contrast to those of a plan sponsor. As such, this is driving the initiative from plan sponsors to implement solutions they feel will insulate them from the conflicting business models.

FIRST-GENERATION VERSUS NEXT-GENERATION DRUG PLAN MANAGEMENT TOOLS

The lack of meaningful reporting in drug plan (and overall health care benefit) experiences led to some very rudimentary and basic first-generation cost-containment approaches being employed by TPPs. In several cases, TPPs have not become much more sophisticated in their plan designs and only a small proportion of Canadian plans have adopted second-generation drug plan management tools, but that trend will continue to change as cost pressures mount.

First-generation drug plan management tools that most pharmacists are aware of include the following:

- dispensing fee caps
- generic substitution provisions in which prescriptions for multi-source brand drugs must be filled with the lower-cost generic equivalent where appropriate
- shifting cost to plan members in an effort to get members more engaged in cost containment (i.e., making the dispensing fee a deductible per prescription, moving to a co-insurance model, instituting a co-payment per prescription)
- excluding certain classes of drugs from coverage (i.e., fertility drugs, erectile dysfunction therapies, cosmetic products)

The second generation of drug plan management tools, which are becoming more prevalent, include the following:

- moving to tiered-plan designs where patients are reimbursed at different levels, depending on what therapy they claim for, to increase awareness of more cost-effective options in key drug classes
- limits to the number of dispensing fees a plan will pay per member per drug per year in an attempt to drive more efficient dispensing practices
- development of PPNs that offer a financial incentive for members to have prescriptions filled by preferred pharmacies
- introduction of mail-order pharmacy into plan designs and the development of financial incentives to use mail-order. While mail-order pharmacy is not new in Canada, previously its use was incredibly poor because there was no awareness and no incentive for members to use it. This has all begun to change, and some very large plans in the country are moving to incorporate mail-order pharmacy that follows the American model, where approximately one out of every six prescriptions is filled by mail.
- introduction of more rigorous prior authorization reviews for expensive biological and non-biological specialty drugs

TRENDS IN TPP DRUG BENEFIT PLANS

The most significant trend in TPP drug benefit plans in Canada is the move toward *active* plan management. In the past, drug plans were very passively managed. Coverage was very generous, plan members had to pay very little out of pocket and there were few restrictions in place. Given the increasing cost burden over the years, the move toward actively managed plans was inevitable, and it is happening at a much more robust pace in Canada than ever before.

OPEN VERSUS MANAGED PLANS

The most common plan design of the past 20 years has been "any prescription-requiring product that has been authorized by a licensed prescriber." Clearly the days of the open-plan design are coming to a rapid end because of the inability to manage costs and the exposure to any new prescription-requiring product approved by Health Canada. This has opened the door to demand for, and acceptance of, managed-plan designs.

The most common managed plans today either use a managed formulary and cover all eligible products at a given level of co-insurance, or a tiered-plan design where eligible drugs are placed into two, three or four different tiers with varying level of coverage. Carriers have jumped into this market in a substantial way because they see the opportunity of developing their own managed formulary as an opportunity to retain clients at renewal and make it more challenging for existing clients to leave because it would be challenging to replicate the same coverage elsewhere.

IMPACT OF CHANGING PROVINCIAL/TERRITORIAL LEGISLATION

The drug benefit plan is becoming more and more complicated for plan sponsors and their advisors to manage every year partly because of changing legislation within individual provinces/territories. For many years, Québec was the lone anomaly because of the rules that existed around plans having to cover anything on the provincial drug formulary. Plan designs had to be created that excluded Québec from many aspects. Most recently, New Brunswick has adopted new regulations that will impact private plans and what must be covered. There are also emerging changes in how the seniors drug plans in regions such as Alberta and Ontario will impact private plans through moves to income-based deductibles.

In addition, the TPP community is well aware of the pricing discrepancies that exist between drugs paid for by provincial/territorial governments and those paid by private plans. The evolution of product listing agreements (PLAs), whereby pharmaceutical companies develop confidential agreements with specific provinces to list their product(s) on provincial/territorial formularies for a negotiated price reduction has led to provincial/territorial governments paying less than non-government payers. This is putting pressure on pharmaceutical companies to offer similar PLA arrangements within the private plan industry. All of this is leading to new programs within the TPP industry aimed at cost containment for expensive products in an effort to level the playing field. This, unfortunately, puts pharmacy right in the middle of the discussion because of pharmacy's role as the distribution channel for these products.

PREFERRED PROVIDER NETWORKS

There has been a longstanding principle within Canada TPP plans that Canadians, unlike Americans, will not be told where they can or cannot fill a prescription. This entitlement is beginning to lose its grip and as such, the TPP market is seeing the emergence of PPNs across the country. For the most part, PPNs are being built into the plan design in such a manner that does not exclude a member from using any pharmacy they wish; it simply provides for a substantial financial incentive to stay within the PPN.

However, for the first time ever, since 2012 the TPP market has begun to see plan designs that require mandatory participation in a PPN and 0% coverage for maintenance (i.e., chronic) medications that are filled outside of the PPN. This is a common American plan design feature but was unheard of in Canada until very recently. This objectively demonstrates how quickly the TPP landscape is changing in Canada.

In addition to brick and mortar PPNs, the uptake in plans adopting mail-order pharmacy as part of their design is notable. The most objective measure of this has been Express Scripts Canada's (ESC) investment into mail-order facilities across Canada and the rollout of its home-delivery pharmacy services. This kind of capital investment would not have been made without careful consideration, so the decision to move ahead in building out a substantial mail-order infrastructure that is independent of the mail-order offerings of large chains such Shoppers Drug Mart and Rexall (who have very little incentive to support mail order and a much greater incentive to drive traffic through their stores) is notable.

SPECIALTY PHARMACY

Figure 17.2 outlines the substantial growth in the approval of specialty (i.e., high cost) drugs in Canada in 2012 and 2013. According to Cubic Health's Canadian Drug Database, in 2013 22% of plan spending for Canadian plan sponsors was related to specialty drugs.[2] Since these drugs typically make up fewer than 1% of all claims, their impact on plan spending is profound. Many plan sponsors have to purchase additional insurance coverage (called stop-loss insurance) to protect themselves from unexpected high-cost drug claims than can cost $25,000 or more per person per year.

Figure 17.2

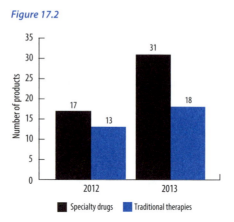

New Drug Products Approved in Canada

Source: Cubic Health Canadian Drug Database, 2014

As a result of the explosion in the approvals of biologic and non-biologic specialty products, and the substantial increase in their use, plans are beginning to turn to specialized pharmacies to help manage their spending and utilization of high-cost products. These pharmacies tend to have close ties to the manufacturers and in addition to assisting in lowering markups on products, they can help coordinate participation in manufacturer-sponsored patient support programs.

Within the past year, all of the largest group health insurance carriers in the country have introduced partnerships with specialty pharmacy vendors. The impact for pharmacy is that high-profit specialty products will continue to be phased out of community pharmacies and into specialty pharmacies.

THREATS AND OPPORTUNITIES FOR PHARMACY

Clearly the threats to pharmacy in continuing on the same course as it has been on for decades as it relates to TPP will be disastrous. The lack of leadership exhibited on the issue by leaders in pharmacy across the country in both community pharmacy and at the advocacy level with provincial/territorial advocacy and national pharmacy groups has been astounding.

Pharmacy's overall lack of success in building meaningful relationships with key TPP stakeholders has expedited the marketplace in taking control of the drug plan benefit, and key stakeholders have not solicited the input of pharmacy in the following areas:

- the move to preferred pharmacy networks, including those that no longer offer members choice in which pharmacy they use
- the emergence of, and TPP support of, mail-order pharmacy
- the emergence of, and TPP support of, specialty pharmacy
- changes to the manner in which TPPs reimburse pharmacies—specifically changes in allowable markups and limits to not only the dispensing fee paid, but the number of fees that are paid

These trends will continue to have an adverse impact on pharmacy's economics. Therefore, the economic threats of the status quo are profound and real.

However, within the dismal state of the economics of simply dispensing drugs, there are profound opportunities for pharmacy to leverage its strengths in the following areas to assist TPP:

- accessibility
- trust
- ability to influence member health and a substantial part of the TPP investment in health care benefits

Pharmacy has the opportunity to move from an economic model of getting paid to dispense a prescription to getting paid to add value as a trusted partner through the provision of medication management services that add quantifiable value for plan sponsors. The opportunity to take advantage of a service-based model will enable pharmacists to be used to their full potential to ensure the following:

- optimal member health that minimizes absence from the workplace, as well as short-term and long-term disability claims for a plan sponsor
- optimal adherence to therapy to ensure the investments TPPs are making in drug plan benefits are having a tangible impact and are not being wasted through poor adherence
- optimizing the therapeutic mix to ensure plans are receiving the greatest value for their investment in drug plan benefits and protecting the sustainability of the drug plan

There is an incredible opportunity for pharmacy to transform its relationship with key stakeholders in the TPP marketplace and play an active role in the health of the members covered under TPP plans. This will only happen by understanding the key players, building appropriate relationships and demonstrating tangibly where value can be added in a language that speaks to TPP.

Pharmacy is uniquely positioned as an accessible health care profession that has direct insight into one of the areas of greatest cost to plan sponsors as it relates to health care benefits. The profession and its members need to work to eliminate misperceptions of the role and value of pharmacists within the TPP community, and educate key stakeholders as to how pharmacy can assist in delivering plan sustainability and better health outcomes, while at the same time helping to contain plan costs and eliminate waste.

REFERENCES

1. Canadian Institute for Health Information. Drug expenditure in Canada, 1985 to 2012. Available: http://publications.gc.ca/collections/collection_2013/icis-cihi/H115-27-2012-eng.pdf (accessed Nov. 9, 2014).
2. Database CHCD. 2014. Available: www.cubichealth.ca.

CHAPTER 18

Hospital Financial Administration

Bill Wilson, *BSP; Director of Pharmacy, Mount Sinai Hospital; Lecturer, Leslie Dan Faculty of Pharmacy, University of Toronto*

Learning Objectives

- Describe the governance and funding of hospitals and other publicly funded health care organizations.

- Describe the budgeting process in the hospital environment and the process of reporting variances to budget.

- Describe the sources of revenue for pharmacy services in the hospital.

- Describe the various aspects of monitoring expenditures including salaries, drugs and other supplies.

- Describe drug use management strategies in hospitals.

In Canada, hospitals are publicly funded and operate under the direction of the provincial/territorial health ministry or similar organization that is not for profit.

Hospitals are also governed by federal and provincial/territorial legislation. In Ontario, for example, this legislation includes the Public Hospitals Act and the Ontario Health Insurance Act. Hospital Pharmacy in many provinces is also accredited by the Provincial Pharmacy Regulatory Authority. Examples include British Columbia and Alberta, and Ontario will be regulated by the Ontario College beginning in 2015.[1–6]

Hospitals also undertake to be accredited by Accreditation Canada. Accreditation Canada develops standards for all aspects of hospital services and accreditation status ensures hospitals meet these standards. Although accreditation is voluntary, the majority of hospitals participate, especially teaching hospitals that require accreditation to maintain their teaching status.[7]

Hospitals are also governed by the same accounting rules as any corporation and their financial reports mimic those of the private sector; however, hospitals' accounting rules are based on their not-for-profit status. Their books are audited and are also subject to audit by government.[8]

There are many similarities in the public system when compared to community pharmacy in terms of budget development, financial reporting as well as adjustments made to revenues and expenses when budget targets are not met.

There are, however, many differences and pharmacists entering into hospitals or other public health care organizations need to be aware of the financial management processes, especially if they will be in a management role.

HOSPITAL GOVERNANCE

The hospital is governed by a voluntary Board of Directors who is responsible to ensure the hospital provides the services they have agreed to provide. They are responsible to ensure appropriate funding and to approve the annual budget before it is submitted to government. In addition, they are responsible for hiring the Chief Executive Officer (CEO) and approving the quality and safety programs of the organization.

The Board is also responsible for approving all Medical staff privileges for the hospital and for overseeing the Medical Advisory Committee (MAC).[3]

MEDICAL ADVISORY COMMITTEE (MAC)

The MAC is the principal policy-making body of the medical staff in the organization and is accountable to and makes recommendations directly to the Board of the hospital. The MAC is responsible for approving all policies related to patient care and documentation in the health record.

The MAC has several subcommittees that support their mandate such as Credentials, Health Records, Infection Control, Quality Management/Tissue Audit and Pharmacy and Therapeutics to mention a few.[3]

Pharmacy and Therapeutics (P&T) Committee

The P&T Committee is a subcommittee of the MAC that is a mandated committee responsible for all aspects of the medication system in the organization.

Every hospital is required to have a committee responsible for the approval of drugs to be used in the hospital and to develop and approve drug use guidelines, etc.

The P&T Committee plays a pivotal role in ensuring the drugs used in the hospital are the most appropriate for the patients of that hospital.

The P&T Committee is a medical staff committee with the majority of members being physicians. There is also a representative from pharmacy, who is most often responsible for preparing agendas, documenting minutes and, most importantly, providing unbiased evidence to the committee when drugs and other drug-related policies are brought forward for consideration.

The membership can also include nursing, hospital administration and in many cases, the committee will invite subject matter experts when a specific topic is being discussed.

All policies approved by the P&T Committee must also be approved by the MAC.

THE HOSPITAL FORMULARY

The hospital formulary contains a listing of drugs to be used in the hospital to meet the needs of the patients of that particular hospital or organization. Each hospital or hospital system will have a formulary that is developed and approved by the P&T Committee and the MAC.[9]

The formulary usually consists of policies on the prescribing and administration of drugs, a listing of drugs approved for use in the hospital and drug use guidelines or prescribing algorithms used to guide the appropriate use of drugs in the hospital. Each organization customizes their formulary to meet the needs of patient care.

Each organization decides if the use of drugs will be limited only to drugs listed in the formulary or if there is some flexibility in acquiring drugs outside the formulary when needed to meet the needs of the patients.

For example, as hospitals move to more short-stay surgeries and other procedures as well as to reduced lengths of stay, the cost of changing a patient from a home medication that is considered non-formulary to a formulary option needs to be reviewed. One has to consider the costs associated in making those changes against the cost of acquiring a non-formulary product. Some hospitals allow nurses to administer the patient's own medications to resolve this issue, but it must be kept in mind that there are costs associated with identifying and perhaps repackaging and relabelling these medications to meet standards.

Hospitals may focus their formulary on medications started in the hospital and those used for treatment only for the hospital stay.

Pharmacy plays a key role in monitoring the pharmaceutical market to determine the potential impact on the drug formulary and, ultimately, the cost of drugs in the hospital. In addition, products may be removed from the market and adjustments have to be made in therapy, especially in the case of pre-printed order forms and drug use guidelines. These changes may have a financial impact on the organization in terms of higher drug costs or in the case of drug shortages, delays in therapy, etc.

HOSPITAL FUNDING OVERVIEW

In Canada, the provinces/territories are responsible for the funding and overall delivery of health care. Hospitals and other public health care organizations are primarily funded through the provincial ministries of health or other organizations that are under the purview of government. Hospitals can also receive funding from other agencies, such as provincial cancer organizations, or through revenue generated by means of parking and other commercial services revenue.

The funding is based upon pre-determined services that the hospitals must provide as part of their agreement with government. In some cases, extra funds can be provided by meeting targets for procedures for which there are long wait times. Governments are looking for ways to fund hospitals based on case costing or other formulas that meet the needs of the province. An example is the new Quality Based Procedures and Health Based Allocation Method that has been introduced in Ontario.

Typically, the provincial government does not directly fund research through the global budgets of hospitals but may do so through research grants separate from global funds. Typically, research dollars are generated by individual grant submissions, industry sponsored research or through separate fundraising activities of the organization.

Capital funding for infrastructure or equipment is partially funded by government; however, the organization must also contribute to the costs through capital amortization or fundraising, typically through the hospital foundation.[3]

HOSPITAL ACCOUNTABILITY

Health care organizations are accountable to government for the services they provide. They are accountable for their spending through numerous reports. This includes financial reports as well as patient activity, workload and in some instances, case costing.[3,4]

The director/manager of the pharmacy service must have knowledge of all these requirements to run a cost-effective department while maintaining a high level of service for the patients.

HOSPITAL ACCOUNTING

Each hospital keeps records according to generally accepted accounting principles (GAAP). These guidelines are published by the Auditing and Assurance Standards Oversight Council and are available from the Canadian Institute of Chartered Accountants.

Each organization develops a chart of accounts that sets the framework for financial reporting. In Canada, a standardized system has been adopted to ensure that each organization reports consistently. The chart of accounts is contained in the management information systems (MIS) guidelines that were developed by the provincial ministries of health in conjunction with the Canadian Institute for Health Information (CIHI).[8]

Budgets and accounting costs are organized around specific cost centres such as 714400000 for pharmacy. Each organization can subdivide each centre based on their reporting needs.

Within pharmacy, for example, drug costs can be subdivided into specific drug categories, such as cancer chemotherapy, for reporting purposes.

PHARMACY SERVICES

Pharmacy services are primarily funded out of the hospital's global budget and are accountable for providing comprehensive services comprised of direct patient care, safe and cost-effective drug distribution services, education and in some cases, research.

SOURCES OF REVENUE

The majority of revenue is derived from transfer payments from the province. In addition, pharmacy services may receive drug cost recoveries from specialty programs such as provincial cancer agencies. The hospital may receive rebates on drug costs based on membership in group purchasing organizations (GPOs) or directly as a result of contracts negotiated with drug suppliers. There may also be contributions on the revenue side from amortization of equipment. In addition, some organizations have opened retail pharmacies located on the premises.

PHARMACY EXPENSES

Salaries and benefits may be broken down into several categories:
- management and operational support (MOS) personnel compensation and benefit compensation
- unit-producing personnel (UPP), workers, compensation and benefit compensation
- benefit compensation for vacation and education
- benefits in lieu of compensation
- maternity leave top-up benefits
- other benefits such as Workplace Safety and Insurance Board (WSIB), group life, employer health tax, extended care and dental insurance, Canada Pension Plan (CPP), hospital pension and Employment Insurance (EI) contributions

These expense lines may vary from hospital to hospital or province to province but are representative of most institutions.

MOS refers to management and operational support staff and includes managers, clerical support staff and others not involved in direct patient care. UPP refers to unit-producing staff who provide direct patient care services, which would include pharmacists and pharmacy technicians. UPP refers to staff who contribute units of work for patient care as per the CIHI workload measurement system.

GENERAL SUPPLIES AND OTHER EXPENSES
This general category can include many different types of expenses and does not include drug or medical/surgical supply costs. This can include, but is not limited to, the following:
- printing and stationery
- housekeeping supplies
- linen supplies
- food and food wares
- general supplies and expenses
- staff training
- travel
- internal laundry processing
- other fees and charges
- delivery and courier
- other fees membership
- other fees subscription
- printing and photocopy services
- audiovisual service
- equipment maintenance external
- equipment purchases

MEDICAL AND SURGICAL SUPPLIES
The items used in the production of medications or packaging supplies, etc., can include the following:
- general medical/surgical supplies
- needles
- syringes
- gloves
- IV solution supplies

DRUGS
In many cases, the cost of drugs will exceed all other costs in the pharmacy portfolio. It is one of the few, if not the only, functional areas in a hospital where the cost of supplies, including drugs, exceeds the other costs, including salaries. Although the cost of drugs may only be a small percentage of the overall operating costs of the hospital, they usually have a high profile with decision makers due to high unit costs for some drugs (e.g., cancer chemotherapy drugs).

The responsibility for the drug budget varies from hospital to hospital depending on the organizational structure of the hospital. For example, in hospitals that use a programmatic structure, the drugs may be charged to the different clinical programs. In other cases, it could be the responsibility of the nursing unit or the pharmacy department. In almost all cases, pharmacy is responsible for monitoring the use of drugs as well as tracking the dollars involved.

Most pharmacy departments utilize a computer system that tracks medications as they are dispensed to the patients according to hospital-based parameters. This could include directly to a patient profile for the purpose of capturing individual patient costs, to a nursing unit cost centre, to a program cost centre, to the pharmacy department or a combination of any of these.

Drug costs can be broken down into different categories based on the need of the organization or for the purposes of reporting to government. For example, drugs could be reported under categories such as cancer chemotherapy, total parenteral nutrition, ward stock or drugs general. Each organization or pharmacy department may choose to subdivide categories based on the needs of the organization.

DRUG THERAPY MONITORING

A key role of pharmacy services is to monitor drug therapy through pharmacists who work in the clinical areas of the hospital or in the pharmacy department. All medication orders are reviewed and verified by a pharmacist and changes are made in consultation with prescribers. The pharmacists perform interventions with the prescriber to ensure the order is correct in terms of dose, frequency, no potential drug-drug interactions, etc. This may also involve making recommendations to change to another medication based upon efficacy and cost according to the hospital's formulary.[9]

Drug therapy monitoring includes the following:
- therapeutic appropriateness of the drug regimen
- therapeutic duplication in the drug regimen
- appropriate route and method of drug administration
- drug-drug, drug-food, drug-laboratory or drug-disease interaction
- clinical pharmacokinetics to evaluate efficacy and safety based on patient's lab values
- monitoring, detecting, documenting, reporting and managing adverse drug reactions
- participation in Drug Use Evaluation (DUE)

DRUG USE EVALUATION

DUE is a structured process to ensure drugs are being used appropriately in the organization. A drug use evaluation is a form of quality assurance that uses current evidence to develop drug use guidelines that can be implemented in collaboration with prescribers and others on the interdisciplinary team.

Typically, the introduction of the DUE program is approved by the P&T Committee to ensure that all prescribers are aware that a review of drug use is being undertaken. The results of the initial review are provided to the P&T Committee, which provides input and approves the next steps. A typical DUE program would have the following steps:
1. Assign responsibility.
2. Perform an overall assessment of drug use patterns.
3. Identify specific drugs or drug classes to be monitored and evaluated.
4. Develop criteria for drug use based on current evidence.

5. Collect and organize the data.
6. Evaluate drug use as compared to the criteria developed.
7. Take appropriate actions to solve problem or improve drug use.
8. Assess the effectiveness of the actions taken and document the results.
9. Communicate outcomes to the key stakeholders.

The main purpose of DUE is to evaluate current prescribing of the identified drugs and provide the prescribers with feedback based on the current evidence. The most important goal in conducting a DUE is to ensure the safe and effective use of drugs. Reducing drug costs is also an important consideration but would not take priority over safety and efficacy.[9]

THE BUDGETING PROCESS

Each organization in the provincial health system must submit a budget to the funding agency. The fiscal year for governments and publicly funded agencies is usually April 1 to March 31 each year.

The budgeting process usually starts four to five months before the start of the next fiscal year. The follow example shows the steps in the process:

1. Budget forms containing actual year-to-date revenues and expenses are provided to the manager. At this time, they may be given a targeted reduction if it is felt that there will be a shortfall in funding.
2. The manager then verifies actual staff in the department and whether they are full time, part time or casual and their budgeted hours and salaries.
3. The manager will also review all supplies and the actual year-to-date and provide a budget for the coming year.
4. The manager will then submit a preliminary budget for consideration.
5. The manager may have to review the budget and make changes based on the hospital's projections of revenue for the coming year.
6. All department or program budgets are rolled up into the overall organization's budget submitted to the Board of the hospital/organization for final approval.
7. The budget is then submitted to the government/funding agency for approval.

BUDGET DEVELOPMENT CONSIDERATIONS

Each manager must be aware of the trends in the organization in terms of patient activity and acuity. Workload measurement can be a valuable tool in determining the resource needs for the coming year including labour and supply costs. If workload is significantly higher than the previous year, it could be part of a case to increase resources. Most hospitals today require a business case be developed to justify any increases in resources unless there is new legislation that mandates changes.

The manager must be aware of any proposed salary increases or other benefits being considered either from finance or through terms in a collective agreement. The manager should be aware of any inflation for drugs in particular, to provide accurate information to the organization as the budget is prepared. The manager should also be aware of changes in prescribing and new drug molecules that may come on the market in the coming fiscal year.

VARIANCE REPORTING

Once the budget has been approved, the manager is responsible for preparing a monthly variance report to advise the organization of any major changes and to forecast the year-end actual costs and revenues.

Each month, the department or service is provided with the current month and year-to-date financials, which include the revenues, expenses and workload. This report data is collected from various sources. Salaries, including benefits, etc., are provided by the payroll system. General supplies and medical surgical supplies are provided by the hospital through the general ledger. In some cases, the pharmacy department may have to provide drug costs and workload data to the finance department that cannot be collected by the computer system.

Upon receipt of this report, the manager must respond with a variance report and provide reasons why the actual numbers vary from the budget. The tolerance may vary from hospital to hospital, but it is important to note that variances of +/− a specific percentage and/or a total dollar threshold must be explained. In addition, the manager is usually required to provide a projection of the year end and to make adjustments to spending or increasing revenues that will bring the actuals in line with the budget if possible.

In the case of salaries and supplies, the manager can make some adjustments to bring the expenses in line. However, it is far more challenging to bring the drug costs in line since the drivers of the drug costs are physicians, the patient volumes and patient acuity. In this case, it is important for the manager to be aware of patient activity and acuity as well as monitoring drug use in the organization to be able to explain the variances.

The hospital collects all patient activity and acuity data and will make it available to the manager as a part of their monitoring function.

WORKLOAD MEASUREMENT

Most organizations require that all workload be measured and reported as part of the overall reports that must provided to the government or other funding agencies. There is a national workload measurement system that has been developed by CIHI that forms the basis for the workload measurement system. The extent of reporting may vary from hospital to hospital and province to province/territory to territory.

The majority of drug distribution workload is captured through the pharmacy computer system using the CIHI workload measurement standards. Each activity is assigned several units that represent minutes to complete the task. This system assigns time values to various drug distribution units such as oral unit doses, IV doses, total parenteral nutrition (TPN) doses and chemotherapy doses dispensed. Details are available in the CIHI workload documents.[10]

The direct patient care activities of pharmacy staff is more challenging to collect since there is no standard time assigned to each activity. This usually requires pharmacists to document the actual time per activity in a separate system that can vary from hospital to hospital.

This information is often used for benchmarking to compare productivity between and across organizations. It can also be used as a tool to justify increased or decreased resources.

PURCHASING PHARMACEUTICALS

Pharmacy services are responsible for the acquisition of pharmaceuticals based upon the decisions of P&T to add the drugs to the formulary. In addition, pharmaceutical products may need to be acquired on a non-formulary basis for patients who are admitted and already stabilized on these medications. It is important that pharmacy services and specifically a pharmacist be the key decision maker in the acquisition of the drugs.

Once there has been a decision on the molecule, pharmacy will determine the brand, if there is more than one supplier, the quantity, etc.

The knowledge and skills of the pharmacist are mandatory in this process to ensure the quality of these products from the aspect of product integrity, packaging and labelling. The day-to-day activities of purchasing and inventory control are usually carried out by trained technicians and other support staff.

The process of acquisition is often facilitated through group purchasing organizations (GPOs) who utilize the product volumes of several member organizations who achieve drug cost savings through economies of scale for multisource products and through volume discounts through single source products from vendors. These GPOs also comply with all fair competition rules such as the broader public sector regulations in Ontario.

GROUP PURCHASING ORGANIZATIONS

Most hospitals participate in contracting through GPOs to achieve economies of scale, not only for pharmaceuticals, but also for a range of other products and services. Advantages include the following:

- lowest possible drug costs
- standardization of drug products
- reduction of contract labour costs for institutions
- enhancement of member institution's purchasing program
- enhanced information sharing
- enhanced purchasing expertise
- achievement of longer contract periods of price protection
- reduced duplication of purchasing efforts among institutions

The success of these group purchasing organizations depends on the commitment of its members to honour the contract awards for the agreed-upon volumes.

These group purchasing organizations usually have a pharmacy subcommittee that makes decisions on which products should be tendered, reviews all responses to the requests for quotation, as well as ensures all products meet a high standard in terms of quality. Usually, the decisions are made first on quality and safety and then on price. Other considerations could include the company's reliability in terms of supply and in some cases, there may be other value adds such as education or research support.

INVENTORY CONTROL

All of the processes described in the previous purchasing pharmaceuticals section are applicable to hospital practice in terms of inventory control.

In addition to fast-moving products, hospitals are also required to carry stock of antidote medications and other emergency medications that will add to the inventory costs and will not be able to be turned at the same rate as the regular medications.

Increased inventory turns need to be balanced with ensuring there are adequate quantities of medications available to meet the fluctuating and sometimes unpredictable needs of patients[9] (see Chapter 22: Inventory Management).

COST-CONTROL STRATEGIES

In all hospitals, there are restrictions on signing authority that limit the amount that various levels of staff can purchase. Through this process, managers will have a firsthand accounting of receipts and expenditures and are able to monitor the actuals against the budget. Each month, the manager is provided with a summary of all of their revenues and expenses as well as the detail behind these numbers.

The pharmacy director/manager can manage the costs directly under their control such as salaries and supplies.

Participation in GPOs is an effective way for hospitals to control acquisition costs of drugs while minimizing the time required to conduct their own contract administration. In addition to the actual costs provided, the manager must be aware of other activities that may explain an increase or decrease in the use of supplies and the increased use of labour.

The manager must be able to monitor activities of the hospital including the following:
- patient activity such as admissions, discharges and acuity measures
- workload measurement statistics including drug distribution and direct patient care activities
- raw counts of production including oral doses, IV admixtures, chemotherapy doses, TPN, ward stock and any compounded items dispensed
- changes in case mix where the organization is undertaking more complex procedures or disease entities
- overtime hours paid due to increased workload (direct salaries can be controlled by limiting the use of overtime unless absolutely needed. If workload increases and more labour is needed, then the manager must use the workload data to be able to justify any overages in wages[10,11])

BENCHMARKING

There are several tools available to managers to allow them to compare their pharmacy services with those in other organizations. In Canada, a benchmarking survey is done every second year that provides a comprehensive list of comparator data (the Hospital Pharmacy in Canada survey). Managers can use this information to compare their own service with those of comparable departments. In addition, provinces/territories may have benchmarking tools that are provided to the institutions to allow for appropriate comparisons of costs and utilization of staff and supplies.

Benchmarking can be a valuable tool in allowing the manager to make decisions and develop strategies to ensure the most appropriate use of the hospital's resources allocated to pharmacy.[10]

RESOURCES AND SUGGESTED READINGS

Gillerman RG, Browning RA. Drug use inefficiency: a hidden source of wasted health care dollars. Anesth Analg. 2000;91(4):921–4. http://dx.doi.org/10.1097/00000539-200010000-00028. Medline:11004049

Hibberd JM, Smith DL. *Nursing leadership and management in Canada*. 3rd ed. Toronto: Elsevier Mosby Canada; 2006.

Longest BB Jr, Rakich JS, Darr K. *Managing health care services organizations and systems*. 4th ed. Maryland: Health Professions Press; 2000.

Miller DE, Fox-Smith K. Pharmacy revenue cycle audits can bring unexpected returns Kristin Healthcare Financial Management; Oct 2012; 66, 10; ProQuest Central pg. 78.

REFERENCES

1. The Canada Health Act. Available: http://laws-lois.justice.gc.ca/eng/acts/C-6/ (accessed Nov. 9, 2014).

2. Federal Narcotics and Controlled Substance Act. Available: http://laws-lois.justice.gc.ca/eng/acts/C-38.8/ (accessed Nov. 9, 2014).

3. Provincial Hospitals Act.

4. Provincial Health Insurance Acts.

5. Provincial Pharmacy Acts.

6. Provincial Regulated Health Professions Act.

7. Accreditation Canada. Available: www.accreditation.ca (accessed Nov. 9, 2014).

8. MIS Standards, 2013

9. Brown TR, ed. *Handbook of institutional pharmacy practice*. 4th ed. Maryland: ASHP; 2006.

10. Canadian Institute for Health Information. MIS workload measurement. Available: www.cihi.ca/CIHI-ext-portal/internet/EN/TabbedContent/standards+and+data+submission/standards/mis+standards/cihi010691 (accessed Nov. 9, 2014).

11. Hospital pharmacy in Canada survey.

V. RISK MANAGEMENT

CHAPTER 19

Managing Risk in a Pharmacy Setting

Michael S. Jaczko, BSc. Phm., RPh, CIM® (Chartered Investment Manager); Partner and Portfolio Manager, K J Harrison & Partners Inc., Toronto, ON

Pharmacists tend to be risk-averse people as a general rule. A pharmacy manager or pharmacy owner may ponder, "Why on earth would I take a chance and subject myself to potential risk? After all, bad things can happen when I stick my neck out!" In practice, most managers and owners accept a certain degree of risk each and every day. Most business operators are inherently prepared to accept some form or level of risk. Conversely, the fact of the matter is that entrepreneurs inherently believe they can take advantage of these risks, build a successful pharmacy practice and ultimately generate value.

Learning Objectives

- Define how the various elements of risk appear in a pharmacy.
- Identify the types of risk to which a pharmacy can be exposed.
- Be able to develop a risk management plan in your pharmacy.
- Identify potential strategies: risk avoidance, mitigation of risk, acceptance of risk and transfer of risk.

Successful entrepreneurs and managers intuitively understand that wealth is made by concentrating risk (taking on risk), while wealth is preserved by diversifying risk. This section introduces the concept of risk as it relates to the factors that can potentially affect a pharmacy business.

WHAT IS RISK?

Risk relates to uncertainty and the variability associated in life and business. A risk is an uncertain event or condition that, if it occurs, can have a positive or negative effect on a person's life or a business.

Risk in the pharmacy business context is defined as the implications of the existence of significant uncertainty about the activities, markets and clinical and business environment a pharmacy operates in.

Depending on people's personalities, a level of risk (the chance of a bad outcome) is accepted because the possible positive outcome is valued. Alternatively, a risk might be considered if the possibility of a bad outcome can be mitigated. The degree to which the possibility of a bad outcome, or its extent, cannot be totally eliminated is by definition the risk people are willing to accept.

TYPES OF RISK

Risk can be sliced and diced in several ways.[1] Think of risk in three distinct categories. First, there are business risks taken by pharmacy owners engaging in the normal course of business, particularly new startups, but risk also lurks in well-established pharmacy operations. The second type of risk refers to financial risks new owners take when they commit their hard-earned money to a new pharmacy practice. This is referred to as placing your capital at risk and defines true ownership. Finally, there are personal risks, which again entrepreneurs take when they commit themselves to a new pharmacy business venture.

BUSINESS RISK

Business risks are those a pharmacy is exposed to because of the commercial and professional nature of the pharmacy practice. These risks have the potential to adversely affect the profitability or even sustainability of the pharmacy practice. Managers and owners must constantly remain vigilant of these risks and be sure to identify them as part of preparing a business plan.

Business risks reflect a combination of revenue risk and operating risk. Such risks combined directly affect the variability of the earnings before interest and tax (EBIT). Because these risks can be identified, managers and owners can modify a pharmacy's business risk through careful decision making; for example, targeting and deploying appropriate resources to customers and patients who actually exist in the market place (i.e., revenue risk).

Business risk is a function of the variability of operating conditions faced by a pharmacy operation. Namely, the higher the degree of variation in operating earnings in the foreseeable future, the higher the business risk. Drug reform currently exerted by provincial/territorial governments is a salient example of business risk.

The wider the variation in a pharmacy business's earnings, the greater the business risk. Understanding the various types of risk is important because each category demands a different (but related) set of risk-management skills.

INTERNAL BUSINESS RISK

Internal business risk, which focuses on the operational efficiency with which a retail pharmacy runs, is referred to as operational risk. This risk relates to how well a store or dispensary is organized. (See Section VI: Operations for topics of discussion involving work flow and dispensary clutter.) A well-designed work flow with minimal distractions and well-organized operational flow tends to attract fewer problems and is likely more successful in coping with the challenges encountered. Furthermore, motivated staff who operate with a coordinated focus tend to handle challenges with considerably less disruption and, resultantly, fewer dispensary errors.

It is important to note that internal business risks are factors that are in the direct control of management. The key to managing operational risk relates directly to the environment created or the culture of an organization. The pharmacy owners are directly responsible for incurring and managing operational risk. Risk management means being aware and challenging what is happening and asking tough questions. It involves constant vigilance and avoiding complacency. The character and environment of a pharmacy operation bears direct resemblance to the personality and character of its owner(s) and/or its manager(s). Culture defines what behaviours are or are not acceptable in the pharmacy work environment. Without a culture that promotes risk management, the operation of the pharmacy is more open to a myriad of issues, misfortune and more risk.

EXTERNAL BUSINESS RISK

External business risk reflects operating conditions imposed upon the pharmacy business that is not under the direct control of the manager or owner. External factors can include the following:

- The *cost of capital*, which is subject to changes in the rate of interest and the ability of a pharmacy operation to service its debt, namely the ability to repay its lenders in a timely, uninterrupted manner.
- The *local business (economic) cycle* is the most pervasive external risk factor, but only if unexpected; otherwise, it is just poor management of costs in relation to expected changes in revenues. Example: a local mill shuts down permanently. But if it shuts down every summer and sales drop, stock and labour can be reduced during this time. The real risk or unknown is whether the decision will adversely affect the store's reputation for things such as selection and service.
- *Demographic shifts* in a community population also influence the economic health of a pharmacy operation.
- *Political policy changes* present a force to reckon with as provincial/territorial government-sponsored drug reform continues to sweep across Canada. In addition, shifts in government philosophy relating to monetary and fiscal policy can have an effect on the cost of borrowing (credit) and an impact on the overall economic environment in which a pharmacy operates.

The implications of external business risks tend to be complex, sometimes unclear and resultantly mixed. Through advocacy efforts, local chambers of commerce and provincial/territorial/national pharmacy associations such as the Canadian Pharmacists Association (CPhA) often seek to mitigate some of these risks on behalf of those they represent. Some of the external factors, however, may represent social trends less susceptible to such efforts.

FINANCIAL RISK

Financial risk is particularly focused on the manner in which a pharmacy finances its operations. Typically, a pharmacy, whether a startup or purchased by new owners through acquisition, can either invest personal capital (referred to as risk equity) or borrow money (referred to as debt capital).

By using debt (a mortgage) to finance a pharmacy, the store is committing to paying a fixed financial charge that must be paid regardless of the level of the pharmacy business's earnings. Conversely, owners who choose to invest their own capital into a pharmacy business will have smaller fixed periodic cash payments to "service" or repay debt.

Financial *leverage* encompasses three elements:

- increases the variability of the pharmacy's net earnings
- affects the pharmacy's expectations of earnings
- increases the risk of potential failure

The greater the use of debt, the greater the financial leverage and, therefore, the greater the risk to which the business is exposed.

PERSONAL RISKS

Risks that relate to the consequences a business failure would have on an investor in a pharmacy business involve many possibly outcomes:

- invested cash money that can be lost
- money borrowed personally may be lost, leading the owner into business bankruptcy
- personal security provided to a financier could lead to personal bankruptcy
- business partners may experience problems such as health issues or divorce
- loss of personal self-esteem or reputation as a result of a bankruptcy

The bottom line is that there is real risk associated with borrowing money or committing to personal guarantees. Those wanting to be owners should retain the services of experienced legal, accounting and business professionals when considering going into business. However, the potential rewards of doing so can make the effort considerably worthwhile.

OPERATIONAL RISK

Operational risk presents itself in many forms.[2]

- *Internal fraud* reflects employees stealing from you or your patients and customers (see Chapter 23: Loss Prevention in Pharmacy). It is the responsibility of management and owners to create a work environment that reduces the temptations associated with a workplace that handles cash and drugs.

- *External fraud* refers to customers and patients committing theft, committing forgeries or participating in a robbery before, during or after store hours (see Chapter 23: Loss Prevention in Pharmacy).

Due to the inherent uncertainty associated with health care and the high performance standards, legal action associated with liability claims for not meeting those standards are common for pharmacies and can affect pharmacy operators and owners. Furthermore, lawsuits can name pharmacy businesses, owners and pharmacists as defendants in legal claims.

Pharmacists remain fortunate to be able to self-govern their profession through the auspices of provincial/territorial colleges. However, pressures associated with rising standards and practice, as well as rapidly evolving roles for pharmacists in the health care system, have the potential for operational mishaps and professional malpractice.

Medication errors occur due to poor or failed processing breakdowns. These errors can be attributed to individual mistakes, poor workflow and less-than-efficient work environments.

System failures attributed to technical challenges, such as glitches in computer hardware or pharmacy practice management software, and failures in telecommunications resources at store level or at server host locations, can all lead to system breakdown and decreased patient service levels. Pharmacists remain vulnerable to the extent that they continue to expand their dependency on such systems.

As a result of certain events, such as the train derailment disaster in Lac-Mégantic, Québec, and the floods in Calgary, Alberta, disaster recovery and business continuity are topics that hit close to home for many pharmacists. Pharmacy managers and owners must be concerned with the pharmacy's ability to recover quickly and completely from these types of disasters and ensure continuity of the pharmacy practice (see Chapter 26: Contingency Planning).

Inappropriate professional and business practices have the potential to haunt any pharmacy practice. The way frontline staff members conduct themselves in business and in their interactions with customers and patients directly reflects on the image or brand of the pharmacy in the community it serves.

Only with careful planning and monitoring can these main operational risks be managed effectively.

RISK MANAGEMENT

Risk is inherent in any business. Managers and owners must assess risks continually and develop plans to address them. The financial risk that arises from uncertainty can and should be managed.

Furthermore, do not think of mastering risk in defensive terms alone.[3] A risk management plan contains an analysis of likely risk with both low and high impact, as well as mitigation strategies. For example, for an entrepreneur, the essence of risk management is not avoiding or eliminating risk but deciding which risks to accept, which ones to pass through to others and which ones to avoid or hedge.[4]

However, remain mindful above all that there is no comfort to be taken in acting in a reckless manner. Pharmacy owners who remain selective as to which risks they are prepared to incur can exploit such risks to their advantage, but pharmacy owners who take risks without sufficiently anticipating or preparing for subsequent consequences can prove to be problematic and in some cases, fatal to the business practice.

The risk management plan is a process and resultant document that a pharmacy manager or owner prepares with a view to anticipating risks, approximating the resultant impact of these risks and ultimately, developing strategies and tactics to respond to potential risks. Figure 19.1 illustrates a sample risk management process that is readily adaptable to a pharmacy environment.

Figure 19.1

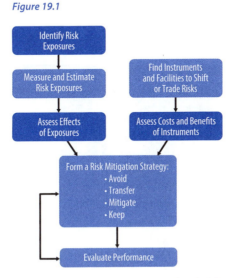

The Risk Management Process (reproduced with the permission of McGraw-Hill Education from Crouhy M, Galai D, Mark R. Risk Management – A Helicopter View. In: The Essentials of Risk Management. NY: McGraw-Hill, 2006)

Much of what distinguishes a modern economy from those of the past is the ability to identify risk, measure it, appreciate its consequences and then take action accordingly. Most critically, a risk management plan includes a risk strategy.

Remaining constantly vigilant to identifying potential exposure to risk remains the key. After identifying potentials risks, it is best to measure and estimate the risk exposure financially, as well as the potential effect of such exposures should the risk materialize. As a result, the pharmacy manager/owner is in a position to form a risk mitigation strategy. Broadly, there are four potential strategies, with numerous variations. Pharmacy managers and owners may choose to do the following:

- Avoid risk by changing plans to circumvent the potential problem and, therefore, choose to head in a different direction.
- Transfer risk by outsourcing risk (or a portion of the risk) to third parties, such as insurance companies, that can manage the outcome. This is achieved financially through the strategic use of insurance products, hedging transactions[5] or operationally outsourcing an activity (central fill, for example).
- Control/Mitigate risk, which reduces the impact or likelihood (or both) through intermediate steps.
- Accept/Keep risk by taking a chance of a negative impact (self-insure to the extent of accepting a higher insurance deductible). These potential costs can be budgeted via a contingency budget line.

Finally, it remains paramount to monitor the risk mitigation strategies employed to ensure the choices made remain appropriate, relevant and effective.[6] (See Chapter 20: Insurance Basics for the strategic use of insurance as a vehicle to transfer risk and the important role a well-constructed shareholder agreement can play in the life of a pharmacy owner partnership.)

REFERENCES

1. Muffee VW. Types of risk. In: *Risk management: theory and practice*. New York: Nova Science Publishers, Inc; 2004. p. 11–25.
2. Dickstein DI, Flast RH. Where we are now. In: *No excuses – a business process approach to managing operation risk*. New Jersey: John Wiley & Sons, Inc; 2009. p. 32–91.
3. Crouhy M, Galai D, Mark R. Risk management – a helicopter view. In: *The essentials of risk management*. NY: McGraw-Hill; 2006.
4. Entrepeneur. Starting a business, business plan risks. Dec. 11, 2004. Available: www.entrepreneur.com/article/49042 (accessed April 29, 2014).
5. Chew DH. Corporate risk management: Journal of Applied Corporate Finance – Columbia Business School Publishing. 2007.
6. Reuvid J. Basic principles of risk management. In: *Managing business risk – a practical guide to protecting your business*. 8th ed. Philadelphia, PA: Kogan Page Limited; 2012. p. 8–13.

CHAPTER 20

Insurance Basics

Michael S. Jaczko, *BSc. Phm., RPh, CIM® (Chartered Investment Manager); Partner and Portfolio Manager, K J Harrison & Partners Inc., Toronto, ON*

Ron Poole, *Risk Management Consultants of Ontario (RMCO) member*

John T. Hunt, *LL.B., LL.M., CFP, CLU*

Learning Objectives

- Understand the various types of insurance a pharmacy business owner needs to consider when managing or owning a pharmacy business.

- Be able to discuss the key aspects about personal professional liability insurance and be in a position to better self-assess their personal needs.

- Be knowledgeable about the application and strategic use of life insurance in a pharmacy business practice.

PHARMACY BUSINESS INSURANCE

Insurance is the transfer of the risk of a loss, from one entity to another, in exchange for payment (see Chapter 19: Managing Risk in a Pharmacy Setting). Insurance is a form of risk management primarily used to hedge against the risk of a contingent, uncertain loss referred to as indemnification. By purchasing insurance, the purchaser enters into a contract with an insurance company for a specific period of time. It protects the customer financially against a loss. Insurance is a mechanism for dispersing risk because it shares the losses of the few among the many.[1]

An insurer, or insurance carrier, is a company selling the insurance. The insured, or policyholder, is the person or entity buying the insurance policy. The amount of money to be charged for a certain amount of insurance coverage is called the premium. The insurance policy details the conditions and circumstances under which the insured will be financially compensated.

TYPES OF BUSINESS INSURANCE

Insurance coverage is available for every conceivable risk a pharmacy business can imagine. The only limit to insurance is the cost and amount of coverage of policies, which vary among insurers. Pharmacists should develop a business relationship with a trusted insurance broker.

General liability insurance

Pharmacy business owners purchase general liability insurance to cover legal circumstances that arise from an accident, injuries and claims of negligence. General liability insurance policies protect against bodily injury, property damage, medical expenses, libel, slander, the cost of defending lawsuits and settlement bonds or judgments required during an appeal procedure.

Commercial property insurance

Property insurance covers everything related to the loss and damage of a pharmacy's company property as a result of a wide variety of events such as fire, smoke, wind and hail storms, civil disobedience and vandalism. The definition of property is broad and includes lost income, business interruption, buildings, computers, company documents and money.

Liability insurance

Liability insurance is designed to offer specific protection against third-party insurance claims and typically would be paid to someone suffering loss while at a pharmacy, such as a customer or a patient. An important form of liability insurance, professional liability insurance (PLI), is discussed later in this chapter.

Commercial vehicle insurance

Depending on the options chosen, commercial auto insurance coverage can include the following:
- bodily injury
- property damage
- personal injury
- collision coverage
- comprehensive coverage

Commercial umbrella insurance

Umbrella insurance refers to liability insurance that is in excess of specified other policies and is also, potentially, primary insurance for losses not covered by other policies. The *umbrella* term is a reference to the broad coverage nature of the policy. When the insured is liable to someone, the insured's primary insurance policies pay up to their limits, and any additional amount is paid by the umbrella policy (up to the limit of the umbrella policy). Examples of liability an umbrella policy may cover include libel, slander and invasion of privacy.

Insurance can be readily purchased through financial institutions, local insurance brokers and provincial/territorial association programs. In today's world, the option not to participate in a business insurance program is not considered a reasonable option, as it is often a condition of being permitted to engage is a particular enterprise.

PERSONAL PROFESSIONAL LIABILITY INSURANCE FOR PHARMACISTS

The majority of the provincial/territorial Colleges and Boards regulating pharmacy in Canada require pharmacists to carry professional liability insurance (PLI) that meet their criteria. The coverage criteria will vary from province to province/territory to territory, but will likely include some, and may impose all, of the following requirements:

Policies are generally written with minimum coverage limits; for example, $2 million per claims occurrence and $4 million in total for all occurrences in the course of a single policy year.

The scope of the professional services covered under the policy must exactly coincide with the practice of pharmacy as regulated by the respective provincial/territorial College. Therefore, as Colleges expand the scope of practice over time, remain mindful that the scope of coverage under PLI should expand commensurately.

A policy must provide full retroactive coverage. This means that all claims that are *first discovered* while the policy is in effect must be insured, even though they may have been *incurred* before the policy took effect.

Legal expenses incurred in the defence of a claim must not erode the limits available for the payment of an award to a plaintiff. For example, a plaintiff's award might be $2 million, and the legal and related expenses might be $400,000, for a total of $2.4 million. If the pharmacist's policy is written with a limit of $2 million, there must be provision for legal expense recovery in excess of the limit—in other words, a recovery of $2.4 million, and not $2 million.

There must be coverage for an extended reporting provision (ERP) for a minimum period of three years. This grants coverage to a pharmacist for any PLI claims incurred during the time they were professionally active but first discovered after they left the profession (e.g., retirement).

The policy must be in the pharmacist's name and provide mobility and coverage wherever the pharmacist practises. This ensures coverage if the pharmacist normally works for more than one employer or changes employment during the course of a policy year.

When requested by the Registrar of the College, the pharmacist must provide evidence of the insurance in the required limits and form. This often occurs at the annual renewing process and in most cases is now conducted online.

The lack of pan-Canadian harmonization in both the scope of practice and the regulation of PLI criteria remains problematic for those who need licences to practice in two or more jurisdictions. It is not uncommon for a practitioner who resides in a border town to cross provincial/territorial boundary lines daily. The National Association of Pharmacy Regulatory Agencies (NAPRA) regularly brings representatives of all Colleges and Boards together for discussion of common issues and coordinated solutions. However, there is currently no public evidence of a NAPRA initiative to bring about uniform risk exposure (for scope of practice) or a harmonized set of national PLI standards.

It is important to remember that not all PLI policies are the same. Even if the policy meets regulatory requirements, the quality of the insurance can vary widely, from best in class to average and seriously defective.

Some pharmacists are encouraged to join programs sponsored by their employers that provide personal PLI. The employer frequently holds the group PLI Master Policy, and the employees receive a certificate, drawn under the master policy, giving them personal evidence of coverage. Master policies arranged by employers may or may not be compliant with provincial/territorial College regulations, and the certificates pharmacists receive from the employer's PLI program are often devoid of any information that would allow the employees to evaluate their coverage with respect to this or any other point of important detail. It is not uncommon for pharmacy practitioners to purchase additional PLI coverage above and beyond corporately sponsored programs.

Having PLI coverage for the following items is important for the employee, but of lesser interest to the employer:

- retroactive PLI coverage for claims incurred before an employee's date of hire, but first discovered subsequently
- coverage while working simultaneously from time to time for another employer
- coverage for claims incurred during the term of employment, but discovered after leaving that employment

These insurance needs should be pursued by employees, whether or not covered by the insurance regulations of their provincial/territorial regulator, and regardless of whether they are purchasing coverage under their employer's program or independently.

PLI is also required by the pharmacy business itself in the event that the store is named in a law suit, separately or as a joint defendant, for professional liability. Accordingly, it is also recommended that a second PLI policy in the name of the commercial entity be purchased.

The standard comprehensive general liability policy issued for commercial operations such as pharmacy businesses always contains an exclusion with respect to professional liability. Fill this gap by purchasing PLI coverage for the pharmacy business. It is not sufficient to remove the professional liability exclusion from the pharmacy's commercial general liability policy (which is seldom possible in any event). Note that most commercial general liability insurance typically only covers liability arising from bodily injury and property damage and will not stretch to include such matters as breaches of confidentiality, lack of product efficacy, defective advice or financial loss not associated with bodily injury. An entity PLI policy, properly written, will cover these latter issues and other problems under the PLI insuring agreement.

Do not accept a Certificate of Insurance as the sole professional liability insurance document—it provides very little real insight into the coverage purchased. Insist on obtaining a full copy of the policy and, over time, become as familiar with its terms and conditions as possible. It can prevent or mitigate financial distress and be called upon to defend one's professional license and reputation. It may be difficult to read, but it is too important to ignore.

Also, do not allow premium charges to be the only criterion in choosing one PLI product over another. Currently, annual PLI premiums range from approximately $90 to $300 depending on the limits selected and quality of coverage. Do not automatically select the cheaper product or assume that the most expensive policy must be best.

In relative terms, the difference in price is inconsequential. Be driven by differences in coverage. Become informed about these differences and of their significance. Remember that insurance is defined as the substitution of a definite but affordable loss (the premium), for an uncertain and unaffordable loss. Make this substitution as reliable as you can.

STRATEGIC USE OF LIFE INSURANCE

For this section, assume that a pharmacy operation is operating as a provincially/territorially or federally chartered corporation.

Life insurance is a contract between an insurance company and the owner of the policy. It provides for the tax-free payment of a specific sum of money to a beneficiary upon the death of the person insured. The owner (also known as the life insured) and beneficiary may or may not be the same person.

Life insurance policies are either term policies that expire after a set term or permanent policies that last for the life of the person insured if the policy premiums are paid. Some permanent life insurance policies have intrinsic cash values that can be accessed before death. Some allow for the overfunding of the policy into an investment account to increase the cash value or to increase the payment upon death. Term policies generally do not have these features.

Pharmacy owners are not much different from other corporate owners when it comes to the strategic use of life insurance. In a corporate setting, the owner of the policy is the corporation. The life insured is typically a shareholder or executive of the company. The beneficiary is almost always the corporation. To make someone else the beneficiary can lead to problems from the point of view of conferring benefits on shareholders or executives who are potentially subject to income tax.

When the life-insured person dies, the insurance proceeds from the policy are paid to the corporation tax free. The company can then pay out these insurance proceeds to the shareholders as a tax-free capital dividend to the extent to which the insurance proceeds exceed the adjusted cost base of the policy. The adjusted cost base of the policy generally diminishes over time and eventually goes to zero. This is a very effective way of getting money out of the corporate structure and leads to tax-planning opportunities that can be undertaken with the pharmacist's team (lawyer, accountant, insurance advisor).

Key person insurance involves the purchase of life insurance to provide funds for the company to operate in an interim period if the pharmacy owner or other key person dies prematurely. The untimely death of a pharmacy business owner or key executive in any business can have a severe financial impact. This is all the more true in a business such as a pharmacy where one person is often the essence of the operation. When a business owner dies, the daily operation of the business is inevitably affected. The key decision maker has been lost, and the more key that person is, the more likely the business will grind to a halt. The morale of the employees will be damaged. Creditors and lenders may get nervous and demand immediate payment of outstanding obligations. A cash infusion to allow the business to stay afloat for long enough to create and implement a plan for the future can make the difference between surviving or not.

Many pharmacists have business loans from banks or other financial institutions. Having an insurance policy to cover the repayment of these debts in the event of premature death is a very good idea in similar fashion to key person insurance. As a practical matter, the creditor may insist on this insurance.

In situations where two or more pharmacists together own a pharmacy, they should enter into a shareholders' agreement that sets out the rights and obligations of each party. Often such agreements will oblige one of the parties to purchase the shares of the company of the other party in the event of death. But where will this money come from? Life insurance is often the best and most cost-effective way to ensure the funds are available when needed. Various arrangements are possible. This life insurance might be owned by the corporation or by the individual pharmacists personally.

The Canadian Income Tax Act deems that every capital asset a person owns—an investment portfolio, real estate, shares in a pharmacy—is deemed to be sold the day before the person dies.[2]

With a few exceptions, such as the house one lived in (the principal residence), one-half of any gain in value on this deemed sale is subject to income tax. Planning should be done to ensure there is money in a person's estate to pay this tax liability. Otherwise, the surviving heirs might face a situation of having to sell off assets they do not want to sell—such as a family cottage, for example—to raise the funds to pay taxes. Life insurance is an effective tool to meet this liability. Life insurance proceeds are paid tax-free and avoid probate where beneficiaries have been named (as opposed to simply naming the estate). Life insurance proceeds are typically paid to beneficiaries within a few weeks of death. Insurance for this purpose might be owned personally or by the corporation depending on the situation and the specific details of the estate plan.

Life insurance can also be used for estate equalization. Parents generally want to be fair to their children. For business owners, normally their first impulse in business succession planning or estate planning is to split the shares of any family business equally among their children—but this might not be the wisest choice in every situation.

Assume that a pharmacist has three children and one child works in the business. The plan is for this child to eventually be the head of the business. These types of family business successions require careful planning and thought. Family meetings and discussions are highly recommended. As part of the business succession or estate plan, it is often a bad idea for the pharmacist or other business owner to transfer or bequeath the shares of the company to all the children if only one child is working in the business. This can lead to conflict between the siblings, and it can lead to financial pressures on the business if any of the children want to sell their shares in the future. Often, a better idea is to transfer all the shares in the business to the one child and to leave the other children other assets or the proceeds of a life insurance policy. In these cases, it should be remembered that fair is not always equal.

REFERENCES

1. Insurance Bureau of Canada glossary. Available: www.ibc.ca/on/business/risk-management (accessed Nov. 9, 2014).
2. Canadian Income Tax Act – ITA 70 (5) (a). Available: http://laws.justice.gc.ca/eng/acts/I-3.3/ (accessed Nov. 9, 2014).

VI. OPERATIONS

CHAPTER 21

Pharmacy Operations

Jody Shkrobot, *B.Sc. Pharm.*

Learning Objectives

- Describe the relationship between the need for efficient pharmacy operations and the patient's needs.
- Explain basic requirements for dispensary flow and dispensary layout.
- Describe how scheduling, workflow and people are connected relative to an efficient pharmacy operation.
- Describe how pharmacy and the pharmacists' needs and systems may change and evolve as the practice of pharmacy changes and new scopes of practice and pharmacy services are incorporated into the daily workflow.

Pharmacy operations play an important role in the success of a community pharmacy practice, but the basis for those operations needs to be measured against the needs of the consumer of the pharmacy's goods and services. Pharmacy operations include everything that goes on behind the scenes to ensure an efficient and profitable business and allows for the patients to be served professionally and in a timely manner. Operations include human resources (HR) management, inventory management, marketing and workflow, as well as all the areas covered in the other chapters in this section. As pharmacy practice continues to evolve toward a more service-based business structure,[1] pharmacy operations must adapt to new reimbursement models that are generally more focused on payments for services as opposed to payment for products. There is a balance between the two, and solid operations must achieve a balance between technical workflow and consistency and execution of professional services; however, this change cannot occur in isolation of the demands of the consumer. For many patients, a more traditional role of dispensing-related activities is in higher demand than clinical services such as extending prescription refills, medication reviews or intramuscular vaccine administration. The physical layout of the pharmacy can be a barrier to this evolution but, if properly designed, can create an efficient dispensary operation that can satisfy many of the patient's needs and the consumer's wants.

The physical layout of a pharmacy helps shape the pharmacy's workflow processes. Many pharmacy locations have physical constraints to their floor plan that are dictated by the leasehold space or structural elements within the floor plan. Over the years, workspaces have adapted to increasing prescription volumes, the integration of new technology, expanding scopes of practice and changes in consumer demands. There is no single workspace design that can be applied for all pharmacies. Linear flow, centre island formats, "bank teller" design and hybrid variations all have their advantages and disadvantages. Their efficiency often depends on prescription volumes, staffing levels and the number and types of services the pharmacy provides. (Specialty areas of pharmacy practice, such as the supply of medications to continuing care type facilities, compounding and telepharmacy services, are usually separated from the common workflow processes within a community environment and will not be discussed in this section.)

Pharmacies are designed to accommodate the needs of their customers and, in many cases, to encourage the retail aspect of the rest of the business that surrounds the dispensary itself. Most consumers come to the pharmacy to have their prescriptions filled. Even with the advent of telephone and e-refill technology, the physical act of presenting to the community pharmacy with a physical prescription or a prescription that has been faxed or telephoned into the pharmacy is the norm. The design of the dispensary must incorporate an efficient physical space where patients can easily access a pharmacy team member. Depending on the patient volume, there must be an adequate number of drop-off points to minimize lineups for patients. Most pharmacies experience peak times within the day where lineups are inevitable, but a bottleneck at drop-off can cause the consumer anxiety or frustration, leading to a loss of sales or the loss of a patient to the pharmacy. When the pharmacy staff can quickly receive the patient's request or be directly engaged with the patient, customer satisfaction rates increase.

There continues to be an ongoing debate as to who should be the individual who engages the consumer first. Should this individual be the pharmacist, pharmacy technician, pharmacy assistant or a customer service agent? Since the current funding models for pharmacy are trending toward decreasing compensation for drug distribution functions and increasing compensation opportunities for more clinical/consultative services, more pharmacies are using pharmacists and pharmacy technicians who are trained to recognize opportunities to provide clinical services at the time the patient presents to the pharmacy. A benefit of this is that more issues (e.g., drug-related problems) can be identified at the initial point of contact before prescription filling has occurred, which saves time correcting filled prescriptions, and that some clinical services (e.g., medication reviews or follow-ups) can occur when the patient is immediately available to the pharmacist. The disadvantage is that many of these interactions take longer and can create a substantial bottleneck for other consumers waiting for assistance from the pharmacy. The other challenge is having the proper personnel in place to engage in this activity. A proper physical design that allows for multiple contact points for consumers creates the most flexibility and can allow the pharmacy team to prioritize consumer requests to maximize productivity. It is also critical that the pharmacy offers adequate privacy for more in-depth patient conversations and that the pharmacist has immediate access to resources required for documenting patient interactions at the point of contact (e.g., patient records, access to provincial/territorial drug information system, clinical decision support tools, private area for more personal conversation or the administration of some drugs by injection, etc.).

Once a pharmacy team member has received the patient's request, the physical preparation of the patient's prescription occurs. Technology plays a huge role in this process, allowing pharmacies to dispense large numbers of prescriptions with low levels of errors.[2] Pharmacy software systems available on the Canadian market are very adept at documenting and managing the prescription transaction. This includes the data entry of the prescription, scanning the physical prescription itself for electronic storage, adjudication processing, inventory management and documenting the final release to the patient. The use of barcode scanning technology allows busy pharmacies to track each step of the prescription's journey through the dispensing process. This allows for more checks and balances to avoid errors, increases employee accountability and performance and allows management to monitor productivity and identify bottlenecks in the system through the use of workflow management software. After prescription drop-off, pharmacies can offer pagers, emails, SMS (text) messaging or automated telephone calls to inform patients when their prescriptions are ready. This minimizes the inconvenience of waiting to the patients, allows them to use their time (perhaps shopping in the other areas of the store) and also allows the pharmacy team to prioritize workloads that can sometimes be balanced across the workday.

The physical design of the dispensary once again plays an important role in determining how efficient the pharmacy can be in preparing prescriptions.[3] The ideal, efficient dispensary would be designed to minimize the number of steps each employee must take to prepare a prescription. For the majority of the fills a pharmacy makes on the average day, the preparation process should not require staff members to have to take more than three to four steps. This can be accomplished by using different individuals through the preparation process so that their work comes to them instead of following through with a process from start to finish. In addition, by physically arranging products that are used more frequently closer to the area where the counting, labelling and packaging actually occur, a pharmacy dramatically increases its efficiency and improves employee working conditions. The use of automated, semi-automated or manual carousels is one solution that can bring the product to the team member rather than having the team member go to the product. Other technology options include "pick to light" high-density storage options that direct staff to the appropriate shelf/cabinet location for the product that needs to be filled and is queued to the appropriate priority for when the patient is expecting to pick up their prescription. This allows products to be stored based on product velocities instead of storing alphabetically.

In addition to physical product storage solutions, several automated filling systems can be used.[4–8] These solutions come in a variety of capacities and are designed to quickly and accurately select, count, label, cap and sort vial-filled prescriptions. These devices are integrated with dispensary software to increase filling accuracy and the speed of prescription preparation. The goal of these systems is to automate at least half of the prescription volume within the pharmacy. Automated prescription filling can occur in about one-quarter of the time that it takes for humans to complete, and the automated solutions can be available 24 hours a day, even operating when the pharmacy is closed. There are several of these devices available in the North American marketplace and they have a proven track record of increasing a pharmacy's productivity. Less automated medication-counting solutions are also valuable devices to improve productivity and filling safety as well. Most have higher accuracy levels than human counting, and many incorporate barcode-scanning technology that adds another verification process that can occur in the filling process. Regardless of the technology used, a well-designed pharmacy needs to maximize the physical positioning of the technology used within the pharmacy. This can be just as critical as integrating these technologies within the dispensing process.

Best practices suggest that throughout the dispensing process, multiple checks at multiple stages within the product preparation process should occur. The pharmacy should instill a culture of safety and have standard operating procedures that require staff to make double-checks throughout the filling process. Again, technology can be an effective tool to decrease the degree of human error that can occur within this process. Most pharmacy software systems use barcode-scanning technology and user-verification functionality to link specific aspects of the dispensing process to a specific pharmacy team member. All of these processes work in concert with a collection system that will remove clutter and can save time throughout the dispensing process. The use of "baskets" or "totes" to retain all products and documentation for a specific patient within the filling process is one best practice that is used frequently. This process allows the individual who is making the final check to have all the information available when making the check, and it keeps all of a patient's orders in one place to prevent potential errors that can occur when multiple prescriptions are separated.

Once the product is prepared, regardless of who or what prepared the medication, a quality assurance and verification process must be performed. The pharmacy needs to be designed so the checking pharmacist, or in some jurisdictions the checking pharmacy technician, has all the information needed to confirm that the final product is prepared correctly. This includes access to computer terminals with patient profile information, images of the product being dispensed, etc. The individual who is making the final check should be located in an area of the pharmacy where there is a minimal level of distraction to maximize accuracy and efficiency. Best practice within this final evaluation is that the individual involved with the checking process is not involved with any other aspect of the dispensing process before this point in time. Operationally, this can be a challenge for many pharmacy environments because the business model does not support having this many staff members within the dispensary, but a well-designed operation will try to facilitate this as often as possible.

Once the final verification process is complete, a patient's orders need to be collated for easy retrieval when the patient arrives for pick-up. Again, workflow management tracking within pharmacy software will allow for barcode scanning of completed prescription orders and can identify bins where completed prescriptions can be placed in anticipation of pick-up. These can be linked to call-back solutions that will advise the patient when their prescriptions are ready. When the patient or a patient's agent does arrive for pick-up, staff must be able to efficiently locate the completed orders and be able to process the final transaction. As a final safety verification step, pharmacy team members should visually inspect the final prescriptions with the patient to ensure the product prepared is indeed the product the patient is expecting.

Regardless of how a pharmacy is designed and how much automation exists, staff must be available to fulfill the regulatory obligations and customer-service-level expectations of the pharmacy. Patient counselling for all prescriptions must be part of the workflow process and can be done upfront, as some pharmacists are now doing, or at the very end. Either way, a clear process must be in place to ensure this key function is not missed and is worked into the dispensary workflow. Workload reporting can help to identify areas that require additional staff time as well as times during the day where resources could be better allocated to other functions. The productivity of the pharmacy must always be measured against the financial model to ensure a sustainable business is maintained. Labour costs need to be managed and assessments of what individual is the most cost-effective individual to perform each function in the dispensary needs to occur on a regular basis. Prescriptions filled per hour and labour costs as a percentage of sales are useful measurements to determine the productivity and profitability of the dispensary. Pharmacists must also be aware of those patients looking for advice or help with over-the-counter (OTC) medications. Again, all pharmacy team members need to be aware of this role of the pharmacist and can help identifying to the pharmacist those patients looking for help.

One of the biggest challenges pharmacies are facing today is finding a way to balance the new services that are offered into the regular workflow while still keeping an eye on the financial bottom line. How much time and additional staffing might be required is certainly one of the questions to address whenever a new service is introduced. One approach to introducing a new service is to look at who provides the service, when they provide the service and how long it will take. Services such as injection that do not require a large amount of the pharmacist's time can be treated in the same manner as a prescription and fit into the regular workflow if the pharmacy is very organized and ready to go. For example, during influenza season a patient asking for injection is screened and the form filled out, with all documentation, billing and workflow done in the same manner as a regular prescription. The pharmacist then moves to the counselling area or other private area where everything is ready to do the injection. In order for this to work, all pharmacy staff need to know their role in the provision of the service. The pharmacist does not need to fill out all the paperwork or the billing, which actually takes longer than the service itself. For services that require a greater amount of time or a specific pharmacist to perform the service, an appointment-based model works. For pharmacies with some pharmacist overlap, this could be the time when pharmacy staff identify patients who qualify for services, such as a medication review, and the pharmacist can then provide the service. While most are still in early days of incorporating the many new services into workflow, there are many pharmacists who have been pioneers in this area. Many of the trade magazines, such as *Pharmacy Business* and *Pharmacy Practice Plus*, highlight these pharmacists on a monthly basis.

An effective pharmacy practice must always be assessing and adapting to changes in the market and consumer demands. Pharmacists and their team members must always analyze and be prepared to make changes to the operations of the pharmacy to improve patient care, consumer satisfaction, productivity and profitability. This allows for the long-term success of a community pharmacy practice.

REFERENCES

1. Alberta Pharmacy Services Framework 2014. Available: www.pbiactuarial.ca/wp-content/uploads/2014/04/Pharmacy-Reimbursement-Changes.pdf (accessed Dec. 10, 2014).
2. Eder R. Chains sharpen pharmacy efficiencies with technology and new designs. Drug Store News. 2002;24(10):63–8.
3. Chi J. Expert gives clues on how to design efficient pharmacy. Drug Top. 2001;145(2):60–6 [cited 2014 Dec. 10]. Available www.questia.com/magazine/1P3-66977969/expert-gives-clues-on-how-to-design-efficient-pharmacy.
4. Script-Pro Perfect integration. Available: www.scriptpro.com/ (accessed Dec. 10, 2014).
5. Skrepnek GH, Armstrong EP, Malone DC, et al. Workload and availability of technology in metropolitan community pharmacies. J Am Pharm Assoc (2003). 2006;46(2):154–60. http://dx.doi.org/10.1331/154434506776180667. Medline:16602225
6. Product Spotlight Kirby Lester pharmacy automation. Available: www.kirbylester.com/news/articles/PPP_Product_Spotlight_Aultman_Hospital_KL60_KL30_Toohey.pdf (accessed Dec. 10, 2014).
7. Thomsen C. Pharmacy automation in retail pharmacies: assessing the right efficiency through technology White Paper March 2013. Available: www.kirbylester.com/whitepaper/Assessing_Automation_TTG_White_Paper_March_2013.pdf (accessed Dec. 10, 2014).
8. Cheung B. Innovation in technology tech talk. Available: www.canadianhealthcarenetwork.ca/files/2009/10/TTCE_May05_Eng.pdf (accessed Dec. 10, 2014).

CHAPTER 22

Inventory Management

Rick Brown, B.Sc.Pharm.; President, Innovative Pharmacy Solutions Inc.

Learning Objectives

- Understand the basics of inventory management in the dispensary and front store.
- Understand financial principles with respect to purchasing and inventory management.
- Identify tools available to effectively manage inventory in a pharmacy operation.
- Explore what to do in case of drug shortages as it relates to patient-centred care.

Inventory management is the process of overseeing the constant flow of products (both dispensary and front store) in and out of existing inventory. This process has an effect on many factors within a pharmacy practice and business. Maintaining consistent levels of inventory while understanding the seasonal fluctuations helps create an efficient pharmacy operation. In this chapter, several progressive management systems are discussed to help maintain adequate inventory levels. The basic concept is not to have too much stock and not to have too little stock. Too much stock will tie up cash and too little stock creates customer issues with not being able to fill their prescriptions.

FINANCIAL IMPLICATIONS

Inventory can tie up a significant amount of a pharmacy's cash. Several factors can play a role in determining how much inventory each pharmacy may carry including location, footprint, type of business, prescription volume, physician prescribing habits and front store sales mix. A pharmacy can range from a small clinic with limited over-the-counter (OTC) products to a large-format pharmacy that includes several front store categories including grocery, health and beauty aids, home health care and giftware. How to determine a specific pharmacy's inventory levels depends on several of these factors.

Controlling cash flow is critical for success in business. Cash flow is the movement of money into or out of a business. The goal is to have a positive cash flow so you can operate your business and cover the debts and loans against the business (see Table 1).

Table 1. Cash Flow Analysis Example

	Positive Cash Flow	Negative Cash Flow
Opening bank balance	$7,500	$4,000
Cash coming in (sales)	$80,000	$65,500
Cash going out (inventory, store expenses, rent, payroll, etc.)	$78,385	$74,775
Total cash at end of month	$9,115	(–$5,275)

A cash flow analysis gives a more realistic picture of whether the pharmacy will have the money to pay its expenses at the end of the month and keep the business afloat. It can be one measure as to the pharmacy's financial health. Inventory is a significant expense to the business and does affect cash flow in a positive or negative way. By managing the pharmacy inventory, cash flow can be positively affected.

INVENTORY TURNS

Inventory turns is a term that relates to how many times a pharmacy sells through inventory in a certain time frame. It is often expressed in terms of the number of turns in one year. The term cost of goods sold (COGS) is the cost of products purchased by the pharmacy from suppliers. Average inventory is the cost of the inventory currently sitting on the shelves. Inventory turns = COGS/average inventory for the period (see Table 2).

A benchmark of 11.7 times/year is common in retail pharmacy.[1] In this example, the pharmacy is below the benchmark and would have to decrease average inventory to $60,000 to reach the industry benchmark. Decreasing the dispensary inventory by $40,000 would create a positive effect on cash flow for this pharmacy.

Other things to consider: too low inventory may result in higher out of stocks, increased balance owings and upset patients. This can create a burden on staff and patients as it relates to optimum patient care. Too high inventory leads to increased burden on cash flow and decreased inventory turns. That is why inventory management is a continuous balance and ongoing process.

Table 2. Dispensary Inventory Turns Example

Yearly pharmacy sales	$1,000,000
Cost of goods sold	$700,000
Average dispensary inventory	$100,000
Cost of goods sold/average inventory = 7 turns/year	

In other words, the dispensary inventory is sold seven times per year.

SOURCES OF INVENTORY

The most common sources for products for pharmacies are either wholesalers or direct from a pharmaceutical company.

Wholesalers are online and will have a window for placing your order for next-day or same-day delivery. The timelines vary mainly due to geography (i.e., more remote regions may require longer lead time of up to a few days and, therefore, the pharmacy will have less frequent deliveries). In the majority of cases, next-day delivery is possible. These wholesalers can be separate corporations or be part of a pharmacy chain's distribution. The wholesalers work on a "markup" basis for their upcharge, which can vary and is somewhat negotiable. Markup is the percentage added to the cost of the product to enable the wholesaler to cover expenses and make a profit. Terms of payment are typically 30 days with discounts being offered for early payments (i.e., 2% off for payments made within 15 days of delivery).

Direct is done by ordering through a pharmaceutical or front store company's order desk. This can be done by phone, fax or online. The markup is eliminated on these orders, but in some cases a separate shipping charge may apply depending upon the company. It is important to include delivery charges as part of your COGS. *Direct orders may also require minimum quantities, which may result in higher inventory than required.* Delivery may take slightly longer than a wholesaler.

Some direct companies for the front store have different services and terms. Examples of these may be magazines/books, greeting cards and beverage companies. They may be serviced within your pharmacy by the company representative.

TOOLS TO MANAGE INVENTORY

Managing pharmacy inventory has evolved over the years. In some pharmacies, it continues to be managed manually as in the past. This tends to be a labour-intensive, inefficient and costly model. The use of technology to manage inventory has and will continue to be a key component in all aspects of pharmacy inventory management. Most pharmacies have embraced technology to optimize inventory management.

The most important aspect of managing inventory is the use of the right resources. Pharmacy assistants and front store managers are key to all the processes of inventory management. The pharmacist will take more of an oversight and supportive role.

PERPETUAL INVENTORY

This accounting system records the sale and the purchase of inventory in real time through the pharmacy operating system in the dispensary or through a point-of-sale (POS) system in the front store. This provides a detailed view of what inventory is in stock (on hand) and what will need to be replenished. This allows for the pharmacy to automatically order inventory the same or next day as the product is sold or dispensed from their supplier. Uploading or receiving of orders from suppliers into the perpetual inventory on a daily basis is important to keeping the inventory current.

DISPENSARY PERPETUAL INVENTORY

Typically, much of the high value inventory is in the dispensary; therefore, the use of a perpetual inventory by the pharmacy software system has the most significance on the pharmacy business and cash flow. There are several parameters to set up in this system initially on implementation; then the ongoing monitoring of order generation and inventory management are necessary to have the system run efficiently.

The software records the dispensing of the product, depletes the inventory and creates a suggested order according to parameters set up in the system. This is automatic replenishment where the computer integrates the use of the product with the parameters set up by the operator and creates an order automatically. The operator sets up a minimum amount of stock to have on hand and a maximum amount of stock to have on hand for each individual molecule or medication. This is also referred to as min/max reorder points. Determining the minimum usage of each product ensures the pharmacy will have adequate stock to dispense for their prescriptions. The maximum level acts as a control so the inventory does not climb above the determined threshold and negatively affect cash flow.

When sending the order into the supplier, one of the key tasks for the pharmacy team is to review the order carefully to make sure there are no anomalies. This will help prevent ordering non-returnable items (liquids, creams and injectables) from a supplier.

Continuous maintenance of the perpetual inventory system is critical to ensuring the integrity of the system. For example, a cycle count is an inventory auditing procedure where a small sample of inventory is physically counted and compared to the current perpetual inventory. The perpetual inventory on the computer is then updated for each item. Cycle counts are scheduled for each section on a regular basis to ensure the accuracy of the inventory. For example, many pharmacies have a schedule and cycle count their entire inventory four times per year. *Discrepancies between the physical cycle counts and the current perpetual inventory should be investigated, recorded and updated on the computer.*

Narcotics and controlled drugs must be part of a self-monitored procedure for the pharmacy manager with a cycle count done a minimum of every three months. The physical count will be compared to the perpetual inventory to determine any discrepancies. Any significant discrepancies should be investigated by the pharmacy manager to determine the cause (i.e., drug diversion, theft or receiving procedures mistakes).[2]

FRONT SHOP PERPETUAL INVENTORY

A POS system is used in the front shop where each retail transaction is recorded and the customer pays for the product(s). Perpetual inventory can be set up similarly on this software system where it can order products according to the min/max set up by the retailer. Once again, continuous monitoring and maintenance of the inventory system is important ensuring the integrity of the process. This can be especially important during a flyer program where the customer expects the product to be on the shelf for purchase. Not monitoring the stock levels and being out of stock creates a loyalty and trust issue with customers.

OUT OF STOCKS DUE TO INVENTORY MANAGEMENT

Managing the inventory too tightly (i.e., keeping below minimum stocks) creates a problem for the patients. This can range from not having enough supply to fulfill the complete prescription (which creates a balance owing) to having no stock on hand to fill any of the prescription (which can create a hardship on the patient). This puts a strain on the patient-centred care for the pharmacy. Constant monitoring is important to correct such situations as a critical part of inventory management.

OVERSTOCKS DUE TO INVENTORY MANAGEMENT

Overstocking creates an extra need for cash that will be tied up in the business. Having large overage of products creates a strain on financing the inventory. Higher-than-needed inventories can create an increase in expired products, which in turn, may become a loss to the business. Suppliers will take back several expired products for credit. However, several companies will only give a certain percentage, while others offer no compensation for expired products. Suppliers all have information online to help pharmacy staff determine which products are returnable for credit and which ones are not.

SEASONAL INVENTORY

At certain times of the year, inventory fluctuates up or down. In some cases, the pharmacy inventory may increase above the maximum during the peak season. An example may be allergy season where the inventory of antihistamines will increase over the spring and summer. In other cases, the pharmacy inventory may decrease below the minimums. The demand for cough and cold products decreases over the summer and ramps back up in fall. By monitoring these seasonal fluctuations, the front store manager can determine the correct stock levels.

EXPIRATION DATES

All products in the pharmacy have an expiration date, from potato chips to medications. It is important to have a system to capture these products before they get into the public's hands. Dispensary inventory should be physically reviewed every month to determine medications that will be going out of date. Placing a sticker or a note on the product ensures that expired product will never be dispensed. All expired drugs should be taken off the dispensary shelf and put into a secure area; then it should be determined if a credit is available from the supplier. If not, they should be disposed of according to the accepted destruction practices of the province/territory.

Front store products can be handled similarly. However, in the front shop there is an opportunity to discount and sell the product before their expiration dates to help reduce the pharmacy's loss. Once the product has expired, remove from the retail shelf and place into a secure area to determine if any credits are available from the supplier. Remaining products must be disposed of according to the accepted destruction practices of the province/territory.

ANNUAL INVENTORY COUNT

This is an important process that is done each fiscal year end for the business. An annual inventory count helps determine the year-end income statements with the accountant. Accurate COGS will be used to determine the final margin for the business. The annual inventory count can be done in a few ways as outlined next but no matter what the method, this remains one of the most important days in the lifecycle of a pharmacy.

PHYSICAL COUNT

This is typically done by an outside inventory company who will supply a team to come in and count the inventory on a specific day. Some smaller independent pharmacies may do it with existing staff at close of day. In the dispensary, each medication is counted either by each individual tablet or by part bottles. The cost is calculated by multiplying the number of tablets, creams or bottles by the supplier cost.

An important step to do ahead of time is to make sure all products are priced either on the shelf or on the product itself. All outdated products must be removed from the shelves and will be counted as a loss. *Outstanding balanced owings need to be taken into account.*

In the front store, each item is counted and multiplied by the cost found in the cost file of the supplier. Damaged or expired stock needs to be accounted for and will be separated and counted as a loss (shrinkage).

PERPETUAL INVENTORY ANNUAL COUNT

If the dispensary and front shop are on perpetual inventory, the process is simplified for the annual inventory count. The importance of carefully maintaining the perpetual inventory over the year with cycle counts and updates is critical. At the end of the day, the perpetual inventory should be very close to the physical inventory. An inventory summary report will be run at the end of day for the front store and dispensary. Physically spot-checking several items from the inventory summary report to compare to the perpetual inventory database is important to ensure confidence in the inventory count. Adjustments will be made to account for products not in the perpetual inventory. Examples may be the cost portion of the patient pick-up prescriptions and/or pre-filled (not billed) compliance packages.

DRUG SHORTAGES

Drug shortages have become a common issue with pharmaceutical manufacturers and wholesalers. Active pharmaceutical ingredients (API) are now sourced and manufactured around the world and with globalization of pharmaceutical manufacturing, the Canadian supply chain can experience drug shortages. There can be several simple and/or complex reasons for drug shortages in the drug supply chain. Some causes may be government intervention due to plant inspections or shutdowns, natural disasters, re-tooling of manufacturing plants, labour shutdowns and unavailability of raw materials. Shortages can last a few weeks to several months. This can be a significant issue as pharmacists need to deal with drug shortages when it comes to patient-centred care.

As the key health care professionals in drug distribution, pharmacists must be able to review all options to deliver the correct medications to their patients. The key to managing drug shortages is communicating with patients and keeping them informed as to the progress.

DRUG SHORTAGE COURSE OF ACTION

The first option may be as simple as changing brands to an interchangeable product. It is important to inform patients of the change as the drug may not look exactly like their previous brand. The next step is to check with other retail and hospital pharmacies in the community to see if they have any product available to purchase. Check with other wholesalers and suppliers to determine if they have any stock available and/or what date it may be available. Wholesalers and suppliers may have websites that can be accessed to determine the best availability date for each drug. A website set up by The Multi-Stakeholder Steering Committee on Drug Shortages in Canada is a good resource to track when certain drugs will be released in Canada.[3,4]

Check all possible resources frequently to determine the best available date for each drug. If all sources are exhausted, contact the physician directly to explain the circumstances and have some clinical alternatives ready to discuss. Once a decision is made, follow up with the patient to discuss the medication or therapeutic changes that will be done going forward. It is important, as mentioned earlier, to keep the patient informed throughout the process of a shortage.

Inventory management is an important aspect in the practice and business of pharmacy. Pharmacists play a key role in developing and implementing processes to control and maintain this asset. By understanding the importance of proper inventory management, the pharmacist can oversee and play a supportive role to the front store manager and pharmacy assistants as they deal with the mechanics of inventory management. This will help maintain the viability of the business and promote optimum patient care. Tools are available to control and maintain the pharmacy inventory, and new processes will continue to evolve to help optimize the inventory while furthering automation of the process. Drug shortages will continue to be a challenge; however, it is important for pharmacists to be able to deal with them and determine the right course of action for their patients. As processes continue to change and evolve in pharmacy inventory management, pharmacists will need to continue to embrace the changes and develop processes that will help optimize patient-centred care in their practice.

REFERENCES

1. 2009 National Community Pharmacists Association Digest. Available: www.ncpanet.org/pdf/digest/ExecutiveSummary09Digest.pdf (accessed April 8, 2014).
2. Narcotic and Controlled Drug Accountability Guidelines. Available: www.napra.ca/Content_Files/Files/Manitoba/current%20web%20site/ncd_accountability.pdf (accessed Aug. 30, 2014).
3. Canadian Drug Shortage Database. Available: www.drugshortages.ca/drugshortagehome.asp (accessed April 8, 2014).
4. Multi-Stakeholder Steering Committee on Drug Shortages. Available: www.drugshortages.ca/CMFiles/MSSC_Multi-Stakeholder_Toolkit_EN.FINAL.pdf (accessed April 22,2014).

CHAPTER 23

Loss Prevention in Pharmacy

Leigh Jones, *Loss Prevention Coordinator, Shoppers Drug Mart, Eastern Ontario*

Learning Objectives

- Define loss prevention and identify areas in pharmacy operations that require prevention.
- Describe the difference between internal and external loss.
- List the systems and technologies that can be used to minimize risk.
- Describe the responsibilities of staff in a loss prevention program.
- Outline the responsibilities of an owner/manager in a loss prevention program.

Retail loss prevention is a set of practices and procedures organizations follow to protect their assets and preserve profit. Assets are everything from a company's employees, buildings and merchandise, to IT infrastructure and products they sell. Profit preservation is any business activity specifically designed to reduce preventable losses, also known as shrink. Shrink or shrinkage is the difference between recorded inventory and actual inventory on hand. The difference in these numbers would be considered shrink. Preventable loss (shrink) is loss caused by deliberate or inadvertent human actions. Deliberate human actions that cause loss to a retail company can be theft, fraud, robbery, vandalism, waste, abuse or misconduct such as time theft (wasted time). Inadvertent human actions attributable to loss are poorly executed business processes, where employees fail to follow existing policies or procedures. Loss prevention is mainly found within the retail sector but also can be found within other business environments.

Traditional approaches to retail loss prevention have involved visible security measures, such as uniformed security guards or plain-clothed loss prevention officers, and then matched with technology such as closed-circuit television/security (CCTV) cameras, physical security and electronic article surveillance measures. Most companies either have their own in-house loss prevention team or use external security agencies.

Figure 23.1

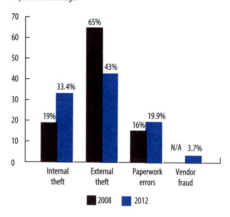

Retail theft
Q: From the following categories, what portion is attributed
to your total shrinkage?

Sources of Shrinkage[1]

Sources: PWC, Retail Council of Canada, Andrew Barr/National Post

INADVERTENT CAUSES

Poorly executed business policies and procedures contribute to loss either via the lack of training or the lack of compliance. Retail procedures vary from an internal employee bag check program to external visitor sign-in and sign-out policies.

Poor inventory management, such as failure to accurately receive product either through vendors or from a company's own distribution centre, can also cause loss. This includes building or creating incorrect products in the company's inventory management system.

Another cause of loss is processing errors such as not ensuring the product being sold to a customer or patient matches the store's inventories item of the same product. An organization that still uses a manual method of inventory control will increase their risk of incorrect receiving and selling of product. Human error is more common than electronic error.

Incorrect accounting can range from missing invoices to inaccurate claims (e.g., damaged and expired product not being returned). This can result in inaccurate billing and payments to and from vendors.

DELIBERATE CAUSES

Deliberate criminal activity such as robberies, break and enters and fraudulent prescriptions are explained in Chapter 24: Safety and Security in Pharmacy.

Prescription fraud, both internal and external, is more common than one would expect. Checks and balances need to be in place to ensure that all prescriptions are legitimate and physically accounted for. Insurance fraud can be another factor surrounding this. Pharmacy staff manipulating the system to submit false claims can happen, so a pharmacy manager or owner should review available pharmacy dispensing reports for any anomalies, checking pending, dispensed and cancelled prescriptions. Running this type of report alphabetically by patient or drug type on a weekly basis can show reoccurring patterns that may indicate fraudulent activity.

Customers can make up a significant portion of loss through shoplifting. There is no specific look or individual type that stands out as a shoplifter. Men, women, children, teens, young and old have all shoplifted. A well-trained staff and a strong customer service environment can greatly reduce these losses. Deploying either uniformed security guards or undercover security officers has a noticeable impact reducing shoplifting in a retail location that is being targeted for shop theft. In extreme cases of shoplifting, both types of guards can be deployed to work together in the store.

Inappropriate ordering and lack of attention to detail can lead to waste and damage. Lack of precision and caution in prescription filing may also be a cause of waste (e.g., spilling a bottle of pills on a pharmacy floor or pills coming into contact with other product that may contaminate the drug, pill or liquid). Neat, clean and organized (NCO) should be a standard in reducing loss.

Internal vandalism may be an employee deliberately trying to deface a product for the purposes of stealing it. This may also include damaging the narcotic lock-up and/or other types of storage units to gain access. In some locations, there are robots to assist in dispensing. Another example of such vandalism has occurred with employees kicking the robot out of frustration or anger, resulting in high repair costs.

In any organization, employee relations could result in lost productivity, referred to as intentional delinquent behaviour. When employees choose not to follow procedures and policies set forth by their company and/or their department, as a best practice their leader must manage that misconduct. When managing employees' performance, a leader uses valuable time to coach and mentor them to bring them back on track for their roles' expectations. During this performance management stage, employees' productivity drastically diminishes as their effectiveness of delivery and execution of tasks are problematic. Examples of such misconduct can be any breach of a company policy. For example, not following a bag check policy (a procedure that is in place where staff submit their bags, backpacks and purses for a search by management at the end of the shift) or misusing privileges related to employee company discounts (e.g., sweet-hearting, which is offering a discount or markdown of a product without authorization to a friend or family member), fraud and breach of confidentiality.

PHARMACY OPERATIONS REQUIRING PREVENTION

Inventory counts are crucial in pharmacy operations to deter both inadvertent and deliberate causes of shrink. To avoid discrepancies, periodic counts of controlled substances should be completed as part of the pharmacy's business model. Such tasks ensure accuracy of inventory and help to identify and minimize losses. Incorporating this into best practices on a regular basis allows management to further investigate concerns in a timely manner through recognizing common denominators. Regular inventory counts on all inventory is a good practice, as is bringing in an outside inventory company to audit internal inventory accuracy annually (see Chapter 22: Inventory Management).

It is strongly encouraged that the pharmacy owner or manager review all prescriptions. Should the pharmacist fail to follow such guidance, one's integrity of procedures and policies could be questioned. If fraud were to take place, these documented formalities become the evidence needed to pursue an investigation. In turn, this documentation may also be required by authorities during investigations.

Due to the sensitivity of narcotics and controlled substances (which have the potential for abuse), it is important to ensure the accurate retention of the hard copy of the prescription for audit purposes. It is also a requirement by most College of Pharmacies. Some locations may have computer scanning for document retention.

THE DIFFERENCE BETWEEN INTERNAL AND EXTERNAL LOSS

Internal loss is shrink that can be created on purpose or by mistake. Vendors, employees and lack of proper inventory management are all potential sources of internal loss. Vendor loss can occur when a vendor holds back merchandise to be delivered to a store. Should the receiving employee not detail what is received, a vendor may easily be able to keep merchandise for personal use or to gain monetary profit. On this occasion, the store still pays for the product yet does not physically receive it. If and when an employee does not follow inventory management, once the product is part of the pharmacy inventory, the employee may also hide and keep the product to sell and/ or share with family and friends. Employees also have direct access to product, enabling them to misuse their access, resulting in loss.

Another internal example involves coercion. Recently, the author experienced an investigation into losses surrounding OxyContin that revealed a pharmacy employee had been stealing merchandise and narcotics from her place of employment. During the investigation, the employee had been captured on CCTV surveillance concealing the product without paying for it and then exiting the store. When the employee was arrested by loss prevention investigators, she explained how she had been approached one day before her shift while she was in the laundry room of her apartment building. The person who approached her was tied to organized gang activity and the distribution of narcotics. He was able to identify this employee and where she worked by her name tag and business uniform she was wearing while on her way to work. Intimidation, vandalism and threats of violence were used against this employee and her child to persuade her to steal OxyContin and various other items from her place of employment. Out of fear for her safety and that of her child, she complied with the demands and continued to do so until she was caught. The story was further verified by police and protective measures were taken to protect her and her family. Without policies and procedures in place, this activity could have continued, creating further losses, as well as allowing prescription narcotics to be sold on the street. Accurate periodic counts of narcotics and controlled substances at this pharmacy were able to identify the loss quickly, and measures were put into place to identify the common denominator.

Another form of internal theft could be time theft. It occurs when an employee misuses company time during their planned shift, such as swiping in from an unpaid break but not actually returning to work on time and receiving pay for it. A workforce management system (WFMS) to monitor employees swiping in and out for their shifts is a way that businesses manage schedules to ensure that proper shift coverage is in place and employees receive their pay for hours worked. Employees swipe in for the beginning of their shift, swipe in and out for unpaid breaks and swipe out at the end of their shift.

External losses are typically from criminal activity targeted against the business by non-employees. Robbery, break and enter and shoplifting are external acts of loss. In a robbery setting, it is common for the robber to enter the premises wearing a disguise and brandishing some form of weapon. It is also common for a robber to quietly approach the pharmacy counter and pass a note demanding various narcotics. By having an effective robbery prevention program in place, any harm to employees can be minimized dramatically. Complying with a robber's demand has been shown to be the most effective way to prevent injury to employees. When robberies take place, the effects on employees can be very traumatic so it is imperative that a good counselling program be available to help with their needs. Ensuring that other security measures, such as CCTV, are in place and functioning allow authorities to have a better chance of identifying the suspects. Many times when robberies have taken place, silent alarms (also known as panic buttons) seem to be forefront in the minds of many employees. These types of measures are discouraged due to the fact that they could cause a potential hostage situation. Waiting until a suspect has left the premises before calling 911 or a local emergency number is a best practice, as this avoids any confrontation between police and suspect within the pharmacy.

Having an emergency procedures binder in place to help educate and guide staff in the event of a robbery is a great tool. All new employees should be trained on the contents of this manual and its procedures before entering into the work environment. A clear understanding of where this manual is kept and how to access it during an emergency will help ease the robbery situation when it arises. Keeping the binder near the phone in the pharmacy would be ideal, as information would then be readily available for the staff member to communicate to police. The manual should contain key information such as location address and telephone number, emergency contact names and numbers. It can also be expanded to cover other emergencies such as threats, bomb scares, earthquakes and floods (see Chapter 26: Contingency Planning).

SYSTEMS AND TECHNOLOGIES TO MINIMIZE RISK

Depending on the retailer and retail location, technologies to minimize risk will vary.

CCTV is recommended for all pharmacy operations and other areas of a business to help monitor external and internal theft. Strategic positioning of cameras can help in the protection of staff on the job by identifying health and safety violations or protecting staff members' personal belongings. These systems are instrumental in finding out what happened, aiding in an investigation and protecting a company's assets.

GPS trackers recently adapted to pharmacy to help reduce the risk of pharmacy robberies and apprehending the offender. A device that is concealed within a product in a narcotics safe and handed off to suspects during a robbery can be tracked remotely by satellite and cell phone towers to accurately identify direction of travel, speed and location of stolen merchandise.

Security gates can be installed so they can be pulled across doors and windows at store closing are designed to deter break and enters. They are fitted on the inside of the window and typically operate on a track like a giant curtain. These have helped dramatically to stop break and enters where objects have been used to smash out windows so that entry can be gained.

Alarm systems similar to home alarm systems are recommended in all retail locations. These systems have motion sensors within the location, glass-break sensors aimed at windows, and points of contact on all doors and safes. These systems are monitored remotely by a monitoring company and when triggered, police are notified.

Safes or vaults are becoming widely used to protect narcotics and controlled substances within pharmacy. Safes can be of different sizes and can operate from a key lock, combination dial or an electronic key pad. The electronic key pad allows individual codes to be given to those allowed to access the safe. Each code can be monitored for time of entry and by whom.

STAFF RESPONSIBILITIES IN A LOSS PREVENTION PROGRAM

It is not just the responsibility of management in a business to educate employees about policies and procedures. Staff should also educate themselves about the business policies. During the hiring stage in many businesses, new employees will be asked to sign documents and watch videos stating that they understand and will comply with the policies and procedures outlined in their hire package. Staff should be encouraged to ask questions, and management should have an open door policy with staff about loss prevention practices in the workplace. Staff should feel comfortable with approaching management about situations they see that could affect the safety and security of fellow employees or the brand and business directly.

Staff can play such a vital role in shrink reduction when they are engaged in a strong loss prevention program. Greeting customers when they enter a store, making eye contact and interacting with them could just make the difference if someone were going to shoplift.

OWNER AND MANAGER RESPONSIBILITIES IN A LOSS PREVENTION PROGRAM

It is an owner's or manager's responsibility to not just manage policies and procedures through follow-up and example, but to also be an ambassador for the loss prevention culture within their business. Employees within a business that displays a strong loss prevention culture should be encouraged and educated by team leaders to adopt a loss prevention way of thinking. Leaders in the business should speak about the policies and procedures on a regular basis or show leadership by following these policies in their day-to-day practices. Updating staff on any events that have taken place within the store, such as shoplifting incidents, is a great way to build awareness and encourage staff to think about consequences, not only of how it affects the business but how it can also affect them. There is a strong correlation between a strong loss prevention culture and low shrink. Employees should be made aware of the loss prevention tools being used in the business and what the functions of these devices are. Managers should ensure staff that they are providing a safe and secure workplace and clearly define how these tools work into that safety. Involving employees will help them understand that loss prevention success is a team effort.

REFERENCE

1. Shaw H. Workers steal 33% of all goods that go missing at retailers: survey. National Post. Oct. 31, 2012. Available: http://business.financialpost.com/2012/10/31/workers-steal-33-of-all-goods-that-go-missing-at-retailers-survey (accessed Oct. 29, 2014).

CHAPTER 24

Safety and Security in Pharmacy

David Toner, *Loss Prevention Coordinator, Shoppers Drug Mart, Burnaby, BC*

Learning Objectives

- Explain the legislated requirements for safety and security.
- Describe how a pharmacy's operations safety and security needs will differ from other operations.
- Describe the similarities between loss prevention and safety and security measures and programs.
- Outline the responsibilities of staff in a safety and security program.
- List the responsibilities of an owner/manager in a loss prevention program.

Chapter 23: Loss Prevention in Pharmacy focuses on prevention of loss and inventory management. Many of the concepts discussed in relation to loss prevention are also inherent in protecting the safety and security of staff and personnel. This chapter covers the fundamentals of the safety and security that pharmacists and pharmacy owners/managers need to know.

Loss prevention security is defined as the protection of people (staff), the property (the business and assets) and information (patient information and IT). The operation of a pharmacy invites, by its very nature, interactions with members of the public. In some cases, these interactions can expose staff to confrontational situations and, possibly, belligerent and aggressive behaviour from customers/patients. In some cases, retail pharmacies are open for business 24 hours per day. Whether in a retail outlet or a hospital setting, very similar concerns arise.

PHARMACY OPERATIONS: THE THREATS

Loss prevention provides guidance related to the threat of internal loss and to the safety and security concerns experienced in pharmacy such as external threats. The primary external threats to a pharmacy operation include the following:

Patient interactions, even difficult ones, can generally be managed by a professional and experienced staff. When faced with belligerence, a firm policy regarding harassment and aggressive behaviour should be established and communicated to the patient/

customer. More junior staff should defer to the senior staff member or owner for support and direction, but nonetheless be trained in what the business standards of practice or operational policies state with regard to these situations. It is sometimes advisable to post signage indicating a "no-tolerance" policy regarding this type of behaviour.

Pharmacy delivery is a common retail pharmacy practice to offer patient services to those who may not be able to come into the store to pick up their medications on their own. Special attention and safeguards need to be taken to ensure a proper delivery log is in place to ensure all prescriptions are delivered. Care and attention needs to be taken by the delivery driver to reduce the risk of a robbery while prescriptions are being delivered.

Drug diversion involves patients attempting to pass forged or altered prescriptions to obtain drugs, often as a result of personal addiction and desperation. Pharmacy staff must have clear protocols for dealing with suspicious scripts. Any script that appears to have been altered (e.g., had drug/brand name changed, dosage or quantity changed) should be questioned. Verification with the prescribing doctor for all controlled and narcotic drugs in this situation is recommended.

Break and enter with intent to steal from a pharmacy occurs after hours and is not generally a safety issue as this happens when staff members are not present. The risk here is more to the profitability of the business. Various physical methods of deterring a break-in will be discussed later in this chapter.

Robbery of drugs is the most serious threat to safety a pharmacy faces, when the threat of or use of force is used to elicit cooperation from the victim. Unlike break and enter, which is a property crime, robbery is a crime against a person.

In recent years, a drastic increase in robberies of pharmacies for OxyContin and other opiates has highlighted the need to address security issues. Pharmacy staff are the "gatekeepers" of drugs that can be worth 10 to 30 times on the street what they will be sold for at retail.[1] The criminal element is well aware of this, and this creates a significant motive for robberies to occur. In the city of Vancouver, there has been a staggering 214% increase in pharmacy robberies between 2011 and 2013.[1]

Many criminals view pharmacies as an easier target, as there is a disparity in the level of security measures and practices between one pharmacy and another, particularly in the retail sector. For example, small independent operations may have far more limited staffing, resources and visibility than larger chain stores.

LEGISLATION

Similar to many other professions, there are legislated requirements designed to address the safety and welfare of practitioners. Provincial/Territorial legislation governs occupational health and safety requirements laid out for employees and staff. In British Columbia, for example, WorkSafeBC requires that retail operations perform risk assessments to determine the dangers and have written policies to address these. There is also specific legislation that speaks to minimum staffing levels, availability of cash or other goods and training for employees on violence prevention in the workplace.

Federal legislation under Health Canada stipulates how narcotics and controlled drugs are dispensed and requires reporting to Health Canada any missing or stolen drugs. Federal law also requires secure storage and safeguarding of confidential patient files and document retention. Although not a direct threat to staff safety, confidentiality of patient information is an additional security concern. All staff should sign a confidentiality agreement (re-signed annually) stipulating the importance of safeguarding patient medical and financial information. Best practice would be to have all new employees complete this as part of their orientation and then re-sign as part of an annual refresher. All sensitive documents should be shredded off site by a professional destruction service.

In addition to federal and provincial/territorial legislation, regional Colleges of Pharmacy in each province/territory establish regulations and by-laws to ensure safe practice by licensed members.

ADDRESSING THE THREATS: WHAT CAN BE DONE?

Several steps can be taken to reduce the risk of criminal threats. Reducing the risk to increase likelihood of detection or capture, or effort to overcome obstacles is seen by criminals as greater than the potential reward.

PHYSICAL LAYOUT/DESIGN

One of the most elemental steps in ensuring a safe work environment is the physical layout of the workspace. Safety and security can be addressed through the use of principles known as Crime Prevention Through Environmental Design (CPTED).[2] The premise of this concept is that the movement of people, and to a large degree their behaviours, can be influenced by the physical design of a space.

The physical evolution of pharmacy can be seen in the way positioning of the workspace has changed. In years past, the pharmacist was on an elevated platform, often behind a high shelf and glass barrier. This severely limited the view of the sales floor from the pharmacist's position. In more contemporary designs, the pharmacy is on the same level as the customer, with only a low counter between the pharmacist and the patient. This approach facilitates more open customer interaction and patient care and creates open sightlines and visibility—a key component of the aforementioned CPTED.

Further measures for preventing crime include proper exterior and interior lighting, physical barriers to pedestrian movement such as gates, turnstiles and walkways, and barriers to vehicle breach such as bollards placed in front of doors and windows.

Failure to plan for all security contingencies can be quite costly. One retail pharmacy was compromised by a break and enter when thieves removed the entire floor-to-ceiling glass wall in the building and made off with thousands of dollars in drug inventory and caused significant damage. This was made possible by a design flaw as the glass was removed intact and not broken.

SECURITY HARDWARE

Door locks must be of high grade and designed to withstand a break-in attempt. Two-inch deadbolts are recommended for exterior doors and anti-pry plates over the door seem to further protect the bolt.

Key control is often overlooked. A list of key holders should be created and kept securely. Copy-protected keys or a patented key system should be used to prevent any unauthorized duplication of keys. Copy-protected keys are stamped "do not copy" and require written permission from the owner to duplicate. Patented keys are supplied by licensed locksmiths and cannot be duplicated; additional keys can only by obtained from the original company supplying them.

The lock is only as strong as the door it is mounted on. Solid-core steel doors are the most secure, although not aesthetically appealing. These are recommended for fire exits and back/receiving area doors.

In store front areas where plate glass doors or windows are common, it is highly recommended that security laminate or film be used to prevent entry by smashing the glass. High-risk locations or those that have had previous burglary attempts should use steel shutters or expandable security grills to cover windows and glass doors when the business is closed.

TECHNOLOGY

The pharmacy should make use of various types of technology available to protect the staff and the business. Break-ins and robberies can be curtailed by using closed-circuit television cameras (CCTV), burglar alarms and safes.

The use of surveillance cameras to monitor areas has been shown to reduce the likelihood of crime. Further, if a crime does occur, the footage from video cameras provides excellent evidence for investigators to help identify suspects and successfully prosecute them.

A CCTV system should consist of a digital recording and storage unit capable of at minimum 90 days of memory retention. Cameras should be strategically placed to cover all entrance and exit points, points of sale and critical drug storage areas such as narcotic safes. The ability to save data to CD or other media is also needed, as police will often require footage of an incident. The terminus or "head-end" of the unit should ideally be secured in an area out of public view and restricted as to which staff members are permitted to access the unit to prevent any attempt at tampering.

An integrated burglar alarm system should be standard for all pharmacies. In many cases, business insurance policies will require an alarm system as operating the business without one simply invites too much risk.

A system should include protection for all doors, windows, roof hatches and other sensitive areas of the business. Consultation with a loss prevention specialist is recommended. Motion sensors should be used in open spaces, hallways and corridors within the premises, and safes should be alarmed. As well as break-ins, motion sensors will alert staff closing a business to the presence of after-hours intruders hiding within the premises, common in break-out type scenarios. The alarm system should be monitored by an outside agency responsible for responding to alarm situations and dispatching police as required.

To deter pharmacy robberies, police agencies and private security firms have begun deploying GPS tracking units to assist in apprehending suspects in narcotic robberies. These units are decoy bottles, labelled to look like OxyCodone or other desirable drugs. The device is placed in the safe where it can broadcast a GPS signal when moved. The bottle is given or taken along with other drugs in the event of a robbery to the suspects. These units have proven very effective and have assisted in the recent arrest of suspects wanted in connection with a string of pharmacy hold-ups.

Reliable safes for the secure storage of narcotic and controlled drugs should be used. Safes are available in a spin style combination dial, keyed or electronic dial. It should be noted that the electronic dial combinations are generally more user friendly and can be re-programmed by the user when it is deemed prudent to change the combination, rather than having the additional expense of a locksmith. Safes should be large enough to hold all narcotic inventories and be bolted to the floor to prevent any attempt at removing the entire unit.

When in doubt, it is always recommended that the pharmacy owner obtains a professional assessment by a qualified security consultant. A risk assessment can generally pinpoint what the weaknesses are in the specific location, and recommend solutions for mitigating them as well.

SECURITY PROGRAM RESPONSIBILITIES

The education and training of pharmacy staff in how to deal with situations are crucial to any program's success. From the loss prevention or safety and security perspective, proper training and staff awareness are critical. It is recommended that staff be trained immediately upon hiring, before being placed in regular operations and potentially put at risk. A comprehensive training package would include some form of instruction (either written or video) in safety and security, a written test of the staff member's knowledge and understanding after the training is delivered and a signed acknowledgement form placed in the employee's personnel file acknowledging completion of the training. A best practice for HR would be to have this training revisited and the acknowledgement form re-signed annually.

Owners and managers of pharmacy operations have legal responsibilities to their staff, both to maintain a safe work environment and to provide specific training and operating policy related to this.

Following all recommendations will minimize criminal activity against the pharmacy business; however, it is important to note that all crime cannot be prevented.

Staff members are responsible for following policy and reporting to their manager/employer any situation they feel negatively affects their safety or security. In the event of a robbery, compliance is always the best course of action. Employees should never place themselves or their coworkers in jeopardy by attempting to stop or foil a robbery.

It should be pointed out that even the most robust security or loss prevention program can be undermined or defeated by lack of engagement from staff or management. Safety and security is everyone's responsibility.

RESOURCES AND SUGGESTED READINGS

Department of Justice. Building a safer Canada: a community-based crime prevention manual. 1996.

Insurance Bureau of Canada. Loss prevention. Available: http://www.ibc.ca/on/business/risk-management/on-premise-loss-prevention (accessed Nov. 9, 2014).

Ontario Ministry of Labour. Health and safety awareness training for workers and supervisors. Available: www.labour.gov.on.ca/english/hs/training/ (accessed Nov. 9, 2014).

Wekerle G, Whitzman C. Safe cities: guidelines for planning, design, and management. New York: Van Nostrand Reinhold; 1995.

REFERENCES

1. Det. Stephen Thacker, Vancouver Police/RCMP presentation to BC College of Pharmacists, April 2014.

2. International CPTED Association. Available: www.cpted.net (accessed Nov. 9, 2014).

CHAPTER 25

Pharmacy Services

Stacy Johnson, *B.Sc.Pharm; Director of Pharmacy Professional Services, Pharmacy Department, Safeway Operations, Sobeys Inc.*

Learning Objectives

- Discuss how different pharmacy services may be available at different pharmacy practices.
- List the various pharmacy services available.
- Define the term *niche services* and outline the advantages of niche services.
- Identify the reasons for marketing a new or specialty service.
- Discuss the criteria for choosing a particular service or specialty to market.
- Outline the steps that need to be taken to market a service.

Pharmacy services are the patient-focused services that primarily encompass the enhanced medication-related services[1] or the expanded patient care services[2] of the care provided by pharmacists. These services include value-added services, clinical pharmacy services and specialty or niche services.

For many years, the pharmacist's role evolved slowly and gradually and value-added services were the most common services provided by pharmacists to patients. In 2007, Ontario launched the MedsCheck program and Alberta adopted legislation that enabled pharmacist prescribing and administration of injections. Since then, almost every Canadian province and territory has enabled clinical pharmacy services to some degree. In addition, many governments and third-party payers are also remunerating pharmacists for the provision of these services.

To address the rapidly changing pharmacy environment, the Canadian Pharmacists Association led the development of the Blueprint for Pharmacy, which "... is a long-term initiative designed to catalyze, coordinate and facilitate the changes required to align pharmacy practice with the health care needs of Canadians."[3] The Implementation Plan was released in September 2009. This plan included the following deliverables under Financial Viability and Sustainability:[4]

- 3.2.1 A framework for professional pharmacy services to provide a method and rationale for establishing fees.
- 3.2.2 Compensation models to support the services in the framework, and emerging services.

To achieve these deliverables, the Canadian Pharmacy Services Framework (CPSF) was completed. This work, "...outlines a roadmap to deliver expanded patient-centred pharmacy services that are cost-effective and based on both the needs of Canadians and value to the health care system."[5] The CPSF categorizes services with relation to core dispensing, enhanced medication-related or expanded patient care services.

The goal of delivering pharmacy services is to achieve the Vision for Pharmacy, as defined in the Blueprint for Pharmacy: "Optimal drug therapy outcomes for Canadians through patient-centred care."[6]

While basic service has always been an integral part of the care that pharmacists provide to patients, pharmacy services are increasingly expanding to include those that provide an additional level of patient-centred care. This care may not necessarily be provided during the product-centred service of dispensing a particular medication. For example, a patient may present independently to receive medication management services or niche services such as travel medicine consultation.

Community pharmacies across Canada provide a variety of pharmacy services; however, not all pharmacy services are available at every community pharmacy. Contributing factors may include the following:

PHARMACIST FACTORS
- composition of primary pharmacy education
- on-the-job training
- number of years of experience as a pharmacist
- additional certifications or authorizations (e.g., immunization/injection administration, Certified Diabetes Educator, additional prescribing authorization)
- varying levels of personal competency, experience and confidence in specific practice areas

PHARMACY FACTORS
- professional philosophy and/or business strategy of owner/manager
- technology systems
- physical work environment (counselling windows or rooms, place for patients to wait)
- support personnel (e.g., regulated pharmacy technicians, pharmacy assistants)

EXTERNAL FACTORS
- provincially/territorially specific legislation or regulations
- patient awareness
- public or private remuneration
- patient interest/need/demand
- collaboration (or lack thereof) with or by other health care professionals

VALUE-ADDED SERVICES

In general (although with some exceptions), these services are provided as part of the core dispensing service.[7] They are generally provided at no extra charge (e.g., provide additional value for the same price) although occasionally with a small fee. These services include the following:

TELEPHONE FOLLOW-UP

In addition to standard monitoring and follow-up processes, a pharmacist will telephone the patient after several days have elapsed to assess efficacy, side effects and answer questions related to a specific prescription. It can also be used to assess adherence. This service is most commonly provided for antibiotic prescriptions or for medications that are new to the patient but will be taken long term.

COMPLIANCE PACKAGING

Patients who use multiple medications or have trouble remembering to take their medications can have their prescriptions prepared in "bubble" or "blister" packaging. The pharmacy packages the medications into compartments unique to time of day and day of week. This service may be funded to some degree and may also be known as "multi-drug unit dose" packaging.

AUTOMATED REFILL AND REFILL REMINDER SYSTEMS

A variety of systems exist. Most commonly, patients sign up to have their chronic prescriptions automatically renewed and prepared for pickup on a particular day of the month. Additional refill reminder systems place a call, email or text to advise the patient that their refill is either due or is ready for pickup. Medication synchronization is a related service, in which all the patient's long-term medications are aligned in terms of refill cycles.

FLAVOURING

A patented system is available that enables pharmacists to provide flavour customization for liquid medications to increase palatability and, therefore, adherence for children.

RESOURCE MATERIALS

In addition to the standard, required written patient information provided when dispensing medications, most pharmacies have supplemental resources available, in print or online, to provide extra information. These materials may be in languages other than English to further meet the needs of a particular clientele.

SCREENING OR CLINIC DAYS

Where allowed by regulation, the pharmacist or other appropriate health care provider hosts a discrete event that addresses awareness, prevention or management of a specific disease state or condition. Examples include blood pressure, cholesterol, bone density or blood glucose screening.

CLINICAL PHARMACY SERVICES

These services are the enhanced medication-related services or the expanded patient care services. These services generally require enabling legislation or regulation. They may be reimbursed in part or in full by the respective provincial/territorial government or private drug plans who then may also have specific definitions of elements such as patient eligibility, maximum billings per day, an annual budget for delivery of the service, types of services allowed, required documentation, how to bill, etc.

ENHANCED MEDICATION-RELATED SERVICES

These services are additional interventions generally provided at or around the time of dispensing a medication. These services require additional time and additional skills, knowledge and abilities on the part of the pharmacist. Some require prescribing authority on the part of the pharmacist. They also require additional documentation as per provincial/territorial regulatory standards, with which a pharmacy assistant or pharmacy technician may assist. These services include the following:

ADAPTATION

Adaptation services may include renewing existing prescriptions, altering the dose, dosage form, regimen or route of administration; prescribing in an emergency; or therapeutic substitution. Therapeutic substitution is provided when the pharmacist substitutes another drug that is expected to have similar therapeutic effect; it is sometimes funded at a slightly higher rate than other adaptation services. In some provinces/territories, prescription renewal (sometimes called continuing care) and therapeutic substitution are separately defined as a service that is distinct from adaptation. Not all provincial pharmacy regulators have enabled all services included in adaptation.

PHARMACEUTICAL OPINION

The pharmacist provides an opinion to the physician on interventions such as therapeutic duplication, suboptimal response to a drug, adherence issues, adverse drug reactions or other. The response is documented. Some provinces allow for reimbursement for this service regardless if the physician accepts the opinion or not. Pharmaceutical opinion programs are useful when pharmacists do not have the regulatory authority to address these problems independently.

REFUSAL TO FILL

A pharmacist assesses a prescription and chooses not to dispense it when it is not in the patient's best interests. Reasons may include significant drug interaction, prior adverse reaction, potential overuse/abuse, therapeutic duplication or other.[8]

ADMINISTRATION OF IMMUNIZATION OR INJECTION

Upon assessment of appropriateness, including contraindications and/or precautions, a pharmacist administers a medication or vaccine by injection by intramuscular, subcutaneous or intradermal routes. The patient is monitored for adverse events, which the pharmacist must be prepared to address, including urgent health issues such as severe allergic reaction (anaphylaxis) to a vaccine. There is currently a high degree of variability across Canada in the scope of authority to administer injections. Some provinces/territories allow for immunizations only (including possibly for influenza immunization only), whereas others allow pharmacists with the required training and knowledge to administer any medication by injection.

TRIAL PRESCRIPTION

This service is provided to patients who have been prescribed a new medication. After assessment, the pharmacist dispenses an initial "trial" quantity (usually 7 to 10 days but can be up to one month) to enable the patient to determine tolerance, assess side effects, etc. The pharmacist follows up with the patient after the trial quantity is completed and assesses for efficacy, tolerance and adherence and determines if the therapy should be continued. Typically, only one dispensing fee is earned (usually on the trial portion) and an assessment fee is earned upon the decision to provide the balance or not.

PERSONAL MEDICATION RECORD/MEDICATION RECONCILIATION

The pharmacist interviews the patient, family and/or other health care providers to create the Best Possible Medication History. This BPMH is a comprehensive list of all prescription, non-prescription and complementary medications the patient is using. The pharmacist verifies with the patient and documents how, when and why the medication is being used. The BPMH can also include a list of discontinued medications.

EXPANDED PATIENT CARE SERVICES

These services are most commonly provided independently from the core dispensing service. They may be initiated during the core dispensing service but may also be initiated independently from dispensing. Expanded patient care services include the following:

COMPREHENSIVE MEDICATION MANAGEMENT

This service may be known as medication therapy management, standard medication management assessment, chronic annual care plan, medication assessment program or other. The core activities include assessment, identification of drug therapy problems, development of a care plan and evaluation/follow-up.[9]

During the assessment, the pharmacist gathers information from the patient including demographic, past medical history, current and discontinued medications, allergies, over-the-counter and natural medicines, smoking history and any other relevant information. The pharmacist may also conduct a physical assessment to obtain additional information. The pharmacist completes a BPMH. During or after the completion of the BPMH, the pharmacist identifies any drug therapy problems (DTP) and develops a plan to address them. The care plan is a summary of the BPMH, any DTP and the plan for resolving, lifestyle or other recommendations (an action plan) and referral notes. Follow-up is conducted at appropriate intervals to monitor response to DTP or lifestyle interventions.

This service is reimbursed to varying degrees by provincial/territorial governments and private drug plans across Canada. Eligibility criteria range from number of medications, number or type of chronic disease conditions, age or type of medications (e.g., medications considered at high risk). There may be maximums placed on the number of billable follow-up services as well.

SMOKING CESSATION

A pharmacist identifies a patient who uses tobacco and has considered or wishes to quit. The intervention is tailored to the particular stage of change that the patient is experiencing. If the patient is in the contemplation or action stage, an appointment is made for an initial consultation. History is taken and risk factors and triggers identified, and the pharmacist develops a quit plan in collaboration with the patient. The pharmacist may have the authority to prescribe medication to aid in the cessation attempt. A series of four to eight follow-ups are made after the quit date—either by telephone or in person—to provide support throughout the quit process. If the patient relapses, the sequence can be started over again.

INDEPENDENT PRESCRIBING

Where relevant provincial/territorial legislation enables such activity after completing a series of requirements, an application can be made to the regulatory body for Advanced Prescribing Authority, Level 1 Prescribing or other. The pharmacist may be required to take additional training, document his/her patient care process, collaborate with other health care providers or describe how he/she makes patient care decisions. Upon approval, a pharmacist can independently initiate Schedule 1 medications for patients. Restrictions may include narcotics or controlled drugs, and/or prescribing only in areas in which the pharmacist can ensure personal competence, hold additional certification in and/or practices in particular settings. Pharmacists must assess the patient, develop a treatment plan, document and follow up when prescribing. Communication to the primary care provider about the prescribing decision is required.

MINOR AILMENTS

After meeting regulatory requirements, which may include additional training, pharmacists are enabled to prescribe to treat a specific set of minor ailments. The ailments may include conditions such as oral thrush, diaper dermatitis, insect bites, acne, oral aphthous ulcer, allergic rhinitis and/or others. Pharmacists are expected to follow established treatment guidelines and may be restricted to prescribing from a set list of medications (including Schedule 1 medications). The pharmacist must assess the patient, develop a treatment plan (that may include following a service protocol), document, communicate to the patient's physician and follow up. This service enhances the ability of patients to manage minor ailments themselves and improves access to a health care provider for minor conditions.

SPECIALTY OR NICHE SERVICES

Pharmacies may also provide additional specialty or niche services. More often than not, these require investment from the owner for additional training, physical layout additions or modifications, specialized equipment and often, additional staff. Examples of these services are long-term care, infusion, travel health, women's health, natural medicine or specialty compounding. These services are unique, specialized and differentiate the pharmacy apart from others. For some of these services, there may be less competitive pressures due to fewer pharmacies providing them. However, in some cases (such as long-term care), there may be heightened competition due to the volume of business to be gained. Investing in the development of niche services often enables the pharmacy to bid for contracts that may extend for several years, therefore improving the stability of the business model.

MARKETING SERVICES

When a pharmacy decides to start offering pharmacy services of any sort, it is important to develop a marketing plan. Many of these services are new or not yet widely available and are, therefore, often unfamiliar to patients. Often, complicated eligibility criteria make it difficult for patients to know they are eligible for a service. One of the most important reasons to market the service is to increase patient awareness and demand for the service. Gaining referrals from other health care professionals (physicians in particular) is another reason to market the availability of new pharmacy services (see Section XI: Marketing, Promotion and Customer Service for more information on marketing).

Criteria for choosing a particular service to market may include the following:

- priorities of the owner/manager
- amount of investment already made in starting a particular service
- readiness of pharmacy staff to consistently provide the service at a high quality
- seasonal determinants (e.g., influenza vaccination season)

When deciding to market a particular service, the first step is to research the market. One way of doing this is to conduct a SWOT analysis. In this method, the pharmacy will list strengths, weaknesses, opportunities and threats regarding the given service. This will help to determine which service to market and where to position the marketing.

Another way to do this is to ask and answer a series of questions such as the following:

- Why are you offering this service? What needs does it meet?
- What will set you apart?
- Who is your target population?
- What are the needs specific to your community?
- Who are the other health care professionals in your area?
- What are your competitors offering that is similar and different?
- Is there room in the market for your service?

Once the service to market has been chosen and the needs of the marketplace narrowed down (along with the business case to support implementation), the next step is to determine the marketing medium or channels. There is a variety of options to choose from and the choice can depend on the demographic of the target audience, budget or the availability of resources such as technology. Examples include newspaper, radio, television, posters, bag stuffers and point-of-sale (POS) flyers, telephone calls (with appropriate consent), social media and word of mouth. It may also include in-store signage such as messages at POS, buttons or ribbons worn by staff, intercom announcements or display tables, cold calls and notifying physicians in the area or the local health unit of the new service, if appropriate.

While you are developing your marketing plan, it is also important to train the pharmacy staff on expectations for the execution of delivery of the service. How will they identify eligible patients? What will they talk to them about? Are there automated messages, pop ups, forced printouts, etc., that will assist them? When will they provide the service? Where will the service be provided? How will they be evaluated on the provision of the service (e.g., with quantitative or qualitative measures, both or none)?

A plan to evaluate the marketing is also important. Was the method

> Activity: Compare and contrast the services available in at least three provinces/territories. In particular, examine which services are enabled through legislation compared to those that are publicly funded.
>
> Activity: Compare and contrast the services provided in at least three community pharmacies. Define if they are value added, enhanced medication, expanded patient care or specialty/niche services.

chosen a successful one? Did demand for the service meet expectations? Did the money spent deliver a return on investment?

(See Section IX: Developing, Implementing and Managing Clinical Pharmacy Services for more on choosing a pharmacy service to pursue and then developing, planning and implementing it.)

RESOURCES AND SUGGESTED READINGS

Canadian Pharmacists Association. Blueprint for Pharmacy implementation plan. 2009. Available: http://blueprintforpharmacy. ca/docs/pdfs/blueprint-implementation-plan_final---march-2010.pdf (accessed Nov. 1, 2014).

Canadian Pharmacists Association. Canadian pharmacy services framework. 2011. Available: www.pharmacists.ca/index.cfm/ pharmacy-in-canada/advocacy-government-relations-initiatives/canadian-pharmacy-services-framework/ (accessed April 1, 2014).

Houle SK, Grindrod KA, Chatterley T, et al. Paying pharmacists for patient care: A systematic review of remunerated pharmacy clinical care services. Can Pharm J (Ott). 2014;147(4):209–32. http://dx.doi.org/10.1177/1715163514536678. Medline:25360148

REFERENCES

1. Canadian Pharmacists Association. Canadian pharmacy services framework. 2011. Available: www.pharmacists.ca/cpha-ca/ assets/File/cpha-on-the-issues/CanadianPharmacyServicesFramework.pdf (slide 10, accessed April 1, 2014)

2. Canadian Pharmacists Association. Canadian pharmacy services framework. 2011. Available: www.pharmacists.ca/cpha-ca/ assets/File/cpha-on-the-issues/CanadianPharmacyServicesFramework.pdf (slide 11, accessed April 1, 2014)

3. Canadian Pharmacists Association. Blueprint for Pharmacy implementation plan. 2009. Available: http://blueprintforpharmacy. ca/docs/pdfs/blueprint-implementation-plan_final---march-2010.pdf (page 5, accessed November 1, 2014)

4. Canadian Pharmacists Association. Blueprint for Pharmacy implementation plan. 2009. Available: http://blueprintforpharmacy. ca/docs/pdfs/blueprint-implementation-plan_final---march-2010.pdf (page 33, accessed November 1, 2014)

5. Canadian Pharmacists Association. Canadian pharmacy services framework. 2011. Available: www.pharmacists.ca/index. cfm/pharmacy-in-canada/advocacy-government-relations-initiatives/canadian-pharmacy-services-framework/ (accessed November 1, 2014)

6. Canadian Pharmacists Association. Canadian pharmacy services framework. 2011. Available: www.pharmacists.ca/cpha-ca/ assets/File/cpha-on-the-issues/CanadianPharmacyServicesFramework.pdf (slide 2, accessed April 1, 2014)

7. Canadian Pharmacists Association. Canadian pharmacy services framework. 2011. Available: www.pharmacists.ca/cpha-ca/ assets/File/cpha-on-the-issues/CanadianPharmacyServicesFramework.pdf (slide 9, accessed April 1, 2014)

8. Canadian Pharmacists Association. Canadian pharmacy services framework. 2011. Available: www.pharmacists.ca/cpha-ca/ assets/File/cpha-on-the-issues/CanadianPharmacyServicesFramework.pdf (slide 31, accessed April 1, 2014)

9. Canadian Pharmacists Association. Canadian pharmacy services framework. 2011. Available: www.pharmacists.ca/cpha-ca/ assets/File/cpha-on-the-issues/CanadianPharmacyServicesFramework.pdf (slide 40, accessed April 1, 2014)

CHAPTER 26

Contingency Planning

J. Reddy Bade, *B.Sc.Pharm, Certified Diabetes Educator, Certified to Administer Medication by Injection; Shoppers Drug Mart 2401*

Anita Brown, *Bsc Pharm, Certified Diabetes Educator, Additional Prescribing Authorization, Certified in Patient Care Skills; Shoppers Drug Mart 2401*

Bob Brown, *Bsc Pharm; Owner Associate, Certified to Administer Medication by Injection; Shoppers Drug Mart 2401*

Aleksandra Trkulja, *BScPharm, Additional Prescribing Authorization, Certified to Administer Medication by Injection, Certified in Travel Medicine, Certified in Patient Care Skills; Shoppers Drug Mart 2401*

A contingency plan is an activity undertaken to ensure that proper and immediate follow-up steps will be taken by management and employees in an emergency. Its major objectives are to ensure containment of damage or injury to, or loss of, personnel and property and continuity of the key operations of the organization.[1]

Most often, it is impossible to predict when an emergency situation may arise such as a natural disaster, man-made disaster or communicable disease outbreak. As direct patient care health providers, pharmacists, especially those in community practice, are often the first contact for patients. This will result in increased demands placed on pharmacists to provide advice to the public related to the situation and to ensure the distribution of patient medication during the emergency. At the same time as these increased demands, pharmacy staff absenteeism, drug supply chain interruptions and other concerns may arise that will impact the ability of pharmacists to maintain essential pharmacy services and continuity of care.[2] Developing a contingency plan involves making decisions in advance about the management of human and financial resources, coordination and communications procedures and being aware of a range of technical and logistical responses. Time spent in contingency planning equals time saved when a disaster occurs.

LESSONS LEARNED FROM THE ALBERTA FLOOD OF 2013 – ONE PHARMACY'S STORY

This chapter is written as an example of contingency planning. On June 20, 2013, a catastrophic flood devastated High River, Alberta. The whole town was evacuated, with many people and businesses being given only minutes to abandon their premises. More than 14,000 people were displaced. The acute and long-term care hospital and several long-term care and assisted-living residences were also evacuated with virtually no warning or preparation time. Physician offices, pharmacies, dentist offices and all medical services were shut down within hours.

At the same time, 25 minutes north of High River, the city of Calgary, population 1,000,000, also suffered from catastrophic flooding. It was called the worst flood in 1,000 years. The downtown of Calgary was evacuated. Emergency services in southern Alberta were stretched to the limit. Communication and transportation throughout Calgary and the High River area were disrupted.

Okotoks is a small town located in between High River and Calgary. Second to Calgary, we are the closest community to High River with services and resources capable of helping manage the chaos that accompanied High River's evacuation.

We had no plan in place! Never in a million years would we have anticipated being thrust into this situation. Within hours of the first evacuations, our pharmacy was inundated with evacuees seeking provisional medications. It felt like we were working in a MASH unit. The patients we met within the first days of the flood were the most ill. They had multiple chronic health conditions, requiring numerous medications, such as palliative patients requiring narcotics and several methadone patients requiring assistance with their methadone needs. They were evacuated so quickly they were lucky to have their wallets and any form of identification, let alone a detailed record of their medications. Their pharmacies, also located in High River, were under water and were unavailable to contact to confirm and/or clarify medication histories for us. Their physicians from High River were also evacuated, their offices closed and records and files unavailable.

The flood happened during the evening on a Thursday. By 9:30 am Friday morning, we had a lineup of people almost to the front of the store. Everyone was anxious and traumatized by the catastrophic damage to their homes, businesses and livelihood. Unfortunately, Okotoks was not immune to the flooding. Resources in Okotoks were stretched to the limits. The flooding closed one of the two main bridges. We had 14,000 extra people seeking refuge in town, and one of our main roads was shut down. At 1 pm, the power in Okotoks went out. The store was full of people, waiting for medications. We had staff collecting flashlights and our pharmacy team continued to work in the dark. Patients whose medication needs were not urgent were escorted from the building. Those who had nowhere to go, or who felt they needed to wait, were asked to sit in the waiting area until their medications, which were already started, were completed. The store was locked. We had a pharmacist at the front of the store triaging patients' requests outside. Urgent needs such as insulin, fever and pain medication were addressed as best as we could, documented and supplied at pharmacist discretion.

All of this occurred on a Friday afternoon with no more orders for replenishment until Monday. With our prescription volume more than doubling in hours, we realized that medication supplies were going to become a problem. Although High River and Okotoks are only minutes away from each other, the demographics of the towns are very different. The prescribing habits of physicians in High River are different from those in Okotoks. We were scrambling to secure medication to meet the needs of our displaced High River patients.

Our prescription volume was shocking, but also shocking were the scenarios that we were faced with, and that we were required to deal with on the fly:

- methadone patients
- palliative patients
- cancer patients

- intravenous (IV) medications
- nursing home patients requiring emergency supplies of medication in compliance packages
- people not having anything, including money, credit cards or access to banking information: Often we trusted that a patient would return at a later time to pay. We established charge accounts and were prepared to absorb some losses to ensure patient care.
- multiple evacuation centres: We had at least three separate evacuation centres for which we supplied baby formula, insulin, inhalers, self-monitoring blood glucose supplies, toilet paper and other aids to daily living.

What we did for three months was run our business as best as we could in the midst of one of the worst natural disasters in Canadian history. We did what we were trained to do; we used the resources that were available to us. We had policies and procedures in place that we adhered to as best as possible. We practised pharmacy the way that the legislation allowed. We had warm and dry beds to go home to every night. Our patients were displaced and scared and uncertain of their future. We did what we could do to reduce their stress. If we were faced with such a calamity again, what would we do differently, and what systems did we have in place that allowed us to operate as business as usual?

SOME AREAS TO CONSIDER IN PHARMACY CONTINGENCY PLANNING

Emergency planning procedures that could be implemented in the event of a natural disaster (weather-related, power outages, floods, explosions) or other types of unforeseen emergencies would be important to consider for any business, but certain issues are unique to a pharmacy. The Manitoba Pharmaceutical Association has assembled an Emergency Preparedness Resource Kit for Pharmacists. The following are key points:

- Ensure the pharmacy's emergency preparedness plan is comprehensive and addresses drug supply chain interruptions at the pharmacy site.
- Strengthen emergency communication protocols among staff and with government, public health offices and regulatory authorities.
- Depending on the type of emergency, ensure all pharmacy staff are knowledgeable and frequently updated on provincial clinical management guidelines for direct patient care.[1]

As direct patient care providers, it would be an excellent exercise for any pharmacy team to review their practice site emergency preparedness.

EMERGENCY ACTION BINDER

These are key points to be considered when planning for unforeseeable emergency situations: robberies, power outages, fire, natural disasters, etc. Based on our experience, we suggest an Emergency Action Binder as described in Table 1.

STRENGTHEN EMERGENCY COMMUNICATION PROTOCOLS AMONG STAFF AND GOVERNMENT, PUBLIC HEALTH OFFICES AND REGULATORY AUTHORITIES

In Alberta, as part of a pharmacy standard of practice, a pharmacy must ensure that a licensed pharmacy has an adequate number of staff to provide professional services safely and effectively.[3]

Table 1. Emergency Action Binder

Staff	Current list of staff with more than one contact number Put all regular staff on standby for extra hours. What additional staff resources are available and how can we get these set up?
Person in charge	Who makes decisions? Who is second in command if the person in charge is not available?
Emergency supplies	Flashlights and cell phone access, water, food for staff/patients if needed
Medication supply	Plan in place to procure additional medication—who to contact, wholesale emergency contacts, delivery persons to pick up Communicate within the pharmacy team—limit supplies of medication to absolutely what is necessary until plan for additional medication orders can be made available.
Designation of roles	Put the right people in the right place; have a plan, look at the strengths of staff members and put them in that position. Train staff to take on roles during a disaster and be comfortable making decisions.
Patient care/best practices	Ask your patients: What did the doctor tell you this medication was for? How do you take this medication? Just want to make sure, this medication looks the same as before?
Documentation	If you didn't write it down, it didn't happen.
Out-of-the-box thinking	We adapted our solutions to the resources we had available: One-week supply of medications to patients we had never met before, at no cost, until patient could organize their finances One-week supply of narcotic/controlled substances until we could obtain physician signatures on prescriptions
Professional/stakeholder relationships	Foster collaborative relationships with those prescribing medications. Make sure your prescribers know what you can do for their patients. Work with other stakeholders in health care/public health, community disaster planning groups.
Cold chain	See the Cold Chain section in this chapter.

In the attempt to be ready for this type of disaster in the future, it would help to have your staffing organized. During the Alberta 2013 flooding, we were so overwhelmed in the first few days of the flood that we didn't have time to think about securing extra staff. We knew we needed more help, but we didn't have people we could call and didn't have the time to start looking. A list of relief pharmacists and relief assistants would have been helpful. In the future, we will have an action plan to quickly access the highly trained staff required to manage a dramatic change in prescription volume associated with this type of emergency.

Key points:

- Have a current list of staff with more than one contact number.
- Put all regular staff on standby for extra hours.
- Find out what additional staff resources are available and how to get them set up.

At the height of the flooding, pharmacies and physicians throughout the region were overwhelmed. There had to be trust between health care professionals that decisions could be made in the best interest of patient safety without waiting for responses. Our urgent care department had wait times exceeding eight hours for medical emergencies; they had to have trust in us and the other pharmacies that their patients' drug-related problems would be addressed. When we were faced with the need to provide narcotics or controlled medications, we needed to know that we would have the support and trust of the local physicians to get the job done. We had their support. We continue to have their support.

Our community partners, public health and town officials, did not hesitate to contact us in the first hours of the flood to obtain provisional supplies to help evacuees. We supplied diapers, baby formula, toilet paper, water and some less urgent medications to three different evacuation centres. We quickly established a billing system where supplies could be obtained efficiently, and billing and payment for supplies were taken care of after the fact.

Corporate resources and professional supports were excellent, quickly assisting us with minor renovations to the store to help us deal with patients, including an additional cash register and computer. They checked on us regularly and provided moral support. Our biggest deficiency was not asking for something earlier.

DEPENDING ON THE TYPE OF EMERGENCY, ENSURE ALL PHARMACY STAFF ARE KNOWLEDGEABLE AND FREQUENTLY UPDATED ON PROVINCIAL CLINICAL MANAGEMENT GUIDELINES FOR DIRECT PATIENT CARE[2]

Someone from head office asked us, "How many prescriptions did you fill during those first few days of the flood?" We didn't understand the question. So many of the patients we were seeing did not have prescriptions. The pharmacist was often required to conduct a medication review without any of the patients' medications, and issue an extended prescription. We used the full scope of practice for pharmacy in Alberta! One of the advantages that our pharmacy had is that we were very familiar and comfortable with using the full scope of our practice. It wasn't difficult for us to step up and help our displaced patients with their medication needs. A pharmacy team must have an excellent understanding of their jurisdiction's scope of practice.

PRESERVING THE COLD CHAIN

During the flood, our pharmacy was without power for almost two hours, which gave us a strong consideration to have back-up options to handle emergency situations in the future. Generators are expensive, may only be able to manage a limited number of appliances and have to be ventilated to the outside because of exhaust. Though a generator may be very helpful during a lengthy power outage, the more important and essential operating question would be how to manage the cold chain to prevent your fridge items from being compromised.

It is reasonable to consider purchasing a back-up generator to use in the case of an emergency. The first question for your team is, what is the generator for? Would it be required to just support the pharmacy fridge? Or are you looking for something to back up the entire store? If you are looking to back up the entire building, can you afford to buy a generator? How do you access a generator at the peak of a natural disaster, when all the local resources are stretched to the limit?

The *National Vaccine Storage and Handling Guidelines for Immunization Providers (2007)* is an excellent reference to help guide your pharmacy team in how to manage inappropriate vaccine storage requirements and ensure that the cold chain is maintained for all your refrigerated items. This information is certainly important during a power outage related to an emergency, but it is also very useful in your everyday practice (e.g., the fridge is left open overnight, the fridge is accidently unplugged).

Our experience taught us that the best resource to determine the viability of a compromised cold chain medicine is to contact the manufacturer directly for recommendations. A list of phone numbers that could be accessed during an emergency would be helpful, as would a chart listing how long items can be safely left unrefrigerated.

A WORD OF CAUTION

Do not discard vaccines or diluent before determining their integrity. When a cold chain break is suspected, consult your local public health office, immunization program and manufacturer because their resources may maintain more detailed stability guidelines to aid in the assessment of cold chain breaks.[4]

STEPS IN HANDLING INAPPROPRIATE VACCINE STORAGE (LIGHT AND TEMPERATURE)

If you become aware of inappropriate vaccine storage conditions, take the following steps immediately:

- Notify the designated vaccine coordinator.
- Record the following information:
  - date and time of incident
  - the issue (e.g., inappropriate temperature and/or exposure to light)
  - length of time the vaccine may have been exposed to inappropriate conditions
  - the room temperature where the vaccine storage unit is located
    - A standard household thermometer may be used.
    - Do not use the thermometer from the vaccine storage unit.
    - Do not rely on the temperature displayed by the room thermostat.
  - current temperature inside the vaccine storage unit (and freezer)
  - minimum and maximum temperature readings inside the vaccine storage unit (and freezer)
  - presence of water bottles in the refrigerator
  - presence of frozen packs in the freezer
  - action that has been taken to protect the vaccines
  - action that has been taken to correct the issue
- Document the inventory of the vaccines affected by this event. Include vaccine name, lot number, expiry date and quantity.
- Isolate and quarantine the affected vaccines and mark them as "DO NOT USE."
- Store the affected vaccines under appropriate conditions until the integrity of the vaccine is determined if possible.
- Do not assume that vaccine inappropriately exposed to light or to excessive temperatures cannot be salvaged.

DEALING WITH MALFUNCTIONING VACCINE STORAGE UNITS

The most important step to take if the vaccine storage unit is not working properly is to protect the vaccine supply. Do not allow the vaccine to remain in a non-functioning unit for an extended period while you attempt to correct the problem. If the power in the building is compromised, can you move the affected medication into coolers that are packed with ice? Ensure that temperature continues to be monitored.[4]

IDENTIFY THE STEPS INVOLVED IN EVACUATING THE BUILDING

It is very important to discuss with your staff an evacuation plan and strategy. Sometimes it will be necessary to evacuate your building as a result of situations occurring either inside or outside the premises. Over the years, we have had to evacuate because of power loss, flooding, robbery and the threat of robbery. Regardless of the reason for the evacuation, there needs to be a plan:

- Establish the threat/concern/problem/issue.
- Escort your patients out of the store.
- Have a supply of flashlights readily available.
- Have a staff member tend to the front door; delegate a reliable staff member at the main entrance to stop patients from entering, explain what the emergency is and where the closest pharmacy is if prescriptions are an emergency.
- Account for all staff once safely outside the building.
- Contact appropriate authorities and anyone else who needs to be aware of the situation (head office, owner of store, stores in the area as they will need to help patients).

If at all possible, have a pharmacy staff member at the front of the store helping to triage patient medication needs.

THE IMPORTANCE OF STORING INFORMATION OFF SITE

The disaster in High River reminded us of the importance for off-site storage of information and having access to it. It also reminded us of the importance of entering prescription information into the computer immediately. We did not require hard copy off-site information; it was electronic records that we needed. All pharmacies should strongly consider copying and storing their electronic records at a secure location off site. In our experience, it was 7 to 10 days before the buildings in High River could be accessed and the electronic storage devices retrieved, with no guarantee there was no water damage. We had multiple situations where patients had left new prescriptions with their pharmacy, but these prescriptions were not entered into the system, and subsequently lost with no record. Store electronic records off site and make sure all new prescriptions are entered into the computer in a timely manner.

HANDLING PATIENT CARE IN EMERGENCY SITUATIONS

During the flooding, our pharmacy was overwhelmed by the number of patients seeking assistance with emergency provisional supplies of medication, and by the number of patients seeking assistance with over-the-counter (OTC) assessments. From our experience, the most invaluable pharmacist service during the disaster was providing emergency prescriptions. As direct patient care health providers, however, we found that we were the first contact for many patients seeking OTC treatments. In Alberta, it is within the scope of *all* pharmacists to prescribe provisional medication for continuity of care. At our pharmacy, we have several pharmacists with additional prescribing authorization. At the height of the flood, in an attempt to help relieve the burden on our already strained medical resources, our urgent care centre referred some patients experiencing minor ailments to our pharmacy for assessment. Our additional prescribing authority gave us a greater opportunity to assist some patients with self-limiting, self-diagnosed conditions.

What was unique about the flooding situation was the length of time that medical and pharmacy services were disrupted in High River. Once it was clear how long it was going to take for some sort of the normality to return for our High River patients, some of our prescribing activities became managing ongoing care. In Alberta, a pharmacist with additional prescribing authority is authorized to manage medication changes. Negotiating therapeutic goals was of great importance for the patient, especially during critical times. For example, we met patients who had blood work done before the flood. A discussion had already been had with their physician about possible medication changes, pending blood work. The patient was unable to follow up with the physician. The pharmacies were unable to contact the physician. The solution was for the pharmacist to review the blood work through Wellnet medication records and to initiate the necessary changes. Examples include synthroid, warfarin, diabetes medication and blood pressure medication.

It was very difficult to communicate to other health care professionals what we were doing to help manage their patients' needs. By using standardized subjective, objective, assessment and plan notes (SOAP) during consultations, the pharmacist was able to properly document changes to a patient's care plan. The patient was provided a copy of the documentation and instructed to present the information to the physician at the next visit.

Of course, *do no harm*. Our prescription volume more than doubled overnight. We had relief staff helping our regular staff. We were dealing with patients with whom we were unfamiliar and vice versa. This was a transition point in patient care, an environment very vulnerable to medication error. To protect our patients, old and new, we focused on very basic but sound pharmacy practice. All original paperwork (Wellnet medication records and relevant blood work) travelled with the medication until it was picked up by the patient. The communication to the entire pharmacy team was that, for any prescription for which the pharmacist has done an assessment for continuity of care, the pharmacist must speak with the patient before medication could leave the building. "Mr. Smith, I know you have used this medication before, but it is new here. We just want to look you in the eye and ensure everything with the medication looks the same as before!"

To manage patient care during a disaster, it is necessary to complete an efficient assessment and triage of the patients, determining if the patient can be postponed a few days and allow access to those who need the care immediately. Pharmacy assistants and technicians can help triage priority by determining what supplies, if any, the patient may have. Pharmacists should decide on priority based on the type of medication therapy, patient's condition and current needs.

Pharmacists are dealing with emergencies and micromanaging similar types of challenges in their everyday practice. During critical times, pharmacists may be faced with increased numbers of patients plus increased number of ethical dilemmas and uncertainties about different clinical issues. It is important that all pharmacy staff are aware that disasters present with an increased potential for adverse effects due to improper nutrition and hydration as well as improper conditions for medication storage. Experience plays a significant role and alleviates a part of the burden when making decisions and finding quick, efficient and safe solutions for patients.

Assertiveness and good listening skills are essential when trying to provide patient-centred care under any circumstances.

The supply of medication should be rationed to amounts necessary to meet the patients' immediate needs. Patient needs varied as some had been evacuated to distant locations, their mobility greatly limited. Volume of prescriptions increased so dramatically that regular replenishment schedules were insufficient. It is important to coordinate patient needs with their ability to travel and with replenishment. Can your suppliers provide delivery on the weekend? What happens when the highway closes?

Disasters can happen at any time. Being successful during critical times such as a natural disaster, requires adherence to good habits during the normal times. Does your pharmacy staff practise the full scope of practice allowed within your jurisdiction? Is your pharmacy staff aware of the various health care resources available in your community? Does your pharmacy practise in a cooperative and collaborative way with your neighbouring health care professionals?

RESOURCES AND SUGGESTED READINGS

Canadian Pharmacists Association. *Compendium of pharmaceuticals and specialties.* 41st ed. Ottawa, Ont.: Canadian Pharmaceutical Association, 2006.

Friedman E. Coping with calamity: how well does health care disaster planning work? *JAMA* Dec 21, 1994, Vol.272(23), p.1875(5). Available: www.ncbi.nlm.nih.gov/pubmed/7990224 (accessed Nov. 23, 2014).

McConnell A, Drennan L. Mission impossible? Planning and preparing for crisis. J Contingencies Crisis Manage. 2006;14(2):59–70. http://moodle.coatbridge.ac.uk/multimedia/ARM/wk4/Mission%20Impossible.pdf. http://dx.doi.org/10.1111/j.1468-5973.2006.00482.x.

World Health Organization. *Thermostability of vaccines.* Geneva, World Health Organization, 1998. (WHO/GPV/98.07)

REFERENCES

1. BusinessDictionary.com – Contingency plan definition.
2. Manitoba Pharmaceutical Association. Emergency preparedness resource kit for pharmacists, p. 2.
3. Standards of practice for pharmacists and pharmacy technicians, July 2011.
4. National Advisory Committee on Immunization. *Canadian immunization guide.* 7th ed. Ottawa, Ont.: Public Health Agency of Canada, 2006. (Minister of Public Works and Government Services Canada. Cat. No. HP40–3/2006E).

CHAPTER 27

Legal Considerations for Pharmacy Operations

A: The Pharmacy Regulatory Environment

Della R. Croteau, *RPh, BSP, MCEd*

B: Contracts and Agreements

Mark N. Wiseman, *B.Sc., M.Env.Sci., LL.B.*

A: The Pharmacy Regulatory Environment

Learning Objectives

- List the federal and provincial/territorial legislation under which pharmacies operate.
- Explain the regulatory requirements around a self-regulated profession and aligning pharmacy practice to the regulations and the standards of practice.

OVERVIEW OF LEGAL CONSIDERATIONS

Operating a pharmacy is distinctly different from operating another retail business because pharmacists are responsible for the safe distribution of drugs and for provision of patient-focused care. One of the responsibilities in operating a pharmacy is to meet the many regulatory requirements that support a safe and effective pharmacy practice. A simple approach to looking at all the legal considerations is to consider the three different areas covered by legislation, which include the products (medications), the places (pharmacy practice sites) and the people (pharmacists and pharmacy technicians).

There are several laws, both federal and provincial/territorial, that affect the practice of pharmacy and have been set up to protect the public by ensuring the safety and quality of pharmacy services. Legislation is in place for the distribution of medications, special considerations for narcotic and controlled drugs, the operations and inspections of a pharmacy, and requirements for a dispensary. There are also laws that dictate coverage and payment for medications. Some provinces also have legislation governing the licensing, requirements and inspections for hospital and/or institutional pharmacies. In addition, there are laws and requirements around the practice of pharmacy, including the responsibilities of the pharmacist and pharmacy technician in providing patient-focused care, which also must be considered in the operation of any type of pharmacy.

DRUG DISTRIBUTION

Federal legislation governs which drugs are licensed for sale in Canada. The Food and Drugs Act[1] contains overarching information about distribution and manufacturing of drugs as well as the list of drugs, but the Food and Drug Regulations, especially Part C,[2] give more specific information regarding the responsibility of a pharmacist. The Natural Health Product Regulations[3] are also part of this Act.

The Controlled Drugs and Substances Act[4] sets out the schedules or list of drugs and substances that are restricted and enforcement and punishment regarding their use or misuse. The Narcotic Control Regulations[5] to this Act set out the duties of a pharmacist with regard to the handling and dispensing of narcotics as well as the restrictions on prescriptions. Also attached to this Act are the Benzodiazepines and Other Targeted Substances Regulations,[6] the Marihuana for Medical Purposes Regulations[7] and the Precursor Regulations,[8] which restrict the sale of large quantities of substances used for making illicit drugs and substances.

Traditionally, each province also had drug schedules, and individual decisions were made by each as to the listing of a drug. In an effort to provide consistency from region to region, the National Association of Pharmacy Regulatory Authorities (NAPRA) worked with the federal government to form the National Drug Schedules Advisory Committee (NDSAC).[9] This committee is made up of drug experts who, upon request from a manufacturer, consider the action of a drug and its safety profile and make recommendations as to whether a drug should remain on prescription (Schedule 1), should be moved to behind the counter and only sold with pharmacist advice (Schedule 2), should be sold only in pharmacies with a pharmacist available for advice (Schedule 3) or can be sold anywhere (Unscheduled). This list of drugs makes up the National Drug Schedules, which can be found on the NAPRA website.[10]

Each province/territory maintains its own drug schedule, but Manitoba, New Brunswick, Nova Scotia, Ontario, Prince Edward Island, Northwest Territories, Nunavut and Yukon all refer to the national schedules by reference, which means that once NDSAC has made a recommendation for the listing of a drug, the province/territory adopts that listing. Alberta has some slight differences due to products offered in non-pharmacy outlets before adoption of the national process but now follows the NDSAC recommendations. British Columbia, Saskatchewan and Newfoundland and Labrador still require a provincial approval process before adopting the recommendations. Québec does not use the national drug schedules, but rather maintains a provincial schedule.[11]

The schedules are important as legislation refers to them in determining the storage and location of drugs for sale in the pharmacy as well as the prescription and record-keeping requirements. The legislation is written to make this the responsibility of the pharmacist, but the pharmacy operation needs to be set up in such a way as to facilitate all pharmacists and pharmacy technicians working within a pharmacy to meet these requirements.

MONITORING OF NARCOTICS

Most provinces have a prescription monitoring program to monitor narcotics and controlled drug use.[12] The programs have been put into place to reduce the misuse and abuse of targeted medications by patients, and to monitor prescribing and dispensing practices of health care professionals. The programs usually involve the regulatory bodies for pharmacy, medicine, dentistry and veterinary medicine, as well as the provincial Ministry of Health. Some regions use a triplicate prescription system and others incorporate the program within their prescription drug plan billing system. The monitoring programs in many places began as joint policy between regulatory bodies to address the growing concerns of narcotic misuse and abuse, but in many cases they have become embedded in provincial legislation.

PRIVACY OF HEALTH INFORMATION

With increasing technology and the ease of sharing and circulating information, the federal government introduced the Personal Information Protection Electronic Document Act (PIPEDA).[13] This Act was the first to provide for restrictions on the collection, use and disclosure of personal information and address electronic alternatives to processes using paper records and transactions. The legislation was introduced mainly to address business transactions and was followed by privacy legislation in each province. Some provinces address personal health information specifically, as well as the responsibilities of health care custodians such as pharmacists and pharmacies on collecting, using, disclosing and disposing of personal health information, as well as guidelines for sharing of information within the health care team to optimize patient-focused care. Those provinces with provincial health information networks have additional policies or regulations that outline requirements for protection of personal health information within the provincial network. Pharmacy operators (owners and managers) share the responsibility with staff members for creating and maintaining systems to protect the personal health information of their patients.

PHARMACY OPERATIONS

Each province has separate legislation governing pharmacy operations. Some have a separate act, and in others, the legislation is embedded within the Pharmacy Act. The Acts contain the overarching enforcement and inspection pieces but allow the development of regulations or by-laws that outline areas such as owning and operating a pharmacy, physical facilities and space requirements, the handling and sale of drugs, record keeping, the dispensary area, patient services area, prescription labelling requirements, and lock-and-leave provisions. Ownership provisions and requirements for opening and closing a pharmacy are also found in the Act or accompanying regulations or by-laws.

To supplement the legal requirements, provincial regulatory authorities have developed policies, guidelines or by-laws to provide more detail about operational processes or to address issues that have arisen for which there is no specific legislation. These additional documents provide direction in areas such as distribution of medication samples, faxing prescriptions, electronic signatures, managing drug errors, required references, central fill, remote dispensing, compliance packaging or sale of needles and syringes. An advantage of addressing issues in this manner is that the policies can be updated by the regulatory body as practice changes, rather than requiring a legislative change by government.

DRUG PLAN BILLING AND INTERCHANGEABILITY

Each province/territory also has a drug plan, usually providing coverage for seniors, those on social assistance or those patients with illness requiring drugs with astronomical costs. Although there has been much discussion about a Canadian formulary or list of drugs covered by these plans, the current system is a formulary in each province/territory. Along with that formulary, provincial/territorial governments have introduced legislation on products covered, interchangeability of products and billing parameters. This is strictly provincial/territorial legislation and must be reviewed region by region. Operators of pharmacies must work with their technical support to ensure these changes are reflected in the pharmacy's billing systems.

THE HEALTH CARE PROFESSIONALS: PHARMACIST AND PHARMACY TECHNICIAN

The Pharmacy Act and associated regulations or by-laws in each province/territory outline the requirements for becoming a pharmacist, the scope of practice of a pharmacist and responsibilities for maintaining a licence to practice. In those provinces with regulated pharmacy technicians, similar legislation has been introduced. There have been many changes in the scope of practice for both of these practitioners and legislation is still changing in many regions.[14] Although the pharmacist and pharmacy technician are responsible for maintaining their competency to practise, pharmacy operations must also be organized to support the health care professionals in providing patient-focused care.

ALIGNING PRACTICE TO LEGISLATION AND STANDARDS OF PRACTICE

Pharmacy, like many other health care professions in Canada, is considered a self-regulating profession. Self-regulation is a model in which government has given a professional group, such as pharmacy, medicine or nursing, the responsibility of overseeing the profession to ensure good health care is provided to the public. Self-regulation tends to be the model for professionals where the specific body of knowledge necessary to practice the profession makes it difficult for external bodies to regulate.[15] Government sets up a statute to ensure protection of the public, while allowing the profession itself to set ethical and practice standards; however, governments are increasingly expecting that legislation proposed by the regulatory bodies must be in the public interest, rather than solely for the benefit of the health care professional.

In addition, self-regulating professions are also responsible for ethical conduct[16] and have an established Code of Ethics for members. Pharmacists and pharmacy technicians are expected to act within this code, and operators should be aware of the ethical code and the obligations of practitioners within the pharmacy to practise by this code.

Every profession also has standards of practice that have been described as, "the generally accepted consensus of right-thinking members of the profession."[17] Some of these standards are even unwritten but expected by the profession. Pharmacy regulators have tried to assist members by publishing documents to describe minimal practice expectations. The Model Standards of Practice for Canadian Pharmacists[18] developed by NAPRA reflects the range of responsibilities of a pharmacist depending on the role in which they are practising. The standards of practice outline what applies to pharmacists in all situations: when pharmacists are providing drug distribution services, when pharmacists are providing care and when pharmacists are managing the pharmacy. Most provinces/territories have adopted these standards of practice, or standards that are very closely aligned to this model. Similarly, as pharmacy technicians are becoming regulated in more regions, NAPRA has also developed Model Standards of Practice for Canadian Pharmacy Technicians.[19]

Pharmacy is a profession in which the regulatory body has jurisdiction over the place of practice (the operation of the pharmacy), the distribution of drugs and regulation of the health care professional. As pharmacists have overall responsibility for a safe drug supply and for patient-focused care, these two aspects of practice are intertwined. The skill and knowledge of an experienced practitioner are not optimized if the pharmacy operation is not set up to support best practice. Likewise, there can be a very well-organized and maintained pharmacy operation, and the practitioner needs support with the knowledge and skills to maintain a quality practice. From a legal standpoint, many of the laws state what a practitioner can or should do, but a well-organized pharmacy operation is necessary to support the practitioner to meet the legal obligations.

For example, the pharmacist is obliged to provide injections in an appropriate environment for the patient; this requires pharmacy operators to create a private physical space for this to happen. Another example would be in the narcotic control regulations that address the pharmacist's responsibility for maintaining a special narcotic prescription file. Although the pharmacist is obligated by the legislation, pharmacy operations must be set up and managed in a way that provides an efficient method of record keeping for any pharmacist or pharmacy technician who works in that pharmacy.

Pharmacists, pharmacy technicians and pharmacy operators have an opportunity to contribute to setting the standards and guidelines for good practice, as well as helping to form legislation. Pharmacists and pharmacy technicians can provide their expertise at the council or committee level of the regulatory body and also have the opportunity to input on development of standards, guidelines and legislation that are circulated for feedback during the consultation stage. New legislation, standards of practice and policies or guidelines are developed to ensure practice is safe and effective, especially in light of the recent changes in scope of practice for pharmacists and the regulation of pharmacy technicians.

To ensure the public is protected, pharmacy regulators have developed continuing quality improvement processes. These include inspections of the pharmacy operations themselves, which have been in place across Canada for many years. More recently, this quality assurance approach has expanded to review the practice of the practitioner and the care provided to the public. It would also be prudent for pharmacy operators to have a continuous quality improvement process in place to ensure compliance with legal and practice requirements and to ensure

Table 1. Regulatory Body Websites

Alberta College of Pharmacists: https://pharmacists.ab.ca/
College of Pharmacists of British Columbia: www.bcpharmacists.org
College of Pharmacists of Manitoba: http://mpha.in1touch.org
New Brunswick College of Pharmacists: www.nbpharmacists.ca
Newfoundland Labrador Pharmacy Board: www.nlpb.ca
Northwest Territories Health and Social Services: www.hss.gov.nt.ca
Nova Scotia College of Pharmacists: www.nspharmacists.ca
Nunavut Department of Health: www.gov.nu.ca/health
Ontario College of Pharmacists: www.ocpinfo.com
Ordre des pharmaciens du Québec: www.opq.org
Prince Edward Island Pharmacy Board: www.pepharmacists.ca
Saskatchewan College of Pharmacists: www.saskpharm.ca
Yukon Department of Community Services: www.community.gov.yk.ca

the quality of the patient-focused care provided to the public (see Chapter 28: Medication Incidents and Quality Improvement).

For legislation, regulations, policies, by-laws, standards of practice and codes of ethics governing pharmacy in each province/territory, it is most efficient to visit the website of the appropriate regulatory body, which also provides a link back to the federal legislation (see Table 1). Pharmacy owners and managers should familiarize themselves with the requirements in their province/territory.

B: Contracts and Agreements

Learning Objectives

- Discuss the contract law that pharmacies are bound by, including contracts with third-party insurers, partners and vendors.
- Describe the risks and benefits of agreements and contracts with stakeholders.

In addition to being subject to federal and provincial/territorial legislation and professional college regulations, every pharmacy must enter into agreements with third-party prescription plan providers to bill prescription services to their plans. These agreements range from acquiring pharmaceutical supplies to establishing the pharmacy business. In general, it is important for pharmacists to understand the underlying principles behind each agreement and to recognize when legal support is necessary from a legal professional.

CONTRACT BASICS

It is important for pharmacists to recognize that a contract, or interchangeably an agreement, is any common intention between two or more parties where one party provides something to the other in exchange for something else. Both parties must give up something to receive something in return. With this in mind, before entering into any agreement, it is important to first ensure that the facts included in the agreement are accurate and applicable to the situation at hand. Keep in mind that if a contractual dispute later arises and a court is required to interpret the agreement, the court's initial determination will be based on a straightforward interpretation of the text, read in context of the entire agreement. The court will interpret the contract from the standpoint of when it was made (the date of the agreement) and will look to ensure interpretations that are commercially absurd are avoided. If the text of the agreement provides a clear interpretation of the contract, the court may not provide parties with an opportunity to explain what they believed the contract to mean at the time of signing, even if one party had a different interpretation of some provisions. As a result, it is important to read each clause in an agreement and openly discuss the intended meaning to ensure no ambiguity exists. It is appropriate, and moreover beneficial, for both parties to enter into a binding relationship knowing exactly what is expected of themselves and the other party.

As such, when drafting an agreement, it is essential that parties mean what they say, and say what they mean. Avoid ambiguous language. Pharmacists should not agree to provisions or terms that are clearly inapplicable to the situation in question. Often, pharmacists are presented with standard agreements that contain standard clauses to cover multiple situations. However, if any of these clauses do not apply to the situation, pharmacists need to insist they be stricken and initialed, before signature. The other party should not be concerned by the removal of such unnecessary clauses. Before executing an agreement, pharmacists should address the following considerations.

When reviewing a contract, pharmacists must ensure the date the contract is made is easily referenced. The parties must be properly identified, with names spelled correctly and accurate addresses listed. Each party must be named using the appropriate legal name so it is obvious who is responsible for performing the obligations outlined in the agreement. For example, if the pharmacy is a corporation, then its legal name should include "Inc." or "Ltd."[1] (See Chapter 14: Financial Statements and Forms of Business Ownership for more information from an accounting point of view.) This is important, as instances may arise where an individual pharmacist is added as a party to an agreement. Should this occur, legal liability to fulfill the terms of the agreement, and more importantly damages should the terms of the agreement be breached, may fall to the pharmacist personally. It is important that the individual executing the agreement be named as a signing agent on behalf of the pharmacy, and not named as a party to the agreement. This potential risk is resolved by ensuring that the pharmacy's proper legal name is the listed party on all agreements.

Pharmacists must thoroughly read the contract and if they have any questions, they should take the time to review the contract with legal counsel to understand legalese before signing. Lawyers can answer questions, interpret "boilerplate" (form) language and alert pharmacists to hidden risks within the contract language. Pharmacists should not assume that the use of a standard contract eliminates the need for a lawyer's review.[1]

In addition, pharmacists may consider retaining a lawyer to assist with contract negotiations. If the negotiations are complex and/or tensions run high between the parties, there is benefit in having a lawyer who can provide distance and objectivity to the discussions. Pharmacists can communicate their priorities, goals and financial budget (for both the agreement and legal services) to their lawyer before negotiations start to ensure the agreement aligns with the pharmacy's operational objectives and that legal fees are provided in an efficient and cost-effective manner. Having such direct communications up front will increase the likelihood that the process runs smoothly and unexpected issues do not arise.

Pharmacists should insist on amendments if they are necessary to ensure their ability to comply with the terms of the agreement. After reading the contract, if a pharmacist disagrees with a key provision (particularly those regarding the pharmacist's obligations), the pharmacist can present a proposed amendment and not sign the contract until it is included. It is not enough that the other party agrees to the amendment via written correspondence or oral discussions; the contract must specifically include the amendment, as most contracts include an integration clause that states the contract supersedes any prior written or informal agreements. The contract is the final word.[1] In the event that a pharmacist is unable to amend an agreement, it is important that he/she understands his/her obligation and is able to fulfill its requirements. Pharmacists should not enter into an agreement knowing they will be unable to fulfill a term, nor should they accept the other party's assurance: "Do not worry about that clause; we never enforce it." Spoken statements during negotiation that are not reflected in the agreement are not applicable.

There can be no ambiguity. Pharmacists should not accept the other party's spoken explanation of a perplexing term or provision, nor assume that the other party defines terms in the same manner in which they would define terms. If there is uncertainty, the agreement can include definitions and additional language to ensure clarity and thoroughly articulate each party's obligations. In some instances, it is helpful to affix attachments or exhibits to the contract to demystify complex issues.[1] Additions should be welcomed to ensure there is no ambiguity as to the terms of the agreement.

Pharmacists need to be sure they are negotiating with the right individual, the person with the requisite authority to extend the final decision on negotiations and execute the contract. Otherwise, pharmacists will be squandering valuable time and money. The individual with the proper authority will have a vested interest in ensuring the contract is negotiated, executed and performed appropriately. To make sure they have the right person, pharmacists can inquire about the individual's ability to make the third party fulfill obligations and live up to the terms of the contract.[1]

Pharmacists should scrutinize clauses that pertain to termination. The contract should define the circumstances by which the parties can terminate the contractual relationship. If one party does not perform according to the other's expectations as outlined in the contract, the other party should have the right to terminate without being held responsible for breaching the contract. The contract should note the grounds, process and timeline for termination from the perspectives of both parties. In this same context, scrutinize the duration of the contract. What are the timing expectations for performance? Is time of the essence? When does the contract expire? One year? Five years? Does the contract renew annually automatically or does it require a written notice? It is a complicated, expensive and stressful process to extricate a party from a contract when the other party is properly performing according to the terms. Pharmacists should not bind themselves for an extended time period unless they have considered things carefully.[1]

It is essential for pharmacists to retain the original contract, amendments, supplements and other communication pertaining to the contract. Again, pharmacists should not agree to a modification of the terms without a written and signed amendment to the original contract.[1]

In the event that pharmacists are presented with an agreement to which they have little to no opportunity to make modifications, it is very important to understand the obligations placed upon the pharmacist and the pharmacy. In the event of a breach, the damages could be much more than simply terminating the agreement. Many agreements have predefined damage provisions in the event of a breach. In these cases, pharmacists should review the agreement with a lawyer so they can identify the obligations and the consequences of any breaches. If pharmacists are unable to fulfill the terms of an agreement, they must force negotiation with the other party or make arrangements to meet the terms.

TYPICAL PHARMACY CONTRACTS

With the above basics in mind, pharmacists will be presented with the following typical contracts.

PHARMACY PROVIDER AGREEMENTS

To provide service to certain customers, pharmacies must enter into pharmacy provider agreements with third-party payers (see Chapter 17: The Canadian Third-Party Payer Market). These third-party payers administer, adjudicate and pay claims submitted by pharmacies on their customers' behalf. To submit claims, pharmacies are provided standard forms and specific instructions. In the event the pharmacy fails to follow the standard processes set forth in the pharmacy provider agreement, the pharmacy risks not being compensated for the submitted claim. The pharmacy provider agreement defines the dispensing fee that can be charged to an individual covered under the agreement, which prescription and over-the-counter (OTC) medications are covered, whether rebates or incentives may be offered and how generic or therapeutic substitutions may be made. Third-party agreements also speak to allowed drug cost and the allowed markups, and whether any fee or cost differences from the pharmacy's usual and customary fee and the fee and cost paid by the third party can be passed on to the patient. Third-party payers will require the pharmacy to retain records of transactions for the purpose of future audits that check to ensure the pharmacy submits appropriate claims only. It is important for the pharmacy to understand the obligations placed upon it by the third-party payer and to ensure it can meet them before executing the document.

WHOLESALE SUPPLY AGREEMENTS

In the event a pharmacy enters into a supply agreement with a wholesale distributor, it is important to first understand whether the distributor can supply all of the pharmaceuticals required. Many wholesale supply agreements are exclusive in nature; that is, the pharmacy is required to purchase 100% of its pharmaceuticals from the wholesaler. In the event a pharmacy purchases pharmaceuticals from another third party, the wholesaler may terminate the wholesale supply agreement or apply damage provisions set forth in the agreement. Pharmacists need to be aware of the wholesaler's right to penalize. Penalties are often punitive in nature and the decision to impose a penalty is at the wholesaler's sole discretion. It is important to note that many wholesale agreements are presented to a pharmacy owner as part of an overall banner agreement.

FRANCHISE AND BANNER AGREEMENTS

In today's Canadian retail pharmacy environment, most pharmacy owners choose to join a banner group or buying group. Examples of banner programs include (but are not limited to) Drug Trading Co. Ltd. (which operates the Guardian and IDA programs), Pharmasave™, PharmaChoice™ and Remedy's Rx™. These relationships provide significant benefit to the pharmacy owner but commensurately contain conditions and create expectations that the pharmacy owners need to fulfill. In essence, a banner agreement is an agreement whereby a banner permits the pharmacy to display its brand and trademarks in exchange for being the pharmacy's wholesale supplier. The banner agreement will place strict requirements upon the pharmacy regarding the use of the banner's trademarks and will outline penalties should the pharmacy breach their obligations. It is important to be fully aware of and discuss the branding expectations with the banner before executing the banner agreement. Furthermore, pharmacy owners are best advised to have an experienced lawyer, familiar with such agreements, review the proposed banner agreement.

In the event a pharmacist decides to become a franchisee of an established pharmacy chain, it is important to understand that the pharmacist will be the public representation of the franchisor. As a result, the franchise agreement will focus on ensuring the pharmacist acts in a prescribed manner that is consistent with the franchise model. Franchise agreements provide pharmacists with the benefit of a known brand, established supply chains, advertisement, point-of-sale (POS) systems and ongoing help with business operations. In exchange, the pharmacist is expected to meet specific obligations. In the event the pharmacist does not fulfill the obligations set forth in the franchise agreement, the franchisor will have pre-determined damage rights outlined in the agreement. The franchisor will likely have sole discretion in determining whether the pharmacist has fulfilled his/her obligations, so it is important for pharmacists to fully understand all obligations and discuss them with the franchisor before executing the franchise agreement.

As with most agreements, the franchise agreement will have a commencement date and a termination date. The franchisor will likely have an option to renew the agreement at the end of the first term. The pharmacist should be aware of this. His or her ability to walk away at the end of the term, or earlier, may be highly dependent upon the franchisor.

The franchisor will provide the pharmacist with access to a supplier for pharmaceutical and front-store products. In most cases, the franchisor will have negotiated an agreement with the supplier whereby pricing benefits are obtained as a result of being part of a larger group of pharmacies. In exchange, franchisees are often required to purchase all of their products from the designated supplier. Franchisees can ask whether any leeway exists in this area (e.g., to procure products from local suppliers).

Being part of a franchise, the franchisee will be required to contribute a monthly amount toward brand recognition initiatives such as advertising. As a result of its branding and marketing preferences, the franchisor will provide franchisees with specifications regarding signage. In the event a franchisee wishes to make a change to signage or advertising material, he/she will be required to first obtain permission from the franchisor. The franchisee will be required to follow any merchandising programs established by the franchisor, such as dispensing fees or sales on merchandise. In all cases, the franchise agreement will broadly describe the penalties for any breaches to the franchisor's instructions. With that in mind, it is very important for the franchisee to discuss penalties with the franchisor before executing the franchise agreement.

SERVICE AGREEMENTS

Pharmacies will be called upon, or have the opportunity, to provide services to third parties such as long-term care facilities, prisons and group homes. Prior to providing services, the pharmacy needs to execute a service agreement that confirms the term or duration of the agreement and the services to be provided by the pharmacy. It is important that all services to be provided by the pharmacy are explicitly outlined in the agreement. The agreement will also outline the obligations of the parties, such as abiding by applicable facility policies and procedures, providing services on an emergency basis, after hours, etc. It will also outline the consequences if one party breaches their obligations, which may include pre-defined damages.

LEASE AGREEMENTS

Pharmacy owners require a location from which to operate. When the option of owning the commercial property is not available, most pharmacy owners will lease space from which to operate their pharmacy. Lease agreements can be very complex contractual agreements and as such, should always be reviewed by a lawyer with experience in negotiating commercial retail leases. Important areas of negotiation include the term of the lease, meaning the length or period during which the pharmacy operator can continue to use the leased space, as well as renewal clauses that dictate the terms to which a lease would be subject to be renewed. Other important aspects of a commercial retail lease include the amount of rent to be paid and the common area costs (CAM) for which the lessor (the pharmacy operator) is responsible, in addition to the base rent set out in the lease.

To successfully operate a pharmacy, it is important for pharmacists to fully understand the contents and resultant implications of each agreement they enter into with third parties. Prior to executing any agreement, it is incumbent upon pharmacists to enter into candid discussions with the other party regarding interpretation, and to recognize when legal advice is necessary. Should pharmacists fail to appreciate the complexities and interpretation of each clause, they may spend more time and effort dealing with misunderstandings than they do practising the profession of pharmacy.

REFERENCES TO PART A

1. The Food and Drugs Act. Government of Canada. Ottawa, 1985, last amended 2013–06–19. Available: http://laws.justice.gc.ca/eng/acts/F-27/ (accessed June 5, 2014).
2. Food and Drug Regulations. Government of Canada. Ottawa, last amended 2014–01–29. Available: http://laws-lois.justice.gc.ca/eng/regulations/C.R.C.%2C_c._870/ (accessed June 5, 2014).
3. Natural Health Product Regulations. Government of Canada. Ottawa, 2003, last amended 2008–06–01. Available: http://laws-lois.justice.gc.ca/eng/regulations/SOR-2003-196/ (accessed June 5, 2014).
4. Controlled Drugs and Substances Act. Government of Canada. Ottawa, 1996, last amended 2012–11–06. Available: http://laws-lois.justice.gc.ca/eng/acts/C-38.8/index.html (accessed June 5, 2014).
5. Narcotic Control Regulations. Government of Canada. Ottawa, last amended 2014–03–31. Available: http://laws-lois.justice.gc.ca/eng/regulations/C.R.C.,_c._1041/index.html (accessed June 5, 2014).
6. Benzodiazepines and Other Targeted Substances Regulations. Government of Canada. Ottawa, 2000, last amended 2012–12–19. Available: http://laws-lois.justice.gc.ca/eng/regulations/SOR-2000-217/index.html (accessed June 5, 2014).

7. Marihuana for Medical Purposes Regulations. Government of Canada. Ottawa, 2013, last amended 2014–03–31. Available: http://laws-lois.justice.gc.ca/eng/regulations/SOR-2013-119/index.html (accessed June 5, 2014).

8. Precursor Control Regulations. Government of Canada. Ottawa, 2002, last amended 2013–12–19. Available: http://laws-lois.justice.gc.ca/eng/regulations/SOR-2002-359/index.html (accessed June 5, 2014).

9. National Association of Pharmacy Regulatory Authorities, and the National Drug Scheduling Advisory Committee. Ottawa. Available: http://napra.ca/pages/Schedules/Committee.aspx (accessed June 9, 2014).

10. National Association of Pharmacy Regulatory Authorities. National drug schedules. Ottawa. Available: http://napra.ca/pages/Schedules/default.aspx (accessed June 9, 2014).

11. National Association of Pharmacy Regulatory Authorities. Implementation of the national drug schedule model across Canada as of 2013. Ottawa. Available: http://napra.ca/pages/Schedules/Overview.aspx?id=1926 (accessed June 9, 2014).

12. Richard G, Ojala V, Ojala A, et al. Monitoring programs for drugs with potential for abuse or misuse in Canada. Can Pharm J (Ott). 2012;145(4):168–71. http://dx.doi.org/10.3821/145.4.cpj168. Medline:23509545

13. Personal Information Protection and Electronic Document Act. Government of Canada. Ottawa, 2002, last amended 2011–04–01. Available: http://laws-lois.justice.gc.ca/eng/acts/P-8.6/index.html (accessed June 9, 2014).

14. Blueprint for Pharmacy. Environmental scan: pharmacy practice legislation and policy changes across Canada May 2014. Ottawa: Canadian Pharmacists Association, 2014. Available: http://blueprintforpharmacy.ca/docs/kt-tools/environmental-scan---pharmacy-practice-legislation-and-policy-changes-may-2014.pdf (accessed June 9, 2014).

15. Baggott R. Regulatory politics, health professionals and the public interest. In: Allsop J, Saks M, editors. *Regulating the health professions*. London: Sage Publications; 2002. p. 31–46. http://dx.doi.org/10.4135/9781446220047.n3.

16. Stone J. Evaluating the ethical and legal content of professional code of ethics. In: Allsop J, Saks M, editors. *Regulating the health professions*. London: Sage Publications; 2002. p. 62–76. http://dx.doi.org/10.4135/9781446220047.n5.

17. Steinecke R. Types of standards and guidelines. Grey areas. Toronto: Steinecke, Maciura, LeBlanc, Barristers & Solicitors, April 2004. no. 74, p1.

18. National Association of Pharmacy Regulatory Authorities. Model standards of practice for Canadian pharmacists. Ottawa. March 2009. Available: http://napra.ca/Content_Files/Files/Model_Standards_of_Prac_for_Cdn_Pharm_March09_Final_b.pdf (accessed June 9, 2014).

19. National Association of Pharmacy Regulatory Authorities. Model standards of practice for Canadian pharmacy technicians. Ottawa. Nov. 2011. Available: http://napra.ca/Content_Files/Files/Model_Standards_of_Prac_for_Cdn_PharmTechs_Nov11.pdf (accessed June 9, 2014).

REFERENCE TO PART B

1. Fields AC. Contracting tips for the independent pharmacist. Available: www.aprx.org/templates/aprx/Assets/aprx-advisor---contracting-tips.pdf (accessed Dec. 13, 2014).

VII. QUALITY CONTROL, QUALITY ASSURANCE AND CONTINUOUS QUALITY IMPROVEMENT

CHAPTER 28

Medication Incidents and Quality Improvement

Todd A. Boyle, *PhD; Professor and Canada Research Chair in Quality Assurance in Community Pharmacy, Gerald Schwartz School of Business, St. Francis Xavier University*

Certina Ho, *RPh BScPhm MISt MEd; Project Lead, Institute for Safe Medication Practices Canada; Lecturer, Leslie Dan Faculty of Pharmacy, University of Toronto; Adjunct Clinical Assistant Professor, School of Pharmacy, University of Waterloo*

Learning Objectives

- Develop an understanding of medication incidents, their causes and how they are categorized.
- Describe the role of continuous quality improvement (CQI) in enhancing medication incident reporting and learning.
- Understand pharmacist expectations (e.g., standards of practice) with respect to the reporting and disclosure of medication incidents.
- Become familiar with software and tools that can be used to support CQI in Canadian pharmacies.
- Identify system improvements that can be implemented to help prevent the future recurrence of a similar medication incident.

Although there have been significant advances in technology and process automation, pharmacy practice remains a profession in which there are many opportunities for human error to occur. Medication incidents, such as dispensing errors that lead to the patient receiving an incorrect drug, dose or quantity of medication, can have significant negative implications for a wide range of pharmacy stakeholders. For example, while an incorrect drug being dispensed may result in patient harm, there are also other negative outcomes such as possible litigation, harm to the pharmacy's reputation and decreased staff morale.

Despite the negative impact that medication incidents can have on patients, pharmacy staff members and the reputation of the pharmacy, many pharmacists are reluctant to acknowledge and discuss medication incidents. When an error occurs, there is a tendency both within the profession and the public at large to look for someone to blame and punish for the error. Yet only by adopting a non-punitive systems-focused process for openly discussing errors can their causes be identified and changes made to enhance the quality and safety of the medication management system.

MEDICATION INCIDENTS

The Institute for Safe Medication Practices Canada (ISMP Canada) defines a medication incident as, "any preventable event that may cause or lead to inappropriate medication use or patient harm while the medication is in the control of the healthcare professional, patient, or consumer."[1] Medication incidents can originate at any stage of the medication-use process. Some of the more common types of medication incidents include incorrect patient, incorrect drug, incorrect dose, incorrect frequency of administration, incorrect duration of treatment, improper storage of medication and incorrect route of administration.

Medication incidents are preventable. However, attributing the incident to an individual pharmacist, technician or other staff member fails to recognize the system deficiencies that may be the root cause of the error. The high profile Cropp case in the United States[2,3] highlights how process and system factors often play a significant role in a medication incident. Eric Cropp was a pharmacist at an Ohio hospital who failed to identify that a pharmacy technician under his supervision had made a chemotherapy solution that contained dangerous amounts of sodium chloride.[2] Specifically, the final solution contained more than 20% sodium chloride when it was supposed to contain only 0.9%.[2] It resulted in the death of a two-year-old, Emily Jerry.[3]

As the pharmacist who was responsible for the final check of the prepared product, Cropp was convicted of involuntary manslaughter and sentenced to six months in prison, six months of home confinement, three years of probation, 400 hours of community service, payment of court costs and a $5,000 fine. In addition, he was permanently stripped of his licence by the state pharmacy board.[2,3] However, several human, process and system failures occurred that day that contributed to this tragic error: the computer system in the pharmacy was not operating in the morning, leading to a backlog of orders; the pharmacy was short-staffed; given the workload, normal rest or meal breaks did not occur; and although the chemotherapy solution was not needed until hours later, Cropp received a call from a nurse to dispense it immediately.[2]

Many of the contributing factors in the Cropp case are among the common causes of medication incidents. See Table 1 for common factors that increase the risk of medication incidents.[4–8]

Table 1. Common Factors that Increase the Risk of Medication Incidents[8]

Staff shortages
Noisy or cluttered workplace settings
Poor lighting
Interruptions
Lack of policies or procedures
Missing or insufficient documentation
Miscommunication
Missing patient information
Missing drug information
Labelling and packaging issues (e.g., medications with similar labelling or packaging, or medications with look-alike or sound-alike names)
Drug storage or delivery problems
Staff education deficiency
Patient education deficiency
Quality control or independent check system deficiency

An error need not cause harm to invoke changes in the pharmacy. Near misses (e.g., events that did not reach the patient as a result of chance or through timely intervention[1]) and no harm events (e.g., events where the medication has been dispensed and may have been consumed, but the patient presents no symptoms or does not require treatment) offer the opportunity to identify and correct the causes of errors before they result in the type of outcome that occurred in the Cropp case. Regardless of the patient outcome, learning from medication incidents and formally planning, implementing and monitoring subsequent changes are steps that many pharmacies are now being required to undertake by their provincial/territorial regulatory authority.[9]

CONTINUOUS QUALITY IMPROVEMENT

The exact number of medication incidents that occur in Canada each year is unknown. However, if the results of international studies[10,11] are applied to the approximately 574 million retail prescriptions dispensed in Canada in 2013,[12] it is estimated that between 1.3 and 16.3 million medication incidents, including near misses and no harm events, occur in Canadian community pharmacies every year. As a result, learning from medication incidents and taking steps to reduce or prevent incident reoccurrence can have a significant impact on the safety of pharmacy practice. Continuous quality improvement (CQI) is a management philosophy focused on enhancing various aspects of performance and quality through an ongoing and incremental approach. In the pharmacy setting, CQI uses teamwork and problem solving to achieve performance improvements such as improved customer service, the addition of new patient-centred services, removing process inefficiencies and reducing medication incidents.

Within a medication incident context, formal CQI programs shift the focus away from the individual who committed the error (a culture of blame and shame) and onto the medication-use processes in the pharmacy. This shift in focus is critical. Removing the individual who was most closely associated with the medication incident may do nothing to prevent recurrence of a similar incident. Identifying and rectifying the root causes of the incident are likely to be far more effective means of preventing a recurrence. CQI programs provide pharmacies with the tools, training and support needed to undertake this systematic evaluation and implement the needed change. The changes made also need to be monitored over time to ensure they are maintained and achieve their intended outcome.

Given the important role that CQI programs play in improving patient safety, many pharmacy regulatory authorities throughout North America now require that pharmacies have a CQI program in place.[13] However, a large degree of variation exists in CQI program requirements from one regulatory jurisdiction (province/territory or state) to the next. Mandated CQI program requirements across North America range from simple paper-based documentation programs to those with significant technology and web-based analytic components.[9,14]

APPLICATION OF CQI

An example of a comprehensive community pharmacy CQI program in Canada is the one developed by the Nova Scotia College of Pharmacists (NSCP). Under the NSCP Standards of Practice for Continuous Quality Assurance Programs in Community Pharmacies,[15] all Nova Scotia community pharmacies are required to do the following:

- Have a formal, documented CQI program in place
- Anonymously report medication incidents and near misses to an independent and objective national third party

- Perform annual safety self-assessments to track quality improvements over time
- Conduct quarterly staff meetings to examine medication incidents that have occurred
- Plan and implement quality improvement changes

While Nova Scotia community pharmacies are free to develop their own CQI program, the NSCP, in partnership with university researchers, pharmacists and ISMP Canada, developed the SafetyNET-Rx CQI program as an option to meet the NSCP standards of practice. Although originally developed for Nova Scotia pharmacies, SafetyNET Rx is applicable to most Canadian pharmacies and has been adopted in various forms by pharmacies throughout Canada. As presented in Figure 28.1, key components of the SafetyNET-Rx CQI program include training of

Figure 28.1

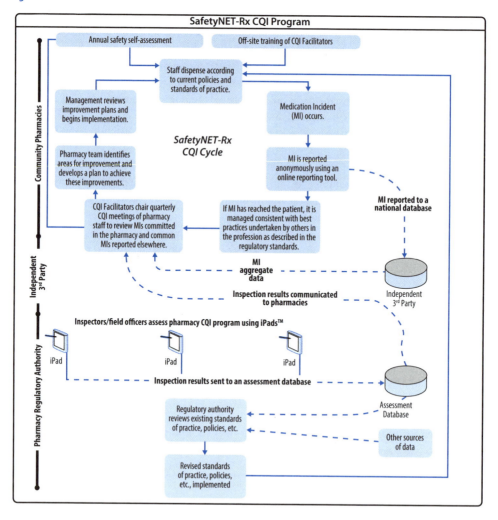

SafetyNET-Rx CQI program (used with permission)[16]

CQI facilitators, annual medication safety self-assessments, a formal CQI cycle to allow pharmacy staff to identify the root causes of medication incidents, anonymous online reporting of medication incidents to a national database, tools to support quarterly CQI meetings, access to aggregate analysis on common medication incidents occurring in other pharmacies and a platform to allow the pharmacy regulatory authority to provide feedback to pharmacies on the completeness of their CQI program.[9,14]

The most common version of SafetyNET-Rx used by pharmacies reports medication incidents to ISMP Canada and uses their reporting and analytic tools. These tools include ISMP Canada's Medication Safety Self-Assessment® for Community/Ambulatory Pharmacy™ (MSSA-CAP)[8] and the Community Pharmacy Incident Reporting (CPhIR) System (an anonymous online incident reporting and CQI system).[17] Pharmacies are also provided with support for quarterly CQI meetings and access to aggregate data on medication incidents occurring at other pharmacies.

Before the SafetyNET-Rx CQI program begins, the pharmacy is required to complete a medication safety self-assessment, such as MSSA-CAP. The MSSA-CAP, completed as a group by pharmacy management, staff pharmacists and pharmacy technicians, assesses pharmacy safety along 10 key elements that range from patient information to quality and risk management. Example MSSA-CAP questions are presented in Figure 28.2.

Figure 28.2

SELF-ASSESSMENT ITEMS		A	B	C	D	E
74	Management actively demonstrates its commitment to patient safety (and safe medication practices) by approving a patient safety plan, encouraging pharmacist/technician error reporting, and supporting system enhancements, including technology, that are likely to reduce errors.					
75	Specific medication safety objectives (e.g., staff reporting without fear of punishment; careful analysis of the system-based causes of errors), are included in the management's strategic plans, directly communicated to all staff, and acknowledged in a positive manner when met.					
	Core distinguishing characteristic #19:					
	Practitioners are encouraged to detect and report errors, and teams (or individual practitioners in small pharmacies) regularly analyze errors that have occurred within the organization and in other organizations for the purpose of redesigning systems to best support safe medication practices.					
76	One pharmacist in the individual pharmacy has responsibility for enhancing detection of medication errors, overseeing analysis of their causes, and coordinating an effective error reduction plan (with corporate support as applicable).					
77	Information is sought annually (e.g., by focus group, individual discussion, questionnaire) to learn about perceived problems with the dispensing system.					
78	The dispensing system (e.g., drug procurement and storage, receipt of prescriptions, obtaining important patient information, prescription filling, patient education, monitoring the effects of drugs) is proactively assessed at least annually to identify potential risk factors that could lead to errors and system changes that would make it less likely for an error to reach a patient.					

SafetyNET-Rx CQI Program MSSA-CAP Sample Survey Items (used with permission)[8]

The SafetyNET-Rx CQI program begins with the off-site training of quality improvement champions in each pharmacy, known as CQI facilitators.[9,14] Each pharmacy adopting the SafetyNET-Rx CQI program must have a pharmacist and a pharmacy technician CQI facilitator. Having both pharmacist and pharmacy technician champions is key to ensuring the perspectives of all pharmacy staff are considered when addressing medication incidents. Key responsibilities of the CQI facilitators include communicating the information they have received from the off-site training and initiating quarterly meetings.[9,14]

As part of the SafetyNET-Rx CQI program, pharmacies are required to complete a medication safety self-assessment annually to track safety improvements over time.

To demonstrate how CQI programs enhance medication incident learning, a medication incident that actually occurred in a Canadian pharmacy is used as an example of how CQI programs can help improve medication safety. A prescription for a patient who was discharged from a hospital was faxed to a pharmacy (Figure 28.3).

Following the SafetyNET-Rx CQI program, pharmacy staff dispensed according to the current policies, standards and best practices of the pharmacy. As a result, Heparin was dispensed and the patient received two doses. Pharmacy staff continued to dispense until a medication incident was identified. A medication incident may be identified by pharmacy staff, patient, customer or health care provider. In this particular case, the medication incident was identified by pharmacy staff when the hospital sent a request for the pharmacy to provide syringes and alcohol swabs for the remainder of the "dalteparin" therapy.[17] Immediate follow-up with the hospital indicated that a prescription for "dalteparin 15 000 U" was actually sent (Figure 28.4). However, the fax transmission received at the pharmacy had the first two letters of the drug name cut off, resulting in the appearance of "heparin." The transmission log from the hospital fax machine indicated that the fax had been sent correctly.

Following the identification of a medication incident, key error details were anonymously reported to ISMP Canada CPhIR system.[17] As presented in Figure 28.5, several key details are provided in the report.

Figure 28.3

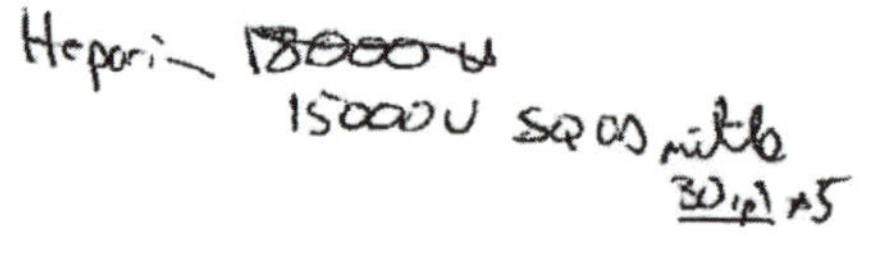

Contents of a faxed prescription received at a pharmacy (used with permission)[18]

Figure 28.4

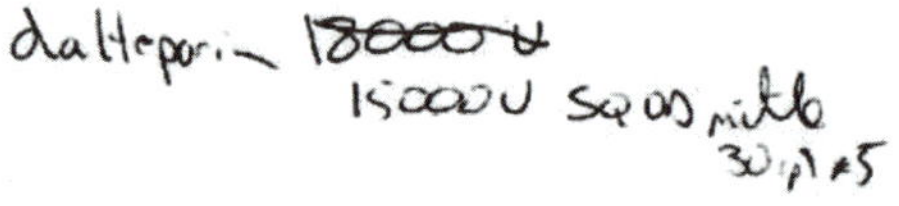

Text from the original prescription (used with permission)[18]

Figure 28.5

Date Incident Occurred	2014-01-10
Time Incident Occurred	Evening (18:00-00:00)
Type of Incident	Incorrect drug
Incident Discovered By	Pharmacist
Medication System Stages Involved in this Incident	• Prescription Preparation/Dispensing • Rx Order Entry
Medications	• FRAGMIN 15000IU(ANTI-XA)/0.6ML • HEPARIN SODIUM INJECTION USP (SINGLE USE VIAL--PRESERVATIVE FREE)
Gender	Male
Age	>65 years
Degree of Harm to Patient due to Incident	NO HARM No Harm (Medication Dispensed) – No symptoms detected; no treatment required
Incident Description/ How Incident was Discovered	A prescription for a patient who had been discharged from hospital was received by fax at the pharmacy. Heparin was dispensed, and the patient received 2 doses. When the hospital sent a request to the pharmacy to provide syringes and alcohol swabs for the duration of the "dalteparin" therapy, we then recognized that an error had occurred. Further investigation revealed that the hospital had in fact sent a prescription for "dalteparin 15 000 U," but during the fax transmission, the first 2 letters of the drug name, "da," were cut off, which resulted in "heparin" being perceived as the prescription order. The hospital's fax transmission log indicated that the fax had been sent correctly, giving no indication of any problem.

Other Incident Info	Rx is from:
	    Hospital
	Rx is presented as a:
	    Hand-written Prescription
	    Fax Prescription
	Type of Rx:
	    Regular
	Rx Order Entry/Dispensing Label Generation
	    New Rx
	Administration
	    Medication was administered

Contributing Factors of this Incident	Miscommunication of drug order
	    Illegible
	    Ambiguous
	    Incomplete
	Drug name, label, packaging problem
	    Look/sound-alike names
	Staff education problem
	    Feedback about errors/prevention
	Lack of quality control or independent check system
	    Equipment quality control checks

Reporting of the medication incident to ISMP CANADA (used with permission)[18]

Medication incidents are discussed at quarterly CQI meetings attended by all pharmacists and technicians. The first goal is to analyze medication incidents that have occurred since the previous meeting. This analysis is done to find out what happened, how and why the incident occurred and what can be done to prevent similar incidents from happening in the future.[19]

There are various methods used for medication incident analysis in different health care settings, depending upon the type and context of the incident and the skills and resources available to the health care team involved. In essence, several key steps should be considered when conducting an incident analysis at a pharmacy. Seven steps recommended by ISMP Canada are applied to the heparin/dalteparin incident[17]:

1. Define and describe the medication incident that occurred in the pharmacy. It is recommended that staff review the original prescription, incident details reported to CPhIR and any other relevant documents.[17]

   In this case: A prescription for a patient who was discharged from the hospital was received by fax at the pharmacy. Heparin was dispensed and the patient received two doses. The hospital's fax transmission log showed the fax had been sent correctly, with no indication of any problem.[18]

2. Try to collect as much information and detail about the incident as possible. It is suggested that pharmacy staff consider the 10 key elements presented in the MSSA: 1) patient information; 2) drug information; 3) communication of drug orders and other drug information; 4) drug labelling, packaging and nomenclature; 5) drug standardization, storage and distribution; 6) medication device acquisition, use and monitoring; 7) environmental factors, workflow and staffing patterns; 8) staff competence and education; 9) patient education; 10) quality processes and risk management.[8,17]

   In this case: The following key elements may have been involved: 1) communication of drug orders and other drug information; 2) drug labelling, packaging and nomenclature; 3) staff competence and education; and 4) quality processes and risk management.

3. Pharmacy staff should attempt to identify all possible contributing factors and potential causes that may have led to the medication incident, using the 10 key elements described in point 2.

   In this case: The following potential contributing factors were identified: 1) miscommunication of drug order (e.g., incomplete, ambiguous or illegible prescription order), use of a handwritten, unformatted document for faxed prescriptions versus a template or form; 2) drug name, label, packaging problem (e.g., look-alike names between dalteparin and heparin); 3) staff education deficiency (e.g., insufficient staff education about possible errors with fax orders); and 4) lack of quality control or independent check systems (e.g., lack of quality control of the fax machine).

4. Pharmacy staff should develop causal statements based on the potential causes identified in the previous step. The relationships between the potential contributing factors should then be mapped. As part of the mapping process, pharmacy staff should discuss why each of the potential causes occurred.[17] ISMP Canada recommends following the ABC format when developing the causal statements:

   • A = Antecedent: This is the set of circumstances, contributing factors or potential causes leading to the incident.

- B = Behaviour/Bridge: This will increase or decrease the likelihood of the occurrence of the incident.
- C = Consequences: This is the result or outcome (the incident).

In this case: The following causal statements were developed based on the potential causes identified[17]:
- The ambiguous or illegible fax prescription order increased the likelihood that the incorrect drug would be entered and dispensed, leading to potential adverse effects in the patient.
- The look-alike drug names between dalteparin and heparin increased the likelihood that the incorrect drug would be entered and dispensed, leading to potential adverse effects in the patient.
- Insufficient staff education and feedback to the pharmacy team about possible errors with fax prescription orders increased the likelihood that the incorrect drug order would be interpreted, entered and dispensed, leading to potential adverse effects in the patient.
- Lack of regular quality control checks of the fax machine increased the likelihood that the incorrect drug order would be interpreted, entered and dispensed, leading to potential adverse effects in the patient.

5. Pharmacy staff should identify and discuss possible solutions that may prevent or reduce the likelihood of the medication incident happening again. Proposed solutions should meet three key criteria[17]:
   - be system-based: Pharmacy staff should develop solutions with a high probability of being effective in preventing a recurrence of the incident.
   - be feasible to implement within the pharmacy, considering the available human resources and any limitations of the physical environment.
   - not have a negative impact on other procedures and activities that are not related to the medication incident.

6. Based on the effectiveness and feasibility of the proposed solutions, pharmacy staff should come up with a suggested ranking for each solution, taking into account any issues related to the pharmacy workflow, policies and procedures.[17]

   In this case: The following possible solutions may decrease the likelihood of similar medication incidents related to fax transmission errors:[18]
   - First, establish a pharmacy policy to conduct regular maintenance and cleaning of fax machines to ensure optimal transmission of prescription orders.
   - Second, remind pharmacy staff members to review all fax prescriptions for quality issues (e.g., truncation of a prescription header, extraneous marks in the prescription body), as well as the legibility of the prescription order.

7. Pharmacy staff should develop an action plan to implement the solution(s) within the pharmacy in such a way that progress can be monitored. Action plans should be SMART (Specific, Measurable, Attainable, Relevant and Time-based). For instance, assign actions to specific individuals with expected timelines; consider possible barriers that pharmacy

staff members may encounter during the implementation of the action plan; stay away from big, bold actions; and use the small cycles-of-change model (plan, do, study, act). Keep in mind that this is an iterative process for implementing and monitoring action plans for continuous quality assurance[17] (see Chapter 10: Change Management).

In this case: The following action plan was developed based on the previous solutions agreed upon by the pharmacy team during the CQI meeting[18]:

- The pharmacy manager will develop a policy by the end of the month where the lead pharmacy technician will conduct weekly maintenance and cleaning of fax machines to ensure optimal transmission of prescription orders. A log book will be available in the dispensary for the technician to document that this task is completed by the scheduled time.
- The pharmacy manager will remind all pharmacy staff members to review all fax prescriptions for quality issues (e.g., truncation of a prescription header, extraneous marks in the prescription body), as well as the legibility of the prescription order. A reminder memo will be placed next to the fax machine by the end of the week.

Further to these suggested solutions for preventing similar medication incidents related to fax transmission errors, the pharmacy team should also consider the following:[18]

- Engage and educate patients throughout the medication-use process, especially at transition points of care. In this case, it was a hospital discharge prescription and it is possible that the patient might have been provided with information regarding discharge medications at the hospital. Engage patients in a dialogue, for example, at the pick-up counter, and show patients their medications so they can serve as an independent double check.
- Consider the appropriateness of the various aspects of the prescription order, such as indication, dose, frequency and route of administration, etc. In this case, unfractionated heparin for subcutaneous administration is usually given every 8 hours or every 12 hours, instead of a once-daily dosing schedule.

The second goal of the quarterly CQI meeting is for pharmacy staff to assess the likelihood that medication incidents that have occurred elsewhere may occur at their own pharmacy and plan changes to prevent these errors from happening to them. SafetyNET-Rx provides pharmacy teams with access to aggregate data on medication incidents occurring throughout Canada. For example, through the CPhIR system, pharmacies can review the type of incidents reported at their own pharmacy and compare it to national aggregate data. In addition, pharmacies can download ISMP Canada Safety Bulletins on common or critical medication incidents occurring throughout Canada.

Through input from the provincial/territorial pharmacy inspectors/field officers/practice advisors, pharmacies are provided with an assessment of their CQI process. The third goal of the quarterly CQI meeting is for staff to examine their CQI process, identify gaps and plan how to close them. Specifically, as part of the SafetyNET-Rx CQI program, pharmacy inspectors using a tablet-based mobile application can provide pharmacies with a real-time assessment of the completeness of their CQI program and areas that need improvement. Pharmacy inspectors assess performance on the basis of four major themes: basic CQI components, medication safety self-assessment, medication incident reporting and medication incident learning. Each of these sections contains multiple choice and open-ended questions that are answered by the inspector after discussion with pharmacy staff. As part of this assessment, pharmacy staff, using the tablet, can comment on the extent to which a safety culture exists in the pharmacy. Results of the assessment are presented to the pharmacy manager, with key gaps discussed at future CQI meetings.

Outcomes from the CQI meeting are suggested changes and an implementation plan to address the key medication incidents discussed. The suggested changes are then reviewed, approved and implemented by pharmacy management. Pharmacy staff then follow the revised medication-use process until a medication incident happens again, at which time the process starts over.

CHALLENGES AND BENEFITS OF CQI IMPLEMENTATION

Despite the potential for enhancing medication incident learning and improving patient safety, pharmacies face significant challenges as they implement and sustain a formal CQI program. Common challenges include finding the time to report incidents when they occur in the pharmacy, apprehension on the part of staff to discuss medication incidents, difficulty in finding ways to have all staff involved and supportive of the key components of the CQI process, and staff unwillingness to accept and fully use the technological components of the CQI program.[9,14]

As pharmacies overcome such challenges and CQI becomes a normal part of the pharmacy workflow, several benefits beyond incident prevention may occur. Key benefits realized by pharmacies that have adopted formal CQI programs include enhanced staff understanding of the medication-use processes within the pharmacy, increased staff openness and comfort with discussing incidents, improved staff confidence and awareness of their individual responsibilities with regard to patient safety in the pharmacy, and a stronger belief that the pharmacy's medication-use system is safer and more reliable as a result of the CQI program.[14]

Medication incidents are an unfortunate part of pharmacy practice. While medication incidents may have significant negative outcomes for the patient and the pharmacy, such errors also represent excellent learning opportunities. Through the process of CQI, pharmacies can identify the root causes of medication incidents and implement process changes to help prevent similar incidents from happening again. However, given the difficulty with openly talking about errors, the development and implementation of CQI programs are not yet universal in pharmacies across Canada. Through the leadership and commitment of pharmacy management, such challenges can be overcome, resulting in enhanced safety, quality and confidence in providing patient-centred care services by the pharmacy.

CONFLICT OF INTEREST DISCLAIMER

Todd Boyle is Team Lead of SafetyNET-Rx, a research and public outreach initiative that encourages and supports an open dialogue among health care stakeholders on issues surrounding medication incidents within community pharmacies.
Certina Ho is a Project Lead with the Institute for Safe Medication Practices Canada, an independent national not-for-profit organization committed to the advancement of medication safety in all health care settings.

RESOURCES AND SUGGESTED READINGS

Church R, MacKinnon N. *Take as directed: your prescription for safe health care in Canada.* Toronto, ON: ECW Press; 2010.
Cohen MR, editor. *Medication errors.* Washington, DC: American Pharmacists Association; 2007.

Dekker S. *Just culture: balancing safety and accountability*. Burlington, VT: Ashgate Publishing Company; 2012.

Institute of Medicine. *Preventing medication errors*. Washington, DC: National Academies Press; 2007.

Institute of Medicine. *To err is human: building a safer health system*. Washington, DC: The National Academies Press; 2000.

MacKinnon NJ, editor. *Safe and effective: the eight essential elements of an optimal medication-use system*. Ottawa: Canadian Pharmacists Association; 2007.

McIver S, Wyndham R. *After the error: speaking out about patient safety to save lives*. Toronto, ON: ECW Press; 2013.

Nova Scotia College of Pharmacists. Standards of practice for quality assurance programs in community pharmacies, Nova Scotia: Nova Scotia College of Pharmacists, 2014. Available: www.nspharmacists.ca/standards/documents/QualityAssurance.pdf (accessed July 22, 2014).

REFERENCES

1. Institute for Safe Medication Practices Canada definition of terms. 2014. Available: www.ismp-canada.org/definitions.htm (accessed Oct. 9, 2014).

2. Institute for Safe Medication Practices Canada. An injustice has been done: jail time given to pharmacist who made an error. 2009. Available: www.ismp.org/pressroom/injustice-jailtime-for-pharmacist.asp (accessed July 22, 2014).

3. Institute for Safe Medication Practices Canada. Ohio government plays whack-a-mole with pharmacist. 2009. Available: www.ismp.org/newsletters/acutecare/articles/20090827.asp (accessed July 22, 2014).

4. Santell JP, Hicks RW, McMeekin J, et al. Medication errors: experience of the United States Pharmacopeia (USP) MEDMARX reporting system. J Clin Pharmacol. 2003;43(7):760–7. http://dx.doi.org/10.1177/0091270003254831. Medline:12856391

5. Szeinbach S, Seoane-Vazquez E, Parekh A, et al. Dispensing errors in community pharmacy: perceived influence of socio-technical factors. Int J Qual Health Care. 2007;19(4):203–9. http://dx.doi.org/10.1093/intqhc/mzm018. Medline:17567597

6. Malone DC, Abarca J, Skrepnek GH, et al. Pharmacist workload and pharmacy characteristics associated with the dispensing of potentially clinically important drug-drug interactions. Med Care. 2007;45(5):456–62. http://dx.doi.org/10.1097/01.mlr.0000257839.83765.07. Medline:17446832

7. Davidhizar R, Lonser G. Strategies to decrease medication errors. Health Care Manag (Frederick). 2003;22(3):211–8. http://dx.doi.org/10.1097/00126450-200307000-00004. Medline:12956222

8. Institute for Safe Medication Practices Canada. *Medication Safety Self-Assessment® Program for Community/Ambulatory Pharmacy*. Canadian Version; 2006.

9. Boyle TA, MacKinnon NJ, Mahaffey T, et al. Challenges of standardized continuous quality improvement programs in community pharmacies: the case of SafetyNET-Rx. Res Social Adm Pharm. 2012;8(6):499–508. http://dx.doi.org/10.1016/j.sapharm.2012.01.005. Medline:22421196

10. Knudsen P, Herborg H, Mortensen AR, et al. Preventing medication errors in community pharmacy: frequency and seriousness of medication errors. Qual Saf Health Care. 2007;16(4):291–6. http://dx.doi.org/10.1136/qshc.2006.018770. Medline:17693678

11. Flynn EA, Dorris NT, Holman GT, et al. Medication dispensing errors in community pharmacies: a nationwide study. Proceedings of the Human Factors and Ergonomics Society Annual Meeting, 2002; 46:1448–1451. http://dx.doi.org/10.1177/154193120204601609.

12. The Canadian Generic Market Year 2013. The Canadian Generic Pharmaceutical Association. Available: www.canadiangenerics.ca/en/resources/market_trends.asp (accessed Aug. 13, 2014).

13. National Association of Boards of Pharmacy survey of pharmacy and law. National Association of Boards of Pharmacy, 2012. Available: www.usc.edu/hsc/nml/assets/pdf/2010%20Final%20Survey%20no%20letter.pdf (accessed July 22, 2014).

14. Boyle TA, Bishop AC, Duggan K, et al. Keeping the "continuous" in continuous quality improvement: exploring perceived outcomes of CQI program use in community pharmacy. Res Social Adm Pharm. 2014;10(1):45–57. http://dx.doi.org/10.1016/j.sapharm.2013.01.006. Medline:23528447

15. Standards of Practice for Quality Assurance Programs in Community Pharmacies, Nova Scotia: Nova Scotia College of Pharmacists, 2014. Available: www.nspharmacists.ca/standards/documents/ QualityAssurance.pdf (accessed July 22, 2014).

16. Reprinted from Res Soc Adm Pharm, 10/1, Boyle T.A, Bishop A., Duggan K, et al., Keeping the "continuous" in continuous quality improvement: Exploring perceived outcomes of CQI program use in community pharmacy, 45–57. Copyright 2014, with permission from Elsevier.

17. Ho C, Hung P, Lee G, et al. Community pharmacy incident reporting: a new tool for community pharmacies in Canada. Healthc Q. 2010;13(Special Issue):16–24. www.ismp-canada.org/download/HealthcareQuarterly/HQ2010V13SP16.pdf. http://dx.doi.org/10.12927/hcq.2010.21961. Medline:20959726

18. Institute for Safe Medication Practices Canada Safety Bulletin Alert. Medication mix-up with a faxed prescription. Institute for Safe Medication Practices Canada, 2012. Available: http://ismp-canada.org/download/safetyBulletins/2012/ISMPCSB2012-06_Alert-MedMixupwithFaxedPrescription.pdf (accessed July 22, 2014).

19. Incident ACP. *Canadian Incident Analysis Framework*. Edmonton, AB: Canadian Patient Safety Institute; 2012. p. 51–5. Available www.patientsafetyinstitute.ca/English/toolsResources/IncidentAnalysis/Documents/Canadian%20Incident%20Analysis%20Framework.PDF, [cited 2014 Dec. 19].

VIII. HUMAN RESOURCES MANAGEMENT

CHAPTER 29

Introduction to Human Resources Management

David Town, *H.B.A., CHRP; President, Your Leadership Matters Inc.*

Learning Objectives

- Define human resources management.
- Explain the importance of human resources management as it pertains to pharmacy.
- Identify factors that can help to achieve effective human resources management.
- Explain the different roles and responsibilities of human resources management based on organizational structures.
- Become familiar with the roles of the Employment Standards Act and Labour Relations Act and how they pertain to pharmacy.

WHAT IS HUMAN RESOURCES MANAGEMENT?

Human resources (HR) management is a business function within organizations that focuses on the effective management of human capital assets (people) to enable an organization to effectively and efficiently achieve its strategic goals and objectives. HR management can be compared to financial management in how it provides support within the organization. Financial management is concerned with implementing processes and systems to manage and control the financial transactions and assets of the organization. Information is gathered to understand the organization's financial health and provide important data that will help the senior management team make decisions that consider the organization's financial capacity to execute the decisions. A company that knows it is financially unhealthy will be restricted in the kinds of activities it can undertake due to constraints imposed by the lack of finances. In contrast, a company that knows it has very strong financial health can undertake a much wider variety of business strategies because of the strength of its finances.

HR management essentially provides the same kind of management support to an organization as the finance function. There need to be processes and systems implemented to manage the human capital assets. To put it another way—to be effective, manage things and lead people. Hiring staff and managing HRs is 10% law and 90% process; the fairness and consistency of the methods determine the results. Manage things such as the law, but lead people through fairness and consistent application of the law.

Examples of HR management processes, in addition to recruitment and selection, include new employee orientation, performance management and succession management. These processes measure the activities of the human capital assets to help managers understand what strengths and limitations exist within the organization with respect to its human resources. The data collected helps senior management make better decisions regarding the organization's ability to execute strategies that the management team may wish to undertake.

Depending on the organization's objectives and strategies, demand for human resources is contingent upon demand for the organization's products or services and on the levels of productivity. After estimating total revenue, management can estimate the number and kinds of human resources needed to obtain those revenues. After it has assessed current capabilities and future needs, management can estimate future HR shortages and over-staffing; then, it can develop a program to match these estimates with forecasts of future labour supply. Many organizations use a skills matrix chart to help monitor the skills mix within the current labour pool to assess where to build additional capability. There are many skills to choose from; the focus should be on skills that are strategically critical to the success of the business. For example, a pharmacy retailer should build a skills matrix that keeps an account of the level of dispensary technician skills within the organization. As with financial assets, the HR assets can be a significant enabler or constraint to the execution of corporate strategy.

The sporting world holds a very good analogy to help in the understanding of HR management. A professional hockey team has a roster of 23 players available for every game. The intention is scoring more goals than the other team. Six players play in the starting lineup and other players enter the game as required. The general manager (GM) must be highly effective at HR management if the team expects to be successful (win a lot of games) over the long term. The GM needs to know who is able to play each of the positions, how well they play the position and how well they should be compensated based on their capability. The GM also needs to know who would replace a player if they get injured or are somehow unable to play. Would the new player come from the bench? A minor league team? From another team? These are important questions that would need to be answered before an injury or absence occurs.

The GM hires a person to manage the team during the game—the coach. The coach focuses on creating an environment for the players that maximizes their performance on the ice. The GM has the final say on the players; the coach plays them to the best of their ability. The coach is on the front line with the players providing feedback and giving them a sense of expectations; the GM is in the background. The coach does any training needed for team performance. The GM sets the business strategy.

In the independent pharmacy, the pharmacy manager has a role similar to the coach and the owner of the pharmacy has a role similar to the GM. In a chain or hospital setting, the pharmacy manager is like a coach and the regional manager, HR manager or hospital pharmacy director all act like the GM.

IMPORTANCE OF HR MANAGEMENT
AS IT PERTAINS TO PHARMACY

HR management is important because an organization's success depends on the level of understanding (alignment) and commitment that employees have with respect to achievement of the organization's strategy. In situations where there is a lack of alignment, organizations find that people are working at different purposes, creating confusion for fellow employees and for customers. When there is a lack of commitment, the organization suffers from greater inefficiencies and weaker financial performance.

Pharmacy focuses on providing professional services using specially trained personnel with a variety of professional qualifications. Effective HR management is even more important because of the impact that individual employees can have on the provision of services and the need to manage highly qualified, specialized resources. Quality of the care and services a patient or customer receives is directly related to the quality and commitment of the people employed by the organization. Effective management of HR can enable an organization to differentiate itself from its competition.

FACTORS TO ACHIEVE EFFECTIVE HR MANAGEMENT

Several factors enable an organization to achieve effective HR management. The first factor—and possibly the most important—is for the organization to embrace the idea that everyone is involved in HR management, not just the HR department. Every employee in an organization knows they are accountable for the thoughtful use of financial capital and company assets. They do not have to be an accountant to know not to spend money recklessly or waste financial resources. Similarly, every person in the organization should own responsibility and accountability for their interactions with other people; it is not up to a specialized department to manage interactions. The HR function can provide leadership and guidance on how to most effectively manage and interact with staff; however, it is most effective when every employee sees it as part of the job.

The second key factor is ensuring that each of the HR planning functions aligns with organizational strategy and culture. For example, if a hotel manager's strategy is to provide five-star service, the manager needs to intentionally explain this to employees and train front desk personnel to answer questions from hotel guests, such as where to go for a good restaurant or entertainment. If the employee cannot deliver quality answers to these questions, it will not be a five-star experience for the hotel guest and the organization has no one to blame but itself for not engaging in appropriate training. Similarly, in a retail pharmacy setting, it is important for HR practices to be aligned with the retail strategy. If the strategy is to provide an exceptional customer experience service, then the HR practices need to support it. The organization's strategy will also provide guidance on the kind of organizational culture the HR practices should support.

An organization's culture is the set of common values and beliefs that drive the actions and behaviours of every employee. Every organization has a culture. The issue is whether it helps or hinders the organization's success. It is important to manage the organization's culture for three main reasons:

- business performance: Companies that align their culture with their strategy will almost certainly enjoy greater financial performance than companies that do not. In their book *Corporate Culture and Performance,* James Heskett and John Kotter cite a landmark study they conducted that documented results for 207 large American companies in 22 different industries over an 11-year period. They reported observing revenue increases of 682% versus 166% and net income increases of 756% versus 1% for companies that managed their cultures well versus companies that did not.[1]

- people: People want to belong to an organization that fits with their values, respects their contributions and allows them to contribute in a meaningful way. Having an intentional culture attracts the type of people who will fit with your culture, and it encourages them to stay because they feel they belong.
- brand: A strong culture that is aligned with the brand promise creates an environment where the brand can come alive internally. Externally, the employees become brand ambassadors in an engaging and authentic way because they are experiencing the brand every day through the company culture.

When done right, culture is the secret ingredient that is hard to replicate and provides a distinct competitive advantage. The HR function can assist in driving the culture the organization desires. For example, if the organization is building a culture of exceptional customer experiences, their recruitment, selection, orientation and training practices must focus on hiring and socializing employees into a strong customer-focused ethos.

For an organization to drive culture that aligns HR management practices with organizational strategy, ideally there should be a person in senior management who has HR management as all of (or at least part of) a job role. In smaller operations, such as an independent pharmacy, the owner usually takes this responsibility. It is very beneficial for this person to have some training or experience in HR management, or to have access to this expertise, to attract and keep the right people who will be critical to the organization's success.

Another key factor is the presence of professional HR management expertise. As with all functional areas within a business, there is professional expertise that enables the effective execution of practices related to the function. There are professional designations, such as the Certified Human Resources Professional (CHRP), that require individuals to meet requirements for education, on-the-job experience and regular recertification. This kind of designation enables organizations to hire professionals with the level of expertise required to effectively manage the HR function. A person would not be allowed to fill prescriptions without the proper education, training and certification, so it follows that an organization should not assign the leadership of the HR function to someone without the proper education, training and certification.

ROLES AND RESPONSIBILITIES FOR HR MANAGEMENT BASED ON ORGANIZATIONAL STRUCTURES

There are many job roles and responsibilities relating to HR management that can exist within an organization. In smaller organizations, the HR function is typically managed by a generalist role staffed by an individual who has education, training and experience in a variety of the HR management functional areas. If necessary, consulting an external lawyer during a termination situation, hiring a recruiter to help find pharmacist staff or subscribing to an HR specialist company for occasional assistance are solutions for lack of internal resources.

In large organizations there can be job specialization, typically in areas such as recruitment, training and development, compensation, etc. The opportunity for specialization occurs because of the volume of work and size of the organization. Ideally, people in the most senior roles would have experience in a variety of the HR management and operational job roles and would be able to focus on how to maximize HR management to support the organization's strategy.

A significant role that is part of the HR function is organizational design and structure, which involves deciding on how to structure, design and coordinate the activities of each of the job roles. How an organization is structured can have a major impact on the behaviour of the individuals and groups within and, therefore, on the behaviour of the organization. An organization's culture should be reflected in its design. Design and structure decisions can ultimately have a significant influence and impact on an organization's success and effectiveness. Organizational design and structure includes decisions on how to organize the various tasks and duties that must be completed.

Talent management is the coordination of a variety of human capital management functions to achieve the organization's strategy. The key roles include development of specific job descriptions; job evaluation and compensation management; recruitment and selection; workforce management; performance management; employee relations; employee development and succession planning.

Developing clear job descriptions is particularly important in a professional environment such as a dispensary where there is a variety of professional responsibilities. For example, certain duties can only be performed by a licensed pharmacist. To manage a dispensary operation effectively, it is critical to understand who does what and why people are assigned the tasks they are assigned.

Job description development should be integrated with job evaluation and compensation planning to avoid perceptions of inequity related to a role's level of accountability and responsibility and the accompanying compensation practices. Job evaluation involves the assessment of the duties and responsibilities of the role relative to other roles within the organization to understand its comparative value. The comparative value is then integrated into a compensation structure designed to compensate job roles according to their relative value and the supply and demand factors in the marketplace. Compensation management also involves the benchmarking of industry compensation standards and the development of a benefits plan that fits with the overall talent management strategy.

With job descriptions in place, the organization must find people with the appropriate skills and desire to fill the various job positions. Recruitment, selection, orientation/onboarding and training are a critical part of the talent management effort required to ensure the achievement of the organization's goals. Depending on the nature of the role, it is often beneficial to hire based on character and motivation and then train for skill. Unfortunately, many organizations spend an inordinate amount of time managing poor performers because of their inability to effectively recruit and select the right people with the right skills and motivation for the various job positions. Managing the orientation/onboarding of new employees is important to any organization that wants to build a strong culture and have employees aligned to the organization's strategy and values. The orientation/onboarding process is often overlooked or poorly executed and should be implemented directly by operational managers with the support of the HR function.

Workforce management involves managing the staffing needs of the operation. A pharmacy can only be open if there is a licensed pharmacist on the premises. There needs to be a certain number of dispensary personnel and, in the case of retail operations, front shop personnel to enable smooth operations. As a result, there is a need for HR management staffing strategies to deal with vacations, unplanned absences, staff departures, etc. Without planning processes, the pharmacy operation risks being hindered by the absence of important skill sets that can affect employee morale, customers' experiences and, ultimately, sales.

For organizations to be successful, they also need to manage employee performance. The approach taken to performance management can impact employee engagement and, in turn, impact quality of service and financial performance. Unfortunately, ongoing performance issues are often a function of the inability or unwillingness of managers to take corrective action with the poor-performing employee. For example, is the poor performance related to an issue of skill or is it an issue of unwillingness to do what is asked? For a skill issue, there could be a plan to provide training targeted at closing the skill gap. If it is a motivational issue, there needs to be some dialogue with the employee to determine if it can be addressed. Either way, if an employee is not meeting performance goals, the manager needs to determine what is going on and take action. In some cases, the situation can lead to discipline measures that should be properly structured (depending on the circumstance it should be progressive in nature) and documented in the employee's file.

In some cases, the poor performance can lead to termination of employment. This necessitates having appropriate employee relations guidelines and strategies for dealing with unacceptable performance. The guidelines should focus on providing a plan for successfully achieving expectations that is clearly communicated to the employee. Ideally, a manager would obtain the employee's written acknowledgement of the remedial plan. To ensure success, the organization's termination practices must be perceived as fair and just by the employee population and must be fully compliant with government legislation.

Conflict management is another area where the development of employee relations guidelines through the HR management function provides support to an organization. Conflict can arise in a variety of circumstances that require specific strategies to resolve the issue and restore organizational harmony (see Chapter 35: Conflict Management and Progressive Discipline).

Another part of effectively managing employee relations is the ability to effectively manage change. The question organizations need to ask themselves is not, "Are we able to change?" It is, "Can we change fast enough to keep up with the competition?" Organizations can deal with change successfully if they learn the principles and strategies associated with effective change management. Most change management failures are a result of the unwillingness of people to adopt new behaviours as opposed to any flaw in the technology or operational process that is being changed. It is this human factor that effective HR management will address (see Chapter 10: Change Management).

HR management also plays an important role in identifying and delivering training needs, identified by each functional area of the business. Identifying training needs is also integrated with employee development strategies linked with performance management and succession planning.

In organizations that are unionized, the HR management function can be integrated with labour relations activities. Alternatively, many organizations separate them into two separate and distinct departments. Either way, it is important to have appropriate expertise to manage the labour relations function as it requires a comprehensive understanding of the specific collective bargaining agreement and the relevant employment legislation in the province/territory where the unionized workforce is located. The company must also have access to skills in negotiating collective agreements and dealing with the potential for employee grievances. Notwithstanding the use of specific expertise, ideally the organization should embrace the idea that everyone in management is involved in HR management, not just the HR or labour relations department. It is an overall mindset, not a department. The best strategy in a unionized environment is to build trust with employees and frontline union representatives to resolve an issue before it escalates into a grievance (see Chapter 36: Managing in a Unionized Environment).

ROLE OF THE EMPLOYMENT STANDARDS ACT, LABOUR RELATIONS ACT AND HUMAN RIGHTS CODE

There are many important pieces of government legislation that impact HR management and most of it is provincial/territorial, so it is important to understand where to find the details, particularly for organizations that operate in multiple provinces/territories across Canada. Each province/territory is different and organizations must follow the appropriate statutes of the province/territory in which they do business, not where their home base or head office is. Relevant legislation in Ontario, as an example, includes but is not limited to the Employment Standards Act (2000), the Labour Relations Act, the Human Rights Code, the Occupational Health and Safety Act, the Workplace Safety and Insurance Act and hazardous material regulations defined under the Workplace Hazardous Materials Information Systems (WHMIS) (see Chapter 37: Legal Considerations in Employment and Labour Law).

There are also Acts that cover privacy, such as the federal Personal Information Protection and Electronic Documents Act (PIPEDA) and provincial Personal Information Protection Act (PIPA)—for example, as it pertains to employee record keeping and the collection of data for recruiting, hiring and reference checks. PIPEDA (or PIPA in some provinces) addresses privacy of personal information collected by organizations. All privacy Acts address the issues of what and when employee information is considered to be personal information that is subject to the provisions of the provincial privacy legislation.

Privacy legislation can impact employee record keeping and the collection of data for recruiting, hiring and reference checks. PIPEDA (or PIPA in some provinces) addresses privacy of personal information collected by organizations. All privacy Acts address the issues of what and when employee information is considered to be personal information that is subject to the provisions of the provincial privacy legislation. Relevant information can include information gathered during the recruiting process; for example, résumés, reference checks or whether the candidate is hired or not.

It is important to understand both the provisions of the Acts and the accompanying regulations. Using Ontario as an example, subjects covered under the Employment Standards Act include posting requirements, record keeping, payment of wages, minimum wage, hours of work, meal breaks, overtime, vacation, public holidays, retail workers, benefit plans, pregnancy and parental leaves, personal emergency and family medical leaves, organ donor and reservist leaves, termination of employment, employee severance, continuity of employment, equal pay for equal work, lie detector tests, reprisals and temporary help. (For more on other provinces/territories, see Chapter 37: Legal Considerations in Employment and Labour Law.)

It is important to note that in Ontario, not all provisions apply to all employees. Pharmacy roles and other roles (e.g., professionals such as IT specialists, lawyers, managers) are exempt. Pharmacy organizations should pay particular attention to regulations identifying which provisions of the Act apply to which roles, as it is different for each province/territory. An important role of the HR function is to consult the regulations to identify which provisions apply and to make sure the organization is aware of their responsibilities. Collective agreements automatically adopt the minimum legislated standards, and the provisions in the agreement apply to all members of the bargaining unit notwithstanding exceptions that may exist in the legislation. (For more on labour relations, see Chapter 36: Managing in a Unionized Environment.)

Human rights legislation has been passed in both the federal and provincial/territorial jurisdictions. The 1977 Canadian Human Rights Act protects individuals and groups against harassment or discrimination when based on any of the 11 grounds outlined in the Act. The Act applies to people in Canada employed by or who receive services from the federal government, First Nations governments or private companies that are regulated by the federal government such as banks, trucking companies, broadcasters and telecommunications companies.

Provincial/Territorial human rights laws share many similarities with the Canadian Human Rights Act and apply many of the same principles. They protect people from discrimination in areas of provincial/territorial jurisdiction, such as restaurants, stores, schools, housing and most workplaces. Human rights law entitles every Canadian to equal opportunity to employment and the right to work each day free of discrimination and harassment.

There are other significant pieces of legislation that impact the management of human resources. For example, in some provinces and territories, employees can exercise the right to refuse to work, as a part of the Health and Safety legislation, if a worker has reasonable cause to believe that to carry out any work process would create an undue hazard. It is also worth noting that legislation governing employees deemed to be part of management is continuously evolving and should be closely monitored. As a final thought, it is incumbent upon the organization to use the appropriate expertise, either an internal or an external resource, to ensure they are compliant with all workplace legislation.

RESOURCES AND SUGGESTED READINGS

Belcour M, McBey K, Hong Y, et al. *Strategic human resources planning*. 5th ed. Toronto: Nelson Education; 2012.

See Chapter 37: Legal Considerations in Employment and Labour Law for additional resources.

REFERENCE

1. Kotter J, Heskett J. *Corporate culture and performance*. New York: Free Press; 2011.

CHAPTER 30

Creating a Desirable Workplace:
The Eternal Circle

Susan E. Beresford, *BScPharm; Pharmacy Manager; ADAPT Moderator*

"You can dream, create, design and build the most wonderful place in the world . . . but it requires people to make it a reality." – Walt Disney,[1] co-founder of the Walt Disney Company, which had annual revenue of approximately US$45 billion in the 2013 financial year[2]

Learning Objectives

- Define what a desirable workplace is and why a desirable workplace is important.
- Identify the criteria that need to be evaluated to create a desirable pharmacy workplace.
- Describe the processes that may be implemented to create a desirable pharmacy workplace.
- Explain the importance, types and barriers of communication.
- Describe effective communication tools and techniques that will help promote the creation of a desirable workplace.
- Describe the term *empowerment* and identify how empowerment can improve staff morale.

MI CASA ES SU CASA—MY HOUSE IS YOUR HOUSE

What is a workplace but a home away from home? Welcoming patients and customers to a practice, making them feel comfortable and valued, listening to their needs as well as their suggestions or complaints—these are all methods to create a positive environment that builds a successful practice. Why would these same characteristics not work for a team and build success from the inside out?

When creating their new work environment for TeamSpace Canada, CEO Michael Johnson said, "We're not creating this space to impress our clients . . . We want something appealing for our staff."[3] Appealing means staff receive laptops, free parking, discounts and an environment close to public transit, coffee shops, restaurants and hiking trails.

Career expectations have changed. A linear authority and communication structure have become a hindrance when appealing to young professionals who are more likely to follow their passion and want to try different things[4]—expanded scope in pharmacy, by any other definition. Balancing a team's expectations with the fiscal reality of pharmacy today can lead managers to become creative in providing the services and support that make staff become more than just employees; they become a team.

What Makes a Workplace Desirable

Workplace benefits: individual and team

Culture: positive team vision in action

Clarity of role: individual and team

Goals defined: short term and long term for individual and team

Communication: open, clear, accessible through multiple formats

Appreciation of creativity/excellence through individual and team incentives

Resources/support

Accountability: the good and the bad by all team members

GEOMETRY VERSUS FLUID DYNAMICS

Organizational structure has been compared to linear layers, triangles standing as a pyramid or upside-down, intersecting domain circles and the more mundane rectangles with arrows (see Chapter 9: Leadership and Management for organizational charts). Experts can define a workplace philosophically and physically, measuring employee engagement and their daily step count, but the bottom line is that clarity is what counts. Do employees understand the business's short-term and long-term goals? Are these goals communicated and then reviewed weekly, bi-weekly, in an annual review? Do employees understand what is expected of them? Do they know the underlying philosophy that will be their guide as they build the business? Could it be shared by something as simple as a bonus structure, creating "our" business? Is there accountability? Do they know what managers do and what it takes to make the business viable, successfully achieving fiscal goals? If a manager does "it" and employees do not see "it" or understand "it," then "it" is not important and does not affect their work life. Good communication creates an understanding that creates value, whether in the work or the workplace. An effective tool to start the conversation is a mission statement for what is to be accomplished today and a vision statement for what is to be accomplished tomorrow,[5] as a team is created that will successfully achieve the business and personal goals.

A mission statement can be as simple as, "Providing patient-centred care in a positive, team-centred environment." Keep it simple enough that it can be remembered and, therefore, used daily as the foundation for the myriad of patient-centred decisions the team will make.

The vision should reflect the leader's passion and the passion inspired within the team as goals are achieved: "Our team will provide all expanded scope services as part of our daily workflow, fulfilling our patients' pharmacy needs." This implicitly requires that team members keep up their education and certifications, become comfortable providing expanded scope services and are accountable to do so while providing excellent customer service.

Fluid dynamics are the "how" of communicating the implicit, developing team-based mission and vision statements and daily workflow. Communication can be formal with a dispensary team meeting quarterly that also encompasses quality assurance. Whole-store team meetings should be held just as regularly with full participation by the dispensary team, whose leader would share information about new projects/clinics, services—what they are, if there is a targeted patient population, tools to invite patients to participate and the expectations for the store team's participation. Fluid means that the workflow and goals can be adjusted to incorporate the team's suggestions. It also means that

Criteria for Creating a Desirable Pharmacy Workplace

Goals are clear, documented, posted

Physical space organized for workflow

Private consultation room

Support from technicians and/or assistants

Up-to-date technology/software

Internet access

Expanded scope services a focus of team

Flexibility in hours/shifts

Professional development encouraged

Individual opinions important while building consensus

Clear communication structure

Clear value of individual to team

Clear team roles

Cushioned flooring over the concrete floor

issues can be addressed as they arise on a daily basis—"open door" informal meetings with team members. An open door policy reflects someone's accessibility and willingness to listen. Remember to document suggestions and either act, put them forward for consideration by the team or share information that helps explain why the suggestion would not be viable at this time. Communicating concerns or ideas brought forward inspires dialogue, creativity and the value felt by team members. This fluid environment encourages the team to engage and build, becoming successful on a daily basis. The team exists in the moment, not the past or the future. Be there with them!

ENTITLED, ENGAGED OR AFRAID?

A pharmacist walks into a dispensary and
   A. waits for the pharmacy assistant to hand over a prescription to check
   B. waits for a regulated pharmacy technician to inform him/her of a patient to counsel
   C. says hello to everyone while walking to the dispensary and checking the communication log, the appointment book and outstanding prescription baskets, then beginning the shift

Which one is a better choice for a team member? Pharmacists are no longer tied to a prescription, and the transition to services based on practice expertise can be challenging. A degree is no longer enough; pharmacists need to have the expertise, confidence and ability to communicate with patients and other health care practitioners (HCP) to provide patient-centred care. Professional growth, not fear of professional inadequacy, is a necessity to successfully implement patient-centred care, and also to successfully grow a pharmacy's patient population, reputation and bottom line. Each pharmacist may have a favoured area of interest or a highly specific expertise as defined by a certificate, but they must all share a base level of expertise. A team of pharmacists will be a peer group defined by the owner/manager, equal in their ability to provide all services daily within their workflow. How high will the bar be set?

WHO ARE YOU? NO REALLY, WHO *ARE* YOU?

Just as managers would know and understand the impact of a team's personal characteristics (i.e., avoids change, craves a new challenge, supportive but not a leader), managers need to understand who they are, their capabilities and areas for personal growth. An amazing resource for this can be found within the ADAPT course offered by the Canadian Pharmacists Association (CPhA). The

As a Manager, Know Yourself

Know your mission and vision—share effectively with team

Encourage positive problem solving

Physical supports in place—do more than pass a provincial/territorial regulatory inspection

Make your workflow effective and efficient—pharmacists doing professional services/counselling; technicians filling, preparing documentation, referring

Clear communication venues/opportunities—regularly scheduled, as well as open door; issues resolved in a timely manner

Support continued education

Support team with opportunities to have fun together

Reinforce goals daily

Encourage the team's collective mind—creativity, problem solving

Support team with regular assessment of the team/individual; annual with quarterly updates, more if needed; encouragement, guidance, motivation

Ensure accountability for actions—positive with guidance; opportunities for growth if success is not up to standard; final option of termination for those who do not engage in supporting team/team goals

Reward excellence

Be receptive to change

Conflict Management Scale takes learners through the process of understanding exactly how they deal with conflict; they can then decide whether to change or optimize their style to reinforce the positive management of their team. ADAPT is a personal journey highlighting the understanding and provision of professional services to the highest standards. Managers need to understand the intricacies of providing a service to plan for and support a team as they provide these services.

Managers must consider their communication skills. The ability to share concerns, *listen*, ask questions, define goals, plan and then follow through on a plan are all impacted by not just the ability to communicate but also the team's ability to share information with a manager, other HCP and patients. Or as Wikipedia states, "Effective communication should generate the desired effect and maintain the effect, with the potential to increase the effect of the message."[6] What effect is being sought? Patient care opportunities? A positive work environment? A successful business? All three?

LEADING BY EXAMPLE

A great communication strategy starts with management. Is the manager willing and able to not just share but to build a team structure that promotes the communication of ideas and solutions, to tend that structure daily to prevent team goals being overcome by individual agendas and to be open to amending that structure in response to environmental variables not within control (e.g., HCP formats necessary for collaboration, government digital information systems)? Communication is verbal and non-verbal, with the clear majority of communication being non-verbal ranging from body language to emoticons. Body language, attitude regarding change and the site's daily workflow set the tone for the team. If managers are not engaged or are seen not to care, staff will not care. If managers do not do the detail work, they will not finish the details. If managers do not respond to valid concerns, dialogue with the team will be adversely affected (see Chapter 9: Leadership and Management).

Barriers to communication can be as diverse as the listener's disinterest or inability to comprehend, inability to effectively communicate an idea or actual fear of what that idea would mean for the individual. Fear of the unknown, the known or the assumed is a chronic barrier to the basic functioning of the individual or the team. Fear is effectively dealt with by open, accessible communication between team members and team leaders.

Education is another powerful tool to address fear and the reluctance to change; when people understand what is needed to provide a service, they will no longer fear the workflow implications of providing that service. Remember, everyone has different experiences that individualize perceptions—someone's "life" filter affects reactions to information and situations. Managers must not just be self-aware, but also team aware, to enhance communications (see Section X: Organizational, Business and Professional Communications).

Communication Tools

Employee handbook

Employee orientation by manager

Quarterly whole-team meetings

Quarterly pharmacy team meetings

Open door policy, daily updates if needed

Accessible communication—shared; electronic message board

Communication board for hard copy updates, new opportunities and ideas

Annual performance appraisal

Quarterly performance appraisal updates

Standards of practice book for pharmacy team

Communication log(s) – whole team, pharmacy team

Appointment book for pharmacy team

THE ETERNAL CIRCLE: MANAGERS, TEAM MEMBERS, PATIENTS AND COMMUNITY

Managers model expected behaviour and abilities; a positive attitude and belief in the mission, vision and team are key to creating a desirable workplace. By being a part of a team, will the individual have the flexibility to make decisions, be confident in management's support and encouraged to seek out new challenges? Will the workplace be a positive environment where not just employees, but also patients and customers, enjoy the atmosphere? Will management encourage and mentor team members toward personal bests? Will management promote a caring and happy workplace based on trust, sincerity and open communication?

Empowerment means giving team members authority and flexibility to make decisions supported by a clearly defined workflow, with the resources necessary to fulfill the expectations of their role. An empowered team works effectively and is not micromanaged, feels valued and not afraid for their job, actively communicates the good and the bad, and understands the value of timely communication and the discovery of new opportunities. The eternal circle is the cycling of information, effort and success that links a manager with the team, patients and community.

Standards of Practice Book (Electronic and Hard Copy)

Emergency contact information for software, hardware, power, city

Employee contact information listing position on team

What to do in an emergency, who to call

Disaster readiness/plan

What to do in case of robbery or theft, including link to or the documents needed

Sign stating "Closed for _____, be back at _____. In case of emergency, contact _____."

Diagram of dispensary layout with information on location of medications, products, supplies

List of professional sites recommended and why

List of passwords and URLs for hardware, professional sites

Cold chain information, disruption plan

FAQ for drug ordering/shortages/preferred suppliers

FAQ for billing issues/credit

FAQ for software/hardware issues

"When all else fails, refer to the Mission Statement. . . . (insert here)"

"Money motivates neither the best people, nor the best in people. It can move the body and influence the mind, but it cannot touch the heart or move the spirit; that is reserved for belief, principle, and morality."—Dee Hock,[7] Founder & Former CEO, VISA, which had an annual revenue of approximately US$10.4 billion in 2012[8]

RESOURCES AND SUGGESTED READINGS

Achor S. *Before happiness: The 5 hidden keys to achieving success, spreading happiness, and sustaining positive change.* New York: Crown Business; 2013.

Adam S. Dilbert – "College humor, dinosaur office: team building." Available on YouTube, posted Aug. 7, 2012.

Buckingham M, Coffman C. *First break all the rules: what the world's greatest managers do differently*. New York: Simon and Schuster; 1999.

Camey BM, Getz I. *Freedom Inc., Free your employees and let them lead your business to higher productivity, profits and growth*. New York: Crown Business; 2009.

Kotter JP. *Leading change*. Boston: Harvard Business Review Press; 2012.

REFERENCES

1. BrainyQuote. Walt Disney quotes. Available: www.brainyquote.com/quotes/authors/w/walt_disney.html (accessed June 16, 2014).

2. United States Securities and Exchange Commission. 2013 Form 10-K, Walt Disney Company. Available: www.sec.gov/Archives/edgar/data/1001039/000100103913000164/fy2013_q4x10k.htm (accessed June 16, 2014).

3. Power B. Generation whippersnapper. The Chronicle Herald. Available: http://thechronicleherald.ca/business/1195107-generation-whippersnapper (accessed March 22, 2014).

4. Ng E, Schweitzer L, Lyons S. New generation, great expectations: a field study of the millennial generation. J Bus Psychol. 2010;25(2):281–92. www.academia.edu/1410939/New_generation_great_expectations_A_field_study_of_the_millennial_generation. http://dx.doi.org/10.1007/s10869-010-9159-4.

5. Diffen. Mission statement vs. vision statement. Available: www.diffen.com/difference/Mission_Statement_vs_Vision_Statement (accessed June 16, 2014).

6. Wikipedia. Communication. Available: http://en.wikipedia.org/wiki/Communication (accessed June 25, 2014).

7. BrainyQuote. Dee Hock quotes. Available: www.brainyquote.com/quotes/authors/d/dee_hock. (accessed June 25, 2014).

8. United States Security and Exchange Commission. 2012 Form 10-K, VISA INC. Available: www.sec.gov/Archives/edgar/data/1403161/000138410812000011/v09301210-k.htm (accessed June 25, 2014).

CHAPTER 31

Effective Management Styles

Billy B. Cheung, *R.Ph., B.Sc.Phm.; Region Director, Pharmacy & Strategic Initiatives, Pharmasave Ontario*

Learning Objectives

- Define the term *management*.
- Explain what makes a good manager.
- Identify the advantages and disadvantages of different management styles.
- Define *leadership*, what does it mean to be a good leader and what are the characteristics of a good leader.
- Describe how effective delegation is part of an effective management style.
- Describe the effective time management and organizational tools that may be used in a pharmacy setting.

The typical community pharmacy operation is complex. It is a unique blend of retail business and frontline health care services. Pharmacy owners and their management staff must have a strong understanding of and effectively manage all the various business and employee aspects of the operation. Key examples include product purchasing and merchandising, retail marketing, dispensary regulations and operations, pharmacy services, staffing and finance, plus the requirements of supporting various technology systems. This is true whether the pharmacy is a small operation or a large pharmacy with multiple departments.

Effective management in community pharmacy can be described as meeting the operational goals and objectives of the pharmacy in an efficient and timely manner. This requires leaders with the knowledge and skills to effectively manage both the business and the human resources effectively. A poorly managed pharmacy operation can result in a financial loss and a work environment in which staff are not productive, do not enjoy their jobs and ultimately, have a negative effect on the service customers receive. This is particularly important as there are currently more than 9,200 pharmacies in Canada,[1] each striving to increase their share of a very competitive marketplace.

In other words, it is in the best interest of pharmacy owners and their management staff to understand and successfully implement good management practices.

WHO IS RESPONSIBLE FOR MANAGING IN A PHARMACY?

A typical community pharmacy will have several different people involved in manager-related roles and responsibilities. This is the case if a person has an official manager job title or if they are responsible for work performed by other staff.

The most apparent person in terms of job title is the pharmacy manager. As an example, in Ontario, the Drug and Pharmacies Regulation Act (DPRA) specifically requires that every pharmacy assign a designated manager who is responsible for and accountable over the decisions and actions that affect the day-to-day operations of the pharmacy.[2] This includes the supervision of both professional and lay staff who work in the store. Other provinces/territories have similar designations, and even in jurisdictions without a formal designation, the person with the title of pharmacy manager would be expected to have these same or similar responsibilities.

Having a pharmacy manager in place, however, does not preclude the need for other staff to have manager-like responsibilities. The pharmacy manager is not likely to be physically in the store for all the operating business hours. It means that staff pharmacists, even those who are newly licensed, are usually in charge to supervise the dispensing operations and, sometimes, the entire store for their particular shift. While they may not be the formal manager by title, they are typically considered the most senior in terms of decision making and as a regulated health care professional, also accountable for the dispensing and pharmacy services provided. Having effective management skills is an important aspect for any pharmacist working in community pharmacy.

There is a growing expectation to better utilize the clinical skills of the pharmacist along with expanded scope activities such as prescribing, immunizations and disease management consultations. As the profession of pharmacy continues to evolve, non-pharmacists will take on dispensary management responsibilities. This evolution is leading to opportunities for pharmacy technicians to be responsible and accountable for the technical aspects of prescription dispensing. According to the National Association of Pharmacy Regulatory Authorities, there are already 2,702 licensed pharmacy technicians in Canada as of January 1, 2014.[3] Some of these newly regulated health care professionals, who work in community pharmacy environments, are finding themselves in roles beyond the previous norm for pharmacy support staff. As dispensary managers, they are responsible for maintaining drug inventory and hiring, training and supervising non-regulated staff. With these enhanced responsibilities, effective management skills are a must.

Aside from the obvious for owners and pharmacy managers, staff pharmacists, pharmacy technicians and others working in the community pharmacy can all have some level of management responsibilities.

WHAT DOES IT MEAN TO HAVE MANAGEMENT RESPONSIBILITIES? TO BE IN CHARGE?

A single individual is not able to effectively do all the work required in operating a pharmacy. The work requires the support of staff and in general, the pharmacy manager is responsible for leading the staff to get the work done. The pharmacy manager must have a clear understanding of desired goals or end points and then work toward these goals with the support of the team. In the case of a community pharmacy, a typical objective is to ensure all prescriptions are dispensed accurately and within a reasonable time frame. In such a case, the manager must work with the staff to ensure they are looking after dispensary inventory, promptly responding to patient requests, prioritizing prescriptions to be dispensed and other dispensary-related activities. What the staff do and how well they do it is strongly influenced by the person who is responsible for managing them. To be a good manager, one should consider the following:

- communication: Ensure staff are kept informed so they understand the background and reasoning for the work they are performing and supporting. Good managers need to be readily available to staff to discuss any and all concerns, issues or ideas. They also need to provide feedback, including recognizing and acknowledging when something has been done well. It helps the staff member understand expectations. Due to the shift work in community pharmacies, there need to be systems in place to share communication regularly between staff and also from the manager. Also suggested are regular staff meetings.

- staff skills and training: It is important to know and account for the skill sets of the person; some tasks may not be suitable for them, while others may require additional training. Good managers need to ensure their staff have access to relevant training so they can effectively do their job. Job functions often need monitoring and further upgrading. This can be done on site or by using training and development opportunities in community pharmacy, such as continuing education sessions and conferences, dispensary software systems training and events available through vendors and suppliers. The manager should recognize a person's strengths and future potential and align the work and opportunities to develop, challenge and train the individual further.

- resources and support: Without proper resources and support to accomplish the work, a manager may be setting a staff member up for failure. The amount of work expected needs to correlate with the timelines and tools available. Pharmacy managers need to constantly review the factors that influence efficiencies, such as scheduling and staffing levels, access to clinical references, whether computer hardware and software are up to date, and even new and innovative technologies that would support the work that needs to be done. Good managers ensure their staff are working hard and to the best of their abilities, yet also ensure they are not overworked.

- delegation: It is key for a manager to delegate and allow others to do the work. It contributes to staff development, training and skills. Allowing others to take on new responsibilities and challenges, make decisions and be accountable is also motivational. Many people enjoy knowing that their contributions to the organization are expanding and valued. This also enables the pharmacy manager to focus on other priorities only he/she can address. A simple example would be the delegation of dispensing to pharmacy technicians. It allows the technicians to enhance their role and in turn, allows pharmacists to focus on their clinical role.

- direction and timelines: Provide clear direction, expectations and timelines; ensure staff know exactly what they are responsible for and what needs to be accomplished. Good managers ensure there is no ambiguity or confusion among the staff with respect to expectations and the work to be done.

This is not an exhaustive list of tips to be a good manager. There are many other things a manager can do that would result in outstanding performance and outcomes from their staff. Some recommended references are listed at the end of this chapter.

THE IMPORTANCE OF TIME MANAGEMENT

Many things can occur simultaneously within a community pharmacy operation, such as multiple staff in the dispensary, phone calls, faxes, emails, patient consultations, interactions with other health care providers and third-party payers, product ordering and receiving, deliveries, staffing issues and maintenance of the physical space. Effective time management requires systems and processes to be in place to ensure all the people working in the pharmacy are working efficiently and accurately.

The workspace of the pharmacy should be clearly defined and supported so the staff know where various dispensing-related activities are to be performed, such as data input, counting, mixtures, prescription checking and pharmacist consultation. Tools, such as a computer system that tracks individual prescriptions from inputting to pickup, add efficiency and clarity to the workflow, and automated phone systems that put prescription reorders directly into the dispensing queue increase productivity. Job descriptions outlining specific roles and responsibilities for each staff member ensure everyone knows what they are supposed to be doing, such as who is performing the prescription intake, answering the phone calls and managing inventory ordering. Sticking to standardized procedures helps eliminate opportunities for errors and enhances job satisfaction.

Since all the staff need to work together as a team, often on different days and times, it is important to have a system to communicate necessary information, coordinate schedules, collaborate and share ideas. This can be accomplished with various tools including email groups, designated notes software and shared digital calendars. Look for opportunities to use available technologies and applications that can help.

Managers are recommended to seek out and learn more about workflow and dispensary efficiency and systems/processes related to their implementation in the pharmacy to enhance time management.

MANAGEMENT STYLES

Managers work with people. These people are staff and each person requires support to do his/her job. It is important to know and understand that there are various techniques when working with staff to get things done. Which technique to use will depend on both the situation and the actual person. Practically for community pharmacy, there are some specific management styles that are useful. (For more on leadership styles, see Chapter 9: Leadership and Management.)

DIRECTIVE

A directive management style is one where the manager very specifically assigns the tasks and responsibilities to everyone involved. There is minimal, if any, input or feedback from the staff. This is the "all hands on deck" style of management. A manager would choose to use this type of style when there is a crisis or when there is a very short timeline for a task that would not be conducive to another style. It may also be a style used for new staff members with very specific task responsibilities.

A community pharmacy example may be one where there is a significant rush of patients needing to have prescriptions filled beyond the regular expected volume. To manage this volume, the manager may very quickly pull all the available staff together, prioritize the amount of work that needs to be completed as efficiently as possible to ensure customers are not left waiting too long, and specifically assign tasks and provide clear direction to each person (one person to do intake and process, another to dispense, a front store staff to handle all phone calls, etc.) until the rush is over.

A directive style of management is not one that should be used regularly, as most people do not appreciate being told what to do, and there are other styles that are more effective. However, it does have a role in certain cases.

COACHING

As the name of this style suggests, the manager is actively working with and supporting staff in their roles and responsibilities. It is a style usually effective for staff members who are new to a role, may not have confidence in a particular task or are failing to perform satisfactorily. The manager provides ongoing and regular feedback on their work and helps them correct or tweak their approach, and ultimately they get to the point where staff are able to carry out their duties independently.

Pharmacy students in community pharmacy work placements have the opportunity to benefit from coaching by more experienced pharmacists. They benefit from the transition of what they have learned theoretically to applying their skills and knowledge practically. In this example, a pharmacy student may be learning about how best to communicate in a language understood by the patient, how to effectively influence a doctor's opinion on therapy or how to handle challenging patients who may be less than cooperative.

COLLABORATIVE

While still working with the staff, this style differs from coaching in that the manager is looking to gain support and consensus related to a particular task, project or work. A collaborative style engages the employees at the beginning of the process, seeking their direct input and buy-in on ideas, approaches and solutions. This style can be very effective, as people in general appreciate being heard and being part of the decision process. The collaborative style can be used individually or with an entire team of people. At the beginning of the process, the manager also needs to ensure staff members fully understand the areas where there may not be collaboration or where decisions may need to be made without everyone engaged to the same degree.

Communication is key to collaborating; the manager needs to provide the background information necessary to help the staff best understand the situation, clarify and answer any questions, listen and respect the input provided and set a deadline for formulating a solution together. Any credit for the success of initiative needs to be shared with the team.

With more jurisdictions allowing pharmacists to provide immunizations, it is an excellent opportunity to use the collaborative style of management. With such a service, it is important for all the staff in a store to be aware of, support and promote it. In a staff meeting, the pharmacist in charge can have the team help develop the plan to implement the immunization service, including how it will be supported and promoted in the community and how logistics will be handled.

VISIONARY

The visionary style of management works best where staff members are already strong, effective and motivated. The manager provides a broad understanding of the vision and overall goal for a particular project, task or responsibility, but does not need to direct, coach or obtain detailed input or feedback. Instead, staff are empowered to make their own decisions on how to achieve the goal or vision. This style requires that staff have a good understanding of the culture of the company, as well as what decisions will or will not be acceptable to the manager or owner. For staff who work well with this type of style, managers need to ensure they are not micromanaging their work. It is not meant to be completely hands off and, typically, the manager will expect to receive progress updates along the way. The manager will also offer to be available and be willing to provide input or support when or if requested by the staff.

A good manager will be able to read the situation and decide which style would be best suited to manage at that particular point in time. It is also important to know when to move back and forth between the various styles to be the most effective in working with staff.

THE MANAGER AS A LEADER

The visionary style of management leads to some considerations for what makes a good manager great—how the actions of a good manager transform to one of leadership. These are managers who can get things done through effectively inspiring and motivating others to support them. The people who work for these managers willingly aim to do their best and in many cases, will go above and beyond expectations. Staff who work for great managers are engaged and actively involved; they want to contribute to the success of the pharmacy as part of their responsibilities. They are proud to be a part of the team and understand their accountabilities. Great managers lead by example and help to set the tone that everyone else follows and supports. Ultimately, the result of a great manager and leader is one where there is a positive work environment, which translates into a positive experience for customers. When the staff are happy, the customers are happy (see Chapter 9: Leadership and Management).

A great manager who is a leader does the following:
- motivates and inspires
- empowers his/her people
- sets clear vision and goals
- makes people accountable
- leads by example

FINAL THOUGHTS

Some tips and techniques for being a great manager will come naturally, while others may take some time and practice to effectively develop. The goal of effective management is to fulfill the priorities and objectives of the organization with team members who accomplish their work efficiently and accept responsibilities beyond expectations. Owners, pharmacists and pharmacy technicians all have a role in effectively managing other people. Understanding the role of a manager, what makes a good manager and different management styles provide a foundation toward successfully operating a community pharmacy.

RESOURCES AND SUGGESTED READINGS

Beck R, Harter J. Why great managers are so rare. March 25, 2014. Gallup Business Journal. Available: http://businessjournal.gallup.com/content/167975/why-great-managers-rare.aspx (accessed Oct. 28, 2014).

Covey SR. The 7 habits of highly effective people. Available: www.stephencovey.com/7habits/7habits.php (accessed Oct. 28, 2014).

Goleman D. Leadership that gets results. March–April 2000. Harvard Business Review. Available: http://hbr.org/product/leadership-that-gets-results/an/R00204-PDF-ENG (accessed Oct. 28, 2014).

Ontario College of Pharmacists. Policy on professional supervision of pharmacy personnel. Available: www.ocpinfo.com/regulations-standards/policies-guidelines/supervising-personnel (accessed Oct. 28, 2014).

REFERENCES

1. National Association of Pharmacy Regulatory Authorities. National statistics, pharmacies (as of January 1, 2014). Available: http://napra.ca/pages/Practice_Resources/National_Statistics.aspx?id=2104 (accessed May 2014).

2. Service Ontario. Drug and Pharmacies Regulation Act. Ontario. Section 146 (1.1). Available: www.e-laws.gov.on.ca/html/statutes/english/elaws_statutes_90h04_e.htm (accessed May 2014).

3. National Association of Pharmacy Regulatory Authorities. National statistics, pharmacy technicians (as of January 1, 2014). Available: http://napra.ca/pages/Practice_Resources/National_Statistics.aspx?id=3072 (accessed May 2014).

CHAPTER 32

Effective Management of Human Resources

R. Mark Dickson, *BSc(Pharm), MBA*

Learning Objectives

- Explain the areas of a pharmacy operation where a manager or owner must effectively manage human resources.
- Describe the process of human resources planning.
- Explain the importance of job descriptions as well as their creation and implementation.
- Identify the steps necessary to evaluate scheduling needs.
- Discuss the importance of change, the process to create change, as well as the implementation of change.

HUMAN RESOURCES MANAGEMENT

At the core of every pharmacy is a team that provides health care products and services to meet the goals and objectives of the operation. These goals and objectives are often dictated by the location of the pharmacy, the services required in that location and the vision of the owner or manager. The personnel in the dispensary and all the other employee groups in the pharmacy must be managed to provide a public experience that is consistent with these goals. Effective human resources (HR) management is essential to achieve effective and loyal staffing, as well as to meet business expectations. Labour cost is typically the largest variable cost within a pharmacy, and effective personnel management is essential to ensure success.

The degree of supervision and management required for pharmacy employees will vary depending on several variables, including department, training, experience, job responsibilities and reporting structures. Different staff groups or departments within the pharmacy will require additional consideration. The following are typical departments:
- dispensary: pharmacists, technicians and assistants
- front shop: cashiers, merchandisers and supervisors
- other: cosmeticians, home health care technicians, delivery personnel, accounting staff

Management of each department may be delegated to team managers, with the managers in turn reporting to the store owner or manager. Specific objectives will be set for each and the staff managed to meet the objectives. In smaller stores, formal groups may not be designated and the store owner or manager may manage the entire staff.

As a distinct group of employees within the pharmacy and likely the highest wage earners, the dispensary staff require some special consideration. Pharmacists, and in some provinces/territories pharmacy technicians, are licensed professionals providing a regulated health care service; however, they too must be managed effectively. Pharmacists are required by law to act in the best interest of their patients. The assumption that all pharmacists perform the same functions and provide the same level of care is a common mistake made by new managers. How the services are delivered, the non-regulated tasks a pharmacist provides and the manner in which services are provided are very much within the management purview of the pharmacy owner or manager. The cost of pharmacists and the critical nature of the service they provide make them a very important group of employees to manage and mentor.

Regardless of what service an employee performs within the pharmacy, the actions of each employee taken collectively are the face of the business to the public and to other health care practitioners. Effective HR management practices are essential to ensure the business prospers.

STAFFING REQUIREMENTS (HR PLANNING PROCESS)

The fundamental principle in establishing a staffing plan is that the mix of staff scheduled must meet the needs of the customer base. Further, the number of personnel scheduled at any given time needs to correlate closely with the work to be done.[1] The goal in developing the staffing plan is to meet or exceed the needs of the customer base at a total labour cost the business can support profitably.

The starting point for HR planning must always be careful consideration of the needs of a given pharmacy's customer base. Here are some questions to consider:
- What are the demographic and socioeconomic mixes of the customer base?
- Where is the pharmacy located and how does the location impact customer demand?
- What goods and services beyond dispensing prescriptions are required or offered?
- What hours is the pharmacy open and do these hours meet the needs of the customers?
- What additional factors will impact customer demand (visiting specialists, local medical clinic hours, delivery schedules, other community health services, etc.)?

After considering these questions, the manager should be able to establish the core product and service demands of the customer base. The success of the business will depend on how closely these demands can be met by the staff.

Customers provide the best information on their service expectations. Many pharmacy chains conduct customer surveys and mystery shopper research to quantify both the demands of the customer and how well these demands are being met by the staff. If this information is available, it should be collected and carefully considered when developing a staffing plan. Conversations with customers can identify their expectations and assist in providing a qualitative measure of satisfaction while potentially highlighting any changes required.

When considering the personnel required for a pharmacy, a common starting point is the dispensary. Most will require a pharmacist on duty for every hour the location is open. Depending on the volume of prescription business, pharmacy technicians, pharmacy assistants and, potentially, clerks may be needed to support the pharmacist. If the store offers any specialty products, such as home health care, cosmetics or electronics, staff will be required to support these product offerings. Additional personnel may also be required, such as cashiers/clerks, merchandisers and supervisors.

In addition to determining the staff mix, it is essential to ensure the number of personnel working at any time is closely matched to the amount of work needing to be done. Staffing levels within each department should be set based on the volume of work and hourly customer service demand. Productivity metrics, such as prescriptions filled per labour hour, sales per labour hour and customers per hour, are helpful tools to quantify the correlation between staff levels and work achieved. These metrics can be benchmarked with industry or corporate targets to help determine optimal staffing levels. The metrics are also instrumental in setting staffing schedules.

When formulating a staffing plan, there are certain minimum standards and guidelines that must be considered and accommodated. For example, provincial/territorial labour statutes and worker safety concerns dictate that a minimum of two staff members be in the pharmacy at all times. This is a consideration for very low-volume pharmacies as well as for pharmacies that are open extended hours. Labour standards establish minimum scheduling, vacation and maternity entitlements that must be accommodated within the staffing plan. In the dispensary, error prevention is a concern and there are standards and guidelines published by NAPRA, provincial colleges and territorial regulatory bodies that will impact the mix and minimum level of staff in the dispensary.

The key outputs of an HR plan are individual job descriptions and staffing schedules. These outputs are achieved from the previously described steps that, for reference, can be simplified as follows:

- Anticipate customer demand for products and service.
- Consider any available direct customer service information.
- Establish staff mix to meet service demand and set job descriptions accordingly.
- Determine optimal staffing levels and schedule to meet anticipated demand.
- Accommodate applicable labour and safety standards within the plan.

HR planning is not a one-time event. All pharmacies operate in a dynamic environment and as a result, managers will need to regularly revisit the staffing plan to align staffing mix and staffing level with demand. In addition, it is important to test and train consistently for staff competencies and productivity.

JOB DESCRIPTIONS

The foundation of good HR management is the job description. This document delineates the needs of the business to be met by a particular employee. When correctly crafted, it will demonstrate the relative importance of the position to the business, define the relationship to other employees and list the required skills and characteristics of the incumbent.[2]

Creation of job descriptions starts with a detailed analysis of the work to be accomplished. What are all the tasks required to operate a pharmacy? Once this list is constructed, there will be some natural groupings of the main components into positions. For example, checking prescriptions naturally falls to pharmacists or regulated pharmacy technicians, while balancing the cash float likely falls to a cashier supervisor. There will be some tasks that will be shared by all staff, while others will be reserved to a smaller number of employees. To create job descriptions, the task list needs to be divided into a detailed, prioritized listing of all the duties and responsibilities for each employee. Collectively, the job descriptions should cover all the tasks required in the pharmacy in sufficient detail to ensure that unnecessary overlap and unintentional omission are both avoided.

There are many formats and templates available for job descriptions. The following are three general features:

- summary statement: brief summary of responsibilities and reporting relationships
- functional listing: detailed list of duties using active language in priority order
- required attributes: list of skills and certifications required for position

Selecting which format to use is largely a matter of personal choice and convenience. Many companies provide standardized templates for use across the organization. Tailoring a template to a specific pharmacy will be much faster than creating job descriptions from scratch. Three sample job descriptions are included for reference at the end of this chapter.

Investing time to customize job descriptions for each employee ensures both that the duties required by the business are all attributed and that the employees are clear on the work that is expected of them.

At a minimum, there should be a job description created for each position in the pharmacy. HR best practice would be that each employee has a job description tailored to the position that is reviewed and updated annually.

Complete and current job descriptions are the starting point for HR management in the pharmacy. They should be the basis of position descriptions used in hiring, an essential piece of the orientation and training process, key to the performance evaluation process and also a component in compensation assessment. Investing time to ensure the document closely reflects and communicates the actual duties and expectations of each employee will establish an excellent foundation for both staff and management to follow.

STAFFING SCHEDULE

The purpose of a staffing schedule is to ensure the appropriate mix of staff is available in the store at any given time to meet the demands of the customers. Wages are the largest single variable cost in a pharmacy, so over-scheduling will result in reduced profitability. At the other end of the spectrum, not having enough staff scheduled will ultimately reduce sales when the expectations of customers are not met in a timely manner. As a general measure, total wage costs should not exceed 12% to 15% of total sales.[1] Specific productivity targets are generally set for sales per labour hour for front store departments and prescription count per labour hour for pharmacy.

To create a staffing schedule, follow the steps below. Note that many pharmacy chains use software programs that utilize a similar process with available sales and schedule data to quickly generate and monitor ongoing staffing schedules.

1. Gather historical sales data for the period to be scheduled by hour by department. This information is generally reported by point-of-sale (POS) systems for sales and by the pharmacy software for prescription count.
2. Gather the historical staffing data for the period broken down by hour by position.
3. Schedule the minimum staff required to open the store (a pharmacist, a cashier, a cosmetician, etc.) based on historical staffing.
4. Use productivity metric targets to add additional staff in each hour based on anticipated sales and prescription count.
5. Allocate available hours to specific staff members based on labour standards (shift length, breaks, etc.) and company policy (full-time employees first, regular part-time and then casual labour).
6. Recalculate anticipated productivity to ensure targets are met.

Scheduling is not an exact science and the daily and hourly fluctuations in workload must be considered. Where possible, cross-training of staff is an excellent method of ensuring the store has the capacity to handle fluctuations in demand. As required, temporarily shift workers from non-service areas (merchandising, clerical, administrative) to customer service. It is also important to consider the mix of staff working at any given time. Generally, there should be an even mix of experienced full-time staff with newer and part-time staff to ensure a consistent level of customer service. Seasonal and weekly fluctuations will occur and the business will evolve requiring ongoing schedule adjustments. There is no such thing as being done with scheduling and managers should expect this to be an area of ongoing responsibility.

Another important variable to consider when creating the staff schedule is staff lifestyle considerations. While the needs of the business must be considered, a schedule dictated only by hourly productivity targets will most certainly be a disaster. Staff members have a reasonable expectation that their shifts will be reasonably consistent and that consideration will be given both to their tenure with the company and special requests. Pharmacies, however, operate in a competitive extended-hour marketplace and no one should reasonably expect Monday to Friday day shifts. Fair rotation of shifts is both equitable for the employees and meets the needs of the business to mix senior and junior staff.

CHANGE

Pharmacies operate in an increasingly competitive environment. Economic constraints and demographic pressures are also increasing the demands on the profession of pharmacy. Employee teams must continually adapt and change in response. Pharmacies that are not able to change in response to the environment in which they operate will ultimately fail.

Change, no matter how small, requires management intervention in the regular routines of the staff. The process for creating change has been well documented by many in the literature. One of the most helpful frameworks for managers to refer to is Kotter's eight steps:[3]

1. Establish urgency.
2. Build guiding team.

3. Get the right vision.
4. Communicate for buy-in.
5. Empower staff action.
6. Create short-term wins.
7. Don't let up.
8. Make it stick.

Store management will be primarily concerned with engaging and enabling the staff (Steps 4 to 6) and then sustaining the change (Steps 7 and 8). Change is more often unsuccessful than not, so getting to Step 8, make it stick, often takes more than one attempt.

An essential piece in managing change is to fully appreciate that for most staff (including the pharmacists), change of any kind is not desirable but is viewed as disruptive and intrusive.[4] Regardless of the overarching imperatives for a particular change or of the communication done, change will temporarily upset the balance and require that staff adapt and find a new balance. Misjudging the gap between managerial expectation and employee resistance and the effort required to win acceptance of change is a common cause of failed change efforts. To be successful, managers must put themselves in their employees' shoes to understand how change looks from that perspective and understand the personal compacts (reasons for working) that drive them. It is extremely rare to find an employee whose reason for working includes the success of the business in any meaningful way.

Change is an inevitable and important piece of business operations. It is important for managers to understand the process of change and to anticipate the impact of change on the employees. Successful managers anticipate and embrace change, ensure the pace of change is reasonable, discuss and plan responses and then take action to implement change. The most important piece of the action will be communication that is thoughtful of employee impact and motivation (see Chapter 10: Change Management).

REFERENCES

1. Bachynsky JA, Nadeau J. Human resource management. In: Bachynsky JA, Segal HJ, editors. *Pharmacy management in Canada*. 2nd ed. Toronto: Grosvenor House Press Inc; 1998. p. 156–93.
2. Howard University. The importance of job descriptions. Available: www.financialwisdom.com/pflsresourcecenter/HowardUniversity/SmallBusiness/JobDescriptions.shtml (accessed on April 11, 2014).
3. Kotter JP. Leading change: why transformation efforts fail. Harv Bus Rev. 2007;(Jan):4–11.
4. Strebel J. Why Do Employees Resist Change? Harv Bus Rev. 1996;(May-June):86–92.

Lovell Drugs – Pharmacist Job Description (used with permission)

Job Title: Pharmacist
Reports to: Pharmacist – Manager and General Manager
Supervises: All personnel working in the store when manager is not available

PRIMARY RESPONSIBILITIES:

- Maintaining customer service levels in the store.
- Pharmaceutical care and all dispensary operations.
- Maintaining the professional image of the store.
- Overseeing store operations while manager or front store manager is not present.

GENERAL RESPONSIBILITIES:
PEOPLE
Responsible for:

- All aspects of dispensing including filling of prescriptions, ensuring correct pricing and following company policy on pricing of prescriptions, and other professional matters included in the pharmacy policy section of the Human Resource Manual.
- Provision of patient care, ensuring systems are in place to make sure all patients are counselled on all new prescriptions and that all OCP requirements are met.
- Ensuring that the standards of practice have been met.
- Working on all company programs such as trial prescription programs and compliance programs.
- Maintaining a professional dispensary environment, ensuring all staff meet professional requirements including attire, confidentiality and general dispensary decorum.
- Maintaining excellent customer service in the entire store.
- Ensuring that telephone service is up to par, quick answer (maximum 3 rings), staff are polite and use their name.
- Promoting an atmosphere of teamwork and positive staff relations.
- Responsible for ensuring that all company policies are being followed.
- Confidentiality in the pharmacy in conjunction with our confidentiality policy.

PLANNING:
Responsible for:

- Reviewing all relevant correspondence from Head Office, as well as notices from the College, third party plans and drug manufacturers.
- Staying current and maintaining the required portfolio of CE learning as per the OCP guidelines
- Management duties in the absence of the manager that require immediate action: e.g., arranging for coverage when an employee calls in sick, completing Prescription Error reports, accident reports, WSIB, dealing with customer complaints, taking action in situations such as theft and robbery.

PLANT:
Responsible for:

- General appearance of the pharmacy.
- Reporting any problems with regard to safety and security.
- Following proper lock up procedures as well as cash handling and safety.
- Following all company policies in the store.
- Computer maintenance, e.g., regular backups, updates and following required procedures.

PROFIT:
Responsible for:

- Dispensing and purchasing according to the Lovell Drugs Formulary.
- Assisting the manager in any of the following: narcotic reports and required month end reports, inventory control, following company procedures for the automated dispensary inventory, expense control including payroll, supply costs, and other general costs.
- Following all safety and security procedures to ensure that we minimize losses both internally and externally.
- Any other job responsibilities as designated by the Store Manager.

Lovell Drugs – Pharmacy Clerk Job Description (used with permission)

Job Title: Pharmacy Clerk
Reports To: Pharmacist Manager, Pharmacist

PRIMARY RESPONSIBILITIES:
- Providing customer service to customers both in person and on the telephone.
- Assisting the Pharmacist in the preparation of prescriptions.
- Clerical activities, including cashier functions, third party drug plan administration, house charge management.
- Follow confidentiality policy; maintain a professional image in both mannerisms and appearance at all times.
- Use tact and courtesy when dealing with difficult customers and the referral of customers to management if a problem cannot be resolved.

GENERAL RESPONSIBILITIES:
DISPENSING
Responsible for:
- Receiving a written prescription or request for a prescription refill from the patient or representative.
- Entering new and repeat prescriptions into computer and checking compliance.
- Filling prescriptions and checking last fill dates.
- Confirming that the original container, its contents and the label are checked and initialled by the pharmacist before releasing to the patient.
- Ensuring completeness of information on the prescription.
- Preparation of prescription labels, establishing and maintaining patient profiles.
- Retrieving, counting, pouring, weighing, measuring and mixing medications.
- Selecting type of prescription container.
- Affixing prescription and auxiliary labels to prescription containers.
- Pricing prescriptions according to the Lovell Drugs Pricing Policy.
- Filing prescriptions.
- Maintaining packaging and dispensing equipment.
- Replenishing medications for nursing units, night cupboards, emergency boxes.

COMPOUNDING:
Responsible for:
- Preparing IV admixtures, TPN solutions, requiring aseptic technique.
- Preparing specialty products.
- Assisting the pharmacist in preparing specialized compounds according to standard operating procedures.

ADMINISTRATION:
Responsible for:
- Preparing and reconciling third party billings.
- Preparing receipts, invoices, letters and memos, and general filing.
- Maintaining drug information files.
- Billing appropriate party for medication.
- Receiving and sending electronic communication.

COMMUNICATION:
Responsible for:
- Communicating with customers, physicians and suppliers, in a professional manner.
- Ensuring that any and all physician inquiries are handled by the pharmacist.
- Emphasis on serving customers first before staff, administration or sales reps.
- Questions relating to prescriptions, drug information, poison information, or any health matter that must be referred to the pharmacist.
- Showing a willingness to assist clients with products outside the dispensary, e.g., OTC, front shop or home health.

MEDICATION MANAGEMENT:
Responsible for:
- Monitoring stock levels to ensure sufficient quantities for optimal operation.
- Preparing and placing orders from specified sources.
- Receiving, checking and pricing supplies purchased.
- Restocking medications and related supplies.
- Maintaining inventory records, including those for narcotics and controlled drugs.
- Rotating stock and monitoring expiry dates.
- Identifying expired products for disposal, destruction, or return to manufacturer.
- Pre-packaging medications (including unit dose and compliance packaging).

OTHER:
Responsible for:
- Adherence to company policies at all times, including Safety and Security, Human Resources, Lovell Drugs Formulary.
- General dispensary neatness and cleaning duties, e.g., replenishing dispensing supplies, emptying garbage.
- Any other task as assigned by the pharmacist or manager.

Note: In stores where Registered Pharmacist Technicians are part of the staff, a separate job description for the Technicians and the Pharmacy Clerks (also called Assistants) will be required.

Lovell Drugs – Cashier/Clerk Job Description (used with permission)

Job Title: Cashier/Clerk
Reports To: Front Store Manager

PRIMARY RESPONSIBILITIES:
Responsible for:
- Providing excellent customer service to customers both in person and on the telephone. Always greet and acknowledge every customer. Emphasis is always on serving the customer before staff, administration or sales reps.
- Handling customers courteously, quickly and efficiently. Call for help when a lineup or delay occurs.
- Answering telephone enquiries quickly and carefully without ignoring in-store customers.
- Providing customers with accurate information on goods and services; seek out the answer if you don't know.
- Using tact and courtesy when dealing with difficult customers and referring customers to management if a problem cannot be resolved.
- Ensuring that all products are rung in correctly under the proper category and that the price is correct. Proper change must be counted back to the customer into their hand.
- Practising selling techniques and closing companion sales.
- Showing a willingness to assist customers with products outside the department and is knowledgeable in all store promotions. Keeping other staff aware of promotions.
- Reporting to the Front Store Manager any unusual occurrences during their shift.
- Maintaining a professional image in both mannerisms and appearance at all times.
- Ensuring that the front work area is clean and neat at all times.
- Maintaining security in the store; be alert at all times. Never leave the cash area without securing your till and maintaining eye contact with the area.
- Developing a clear understanding of store policies. Following the correct procedures for opening, closing and balancing of cash. Cash handling policies must always be properly followed. End all cash transactions with a smile and a "thank you."
- Whenever a product is not available, offering to order it for the customer. Always follow through in getting the customer's name and phone number as well as making sure that the product is ordered and that the customer is called when it arrives.
- Alerting the Front Store Manager whenever you notice products and supplies out of stock or running low.

GENERAL RESPONSIBILITIES:
Responsible for:
- Ensuring that the customer is your number one focus at all times.
- Following all store policies, including all safety and security procedures.
- Accurately recording all cash transactions with a minimum of voids and errors.
- Following store policies with regard to cheques, charge accounts, credit cards and rain checks and voids.
- Handling lottery ticket sales as per store procedures.
- Keeping busy and productive at all times. When on cash identify tasks that can be completed between customers.
- Basic merchandising as requested by the Front Store Manager, including facing up sections, setting up ends, pricing product, decorating the store seasonally.
- Learning basic merchandising such as stock rotation, product placement and facing.
- Maintaining specific sections as allocated.
- Carrying out price changes and ticketing as required.
- General store maintenance as requested by the Front Store Manager or Manager.
- Following all policies and ensuring that you find out the information that is necessary to do your job. Understand the policies in both the Human Resource Manual as well as the Safety and Security Manual.
- Any other jobs as assigned by the Front Store Manager or the Store Manager.

CHAPTER 33

S.H.O.T.: Screening, Hiring, Orientation and Training

Rita E. Winn, *RPh, B.Sc. Phm; COO and General Manager, Lovell Drugs Limited*

Learning Objectives

- Explain the benefits of a structured plan for the recruitment and retention of qualified staff.
- Describe the five steps involved in the screening process.
- Explain the pre-interview, interview and post-interview activities.
- Identify areas that should be reviewed and discussed as part of an orientation plan.
- List the five-step procedure for training new staff members.

Hiring new staff and retaining staff can be a formidable task for a pharmacist owner/manager while trying to balance the everyday wants and needs of a busy and demanding pharmacy business. At the same time, the recruitment, selection and retention of qualified staff are imperative for the success of a pharmacy practice. A structured plan for staff recruitment and retention has many benefits to the present and future needs of a pharmacy business. The benefits include the following:

- opportunities for succession planning
- reduced staff turnover
- better hiring practices by a proactive versus a reactive human resources (HR) strategy
- ability to hire specialists in required areas
- qualified staff to cover vacations and illnesses, and the ability to cross-train staff
- improved productivity in the pharmacy
- improved medication safety
- enhanced customer service and patient care

A methodology that aids in achieving the benefits of a structured recruitment and retention plan is the implementation of an effective Screening, Hiring, Orientation and Training (S.H.O.T.) program.

EFFECTIVE SCREENING AND HIRING

Effective screening and hiring can be broken down into five steps:

1. identifying needs
2. résumé gathering
3. evaluation of résumés
4. interview techniques
5. reference checks

IDENTIFYING NEEDS

The first step is to identify what the needs of the business are before the process of résumé gathering. Decisions should be made as to the type of person and skill set for the position as well as the time allotment required to perform the task. This process is as simple as finding the right person for the right job at the right time at the right price. Planning is also a vital key to effective S.H.O.T. It is always much easier for an organization to find the right person before they are needed, rather than having to hire under pressure.

Before finalizing the process of identifying needs, it is important to review present job descriptions or create a new job description for the position. Job descriptions are vital because they do the following:

- help determine qualifications of a particular job, thus aiding in recruitment and selection for a vacancy (Qualifications can encompass education, experience and personality traits.)
- can be used as an orientation tool to explain a job to a new employee
- aid in developing training programs
- clarify the job, thus helping to eliminate difference in perception between employers, supervisors and staff
- act as a guideline for performance reviews
- help to determine equitable salary/wage administration
- facilitate the communication of department and organization objectives and mission statements

Perform the following after reviewing or creating the job description:

- Reaffirm the necessity and qualifications required.
- Review the entire staff and make any other changes before adding or replacing a staff member. Evaluate whether an existing staff member can move from part time to full time. Are all the present staff efficient and productive? Can some job functions change or switch to other persons? Do not create a job description to fit the individual, but rather one that matches the needs of the pharmacy.
- Review past and future schedules to see if an opportunity exists to refine schedules, therefore reducing the need or the number of hours required for a new recruit.
- Examine if there are any other operational issues such as dispensary flow, store layout or hours of operation that may be inhibiting the efficiency of the pharmacy that can be resolved rather than replacing or recruiting a new staff member.

Only after this process is complete should the decision be made to move forward with the balance of the screening and hiring process.[1]

RÉSUMÉ GATHERING

The second step is résumé gathering. Word of mouth, newspaper advertisements, window signs, employee referrals, internal company HR departments, community colleges, universities, profession-related magazine publications, placement centres and web-based career opportunity sites are all excellent résumé-gathering sources. The choice really depends on key factors such as cost, quality of applicants and type of position available, as well as the time available for recruitment.

For example, recruitment method and the number of sources that are used will be different for hiring a pharmacist or pharmacy technician versus a cashier. The recruitment of a pharmacist or pharmacy technician may include a combination of newspaper advertising, posting the ad on an Internet website or recruiting at a community college or university job fair. Hiring a cashier may involve a newspaper ad along with a posting on the front window of the pharmacy. Résumés for a cosmetician may be gathered through a newspaper ad and a trip to the local community college.

Despite the popularity and increased use of the Internet, newspaper advertising is still a valuable recruitment tool for pharmacies as it reaches a wide audience quickly. Running a newspaper advertisement on Fridays, Saturdays and Sundays, although more expensive, is more effective than running an ad all week.[2] Most newspapers also have a web-based component that is usually included in the cost of the advertisement. If a newspaper advertisement is the preferred method, consider having applications go to a post office box or fax number to avoid being inundated with phone calls and visitors. Job postings should have specific experience, technical requirements and education requirements clearly stated to allow for some self pre-screening by potential applicants. Whatever sources are used for résumé gathering, it is important to remember that the exercise involves public relations. The image of the pharmacy portrayed to job applicants during the recruitment process is the image they will recall as consumers making a buying decision.[3]

EVALUATION OF RÉSUMÉS

The third step is the evaluation of résumés. The number of candidates to interview will depend on the amount of time available to interview as well as the quality of the applicants. Skill, experience and interests that match the career opportunity should be noted. At this point, a second opinion and a helping hand from a trusted key staff member is a valuable resource in trying to evaluate potential candidates. The following factors should be considered based on the applications:

Work experience
- Is the cover letter related to the actual job advertisement or is it a generic cover letter?
- Does the résumé relate to the job description?
- Is his/her work experience stable?
- Are there any employment gaps? Possible reasons?
- Does the candidate switch jobs frequently?
- Is there evidence of decreased responsibility?
- Is his/her pharmacy experience out of province/territory or country, which may require more training?
- Is his/her pharmacy experience recent?
- Does his/her work experience correspond to the salary budgeted for the position?[4]

Education

- Does it indicate over/under-qualification?
- Is there any related pharmacy training?
- Where was the candidate's apparent interest?
- Do grammar and spelling indicate good communication skills?

Interests and activities

- Is the candidate outgoing?
- Have leadership skills been demonstrated?
- Is there too much information or not enough information?

Neatness

The amount of neatness and organization demonstrated in an application or résumé may fore-shadow a person's work habits.

After reviewing the applications and selecting the candidates for interviews, it is important to clearly specify to interviewees where and when the interview is to be held and what the expectations will be. Allow for sufficient time for each interview as well as a gap between interviews to gather thoughts and makes some notes based on observations. It is also important to hold interviews in an area that is free from distraction and confidential for all parties.[3]

INTERVIEW TECHNIQUES

The fourth step of an effective screening and hiring program is the interview process and interview techniques. The same process should be used to interview all candidates to make comparisons between prospective employees. This includes having the same interviewer(s) involved in all interviews for the position. The most important part of the interview process is to explore an applicant's attitude and personality. Successful businesses hire for personality first and foremost and then train the employee to do the necessary skills.

A sample agenda for an interview could include the following:

- Break the ice! Ask the candidate about an activity or interest listed on his/her application or perhaps discuss the weather or some other newsworthy event.
- Ask the candidate what he/she knows about the pharmacy. This will also help to put the candidate at ease and at the same time allows for time to evaluate his/her communication skills. The answer to this question will also indicate if the candidate has done any research about the pharmacy before the interview and if there are any misconceptions concerning the pharmacy.
- Provide the candidate with an outline of the company or pharmacy history, as well as the mission statement. Any misconception or inaccurate information he/she may have will be resolved with this process. The company history and mission statement will also give the candidate a sense of the culture of the pharmacy and may open up some dialogue.
- Outline the job description and salary range for the position. Field any questions from the candidate and ask if this job description and salary range align with his/her expectations and skills. For higher-skill job descriptions such as a pharmacist or a management position, detailed discussion of specific salary offers should be delayed until actually making a job offer. The range should provide sufficient room for negotiation.

- Clarify or verify any details from the candidate's application or résumé. It is important to review all application materials and information supplied before the interview. Highlight and ask any questions or discuss areas that may require clarification.
- Ask questions. Use a similar group of questions for all candidates to ensure consistency. A prepared list of questions, leaving space between questions on separate sheets for each candidate, is the most efficient method. Human rights legislation in all provinces/ territories prohibits questions deemed to be discriminatory such as applicant's age, marital status, spouse's employment, religion and many other areas. Refer to your provincial/ territorial human rights code.

There are many types of interview formats available with today's technology. Common methods include face to face, telephone, Skype or other video technology. Technology formats are useful for prescreening candidates before the more traditional face-to-face interview, saving the interviewer time by eliminating weaker candidates. Depending on the complexity of the position, face-to-face interviews may include several individual interviews followed by a group interview. These sequential interviews allow the interviewer to see the candidate in several different situations. A group interview changes the dynamic of the interview and allows for the initial interviewer to see how the candidates handle themselves with other people and in a different situation. Having several interviewers presents the opportunity for good discussion and different perceptions of the candidates, resulting in a better hiring decision.

The selection of questions used will depend on the position and the specific information required from the candidate. Interview question areas may include the following:
- performance-related skills and experience
- attitude toward work in general, supervisors and/or co-workers
- attitude regarding the job function, pharmacy in general and the candidate's future
- identifying leadership potential, initiative, enthusiasm and self-confidence
- planning and organizational skills
- attitude toward customer service and breaches of policy
- education
- time-management skills
- self-analysis questions relating to a candidate's strengths and weaknesses by sharing real-life examples to illustrate a specific skill set

The following specific key questions may be used to access qualifications and interests of the candidate:
- Why are you applying for this job?
- What were the reasons you changed jobs?
- Describe your previous responsibilities and duties for your last three jobs.
- What did you like or dislike about the jobs you have had?
- Can you give an example where you thought creatively to deliver outstanding customer service?
- Have you worked in a busy environment before? What were some of the skills used to handle these times?
- Have you ever had an issue with a co-worker? How did you handle this?[5]

The number of questions from each area will vary depending on the position being filled. More questions pertaining to education and performance-related skills may be asked of a potential pharmacy technician than a cashier, where additional questions concerning attitudes toward customer service may be asked.

At the conclusion of the interview, always allow the candidate to ask any questions or offer any other commentary. The insightfulness of the questions asked may provide further information regarding a candidate's interest in and fit with the position. Make sure the candidate is clear on how and when they should expect to hear back. Make the candidate aware that reference checks will take place and his/her permission for this process is required. At this point, the interviewer should do a thorough review of all documentation gathered from the interviews. The process of selecting the top two or three candidates should happen at this stage.[6]

REFERENCE CHECKS

The final step is performing reference checks. Although reference checks can be a time-consuming task, they are an invaluable tool to help identify the right person for the job. Much insight can be gathered through the reference-check process that in the long run, will in fact save time and money by providing information to help to make the best hiring decision the first time.

Telephone checks are the best type of reference check. Written references included with an application are useful, but remember that the candidate has had an opportunity to read them and would probably not include anything except a positive assessment. Due to legal and privacy concerns, some employers are reluctant or refuse to provide reference checks and some companies have policies in place that do not allow for providing reference checks. Some companies will only provide verification of the person's name, positions held and date of employment, while others will provide simple yes or no responses to performance-related questions. Although obtaining reference checks has become more difficult, many employers are still willing and able to provide the information. It is best to refer to provincial/territorial legislation for detailed information on laws surrounding personal information protection.

Similar to the interview process, if checking references on more than one candidate, ask the same set of questions to each reference to be able to make comparisons and maintain consistency between prospective employees. It is also important to make notes during the reference-check process to ensure the information about each candidate is clear later on when trying to recall a conversation with the reference. It is a good idea to develop and use a standard template for this process as this ensures the same questions each time, as well as provides a documentation vehicle. Ensure the name of the individual providing the reference, the date of the reference and his/her relationship to the candidate are recorded for future reference.

The successful applicant should then be notified. Such notification should happen before calling the unsuccessful candidates so that if the successful candidate does not accept the position, the next candidate in line could be offered the position. A telephone call and/or an offer of employment letter outlining start date, hours, wages and a brief description of the orientation plan should be confirmed. At this point, there may be a need to negotiate some of these components should the candidate indicate concerns with the offer. The offer should also clearly indicate the length of a probation period if this applies and the expectations and requirements to pass this probation. Upon confirmation of acceptance, the unsuccessful candidates should then be contacted. From a public relations point of view, notification given to unsuccessful interviewed candidates is essential and should be done tactfully.[7]

EFFECTIVE ORIENTATION

The new employee's first day at work is his/her most important day. Managers have an opportunity to create a good impression about themselves, the team and the pharmacy business. The new employee's first impression is indeed a lasting impression. Orientation sets the tone for the working relationship between the parties and when properly done, will help ensure that a new employee will be productive, informed and comfortable right from the initial stage of employment. New-employee orientation may take one day, days or weeks depending on the person, position and number of hours they work.

As the person responsible for hiring new employees, it is important the manager is available on their first day to speak with them as orientation begins. Although various parts of the orientation can in fact be delegated to key staff or the new employee's immediate supervisor, it is significant the manager is seen as the point person for their orientation.

Developing a checklist outlining the orientation areas to be reviewed as well as who is responsible for the orientation of each particular area for a new employee is a useful tool. Review the following areas as part of a new-employee orientation:

- introductions: Introduce the new employee to fellow workers, supervisors, management team and other parties.
- pharmacy walk-around: Spend some time walking through the pharmacy showing the new employee key areas, including common areas such as the lunch room, washrooms and communication boards for schedules and information.
- new-employee documentation: Discuss and help the employee with paperwork pertaining to payroll, benefits and tax forms.
- employee handbooks and manuals: Review and discuss information about privacy laws and confidentiality, company history and mission statement, policies and procedures, codes of conduct, housekeeping policies, communication binders and job descriptions.

Manuals can be reviewed at specified intervals during the orientation period as they may require a considerable amount of time and discussion. After new employees read and discuss the manuals, it is important they sign, date and acknowledge that the manuals have been read and understood. The signed document should be kept in the employee's file to avoid a legal implication if an issue arises at a future date.

Be prepared to have the employees become engaged in the workflow of the pharmacy operation immediately. This will allow them to find a comfort zone and build confidence with a job or task they are familiar with, when everything else around them will probably be very different. Shadowing a high-performance employee for a period of time is another excellent means of orientation for a new hire. Key timelines should also be identified during the orientation process to sit down and discuss the employee's progress. The discussion should be a two-way conversation that includes the following:

- level of job satisfaction
- review of job description/evaluation

- identification of training needs
- other questions, concerns, feedback or ideas

An effective orientation program requires a planned process and time commitment with many checks and balances to guarantee the success of a new employee.[8]

EFFECTIVE TRAINING

The final stage of the S.H.O.T. process is the implementation of a successful training program. Training is a critical opportunity for the employer to instill values of the pharmacy operation to the new employee that are crucial for the success of the overall pharmacy business. Training is as much about the new hire understanding the culture of the pharmacy team as learning the day-to-day operational issues that his/her job description involves. Topics such as teamwork, morale and empowerment should be discussed and demonstrated by the trainers on a continual basis. An effective training program incorporates these five steps:

- Assess training needs: Core training such as health and safety, loss prevention and security, cash handling, customer service, privacy legislation and telephone etiquette should be a requirement for all new employees. Regardless of how long they have been employed in pharmacy, or the position they have been hired for, these core topics need to be discussed so that the new hire understands the fundamental operational procedures of this pharmacy. After core training has been identified, individual training needs of the new hire can be accessed by getting input from the employee concerning what areas he/she thinks will require training, observing the employee's initial hours or days on the job or by following a standardized training plan used for all employees.
- Develop training to satisfy the needs: After discussing with and observing the new employee at work, a training plan should be developed to meet the needs of the pharmacy as well as the progress of the individual. The training may incorporate areas that the new employee needs and requires to fulfill his/her job description, versus having the employee understand something that is not necessarily his/her responsibility but is important to the overall operation. For example, the training plan may have specific areas such as training the new employee on the pharmacy computer system or more general training such as the employee understanding the tools the pharmacy uses to manage inventory.
- Select the method of training: The method of training will vary depending on the task for which the new hire requires training. Training methods may include having the individual shadow another employee, one-on-one training, external training, reading manuals or information or simply just gaining more experience at performing the task. Training programs and their delivery will differ based on the position being trained as well as the background and skills of the individual.
- Design and implement the training activities: A checklist that identifies the areas requiring core, specific and general training combined with a timeline for each training area is the most effective method to design and implement training activities. A detailed review of the job description with the new employee will help to identify and design training opportunities. Training activities will have varying timelines dependent on their complexity. This checklist can also be used to discuss, monitor and follow up on training

activities. Training activities can be implemented by the pharmacy owner/manager, competent staff or any other internal or external sources that may be suitable for the pharmacy operation.

- Evaluate the results of these activities and modify accordingly: An evaluation on the progress of the training activities is crucial to the success of the new employee. Evaluations should take place at prearranged intervals and input should be gathered from the trainers involved as well as the trainee. Training activities can then be modified based on the feedback from all parties and a new plan can be created and a new timeline established.[9]

An effective S.H.O.T. program provides a structured plan for staff recruitment and retention. A structured plan will indeed provide many benefits to the success of a pharmacy practice.[10]

ACKNOWLEDGEMENTS

The author would like to thank countless people from Big V Pharmacies for their contributions and additions to the S.H.O.T. theory over the years. The S.H.O.T. theory originated many years ago and at that time, was primarily the work of Big V's Human Resources Manager, Dave Town. During that time, many managers and directors at Big V had expanded on and used the concept for workshops and various meetings. Twenty years later, I am still adding, updating and using the framework of the program as a valuable human resources tool.

RESOURCES AND SUGGESTED READINGS

Further reading on screening and hiring legislation can be obtained online through provincial/territorial human rights code as well as provincial/territorial Employment Standards Acts.

REFERENCES

1. Winn R. Effective S.H.O.T. Drugstore Canada May 1, 2009.
2. Hancocks D. The human resources advisor. Concord, ON: First Reference; 1993–2005: A301.
3. Winn R. Effective S.H.O.T. Drugstore Canada Aug. 1, 2009.
4. The University of British Columbia. What to look for in resumes. Available: http://hr.ok.ubc.ca/__shared/assets/What_to_Look_for_in_Resumes23172.pdf (accessed June 3, 2014).
5. Hancocks D. *The human resources advisor*. Concord, ON: First Reference; 1993–2005: A411.
6. Winn R. Gearing up for the interview. Drugstore Canada Jan. 1, 2010.
7. Winn R. Making the most of reference checks. Drug Store Canada April 1, 2010.
8. Winn R. Successful orientation. Drugstore Canada May 1, 2010.
9. Hancocks D. The human resources advisor. Concord, ON: First Reference; 1993–2005: D402.
10. Winn R. Successful training. Drugstore Canada Nov. 2010.

CHAPTER 34

Performance Management

Rita E. Winn, *RPh, B.Sc. Phm; COO and General Manager, Lovell Drugs Limited*

Learning Objectives

- Explain why productive performance appraisals are important to the employer, employee and the pharmacy operation.
- Outline the objectives of an annual performance review.
- Describe the typical agenda items for a productive performance review.
- Describe the six steps involved in the coaching process to enhance performance management.
- Define *wage administration* and describe the process by which it is implemented.

Productive performance reviews are critical in achieving effective performance management in the fast-paced, ever-changing pharmacy world. They are important for a pharmacy as they bring out the best in people, identify overperformers and underperformers and allow pharmacy managers to align and communicate their present and future goals of the pharmacy with that of the employee. The performance evaluations should be conducted by the employee's direct supervisor or department head. A formal performance review should take place at least once per year. Employees should have interim performance reviews to monitor their progress, especially if they are a new employee. Results of a review should never be a surprise to employees as they should always know how they are doing and what is expected.

The following are objectives of an annual performance review:

- Provide objective feedback since the last review.
- Acknowledge good performance and, where needed, help the employee to improve productivity/performance during the coming period.
- Review the employee's objectives for the coming period.
- Provide an opportunity to review and update the company's goals and how the employee's job fits the objective.
- Provide the employee with an opportunity to ask questions, voice concerns or offer ideas concerning the pharmacy operation.

- Offer an overall rating to the employee indicating where he/she stands in the supervisor's eyes.
- Discuss the employee's long-term career goals and how to achieve them.

Productive performance reviews should be held in an area that is free of distractions, such as phone calls and interruptions, and scheduled so that adequate time is allowed. Easier reviews with positive staff may be done first to build confidence in the interviewer. The most productive performance reviews are ones that allow employees to understand what the process will be and prepare ahead of time for the review. A posted agenda for performance reviews is an integral part of the process and may contain the following:

PERFORMANCE REVIEW AGENDA

A performance review agenda should include the following:
- the past year's objectives, performance, job description changes
- the working relationship
- working conditions
- future goals for the company and for the employee
- wage review

PREPARING FOR THE REVIEW

The time and effort put into the preparation of productive performance reviews will reflect the success rate you will have in enhancing the pharmacy operation. Preparation, setting clear objectives and delivery of productive performance reviews should include the following:
- Review the employee file. Employee files should contain their résumé, interview notes, job offer acceptance, employment documents, orientation and training checklists, as well as past performance reviews. Past notes and possible counselling sessions should be reviewed. Previous performance review notes should also be evaluated, noting goal achievements, successes and other areas of improvement from the last review.
- It is sometimes beneficial to gather feedback from an employee's colleagues, customers or other store staff and, where possible, cite specific examples.
- Emphasis should be placed on setting clear objectives correctly at the beginning of the process. If set correctly, performance reviews are clear and objective as to whether targets have been met.
- Clear, concise notes in a language that is understandable to employees should be made. Remember that performance appraisals are meant to be a positive reinforcement as much as a review for improvement.
- Have a standardized performance review form that is used for all employees. Such forms will include criteria for evaluation that are related to skill, customers and behaviour. Performance review forms are intended as a summary of the employee's performance evaluation and should clearly outline areas of strength and areas needing improvement. Performance goals for the upcoming period should also be outlined. These checklists also allow areas for verbal and written communication that take place throughout the performance review. Most pharmacy chains, franchises or banners have forms that can

be used or modified for these purposes. If such a form is not available, many types can be found using Internet search engines and can be modified to suit the needs. (See the sample employee performance evaluation form at the end of this chapter.)[1]

CONDUCTING THE PERFORMANCE EVALUATION

- Maintain open and clear two-way communication.
- Review the employee's job description; it may be, in fact, different from what either party believes.
- Discuss problems area(s) frankly and develop corrective actions. Allow a response for criticism, as there may be a reason. Do not make assumptions.
- Avoid ambiguous and vague statements as they are easily misinterpreted. Be specific and stick to performance issues (not personal).
- Emphasize the criteria that are important.
- Adhere to the agenda; however, always allow for feedback and communication from the employee.
- Remember, it is about the quality of the discussion and interaction with the employee. Do not get caught in the trap where the process of filling out forms outweighs the purpose.[2]

This chapter covers the yearly formal performance appraisal process. In situations where an employee is underperforming or not meeting expectations, more attention and a focused progressive discipline process is required (see Chapter 35: Conflict Management and Progressive Discipline).

Although standardized performance reviews are conducted annually, performance management needs to happen on an ongoing daily basis, through effective communication and staff management. One of the approaches to enhance performance management is to implement a coaching mindset. A coach's role is to develop skills in employees and provide an objective point of view of performance. A coach's attention is directed to every level of performer, both the new and weakest, and the stars. The coach is not directly in the game, is not an expert performer in all parts of the game, but is on the sidelines communicating, offering support and delivering the post-game review. The goal is to produce an effective team that works together, creates wins and eventually becomes champions. The coaching mindset can be implemented with an individual member or the entire team. The pharmacy business is no different from this example, and enhanced performance management can be achieved by implementing the following game plan (see Chapter 31: Effective Management Styles).

SET AND CLEARLY COMMUNICATE GOALS

Set clear, relevant and challenging goals for the team to achieve. Determine milestones that can be measured along the path to the goals. Establish priorities along the path and instruct employees to always ask, "Why am I doing this? Is there a better way?" Goals should always be discussed, referenced and visible to all team members. Goals also have to be reviewed to determine if they continue to be relevant, achievable and realistic. If circumstances of the business change such that the original goals are no longer appropriate, they need to be changed to reflect the new environment in which the business is operating.

TRAIN

All pharmacy staff members should be trained and developed to achieve the organization's goals. It is important to remember that all staff members will require different plans based on their skills and seniority. Vital to the process is for staff members to be involved in the development and assessment of their individualized training plan, which is needed to achieve the team goal. Employees need to take ownership of their plan. The simple questions, "What needs to be taught?" "Who can train?" and "When do the training and development need to be done?" for each team member have to be answered.

BUILD RELATIONSHIPS

The pharmacist's role as the coach is to spend time face to face with employees. This is the foundation upon which to build trust and respect, increase morale and ultimately enhance performance. Time spent together can include team meetings, one-on-one interactions and coaching sessions for groups. Coaching techniques may include the following:

- listening to staff members
- avoiding a rigid management style
- reiterating the goals
- communicating openly so all staff feel part of the team
- providing staff with updates and information on the development of the goal
- manage by walking around (MBWA)
- demonstrating confidence in an employee's abilities

At this point in the coaching process, it is imperative to realize that the staff will not always like the decisions made. To avoid confusion, a good coach will clearly communicate what decisions have been made and always ask for positive or constructive input about how to implement or improve them.

MOTIVATE

A coach's role is to explain to players the benefits of the goal and to provide reasons and outcomes that motivate them. The coach can create conditions that allow people to motivate themselves. It is important to use motivators, not manipulators. Manipulation creates "neutral people" and will not enhance performance. Following are some examples of motivators:

- Say, "Thank you." This simple phrase is a number one motivator. It is simple, easy to administer, but widely underused. People just need to feel their work is meaningful.
- Give recognition at a staff meeting or through any other type of communication.
- Focus on what people like to do best.

Rewards are another type of motivator that can be used to enhance performance. Money is not a sole motivation or reward because a manager can never give enough and it becomes an expectation. Effective rewards include the following:

- providing staff lunches on occasion
- outside events and activities
- notes of recognition visible to staff and perhaps customers

- team rewards
- incentive programs that may include discounts, free goods, days off

Rewards should be awarded close in time to when the goal was achieved or the behaviour occurred. The pharmacist should be specific about why the reward was given and make sure that, in fact, there are a multitude of opportunities to be rewarded.

MONITOR PERFORMANCE

Do not allow people to operate in a void. It is important to pay attention to their performance and look for ways to help. Do not wait for a crisis. Offer support on an ongoing basis as part of the coaching process. Always ask the question, "Where does what they do fit into the big picture of the pharmacy operation?"

PROVIDE FEEDBACK

Update staff with the status of the goal and what needs to be finalized to make the goal a reality. Provide feedback as to thoughts and ideas on where to go from here. Listen carefully to their objections and ideas on the plan. This is part of the process of team building and establishing trust. Any change that is needed should be introduced slowly using common sense and communication. The goal as the coach during the feedback sessions is to develop winning attitude, therefore building staff morale. Developing a winning attitude includes the following:
- promoting employee satisfaction and growth within the pharmacy
- preparing employees to meet pharmacy challenges
- demonstrating confidence in their new abilities
- rewarding excellent performance as part of the enhancement of performance and performance management[3]

Wage administration is also an important component and result of effective performance management. Good performance should be rewarded with a fair increase in wages. Wage administration is simply defined as the "administrative procedure of establishing wage levels and operations in an organization."[4]

Pharmacy owners and managers have the responsibility to remunerate individuals for the value they offer relative to their responsibilities. The employee's level of responsibility, job description and how the individual performs those functions would dictate the wage. A wage rate is usually set at entry level for the role and is determined by market competitiveness, as well as part-time versus full-time employment. Generally speaking, employees performing similar job descriptions and responsibilities would receive comparable wages. For example, it would be expected that pharmacy technicians would receive similar wages unless there is a top performer or a weak performer who could then possibly receive more or less dependent on performance. At the same time, cashiers would be expected to receive less in their wage package as compared to pharmacy technicians due to the differences in job descriptions, responsibilities, technical expertise and level of training. One exception is that pharmacies operating in a unionized environment receive similar wages that are classified by job class, job description and/or seniority (see Chapter 36: Managing in a Unionized Environment).

A starting point for wage administration implementation is to create a wage grid listing all the job descriptions of the pharmacy operation and reviewing where the present wages of individuals with similar job descriptions are within the grid. The resulting wage grid will identify each job description and wage range within each job description as well as a time-based wage, which would include a starting wage, a three-month wage and a one-year mark, two-year mark, etc. This wage grid now becomes the focal point for wage administration.

For example, a pharmacy operation may have four pharmacy technicians and an hourly wage range of $16 to $22. Initially, variations in wages could be due to seniority of employees. This variance may disappear with time as long-term employees at the top of the wage range will most likely receive a cost of living increase, whereas individuals at the bottom or middle of the range may receive a higher increase in wages based on their performance to move these employees further up the wage grid.

Many factors determine wage increases and administration, including the following:
- direct competition and marketplace wages
- cost of living estimates
- budget allowances for wages
- financial performance of the pharmacy
- provincial/territorial minimum wage grids

Wage increases are generally reviewed once per year for seasoned employees and more often for new employees as they advance. Wage increases are calculated and expressed as a percentage increase. For example, a wage increase of 3% could be administered by providing all employees with a 3% increase, or a selection of employees at 3%, some employees at 2%, and perhaps some individuals at 1%.

Bonuses, benefits and other incentives such as a parking pass can also be part of the administration of wages and will vary by pharmacy.

A wage review may be part of a performance review, but wage reviews and performance reviews do not have to be done at the same time. In fact, performance reviews separate from wage reviews are more effective as the employee is not worrying or thinking about the wage review but concentrating, listening and participating in the performance review process. If a wage review is part of a performance review, it is important to realize that a message is being sent. The wage increase should be consistent and a confirmation of the overall evaluation of an employee's performance. Be prepared to support the evaluation as part of the journey to effective performance management.

ACKNOWLEDGEMENTS

The author would like to thank countless people from Big V Pharmacies for their contributions and additions to the "Coaching as a mindset" concept over the years. The coaching concept originated many years ago under the title of "Manager as a Coach" and at that time, was primarily the work of Big V's Human Resources Manager, Dave Town. During that time, many managers and directors at Big V had expanded on and used the concept for workshops and various meetings. Twenty years later, I am still adding, updating and using the framework of the program as a valuable human resources tool.

RESOURCES AND SUGGESTED READINGS

Lloyd KL. *Performance appraisals and phrases for dummies*, 2009.

Performance appraisal: expert solutions to everyday challenges. Harvard Business School Press, 2009.

Smart goals guide. Available: www.smart-goals-guide.com (accessed Nov. 15, 2014).

University of Rochester. Writing S.M.A.R.T. goals. Available: www.rochester.edu/working/hr/performancemgt/SMART_Goals.pdf (accessed Nov. 15, 2014).

Whitmore, J. Coaching for performance: growing human potential and purpose. Boston: Nicholas Brealey Publishing, 2009.

REFERENCES

1. Hancocks D. The human resources advisor. Concord, ON: First Reference; 1993–2005: Forms/Appendix.
2. Winn R. People skills: productive performance management. Canadian Healthcare Network. Mar. 1, 2013.
3. Winn R. Six steps to better staff morale. Canadian Healthcare Network. Nov. 1, 2011.
4. Barron's business dictionary. Available: www.answers.com/topic/wage-and-salary-administration (accessed June 10, 2014).

ABC Drugs Employee Performance Evaluation[1]

Employee: _____   Reviewer: _____

Store: _____   Date: _____   Date of last review: _____

	Excellent	Good	Needs improvement	Comments
Ability to work independently				
Appearance				
Attendance				
Communication skills				
Cooperation				
Customer service				
Creativity				
Dependability				
Enthusiasm				
Initiative				
Merchandising skills				
Productivity				
Professionalism				
Punctuality				
Technical skills				
Work quality				
Work consistency				
Working relations				
Other				

Overall performance:

_____

_____

Plans for maintaining or improving performance:

_____

_____

Employee comments:

_____

_____

Signature of employee: _____   Date: _____

Manager: _____   Date: _____

CHAPTER 35

Conflict Management and Progressive Discipline

R. Mark Dickson, *BSc(Pharm), MBA*

Learning Objectives

- Define conflict and be able to identify the causes of conflict.
- Discuss the role of the manager/owner in resolving conflict.
- Describe the general process for managing conflict.
- Explain the process of progressive discipline.

WHAT IS CONFLICT?

Simplistically, conflict can be defined as a disagreement of interests or ideas. More completely it is defined as follows:[1]

- competitive or opposing action of incompatibles: antagonistic state or action (as of divergent ideas, interests or persons)
- mental struggle resulting from incompatible or opposing needs, drives, wishes, or external or internal demands

Notice that the more complete definition contemplates the cause of conflict as incompatibility while also identifying internal as well as external aspects. For managers tasked with managing conflict, the more robust definition is helpful.

Conflict within an organization is inevitable. The impact of conflict on the business can be either positive or negative depending on how conflict is viewed and managed. Conflict channelled positively can result in open discussion, expanded perspective and accelerated change. Disruptive conflict in the workplace can range from tension between two or more employees to vocal or physical confrontation. This chapter discusses identifying and managing conflict internal to the business that is detrimental to operational success.

Internal conflict is a common cause of employee turnover and reduced productivity. Implementation of good human resources (HR) policies and, in particular, good communication with employees will ensure internal conflict is identified and resolved quickly. To manage conflict

Figure 35.1

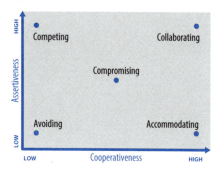

Thomas-Kilmann Conflict Mode[3]

effectively, it is necessary to understand the common causes of conflict. As well, understanding the common responses to conflict will make it easier to manage.

Conflict in the professional or business setting has predictable causes:[2]

- incomplete information most typically caused by poor communication
- different values or beliefs that are not understood or accepted
- competing or different interests that individuals champion
- limited resources and competition to obtain them
- interpersonal differences between individuals
- poor performance by one or more individuals that is not addressed

When faced with a conflict in the workplace, it is helpful to identify the underlying cause both to help defuse the situation and to identify potential constructive resolutions.

In addition to understanding the causes of conflict, it is also important to understand that everyone will respond differently to conflict. When faced with conflict, there are five primary responses that have been well described by the Thomas-Kilmann Conflict Mode: avoidance, collaboration, compromise, competition and accommodation.[3] These responses result from personal predispositions toward assertiveness and cooperation. Each employee will have an innate predisposition to his/her individual position (assertiveness) and to accommodation of the collective (cooperativeness). In any conflict situation, this predisposition will result in behaviours as noted in Figure 35.1.

The most constructive conflict resolutions are achieved through compromise or collaboration where the involved parties balance assertiveness and cooperation to achieve the outcome. Note that avoiding conflict altogether results from a dual lack of cooperation and assertiveness (apathy). Furthermore, in stressful situations (intensity), responses shift downward resulting in avoidance. Conflict, when correctly managed, results in positive solutions through compromise and collaboration.

MANAGING CONFLICT

Within any business, conflict will be a routine occurrence and resolution will normally be reached between the parties without management involvement. Ongoing or unbalanced conflict will require managers to actively intervene. Simply doing nothing or waiting for the conflict to resolve or dissipate on its own (avoidance) is almost never an effective option.

As a manager, it is important to be aware that conflict is a routine occurrence and to be ready for it. Where possible, anticipate situations that may escalate into conflict and minimize them through proactive communication or by making changes before the situation escalates. When conflict arises unexpectedly, it is always important to try to understand all sides of the issues and to initiate dialogue early by asking questions and listening carefully. Once the situation is clearly understood, assess potential options and decide on the best course of action. Seeking some assistance from a third party can be helpful, particularly if the issue is likely to involve the manager or if there is significant emotion involved.[4]

Every situation is slightly different and the intervention required to resolve conflicts will vary; however, the following considerations provide an effective process:[2]

1. Take time for emotions to cool, if necessary.
2. Address the issues in person (not by phone/email).
3. Confine discussion to the current situation.
4. Articulate the cause(s) of the conflict.
5. State why the conflict must be resolved.
6. Communicate how conflict is to be resolved.

Complete resolution of the conflict will typically require some time following an intervention. People will need time to understand and react to the information and resolution presented. Once some time has passed, it is important to reflect on the situation, confirm satisfactory resolution and re-address or adjust if necessary.

In summary, conflict is best identified, discussed and resolved early. Waiting or avoiding a conflict will delay resolution and fosters an unhealthy and unproductive work environment. Delay will typically result in escalation rather than resolution of the conflict.

PROGRESSIVE DISCIPLINE

Conflict arising from interpersonal differences or poor performance can be considered employee misconduct and must be resolved with specific employee intervention. These employees will require coaching and may require discipline to achieve conflict resolution. The formal process of increasingly severe consequences for dealing with issues of misconduct in the workplace is called progressive discipline.[5]

In the area of progressive discipline, avoiding the need for progression is the best possible outcome. The importance of having good HR practices along with written policies and procedures in place cannot be overstated. Clear communication and training on expectations, early informal counselling where needed and more formal coaching or training as required will resolve most situations. In fact, it is a good practice when faced with a potential disciplinary situation to ask these three questions:

- Have the expectations been clearly explained to the employee?
- Have the unmet expectations been pointed out to the employee?
- Has the employee been offered coaching or training to more fully meet the expectations?

If these three questions cannot be answered in the affirmative, then the problem is a communication or training issue and not a matter for progressive discipline at all.

Employee misconduct is the circumstance where an employee is fully aware of what is expected but is not willing or able to comply with the expectations. When considering employee misconduct, it is important to evaluate the seriousness and frequency of the problem, the employee's work history and the impact on the store. Where the misconduct is severe, immediate dismissal may be considered (e.g., theft or fraud). More typically, a process of progressive discipline is undertaken in an attempt to correct the situation and improve the productivity of the employee.[6]

Where progressive discipline is warranted, a formal process will be initiated. Labour laws set forth requirements for any discipline process of an employee by the employer. Corporate policies for stores owned by large chains and collective agreements, where present, will also set out requirements. Complete and accurate documentation throughout the process is essential to demonstrate full compliance with the policies and regulations (see Chapter 36: Managing in a Unionized Environment).

While the specifics vary somewhat, the general process for progressive discipline is as follows:[5]

- verbal warnings: In a timely manner, review the problem with the employee, giving the employee an opportunity to explain the situation from his/her perspective and to describe any mitigating circumstances. Provide the employee with clear instructions on the expectations for improvement. Also inform the employee of specific consequences of not improving and the expected time frame for the improvement. Document the date, expected improvement and time frame in the employee's file.

- written reprimand: Where a verbal warning or repeated warnings do not result in satisfactory resolution of the problem, then a written reprimand should be given. Discuss the problem with the employee in a timely manner and provide an opportunity for the employee to clarify, explain or mitigate. The employee should be provided with a written synopsis of the problem to review, including the required improvements and the time frame for improvement. The employee is required to sign and return a copy of the reprimand within a specific time frame. File the signed copy of the reprimand (or note on the copy that the employee refused to sign) in the employee's file. For serious policy infractions, particularly those involving potential litigation, employee safety or patient safety, a written reprimand may be required without first giving a verbal warning.

- suspension: If the problem has not been resolved within the specified time frame following a written reprimand, a suspension from work without pay may be considered. The process is the same as a written reprimand; however, the employee is sent home from work for a specified period without pay. The letter provided to the employee must clearly indicate the performance expectations, the specifics of the suspension and the future consequences if the performance expectations are not met (e.g., termination). Suspensions are typically only used in instances where there is a labour contract that specifically requires this step before termination.

- termination: Terminating an employee's employment requires a fair process, diligent documentation and considerable caution by the manager. Termination is a process that requires outside counsel from corporate resources, a lawyer or other labour relations specialist. Termination requirements are set out in provincial/territorial employment standards and will almost certainly be subject to review by an external party. Summary dismissal where an employee is terminated for severe misconduct such as theft or fraud is effective immediately and no payment in lieu of notice is provided. Termination for cause following a progressive discipline process will also be effective immediately; however, some payment in lieu of notice is commonly provided simply to avoid costly wrongful dismissal disputes. Payment of at least two weeks' salary or one week for every year of service will likely be required.

It is worth repeating that except in the case of severe misconduct such as theft or fraud, terminating an employee is an undesirable outcome. It is much better for the store to hire well and then develop productive employees through effective training and HR management. When problems arise with employees, they should be dealt with early and as fairly as possible. Where a termination is contemplated for ongoing misconduct, seek external advice early, document extensively and deal with the situation in a timely manner.

The ultimate goal in managing conflict within the business is to achieve timely resolution and ensure a productive work environment is preserved for all employees. As a manager, avoiding dealing with conflict is simply not a constructive option. Understanding the causes of conflict, typical employee responses to conflict and how to respond to and manage conflict in the workplace is essential for pharmacy managers. In the unfortunate situation where progressive discipline is required, early intervention is best. Carefully following a progressive process as described in this chapter will ensure a fair and effective outcome for the business and the employee.

REFERENCES

1. Conflict. Merriam-Webster Dictionary. Available: www.merriam-webster.com/dictionary/conflict (accessed April 16, 2014).
2. University of Colorado Boulder. Resolving workplace conflict. Available: https://hr.colorado.edu/fsap/healthtips/Pages/Resolving-Workplace-Conflict.aspx (accessed April 16, 2014).
3. Kilmann Diagnostics. An overview of the Thomas-Kilmann conflict mode instrument (TKI). Available: www.kilmanndiagnostics.com/overview-thomas-kilmann-conflict-mode-instrument-tki (accessed April 16, 2014).
4. Public Works and Government Services Canada. Eight steps to effective conflict management. Available: www.tpsgc-pwgsc.gc.ca/gcc-bdm/outils-tools-pg1-eng.html (accessed April 16, 2014).
5. HR Council. Keeping the right people. Available: http://hrcouncil.ca/hr-toolkit/keeping-people-discipline.cfm (accessed April 16, 2014).
6. Human Resources and Skills Development Canada. Labour: progressive discipline. www.labour.gc.ca/eng/standards_equity/st/pubs_st/pdf/discipline.pdf (accessed April 16, 2014).

CHAPTER 36

Managing in a Unionized Environment

Tracey Phillips, B.Sc.Phm, MBA; Owner, Westport Village Pharmacy

Mark Coulter, BA, MIR, CHRP; Director, Organizational Development & Talent Acquisition, Rexall

---

Learning Objectives

- Provide an overview of unionized workplaces in Canada.
- Understand why employees join unions and provide an overview of the collective bargaining process.
- Describe the typical provisions included in a collective agreement and how they are different from non-unionized workplaces.
- Describe how the provisions of a collective agreement apply to the management of the pharmacy environment.

Nearly 30%—4.3 million—of Canadian workers belong to unions.[1] While the figures from Statistics Canada suggest the labour movement in Canada is in a 30-year decline, the number of unionized workers has stabilized in recent years, which suggests that organized labour is surviving but not thriving.

Generations ago, unions typically arose in situations where employers were reluctant to establish basic workplace standards (e.g., lack of health and safety rules and regulations in industrial sectors). Today, however, due in large part to the strong influence of unions on standardizing and enhancing workplace conditions for employees, a lot of these issues have been addressed through the development of various federal and provincial/territorial acts, regulations and legislation (e.g., employment standards, human rights, health and safety and pay equity) that govern all employers and apply to all workplaces, whether unionized or not.

Given the diversity and channel blurring of the Canadian pharmacy industry today, it is reasonable to assume that pharmacy managers will one day come into contact with a unionized workforce. Most of the institutional-practice pharmacists in Canada are under collective agreements. Some pharmacies are part of a larger organization and may be only one of many departments that make up that business (e.g., grocery or mass merchants). In these instances, the pharmacy is bound by the same union agreements as the rest of the corporation.

The presence of a union can significantly impact the way in which an organization operates its business and manages its workforce. As such, it is important to understand how unions operate and the provisions contained within a collective agreement to effectively manage in a unionized environment.

WHAT IS A UNION?

A union is an organization that represents the interests of the employees in a particular plant, store, office or industry.[2] Once certified, the union participates in collective bargaining where they bargain with management to negotiate the terms and conditions of employment impacting the policies and procedures that govern these employees in the workplace.

WHAT IS THE DIFFERENCE BETWEEN NON-UNIONIZED AND UNIONIZED WORKPLACES?

Due to regulated employment standards in Canada, unionized and non-unionized workplaces within a particular sector operate very similarly. However, non-union workplaces maintain a unique advantage in that management has the flexibility to more quickly respond to both their business and staff needs without the need for consultation with, and approval from, their employees. They can define and change their employment policies impacting the workplace as deemed necessary and develop unique ways to successfully gather and incorporate employee feedback (e.g., employee committees). Within this environment, non-unionized employees could have little power to influence or change employment policies or broader business decisions that impact their working environment.

Unionized workplaces operate in an entirely different manner. In a unionized environment, the employer does not have the ability to change employment conditions at will. The collective agreement includes several clauses or provisions that have been negotiated and agreed to by both management and the union. The collective agreement defines the parameters governing how management decisions are made in the workplace and in this way, balances power with the employees.

WHY DO EMPLOYEES JOIN UNIONS?

Employees choose to be represented by a union for personal, social and/or economic reasons; however, the desire to be represented by a union is often rooted in the belief that improved wages and benefits, working conditions, job security and workplace policies (e.g., advancement, job transfer, promotion, issue resolution) will result. Some employees also join unions to seek protection from unfair management decisions impacting their workplace. In addition, unions who represent professionals may place equal emphasis on standards of practice, professional development, optimizing their scope of practice and enhancing their professional identity. Finally, some collective agreements contain specific language requiring all employees to join the union independent of their personal desires.

The primary purpose of the union is to engage in collective bargaining on behalf of its membership. Unions were built on the premise that employees acting as a group have more power at the bargaining table and can, therefore, achieve greater results than the individual employee can on his/her own. In other words, there is strength in numbers.

From a historical perspective, unions can be credited with the establishment of minimum employment legislation which has, in many instances, negated the need for employees to seek out third-party representation for the sole purpose of lobbying employers to implement basic workplace standards (i.e., health, safety, employment standards). As such, it is oftentimes real or perceived unfairness that leads employees to seek out union representation in hopes that the balance of power will be met or at the very least, positively influenced through union representation. Employees and unions alike believe that a sole bargaining agent will force the employer to change workplace policies for the good of the entire membership; however, in reality, this is not a foregone conclusion. Once a union has been certified to represent employees, the union and the employer will engage in a negotiation of an initial collective agreement in which existing workplace rules, policies and employment conditions may be negotiated. Unions may promise sweeping changes to working conditions and improvements to wages and benefits, but all issues need to be negotiated and agreed upon by both the new union and the employer before they can take effect in the workplace. That said, once a union has been certified, it can only guarantee three things to their membership:

- Employees will have to pay union dues.
- Employees will have the right to strike or be locked out by the company.
- Employees will have access to formal grievance (issue resolution) procedures.[3]

Collective agreement provisions need to be negotiated jointly by both union and management and as such, either party cannot guarantee the expected outcome before the bargaining process has been completed.

The collective bargaining process results in one agreement for all employees in a specified group. Consequently, individual employees are discouraged from going to management to receive a special arrangement, nor can the company make changes to an individual's pay, benefits or working conditions without first ensuring alignment with the contractual provisions outlined in the agreement.

WHAT IS COLLECTIVE BARGAINING?

A union has a legal right to bargain with management on behalf of the employees in an effort to negotiate a collective bargaining agreement. These agreements, otherwise known as contracts, outline the terms and provisions that govern the workplace for a defined period (term).

Unions have a legal and contractual obligation to fairly represent all employees in the bargaining unit. Notwithstanding this fact, it is important for managers and employees to understand that unions operate just like any other business. Their goal is to maintain and generate additional revenue through union dues paid by their members, while effectively controlling their expenses (e.g., office and administration expenses, strike pay, union negotiations, union drives and arbitrations).

Like all businesses, the union does not want to lose revenue in the form of decreased union dues associated with a decline in membership, nor does it wish its members to be dissatisfied with its services. Therefore, as with all forms of negotiation, management and employees need to agree to a contract that is mutually beneficial for both parties. For management to be successful, it needs to be able to control costs, enhance workplace flexibility and increase productivity, whereas union success is dependent on the degree to which the agreement addresses the specific concerns of its membership.

HOW DO ORGANIZATIONS PREPARE FOR THE COLLECTIVE BARGAINING PROCESS?

Large companies with unionized employees will typically have a corporate department that will prepare for and negotiate new or expired collective agreements. Smaller companies are more likely, and are well advised, to employ the services of a professional labour lawyer to act on behalf of the employer in preparing for and negotiating a collective agreement.

The collective bargaining process generally involves three steps: preparing for negotiations, collective bargaining negotiations and union ratification vote.

To start, the company and union develop their bargaining strategies, conduct background research and prepare their written proposals to share with the other party. The company would review its operational efficiency, examine its labour and benefit costs and prepare proposals that it believes will allow it to meet the needs of its business during the term of a proposed new agreement.

On the other hand, the union would gather information on concerns expressed by its members as well as economic data that might support increases in pay and/or benefits. Union and management then engage in collective bargaining discussions where they share their proposals and negotiate a proposed agreement that includes both non-monetary and monetary provisions and that addresses the unique needs of their stakeholders. Once a proposed agreement has been developed, the union communicates this agreement to their membership and the members have the opportunity to vote on it. A proposed collective agreement is ratified (accepted) if more than 50% of those voting vote in favour of ratifying the collective agreement.[2]

WHAT TERMS AND CONDITIONS ARE INCLUDED IN A COLLECTIVE AGREEMENT?

The terms and conditions in a collective agreement vary based on the unique circumstances of the employer, the industry at large and the specific nature of the union/management relationship. That being said, there are several common provisions, or articles, that are contained in collective agreements independent of the industry or sector.

RECOGNITION AND COVERAGE

This article specifies that the company officially recognize the union as the official bargaining agent of the employees who are covered by the terms of the collective agreement. The definition of the bargaining unit (i.e., the group of employees who are covered under the terms of the collective agreement) is also usually included in this provision. In cases where new employee groups are defined, for example in the case of the pharmacy technician classification, the definition of the bargaining unit set out in the recognition clause will determine whether the new classification is included or excluded from the union. This is certainly still up for negotiation with the union, but success will depend on the stringency of this clause and what other matters either side wishes to negotiate at the time.

It is important to note that certain employees are commonly excluded from the bargaining unit, such as supervisors, security personnel and employees who have access to confidential information pertaining to labour relations (e.g., human resources and payroll departments). Professional staff (e.g., pharmacists) may be either included, as in hospital unions, or excluded, as in retail unions, depending on the recognition clause.

MANAGEMENT RIGHTS

This clause outlines that the rights of management belong to the company, with exception of those outlined in the collective agreement. An example of a management rights clause is as follows:

> *Subject to the provisions of this Agreement, the management and operation of the business and the employment, direction, promotion, transfer, lay-off, and suspension, discharge, or other discipline of employees for just cause shall be vested solely in the Management of the Company.*[2]

In essence, despite the presence of the union, management still has the right to operate its business in an efficient, effective and profitable manner to meet the needs of their customers and stakeholders.

WAGES

This article sets out the rate of pay for each job in each year of the collective agreement. This clause may include the starting rate for each position and/or specific provisions relating to cost of living adjustments.

UNION SECURITY

Once a union has been certified as the sole bargaining agent for the employees, the company is required to collect monthly payments from its members on behalf of the union. These payments are called union dues and their automatic deduction from an employee's pay is called check-off of dues.[2] Union dues are collected from all employees independent of whether the employee signed a union card indicating a desire to be represented by that union.

OFFICERS AND STEWARDS OF THE UNION

A union steward is an unpaid official who represents the interests of union members in the relations with their immediate supervisors and other members of management.[4] Typically, union stewards are elected by union members to represent members within their department and deal with workplace issues affecting employees. The union provides a list of stewards to the company, and the company agrees to recognize these stewards and treat them the same as other employees.

GRIEVANCE PROCEDURE

When an employee believes that he/she is not being managed in accordance with the terms of the agreement, he/she has the right to file a grievance. A grievance is usually considered to be an alleged violation of the collective agreement.[5]

Every collective agreement contains a grievance procedure. The grievance procedure typically outlines how the grievance is to be filed, the number and timing associated with each step in the procedure and the representatives from each side who are involved in each step. The first step of the grievance process typically requires that the grievance be taken to the immediate supervisor for resolution. If the grievance is not resolved at that point, it may be appealed to one or more higher levels of management. In practice, a grievance meeting provides an opportunity to find a negotiated solution that is acceptable to both sides and not necessarily a judgment about which side is "right" and which side is "wrong."

While this is an impartial and formal way of dealing with issues stemming from the collective agreement, it is bureaucratic, expensive and time-consuming.

DISMISSAL OR SUSPENSION

This clause specifies that employees who believe they have been unjustly dismissed or suspended may have their case handled through the grievance procedure.

ARBITRATION

The arbitration article specifies that the company and union agree to settle any alleged violation of the agreement by arbitration.[5] Arbitration is the final stage of the grievance process and requires that a third-party arbitrator or arbitration board investigate a dispute between the employer and the union, and impose a settlement. The decision made by an arbitrator or arbitration board is final and legally binding on both the company and the union. This is an important process because it ensures that all disputes arising during the life of the collective agreement are resolved in a peaceful manner, without resorting to strikes or lockouts.[2]

SENIORITY

Seniority is usually defined in terms of accumulated service in a particular bargaining unit. Seniority may begin when a new employee has completed his/her probationary period (if applicable), and is typically retroactive to his/her start date. Seniority can also be lost if the employee quits, fails to return from leave or recall or has been laid off for a predefined period.

Seniority is often referenced in other collective agreement provisions impacting the workplace. More specifically, it is often used as the key criterion in decisions relating to the allocation of overtime, vacation preference, shift preference and layoffs and recalls.

STRIKES AND LOCKOUTS

Many collective agreements in Canada contain a no-strike clause in which management and unions agree that there will be no strikes or lockouts, otherwise known as work stoppages, during the life of the collective agreement.

Strikes

A strike is the temporary refusal of employees who are part of the bargaining unit to continue working for the employer. Strikes can be used by the union to exert pressure on the employer during contract negotiations due to concerns about wages, pensions, benefits, working conditions, job security, etc., or can result as a protest against unreasonable working conditions.[5]

A union's constitution will outline when and how a strike can happen; for example, a strike cannot happen unless the members vote, by secret ballot, to authorize the union to call a strike if necessary.

Lockouts

Another type of work stoppage that can occur in unionized environments is called a lockout. A lockout is a temporary refusal of a company to continue providing work for its employees.[5]

A lockout is an attempt to force unionized employees to accept the employer's settlement terms, or to try to force the union to make compromises in their current position.

Fortunately, for both parties, there are very few strikes or lockouts in Canada. In fact, more than 95% of all negotiations end in a settlement without a work stoppage. Of the work stoppages that do happen, most last only a short time.[1]

PROGRESSIVE DISCIPLINE

The goal of any organization, unionized or not, is to provide excellent service to its customers, drive operational efficiencies and maximize revenues. As a result, the use of disciplinary action is sometimes necessary to address employee behaviours that contravene established standards. More specifically, disciplinary action is often a required recourse to ensure that employees adhere to established performance standards, follow management direction, work in a safe fashion and maintain appropriate and consistent levels of behavioural conduct.

Although not always a part of every collective agreement, a common area of conflict is the application of the company's right to discipline and discharge. Most collective agreements allow the employer to develop reasonable rules and standards governing the conduct of its employees and to take disciplinary action to enforce these polices if they are contravened.[2] If discipline is not a specific clause of its own in the collective agreement, it will typically be referenced in the Management Rights clause. The union will hold the company to standards and processes in its application of discipline and discharge, which means that a well-thought-out and applied progressive discipline policy is best practice (see Chapter 35: Conflict Management and Progressive Discipline).

Even though employee discipline may be more complex in union environments, managers must hold union employees accountable or respect will be lost for the organizational leadership as a whole. Employees have the right to have a union representative attend and oftentimes speak on their behalf at any meetings involving the discussion or application of discipline. Union representatives may also conduct their own investigations into the allegations of employee wrongdoing or have access to management's investigation. It is important to note that although the company reserves the right to administer disciplinary action as they see fit, in a unionized environment, the employee has a right to file a grievance if he/she believes the disciplinary action taken was unjustified or unfair. Oftentimes, the union will file grievances in situations that involve the suspension or termination of employment.

HOURS OF WORK

Management of any business seeks to ensure that it provides services at the lowest possible cost. Since labour is one of an organization's largest costs, this expense needs to be appropriately managed at all times (see Chapter 32: Effective Management of Human Resources). In unionized work environments, pharmacy managers will need to be intimately familiar with this clause to apply it fairly and consistently.

Most collective agreements contain language that specifies the number of daily and weekly hours employees are expected to work, the start and end times of their shifts, the typical work week, the length of lunch and break periods and, in some cases, the minimum number of days or hours an employee must be available to work. The objective of the company is to ensure it has the requisite number of employees at the required times to maximize productivity, efficiency and quality, while ensuring that customer service targets are achieved. This clause, as well as other non-monetary clauses, is often discussed during collective bargaining negotiations.

One of the ways that organizations have reduced their labour costs is to supplement their full-time workforce with part-time employees who typically have lower wage rates and flexible work hours. The use of part-time employees can reduce the amount of overtime hours that are provided to full-time employees (at a higher wage premium), thereby reducing the company's overall labour expense. In a unionized environment, the collective agreement may contain language on how and to what extent this rebalancing of the workforce may be done.

WORK RULES

Management has regarded speed of work completion, quantity of work, the organization of work tasks and the number of workers who are scheduled within the scope of their decision-making authority. Recently, unions and employees have been trying to make inroads by influencing language that allows more control over decisions impacting their work environment. One example of this occurs when unions restrict the assignment of workers to perform jobs within their classification or prohibit supervisors or employees outside the bargaining unit from performing work within a job classification. For example, a pharmacy manager may not be permitted to ask a cashier from the front shop to help out in the dispensary if this is not considered work within the cashier job classification, despite the fact the person may have the skill set to do so.

TRANSFERS AND PROMOTIONS

Seniority commonly influences the way in which hiring decisions are managed in unionized workplaces. As a general rule, unions prefer the principle of seniority (or length of service) as one of, or the only, criterion in determining job transfers and promotions. This philosophy is based on the premise that long-serving employees should receive preferential treatment in hiring decisions and should also have more protection from layoffs. Management, on the other hand, prefers to maintain control over hiring decisions and select the best person for the job based on skills, knowledge and abilities in relation with the job specifications.

In approximately two-thirds of collective agreements, promotion decisions must take into account some element of seniority.[6] Although a small number of collective agreements contain provisions that include seniority as the sole criteria in hiring decisions, the majority have language pertaining to the use of seniority as one factor (along with skills and qualifications), or the deciding factor if all other factors (skills and qualifications) are considered equal across applicants.

As an example, a pharmacy assistant is working in a pharmacy chain with multiple locations and a vacancy arises in a particular location for a position in the person's specific job classification. The position must first be posted internally so that those interested could apply. The position would then be offered to the most senior qualified person within that particular job classification. This is good succession planning in any organization but is mandatory in a unionized environment.

LAYOFFS AND RECALLS

This article outlines the order of employees who will be laid off in the event that it becomes necessary for the company to reduce the workforce. Seniority often plays a major role in layoffs, and employees who have the least seniority are typically laid off first.

The opposite is true when employees are recalled back to work following a layoff. More specifically, employees who have the most seniority are often recalled first, as long as the senior employee has the necessary qualifications to perform the work formerly done by the junior employee.

OTHER ITEMS OF NOTE

Depending on the specifics of the workplace, the nature of the business or the current political or economic environment, other items of importance to either management or the union might find their way into (or out of) the collective agreement following negotiations. Items such as managed drug plans, sick benefits, eligibility for short- or long-term disability, wage or pension claw backs, and/or attendance policy provisions (to name a few) may be negotiated or renegotiated based on the specific needs of management or the union. It is incumbent upon the pharmacy manager to be aware of all changes to collective agreement language to provide proper guidance to employees and to make fair, consistent and cost-effective decisions.

Although a unionized environment presents some unique challenges for management, it is not an impediment to effectively running a business. In fact, maintaining a good working relationship with union leadership and membership will ensure that managers maintain a productive, engaged workforce who is driven to achieve expected sales, service and revenue targets. The key is to understand the fundamentals of the collective agreement under which everyone is bound, and continuously improve it where necessary, to meet the evolving needs of the business and its employees.

REFERENCES

1. UFCW Canada. Facts about unions. Unions in Canada. What about strikes and lockouts? Available: www.ufcw.ca/index.php?option=com_content&view=article&id=29&Itemid=49&lang=en#link1 (accessed April 1, 2014).
2. Kehoe F, Archer M. *Canadian industrial relations.* 8th ed. Oakville: Twentieth Century Labour Productions, 1996.
3. Field LM. *Unions are not inevitable.* 4th ed. Waterloo: Brock Learning Resources; 2000. p. 27.
4. Belcourt M, Sherman A, Bohlander G, Snell S. *Managing human resources.* 2nd Canadian ed. Scarborough, ON: Internal Thomson Publishing; 1999 p. 566.
5. Kehoe F, Archer M. *Canadian industrial relations.* 11th ed. Oakville: Twentieth Century Labour Productions, 2005.
6. Gunderson M, Ponak A, Taras DG. *Union management relations in Canada.* 5th ed. Toronto: Pearson Addison Wesley; 2005. p. 321.

CHAPTER 37

Legal Considerations in Employment and Labour Law

P.A. Neena Gupta, *B.A. (Hons.), LL.B., LL.M.; Partner, Gowling Lafleur Henderson LLP*

Roger Tam, *B.Sc.Phm., LL.B., R.Ph.; Vice-President, Legal, Hoffmann-La Roche Ltd.*

Learning Objectives

- Describe the different employment and labour legislation impacting the employer-employee relationship.
- Describe how to operate a pharmacy while abiding by all applicable employment and labour legislation.
- Identify employment contracts and what they should include.
- Explain how to manage difficult employee situations such as terminations while abiding with the legislation.

Canada has approximately 33,000 licensed pharmacists, with 24,000 working in 8,600 community pharmacies and 5,600 working in hospitals.[1]

Like all workplaces in Canada, pharmacies are subject to a myriad of employment laws and regulations. Each province and territory regulates employment. In addition, the federal government has its own set of labour and employment legislation. The first step is to determine which set of laws and regulations apply. It is necessary to review the applicable legislation and case law on a regular basis, as the law changes frequently.

Most pharmacies are subject to the laws of the province in which they are regulated. Therefore, this chapter focuses primarily on the provincial laws applicable to most community and hospital pharmacies. Provincial laws are substantially similar across the country, but minor variations regarding minimum wage and hours, vacation entitlements, entitlements upon termination and basic health and safety add complexity to managing a workforce in Canada. If a pharmacy operates under federal jurisdiction (e.g., a military or Veterans Affairs-operated pharmacy or a pharmacy operating in a territory), it will be subject to federal laws, which have some unique aspects discussed below.[2]

The discussion that follows assumes that the employer is not unionized, as there are very different requirements imposed on the employer once a union and a collective agreement are in place (see Chapter 36: Managing in a Unionized Environment). In many cases, the collective agreement imposes its own regime that supersedes the statutory regimes discussed in this chapter.

LEGISLATION GOVERNING THE EMPLOYMENT RELATIONSHIP

Legislation governs specific aspects of the employment relationship in all Canadian jurisdictions. Employment standards, human rights codes, employment equity and employee safety are all discussed in turn below. You should recognize that health and safety are strictly regulated (see Chapter 24: Safety and Security in Pharmacy).

Although the employer and employee often enter into written employment agreements, contract terms that are inconsistent with the minimum statutory requirements will not be enforced.

Finally, in almost all cases, it is illegal to punish an employee for exercising his/her statutory rights. Such conduct is called reprisal and can lead to severe monetary penalties and fines.

EMPLOYMENT STANDARDS

All jurisdictions provide minimum standards with respect to the minimum terms of employment. Typically, employees are not permitted to contract out of the minimum protections afforded by the statute. The specific provisions vary by jurisdiction and change from time to time, but can be easily verified by checking governmental Internet resources or calling the appropriate department's information line.

Employment standards can be quite complex and the legislation can often be varied by obscure regulations that apply to specific industries. It is important to note that pharmacies employ many types of employees, including pharmacists, pharmacy technicians, retail, warehouse and, on occasion, repair and maintenance staff. In each province, different types of employees are treated differently and have different protections under the legislation.

Pharmacists, as regulated health care professionals, are sometimes exempt from the legislative minimum standards. Even in jurisdictions where pharmacists are not specifically exempted from certain types of legislative protections, pharmacists who act as managers are exempt from many of the minimum protections stipulated by law because of their status as a manager.

Furthermore, there are often methods to obtain special permits for exemptions to the minimum requirements by applying to the appropriate ministry or department.

While it is impossible to cover the statutory requirements in detail,[3] it should be noted that legislation in each province typically covers the following.

Hours of work

Statutes will typically provide for maximum hours per day and per week, as well as mandatory intervals between shifts. There are often methods for obtaining exemptions to these rules by applying to the relevant authority.

Overtime pay

The legislation will typically set a threshold of hours per week beyond which employees will be entitled to overtime. The threshold varies across the country but typically ranges between 40 to 44 hours per week. The legislation often establishes methods to average overtime over a longer period to permit different types of scheduling. Time off in lieu of overtime pay at the employee's request is generally permitted, but may require the employee's express written consent.

Public or statutory holidays

Canadians generally enjoy at least eight public holidays: New Year's Day, Good Friday, Victoria Day (last Monday before May 25), Canada Day (July 1), Labour Day (first Monday in September), Thanksgiving Day (second Monday in October), Christmas Day and Boxing Day (December 26).

The first Monday in August is often observed as an additional holiday in many provinces. In certain parts of Canada, the third Monday in February is observed as an additional holiday. Remembrance Day (November 11) is a holiday that is observed by all provinces except Ontario, Québec and Manitoba. In Québec, according to the National Holiday Act, employees are also entitled to a paid holiday on St. Jean Baptiste Day (officially known as Fête nationale du Québec), which is June 24. Businesses are typically required to be closed on statutory holidays, although many exemptions exist. Employers usually have to pay a significant premium to employees who work on a statutory holiday. Because of the importance of pharmacies, there are often exemptions to the closure requirement, but there still may be a requirement to pay a significant premium to employees who work on holidays or the need to provide time off in lieu of the statutory holiday.

Vacation

Employment standards laws generally prescribe minimum vacation entitlements. The minimum vacation entitlement is typically two to three weeks per year, depending on the province. The employer may determine when employees take vacation. In certain provinces, vacation entitlements increase after a predetermined number of years of service.

Pregnancy leave

Most pregnant employees are entitled to 17 to 18 weeks of unpaid leave, depending on the jurisdiction. An employer cannot force or require an employee to go on pregnancy leave early.

Parental leave

New parents and adoptive parents are entitled to take parental leave of approximately 32 to 37 weeks, depending on the jurisdiction. At the end of the pregnancy and/or parental leave, an employee is entitled to be reinstated. The rules regarding the nature of reinstatement differ slightly across jurisdictions. In Ontario, for example, the requirement is to reinstate to the same job if it still exists or to a comparable job if it no longer exists. In Québec, the father of a child is entitled to take a paternal leave benefit, which can only be used by a biological father upon the birth of a child. This is in addition to parental benefits, which can be taken by either parent.

Emergency leave/bereavement

Most jurisdictions permit employees to take a certain number of unpaid days off for personal reasons. Each jurisdiction deals with this issue slightly differently. In some cases, leave due to the death of a family member is dealt with under a specific bereavement leave section, while in other jurisdictions the statute establishes several reasons why an employee can take a limited number of days off without pay. These reasons include the death of a family member, but can also include the illness of the employee or immediate family members, accidents, a household crisis or unexpected interruptions in childcare plans.

Family medical leave/compassionate care leave/critically ill child/family caregiver

Employees who need time off to take care of a seriously ill or dying relative are entitled to leave without pay ranging from 8 to 12 weeks, depending on the jurisdiction. Employees may be entitled to benefits under the Employment Insurance Act during this period.

Military/reservist leave

All jurisdictions provide job-protected leave for members of the reserve forces who are called into active duty or are required to participate in reservist training.

Sick leave/organ donor leave

Depending on the jurisdiction, there may be specific protection granted to employees who need to take time off due to illness. In Manitoba, Québec and Ontario, special protection is granted to employees who need time off to donate an organ.

Jury duty

All jurisdictions provide job protection to enable an employee to serve on a jury. In addition, many jurisdictions will fine an employer significant amounts for not permitting an employee to serve on a jury. Jury duty leave is unpaid, although some of the courts will provide a small stipend to the juror. If an employer chooses to pay the employee, it can ask to be repaid the stipend.

Equal pay for equal work

Canadian employers are prohibited from differentiating between male and female employees who perform substantially the same kind of work in the same establishment, requiring substantially the same skill, effort and responsibility. In such circumstances, different rates of pay are prohibited, except where differences are attributable to a seniority system, a merit system, a system that measures earnings by quantity or quality of production or a differential based on any factor other than sex. The courts and tribunals have established that titles are not determinative and that careful regard should be paid to the actual duties.

Pay equity

Québec, Ontario and federally regulated employers are subject to pay-equity obligations. The scope of obligations differs with the size of the workforce. The legislation is an effort to redress the gender gap in compensation. In essence, it seeks to ensure that there is equal pay for work of equal value. It requires employers to analyze jobs across their organization, review them for value (based on several statutory criteria) and examine whether there are compensation disparities between male-dominated and female-dominated jobs within the organization. This is a complex piece of legislation, and often compensation experts are retained to review the employer's workforce. Where female jobs are underpaid, the legislation prescribes a schedule for pay increments that have to be implemented to redress the balance. Although other jurisdictions have similar legislation, the scope is limited to the public sector.

Benefit plans

Employers are not required to provide employee benefit plans. Spousal plans must cover both common-law and same-sex spouses.

HUMAN RIGHTS

Human rights codes across Canada prohibit discriminatory practices with respect to employment. Generally, these codes provide that every person has a right to equal treatment with respect to employment without discrimination based on race, ancestry, place of origin, colour, ethnic origin, citizenship, creed, sex, sexual orientation, age, record of offences (e.g., a conviction for which a pardon has been granted), marital status, same-sex partnership status, family status or disability. Discrimination on the basis of pregnancy is defined as discrimination on the basis of sex. It should be noted that gender identity/gender expression is a protected ground in several jurisdictions, including Ontario, Nova Scotia, Manitoba and the Northwest Territories.

Employees also have a right to freedom from harassment due to any of the foregoing prohibited grounds in the workplace by the employer, an agent of the employer or by another employee.

At one time, mandatory-retirement policies were very common across Canada. However, mandatory retirement is increasingly treated as a form of age-related discrimination unless the employer can establish a bona fide occupational reason why an employee must retire at a certain age as opposed to undergoing individualized fitness or aptitude tests. There is no legislated mandatory-retirement age. In large part, however, pensions are structured around a presumed retirement date of age 65.

Employers are expected to be vigilant about any allegations of discrimination or harassment. Where there are reasonable grounds to believe a concern exists, employers are expected to investigate fairly, promptly and competently. Depending on the results of the investigation, employers are required to implement appropriate remedial and corrective measures.

Employers should also be aware of the "duty to accommodate." This duty is triggered when a job requirement may end up adversely affecting an employee based on a protected ground. An employee with a disability may not be able to perform all the normal job duties. Careful consideration will have to be given to whether the job can be modified so the employee can perform the essential duties of the position.

While accommodation is a collaborative process, with the employee being required to provide information and consider reasonable accommodation methods, ultimately there is a heavy onus on the employer to originate a solution unless it constitutes undue hardship. The employer should document the accommodation discussions and process to avoid litigation.

EMPLOYMENT EQUITY

The federal Employment Equity Act applies to all federally regulated employers who employ 100 or more people. The Federal Contractors Program applies to suppliers of goods and services to the federal government that have 100 or more employees and are bidding on contracts worth $200,000 or more. It imposes on such private-sector employers obligations to implement employment equity in the workplace. Federal contractors can be audited for compliance and, where the results are unsatisfactory, given a specific time period for remedying any gaps. Québec has also instituted the Québec Contractors Program, which is designed to promote the employment of women, visible and ethnic minorities and Aboriginal peoples.

Most pharmacies will not be impacted by the Employment Equity Act unless the pharmacy is part of a large federal institution, such as a federal penitentiary or hospital, or is a large supplier to a federal department.

OCCUPATIONAL HEALTH AND SAFETY

All jurisdictions regulate workplace health and safety in Canada to ensure employers provide a safe work environment. There are stringent rules requiring the posting of safety legislation, the existence and updating of written policies, the establishment of workplace safety committees, safety training, the use of personal protective equipment and the handling of hazardous materials. Employers, supervisors and workers all share obligations to maintain a safe workplace. It should be noted that a failure to maintain a safe workplace can lead to both civil and criminal consequences.

Many jurisdictions in Canada have tried to deal with workplace violence in a proactive manner. In addition, Ontario also imposes specific obligations on employers to be mindful of the possible impact of domestic violence on workers and the workplace. Employers in Canada, depending on the legislative framework, may have obligations to conduct risk assessments, institute and update policies, train employees and introduce physical and electronic safety measures that help protect the workforce from workplace or domestic violence in the workplace. Where there are reports of workplace violence, employers generally have a duty to conduct a prompt, fair and competent investigation. Furthermore, in Ontario, where there are reasonable grounds to believe that an employee is at risk due to domestic violence, such as stalking by a domestic partner, the employer has an obligation to take active steps to help prevent the employee from becoming a victim.

Québec was the first North American jurisdiction to outlaw psychological harassment in the workplace. The province of Saskatchewan has followed suit. In general, the laws aim to prevent egregious bullying in the workplace and do not protect against the normal psychological stresses in the workplace, such as difficult conversations about performance. Employers in Québec and Saskatchewan have specific obligations with respect to the prevention of psychological harassment in the workplace.

Ontario and several other provinces have enacted specific provisions regarding workplace bullying and harassment in its Occupational Health and Safety legislation. Employers have a specific obligation to have anti-harassment policies, train their employees about the law and investigate allegations of workplace harassment.

Recently, an Ontario employer was required to pay in excess of $400,000 due to workplace bullying/harassment that was not linked to traditional human rights grounds, but rather reflected an egregious example of abuse of supervisory power.

Under the Canadian Criminal Code, directors and executives may face criminal prosecution for negligence that leads to serious injury or death. Under the various occupational health and safety laws across the country, there are significant fines and penalties if an employer fails to comply with applicable legislation. Fines can be as high as $500,000 where death or serious injury occurs, and fines in the range of $100,000 to $150,000 are quite common. Recently, a public school board was fined $275,000 for violation of Ontario's Occupational Health and Safety Act that resulted in the death of a student. An Ontario company was fined $750,000 (plus victim surcharge) for the death of four employees when a scaffold broke and workers did not have proper lifelines. Fines are separately assessed against the corporate entity as well as supervisory employees who were derelict in their duty.

WORKERS' COMPENSATION

Workers' compensation is a system of disability benefits payable to a worker who is injured on the job or while performing job duties. The scheme is intended to relieve the injured worker of the delay, cost and difficulty of suing an employer in a civil action for negligence in the workplace. Compensation is to be provided expeditiously and without proof of fault. In turn, employers are required to fund the system through payroll assessments but are shielded from the risk of lawsuits and damages from employees injured on the job.

In practice, the Canadian schemes operate by having assessments levied upon employers, which are then gathered into a common fund from which benefits are paid to workers who are disabled as a result of workplace injuries or disease. Administration and adjudication are carried out by a statutory corporation known in most provinces as the Workers' Compensation Board, but known as the Workplace Safety Insurance Board in Ontario and the Commission de la santé et de la sécurité du travail in Québec.

Under these programs, injured workers are entitled to income replacement if the injury results in an inability to work. In addition, benefits will cover health care needs arising from the injury, such as prescription drugs, assistive devices and therapy. Workers may also be entitled to a lump-sum amount if the injury results in a permanent impairment.

The legislation also generally requires an employer to re-employ a worker injured on the job either to the pre-injury position or to other suitable employment. This obligation is intended to reduce the accident costs arising from workers' compensation claims as well as to encourage reintegration of injured but rehabilitated workers into the workplace. Where reintegration into the former workplace is not feasible due to the nature of the injury, an employee may also qualify for job retraining.

PAPERWORK – RECORD KEEPING, TAXES, DEDUCTIONS AND REMITTANCES

All employers must ensure that employees' pay is calculated and paid properly. Each jurisdiction has stringent requirements regarding record keeping and information that must be given to each employee on each payday with respect to the calculation of pay and deductions taken from pay. Pay records may be kept electronically.

On a regular basis, the frequency of which is determined by the size of the payroll, employers must remit taxes to the Government of Canada and in Québec, to the Government of Québec. Remittances include income tax installments, Canada (or Québec) Pension Plan, Employment Insurance, workers' compensation and employer health remittances. Records should be kept for 10 years.

THE CONTRACTUAL NATURE OF THE EMPLOYMENT RELATIONSHIPS

Despite the enormous amount of legislative intervention in the area of employment, the relationship of employer and employee is fundamentally one of contract. Parties either explicitly or impliedly agree to an employment relationship. The basic relationship is that the employee attends work and the employer pays an agreed-upon amount. The parties cannot agree to terms that violate the minimum legislative protections outlined previously. Where there is no written contract, a judge will rely on common-law principles to impose a contract on the parties.

In the absence of written contractual terms, the courts will imply a host of contractual obligations on both parties. The general law of contracts (such as offer and acceptance, duress and frustration) also plays an important role in employment law.

While there are some narrow exceptions for certain industries and sectors, most employment contracts are assumed to be of indefinite duration and can only be terminated by specific events such as the following:

- resignation of the employee
- termination *for just cause*
- termination *without* cause
- death
- frustration of the employment relationship

Certain employees governed by federal, Québec and Nova Scotia laws enjoy significant protection against termination without cause not afforded to employees in other jurisdictions. These protections are outlined later in this section.

Limited-term contracts are expected to be the exception to the norm and need to be established on the evidence. The best evidence is, of course, a written agreement. However, the courts have deduced the existence of a term contract from the parties' conduct, job titles and/or the wording in a job posting. Term contracts come to an end at a predetermined point in time or in some cases, when a specific event or milestone is reached. Subject to certain statutory requirements, limited notice or other formalities are required upon the end of a term contract. Nonetheless, great care should be taken in drafting offers of employment for term employment. Many term arrangements morph into contracts of indefinite employment because neither party has attended to the formal renewal terms.

Term employment relationships are appropriate for seasonal employment, maternity leave replacement contract or project work. These types of reasons, however, should be specified in the offer of term employment.

TERMINATION OF EMPLOYMENT – GENERAL

As previously stated, most employment relationships are considered to be of indefinite duration. In the private sector, there is no "at will" employment, except in the case where parties have agreed in writing to a limited probationary period at the commencement of employment. This probationary period usually is limited to three months, although in Manitoba the probationary period is limited to 30 days.

In most cases, to terminate employment without notice or compensation in lieu, the employer must prove *just cause*. Just cause means the employee has breached the employment contract (either written or implied) so seriously that a continuation of the employment relationship is no longer feasible.

TERMINATION WITHOUT CAUSE

In most cases, an employee who is terminated without cause is entitled to notice of termination or pay in lieu of notice. However, certain employees governed by federal, Québec or Nova Scotia laws have special protections against terminations without cause, of which employers need to be aware.

General

An employee's entitlement to notice is derived both from statute and the common law (i.e., "reasonable notice"). The applicable provincial and federal employment statutes prescribe *only* the minimum period of notice or payment in lieu of notice that must be given to a dismissed employee. It is a common and serious mistake to assume that the statutory minimums are the only obligations on the employer in the event of a termination without cause. Statutory minimums usually range from 1 to 8 weeks of notice. In Ontario, some employees are also entitled to an additional lump-sum payment known as "statutory severance," which ranges from 5 to 26 weeks of regular earnings. The severance obligation in Ontario is only triggered if the employer's annual total payroll is $2.5 million or more.

There may be separate and additional obligations in situations involving the termination of a group of employees, including the obligation to provide additional notice and the obligation to provide advance notice to a specific government department.

In the absence of a contractual stipulation to the contrary, judges will routinely imply an obligation on the employer to provide far more generous notice periods than prescribed by the statute. Factors that the courts have reviewed in determining what constitutes reasonable notice include the following:

- years of service
- seniority within the organization
- salary and other compensation
- employee's chances of employment upon termination
- employee's health
- employee's education
- promises of job security, even if not enforceable at law
- whether the employee was enticed from secure employment

There have been cases where employees with long-term service have been awarded 24 months of notice or compensation in lieu of notice. If the employee is successful in finding other employment, the earnings from mitigation will be deducted from any award otherwise payable by the employer, unless there is a contractual provision to the contrary. However, mitigation does not reduce the employer's obligation to provide the statutory minimum notice and, in Ontario, severance if applicable. An employee's failure to act reasonably in terms of mitigation can also reduce damages.

Provincially regulated employees outside Québec can contract out of the obligation to provide reasonable notice at law. However, the contract cannot and should not make any effort to contract out of the statutory minimum notice or severance. Where a contract does not comply with the minimum standards in the applicable statute, the offending provision will be considered void. The courts will not simply impose the minimum statutory notice required by the statute, but will order reasonable notice, which will no doubt be significantly greater than the notice period the employer intended.

Employers in Québec and Nova Scotia and federally regulated employers should be aware that there are significant additional protections given to employees who are facing termination.

TERMINATION WITH CAUSE

If an employer wishes to terminate an employee due to the employee's conduct without providing notice or compensation in lieu, the employer must establish just cause. This is a heavy onus to discharge in the courts and tribunals in Canada. Effectively, the employer must establish that the employee's conduct amounted to a repudiation of the employment contract. Examples of just cause include serious acts of dishonesty, gross misconduct such as violence or harassment, breach of the duty of confidentiality, persistent neglect of duties or gross insubordination.

Mere incompetence is not generally considered just cause, unless it can be shown that the employee is intentionally engaging in poor performance and has been previously warned that their performance must improve.

The onus on the employer is an extremely high one. Most employer-initiated terminations will be terminations without cause, where the employer will provide working notice or monetary compensation in lieu of notice. A lawyer should be contacted when a termination with cause is being contemplated by the employer.

RESIGNATION

Employees may resign their employment. While the law implies a duty to provide reasonable notice, there are very few cases where an employer has been able to obtain redress from the courts or tribunals due to inadequate notice. These cases usually involve highly placed executives or professionals and are often coupled with serious misconduct, such as theft of a corporate opportunity, flagrant solicitation of clients or misappropriation of employer trade secrets.

RESIGNATION BY EMPLOYEE DUE TO CONSTRUCTIVE DISMISSAL

In certain cases, employees may resign their employment on the basis that the employer has made unilateral and fundamental changes to the employment relationship. Examples of constructive dismissal include a significant reduction in pay, changes to the structure of compensation, a relocation outside the normal commuting area or a demotion in the corporate hierarchy (even if pay and job title are grandfathered). In some cases, employees have successfully argued that workplace harassment or discrimination constituted constructive dismissal. An employee who establishes constructive dismissal is able to sue for damages equivalent to the notice the employer would have had to pay upon termination of employment.

Employers contemplating significant changes to an employment relationship should implement strategies to avoid a claim of constructive dismissal, including providing advance notice of any changes. Written contracts of employment may also preserve an employer's right to implement certain types of changes that would otherwise be considered a constructive dismissal.

A WORD ABOUT CONTRACTS

The employment relationship is one of contract. If there is no written document, judges can effectively create a contract based on implied terms. Please note that in most provinces, an accepted offer letter will be treated as a written contract. If the offer is lacking certain terms, a judge will imply contractual terms. Almost invariably, these implied terms favour the employee. Therefore, it is important for managers to ensure they have properly worded contracts for all levels of employees. This avoids misunderstandings and can result in huge cost savings to employers, especially if an employee is being terminated without cause. Appendix B at the end of this chapter contains a checklist the authors use regarding what should be included in the employment contract. Only a few of these terms specifically deserve special mention.

"Consideration" (an exchange of value between the parties) is essential for any enforceable contract outside of Québec. In most cases, this means an employment contract will only be valid if it is entered into *before* the start of employment or before the effective date of a promotion or raise.

RESTRICTIVE COVENANTS

Employers often wish to implement post-termination restrictions on employees' business activities. These types of restrictions are called restrictive covenants. There are two kinds of restrictive covenants:

- non-competition clauses (e.g., Michael agrees not to work as a pharmacist in the City of Regina, Saskatchewan, for a period of 12 months after he leaves the employ of ABC Pharmacy)
- non-solicitation clauses (e.g., Michael agrees not to solicit any clients of ABC Pharmacy for the purpose of providing them pharmacy services for a period of 12 months after he leaves the employ of ABC Pharmacy)

Courts are very reluctant to enforce non-competition clauses. The general rule is that any restrictive covenant 1) must be limited to what is strictly necessary to protect the employer's legitimate interests; 2) must be reasonable; and 3) cannot be contrary to public policy.

In the case of pharmacists, courts will look at the public's interest in having access to a preferred pharmacist to ensure patient continuity of care or the need to ensure a sufficient number of pharmacists in a particular geographic area. In rare cases, courts will enforce a restrictive covenant with an injunction.

Legal advice should be obtained regarding the proper drafting of confidentiality, non-solicitation and non-competition clauses. There are different considerations if restrictive covenants are being negotiated in the context of the sale of a pharmacy business. These business types of considerations are outside of the scope of this chapter.

CONFIDENTIALITY

Even without a contract, the courts recognize the importance of employees keeping business and patient information strictly confidential. Having said that, it is useful to have a written policy or contract that emphasizes the seriousness of maintaining confidentiality at all times, defines the scope of confidentiality and outlines expectations regarding how confidential information is to be protected. Given recent examples of accidental breaches of confidentiality, managers should ensure there is robust training surrounding the issue of confidentiality.

TERMINATION CLAUSES

Almost all employment relationships come to an end. It is important to clarify the entitlements upon termination. An employer will want to stipulate how much notice the employee should give upon resignation. Subject to minimum statutory requirements, an employer will want to limit its exposure to large claims for notice or compensation in lieu of notice upon termination.

It is critical to get a skilled lawyer to draft and review any provisions regarding termination. Note that if the offer is silent as to termination provisions, a court has the right to determine what is fair and reasonable in the circumstances. Courts invariably favour employees in such cases.

A WORD ON MANAGING EMPLOYEES AND TERMINATIONS

In the non-unionized workplace, an employer has the right to terminate an employee at any time, subject to certain human rights and employment standards protections. The only issue will be whether the employer is obligated to provide working notice or compensation in lieu of working notice. If notice is required, the issue is how much notice.

Employers who have properly worded termination clauses will be able to terminate non-performing employees with greater ease and certainty, as the liability will often be limited by contract.

An employer should be aware that there are risks involved in terminating employees who could conceivably claim protection of human rights or employment standards legislation. For example, an employee who has just returned from pregnancy leave may claim that her termination is due to her pregnancy, even though the employer is terminating her for rudeness to customers. An employee with a disability may claim that the termination was related to his/her disability status, even when the real issue is a failure to attend work on a regular basis. These types of cases should be referred to an experienced lawyer before the decision is made to terminate the employee.

Employers should make a habit of treating issues consistently to avoid charges of favouritism or worse, illegal discrimination. Records should be kept of verbal warnings and any progressive discipline (see Chapter 35: Conflict Management and Progressive Discipline). Please note that where a pharmacist or pharmacy technician is being terminated, you may have obligations of reporting to the appropriate licensing body. Please check with your local licensing body regarding such reporting obligations (see Chapter 12: Professional Competence and Ethics).

POLICIES

All employers are required to have certain policies and procedures in writing. Each province requires certain information to be posted or made easily available to employees. Typically, the following information should be posted:
- basic information about employment standards
- basic information about health and safety
- first aid information
- policies regarding workplace harassment, workplace violence and discrimination

More detailed information should be made available to each employee. Most provinces have training requirements regarding harassment, violence and health and safety. It is highly recommended that employers have policies around basic expectations, including the following:
- attendance
- dress code
- vacation
- calling in sick/absences

The list of policies is endless and there are numerous resources available that provide excellent templates that can be modified to meet the needs of the specific pharmacy. Employees should be trained on the policies so there is no misunderstanding regarding management's expectations. It is good practice to have employees confirm in writing their receipt and understanding of important policies and to keep a copy of the signed acknowledgement in the employee's file.

Furthermore, management should be aware that employees have a right to complain about harassment, discrimination and unsafe work conditions. Management should be trained on its obligations when responding to such matters in the workplace, to avoid significant legal exposure, including regulatory penalties and fines.

Management also needs to understand the duty to accommodate and how it is implemented in the workplace. Management should also understand the duty to investigate complaints and how the investigation process works. It is often best to retain an experienced consultant or lawyer in these types of circumstances.

Good employees are a huge asset to any pharmacy. Nonetheless, pharmacists who manage a pharmacy will need to understand that the workplace is heavily regulated. It is important to consult with a good human resources and legal advisor to navigate the complex laws and regulations that govern employers and employees.

REFERENCES

1. Canadian Pharmacists Association. Pharmacists in Canada. Available: www.pharmacists.ca/index.cfm/pharmacy-in-canada/pharmacists-in-canada/ (accessed May 26, 2014).
2. For example, the Canada Labour Code and the federal Employment Equity Act.
3. See Appendix A for a helpful chart regarding what types of protection are provided to pharmacists and pharmacy technicians.

Appendix A: Employment Standards Coverage or Exemption With Respect to Pharmacists[1]

Province/Territory	Minimum Wage	Hours of Work	Daily Rest Periods	Time Off Between Shifts
Alberta Generally covered, unless managerial.	C	C	C	C
British Columbia Generally covered, unless managerial or executive.	C	C	C	C
Manitoba Pharmacists are exempt from some employment standards and covered by others.	E	E	E	E
New Brunswick Pharmacists are exempt from some employment standards and covered by others. Please note also that pharmacists are not entitled to the public holiday provisions of Employment Standards Act. NB Reg. 85-179, s. 3(1)(g).	C	C	C	C
Newfoundland and Labrador There are significant exemptions for pharmacists and their employees	E	E	E	E
Northwest Territories No exemption, unless managerial or executive.	C	C	C	C
Nova Scotia No exemption, unless managerial or executive.	C	C	C	C
Nunavut No exemption, unless managerial or executive.	C	C	C	C
Ontario There are significant exemptions or special rules for pharmacists.	E	E	E	E
Prince Edward Island No exemption, unless managerial or executive.	C	C	C	C
Quebec No exemption, unless managerial or executive.	C	C	C	C
Saskatchewan Generally covered, unless managerial. Note that pharmacists not entitled to overtime.	C	C	C	C
Yukon Generally covered unless managerial or executive.	C	C	C	C

Legend   C = Covered   **E** = Exempt   **SRA** = Special Rules Apply

1 The law is stated as of June 13, 2013.

Weekly Bi-weekly Rest Periods	Eating Periods	Overtime	Personal Emergency Leave	Paid Public Holidays	Vacation with Pay	Notice of Termination	Severance Pay
C	C	C	C	C	C	C	C
C	C	C	C	C	C	C	C
E	C	E	C	E	C	C	C
C	C	C	C	C	E	C	C
E	C	E	C	E	E	E	C
C	C	C	C	C	C	C	C
C	C	C	C	C	C	C	C
C	C	C	C	C	C	C	C
E	E	E	E	SRA	E	E	C
C	C	C	C	C	C	C	C
C	C	C	C	C	C	C	C
C	C	E	C	C	C	C	C
C	C	C	C	C	C	C	C

Appendix B: Employment Contract Checklist

❑ **Conditional or Firm Offer** – are there references, background checks, verification of credentials or proof of right to work in Canada issues?

❑ **Consideration**
- New employment
- Promotion
- Raise/Bonus

❑ **Term** (limited time period or task) or Indefinite? If term, what is the end of the term or project in question? _____

❑ **Scope of Position**
- Job title
- Reporting structure – does employer have right to delegate or change?
- Geographic location – does employer have right to shift/change?
- Scope of position – does employer have right to assign/re-assign duties?
- Executive, management, supervisory, front-line worker

❑ **Probation Clause** – yes or no ?

❑ **Compensation**
- Base
- Bonus
- Profit-sharing plan
- Commission
- Stock option
- Car allowance
- Pension/RRSP

❑ **Benefits** (eligibility for benefits)
- When employee becomes eligible
- Is there a medical qualification or exclusion of pre-existing conditions?
- Premium contributions
- Mandatory or not
- Conversion upon termination
- What happens upon termination?

❑ **Confidentiality Clause**
- Definition of confidentiality
- Prohibition on copying/use outside scope of employment
- Obligation to return confidential or proprietary materials

❑ **Termination of Employment**
- Notice of resignation
- Termination without cause – options include:
  - Statutory (employment standards) minimums
  - Fixed amount greater than statutory minimums
  - Sliding formula that builds on years of service
  - Requirement for mitigation
  - Claw back upon finding alternate employment (employee must always get more than employment standards)
  - Benefits upon termination

- Termination with cause
  - Common-law definition of cause
  - Any additional definition of cause required due to industry issues, e.g. loss of right to practise as pharmacist, regulatory misconduct
- Disability/Absenteeism (note human rights/duty to accommodate issues)
  - Death
  - Definition of compensation if compensation in lieu provided

❑ **Ownership of Intellectual Property**
- Patent
- Trademark
- Copyright
- Moral rights
- Cooperation after end of employment relationship

❑ **Non-Solicitation/Non-Deal/Non-Competition**
- Temporal limits/geographic scope
- Protecting clients
- Protecting prospective clients
- Protecting employees and independent contractors

❑ **Other Matters**
- Layoffs
- Policies
  - Conflict of interest
  - Harassment/workplace respect
  - Expenses

- Boilerplate clauses
  - Integration/excluding parole evidence
  - Stipulation as to court/forum/law
  - Severance of illegal provisions
  - Preserving minimum legislative requirements in lieu of contractual provisions
  - Independent legal advice or opportunity to obtain

IX. DEVELOPING, IMPLEMENTING AND MANAGING CLINICAL PHARMACY SERVICES

CHAPTER 38

Developing Patient Care Services

Alan Low, BSc.(Pharm.), PharmD., RPh, ACPR, FCSHP, CCD; Clinical Associate Professor, Faculty of Pharmaceutical Sciences, University of British Columbia, and Manager, Reimbursement and Medical Affairs, Servier Canada

Learning Objectives

- Develop a needs assessment for a new patient care service.
- Recognize the important factors in developing a successful patient care service.
- Describe a business model in the context of a new patient care service.
- Explain the key considerations in developing a patient care service.

PHARMACY PRACTICE IN TRANSITION

The practice of pharmacy has been in continuous evolution and transition. However, it was in 1990 that a major change in the philosophy of pharmacy practice was introduced with the term *pharmaceutical care*. It involved transitioning from a focus on products to one on patients.[1] Over the last several years, the rate at which the pharmacists' scope of practice is expanding in every jurisdiction in Canada has been rapid.[2,3] The expanding scope supports the pharmacist in more complex interventions in managing medication issues and fosters the delivery of innovative pharmacist-delivered services.

In recent years, competition over the dispensing of medications has increased dramatically and the profitability and costs of generic medications have been declining, reducing the revenue from dispensing medications. Technology, documentation systems and regulated technicians have streamlined dispensing to predominantly a technical function forcing the pharmacist to re-evaluate how best to utilize his/her expertise to help the patient while maintaining a viable and satisfying practice. It seems the natural next step is to develop services that are patient-centred rather than product-focused.

Patient care services is a phrase that has been used in many contexts; it represents many actions and processes performed by pharmacists. Patient care services is defined as *any patient-centred service that is delivered by a pharmacist with the intent to improve health outcomes*. These services incorporate clinical knowledge, expert clinical judgment and an understanding of patient needs and preferences in the delivery of care and education to a patient. Furthermore, the pharmacist has the opportunity to treat the patient as an individual and can exercise the pharmacist's full scope of practice to provide a high level of care and service with respect to optimizing drug therapy.

PHARMACY CLINICAL CARE SERVICES AND PROGRAMS

A systematic review of remunerated pharmacy clinical services reported on 60 programs being carried out by at least three pharmacies receiving reimbursement from government or private payers throughout the world: Canada, the United States, Europe, Australia and New Zealand.[4] Almost three-quarters of the remunerated clinical care services are paid for by government agencies and more than 60% are medication review services with or without a care plan. Other programs ranged in complexity from emergency contraception counselling to minor ailments schemes. This report did not cover services paid directly by patients. The average fee reported in North America for a medication review is $68.86 (converted to Canadian dollar equivalent; can be used as a consideration in the setting of patient care service fees).[4]

Shortly after the introduction of MedsCheck, the medication review program in Ontario, two province-wide demonstration projects were launched and completed in Canada: the Pharmacy Practice Models Initiative (PPMI) in Alberta and the British Columbia Medication Management Project (BCMMP).[5-8] These initiatives and projects allowed pharmacists to demonstrate their ability to provide a variety of medication management services using a patient-centred approach and were linked to remuneration for the services provided instead of dispensing medications. The patient consultations and follow-ups were aimed at identifying and resolving drug-related issues and supported patients to manage their medications. These demonstration projects also evaluated a reimbursement structure based on the Resource-Based Relative Value Scale (RBRVS) rather than the usual strict fee-for-service approach. The RBRVS approach to reimbursement was initially used in the United States to determine payment for physicians and derives the fee by measuring the relative resource cost to produce or deliver the service.[9]

These examples illustrate that pharmacists are capable of expanding their delivery of services that are not solely product-focused. In addition, it is worthwhile to spend time to research local and national services and programs to help gather information on successful approaches and techniques in developing a patient care service.

PATIENT CARE SERVICES

For patient care services to be delivered successfully, the service must be properly developed, planned, implemented and evaluated. This does not only refer to the service itself being provided, but also includes appropriate consideration of the financial viability to deliver the service in a sustainable manner (see Chapter 39: Planning Patient Care Services and Chapter 40: Implementing Patient Care Services).

Although therapeutic knowledge and its individualized application in patient care are very important, management and the business side of pharmacy are as important, if not more important, in the successful delivery and sustainability of services. For example, creating and developing an asthma service where the pharmacist consults with the patient to ensure optimal use, administration, management and understanding of the asthma medications may seem to be the perfect service to offer. However, this service may not generate sufficient revenue to cover the associated costs of delivering it if there is low utilization of this service or high expenses and interruptions in workflow leading to financial losses.

Even an excellent service could fail if the planning process misses a step and there is no assessment of whether there is a real need for this service in the particular location and patient population. The competition must be considered as well. The financial implications of generating forms, implementing processes and developing marketing materials, along with other costs of development and delivery, must be balanced against the fee to be collected. The revenue generated must make financial sense.

Section IX describes patient care services in the context of a community pharmacy practice; however, the same concepts can be applied within a hospital or other health care organization. Patient care services delivered in the hospital by a pharmacist may not be directly reimbursed, but there is flow of funds for the pharmacists' salaries that must be justified and derived from a budget. A service that is not meeting patient needs or does not address a significant issue will not drive value for the investment and the expense it causes. This will result in the discontinuation of the service even in a hospital that is unlikely to go out of business, but still must remain sustainable. The risk to a community pharmacy is more direct, particularly when large losses cannot be afforded.

NEEDS ASSESSMENT

One of the first steps in developing a patient care service is to conduct a needs assessment. The main purpose is to identify and define the target audience, identify and define the needs to which the service will cater and determine if there is a sufficient market (group of individuals who will want, seek and consume the service). The services that are created are more likely to be successful and sustainable if the services are not only needed by the target audience, but also perceived to be necessary. Therefore, assessing the need before creating a service is necessary. Creating and delivering a service based on the premise that it is easily or conveniently developed is unlikely to succeed. For example, building a patient care service around the interest of a staff pharmacist who is up to date on anticoagulation therapeutics and who enjoys working with patients with conditions requiring anticoagulation does not mean it is the best decision for the pharmacy. It would not be a successful undertaking if there is a lower-than-average prevalence of people requiring anticoagulation where the pharmacy is located or if the nearby hospital offers an outpatient anticoagulation service subsidized through the hospital's budget.

A needs assessment begins with defining the target audience. Whether it is carried out by accessing Internet resources that provide demographic information in the applicable neighbourhood or by conducting surveys in the neighbourhood and in the pharmacy, it is imperative to gather as much information as possible to help understand which consumers to target. This data can help identify the best therapeutic area to work in, determine the most suitable service components that the target audience appreciates and other important factors. Statistics Canada has a broad collection of demographic information about Canadians gathered through census reports, whereas local provincial/territorial statistics agencies may have demographical data down to the

Table 1. Needs Assessment – Methods to Collect Data

Patient surveys (e.g., customer suggestion box in pharmacy, targeted questionnaires and surveys, online surveys, mail-in/-out surveys)

Staff surveys (e.g., employee suggestion box in pharmacy, staff meetings)

Pharmacy management software/dispensing software reports (e.g., drug utilization reports, client demographic reports)

Street-corner surveys (e.g., three to five targeted survey questions to random people in the community)

Survey of businesses (e.g., 5 to 10 targeted survey questions to neighbouring businesses)

Interviews (one to one) with knowledgeable stakeholder representatives

Focus group discussions with stakeholders (e.g., group surveys or discussions with or without a facilitator)

Advisory boards of knowledgeable stakeholders to provide key information/questions

Literature search for primary and secondary research (e.g., study report on prevalence of improper inhaler administration)

Internet search for population demographics (e.g., local provincial/territorial statistics websites)

Internet search for treatment and disease-related data (e.g., CIHI)

Discussions with the following:
- National or local provincial/territorial pharmacy/professional advocacy organization
- Local Chamber of Commerce
- Local physicians and specialists
- Local paramedical team members
- Pharmaceutical or wholesale representatives

level of an individual neighbourhood or community, so it is beneficial to search the Internet for the provincial/territorial statistics website. In addition, the Canadian Institute for Health Information (CIHI) gives access to reports on health statistics, which can describe the prevalence of a disease, drug usage and prescribing trends, as well as the number of hospital visits for a particular disease and population. Many reports provide geographical breakdowns and population subgroups that can help group and identify wants and needs. There are many tools and methods that can be used to gather useful information about patient needs, problems and issues to help with decisions about how services can be best provided (see Table 1). It is also important to utilize resources that are right by the pharmacy's location, such as local business owners and health care providers in the neighbourhood, and network with individuals who are experienced and knowledgeable about patient needs and business models.

With so many perceived needs in health care, it may be a daunting task to identify where to even begin. To help define parameters, consider what the pharmacy and staff are capable of delivering in terms of services and therapeutic areas. These could be areas in which the pharmacist or staff have particular interest or expertise, which can be used to produce a short-list of areas where patient needs can be investigated further and better defined. A short-list of needs to focus on may also come from suggestions or discussions with new or existing clients of the pharmacy, especially if the clients express a need or a problem for which they have yet to find a solution or service. It makes the most sense to conduct some research and gather information in areas where there are perceived unmet needs that can link to the pharmacist's or the staff's capabilities, as well as the particular attributes of the pharmacy.

When considering financial viability and sustainability, the volume of service delivery episodes and economies of scale are two of the main drivers. Developing a service in therapeutic areas where there is an expected high volume of clients, with a reasonable amount of capital investment, human resources and a feasible reimbursement model/source, is likely to result in a sustainable if not profitable offering.

The following are fundamental questions that need to be addressed in a needs assessment:

- Who is the target audience or population (their location, demographics, behaviour, etc.)?
- What unmet health care needs does the target audience have that can be addressed?
- What is the scope of the problem or complexity of the issue to be addressed (including the changing trends)?
- How is the unmet health care need currently being controlled or addressed (what has been done before and how was it being done)?

BUSINESS MODEL

The next step is to develop a business model for the patient care service. A business model is part of the development of a business strategy and business plan (see Chapter 14: Financial Statements and Forms of Business Ownership and Chapter 53: Business Planning to Business Plan). In short, success depends on answering the question, "How do you plan to make money?"[10]

A business model in the context of a patient care service is a model or description of how a needed service will be delivered in a manner where revenues exceed expenditures while using current or attainable assets. A business model can be derived by synthesizing the information gathered to develop and produce the patient care service to be delivered. The business model should address the needs identified in a population that has a high likelihood of sustainability or profitability, generating sufficient revenue directly or indirectly, while satisfying the patient's needs. A compensation scheme must be developed that fits the model and also considers comparative fees and services available.

Success of a patient care service also requires the development or identification of critical success factors for a service. These are dynamics or situations that need to be achieved that are indicators of progress. Identifying these milestone measurements moving along the road to a successfully delivered service is important to help with decision making throughout the course of creating and delivering the service. Essentially, consider what the indicators are that demonstrate that the endeavour has been a success. The achievement of these milestones will demonstrate the correct path toward a successful service delivery is being followed.

Successful services are those that are enticing and often different from existing offerings. One approach is to develop a better service than competitors; however, this is often less likely to be sustainable and require constant surveillance of competitors with similar services. A riskier approach, albeit one with greater return, is developing a different service involving something unique rather than just improvements over existing offerings.

SERVICE ATMOSPHERE AND VALUE TO THE PATIENT

Patient care services follow a patient care process and are composed of the following key components: a process for communicating with and assessing the patient, establishing an individualized care plan and preparing a strategy for follow-up and evaluation.[11] The patient should view these components as contributing to their improvement and well-being, which is what makes the service seem valuable to them.

The physical environment and process for assessing the patient and identifying the medication management issues, also referred to as drug-related problems, should be one that is comfortable, non-threatening and in alignment with the patient's values and needs. The assessment processes should be streamlined and incorporate documentation throughout the steps for legal requirements and future reference.

An important aspect of the patient care service that demonstrates to patients that the pharmacist is fully engaged in helping the patient achieve his/her intended health outcomes is the care plan and how it is prepared and communicated. The care plan should be individualized and respect the patient's values, desires and financial situation with the pharmacist working with the patient to make shared informed decisions.[12] Developing a trusting relationship with the patient will improve the value of the interaction and service provided while optimizing the path toward achieving the patient's health-related goals. It should not be underestimated how a well-established relationship with the client leads to client loyalty and return visits as well as referrals and future business.

The relationship with the patient does not end with communicating the care plan. One frequent error is the lack of follow-up by pharmacists after information and recommendations are provided to the patients. A care plan should include a follow-up strategy and re-evaluation to monitor and follow the patient's progress.[11] With the pharmacist taking an active role in following up, the pharmacist proactively seeks communication with the patient, even if the patient does not engage. This approach is not only good patient care, but it is also integral for the sustainability of the patient care service and its profitability. It is the compilation of these interactions and the engagement of the patient that will assist with the desirability and use of the service. The service delivered in the most fitting atmosphere should demonstrate the high value of the service resulting in the patient's willingness to pay. This willingness to pay may be directly controlled by the patient, or it may drive the patient's impetus to cause the public or private payers to provide reimbursement. If patients are not willing to pay for the service, it is likely that the service is perceived to be of little value to them. Therefore, as the service is being developed, delivering high value to the patient must be paramount, and any expense that results in patients accepting a higher price is worthy of consideration.

Pharmacists are among the most trusted health care professionals and possess the expertise to do more than dispense medications to patients to improve health outcomes. For pharmacists to utilize their skills and expertise to help provide patient-centred care, pharmacists will need to develop patient care services that will address the medication and health-related needs of their clients in a financially sustainable manner. By undertaking a process to develop a patient care service that incorporates a needs assessment, a well-thought-out business model and a patient care process, the likelihood of success and professional satisfaction is almost guaranteed.

REFERENCES

1. Hepler CD, Strand LM. Opportunities and responsibilities in pharmaceutical care. Am J Hosp Pharm. 1990;47(3):533–43. Medline:2316538

2. Canadian Pharmacists Association. Summary of pharmacists' expanded scope of practice across Canada. Available: www.pharmacists.ca/cpha-ca/assets/File/pharmacy-in-canada/ExpandedScopeChartEN.pdf (accessed July 31, 2014).

3. Canadian Pharmacists Association. Our Way Forward: Optimizing drug therapy outcomes for Canadians through patient-centred care. Available: http://blueprintforpharmacy.ca/docs/pdfs/blueprint-priorities---our-way-forward-2013---june-2013.pdf (accessed July 31, 2014).

4. Houle SKD, Grindrod KA, Chatterley T, et al. Paying pharmacists for patient care: A systematic review of remunerated pharmacy clinical care services. Can Pharm J (Ott). 2014;147(4):209–32. http://dx.doi.org/10.1177/1715163514536678. Medline:25360148

5. Ontario Ministry of Health and Long-Term Care. MedsCheck. Available: www.health.gov.on.ca/en/public/programs/drugs/medscheck/medscheck_original.aspx (accessed Aug. 5, 2014).

6. Canadian Pharmacists Association. News Story: Alberta – Alberta Pharmacy Practice Initiative explores pharmacist remuneration. Available: http://blueprintforpharmacy.ca/news/news-story/2011/04/13/alberta---alberta-pharmacy-practice-initiative-explores-pharmacist-remuneration (accessed Aug. 5, 2014).

7. Alberta Pharmacists Association. Alberta Pharmacy Practice Models Initiative: evaluation report March 28, 2010. Broadview Applied Research Group, April 9, 2010.

8. Davidson K. BC Medication Management Project: BCMMP paves the way for future of pharmacy. Tablet. 2012;20(7):18–21.

9. Hsiao WC, Braun P, Dunn DL, et al. An overview of the development and refinement of the Resource-Based Relative Value Scale. The foundation for reform of U.S. physician payment. Med Care. 1992;30(11 Suppl):NS1–12. Medline:1434963

10. For Dummies, by John Wiley & Sons, Inc. Defining your business model. Available: www.dummies.com/how-to/content/defining-your-business-model.html (accessed Aug. 30, 2014).

11. Cipolle RJ, Strand L, Morley P. *Pharmaceutical care practice: the patient-centered approach to medication management.* 3rd ed. New York: McGraw-Hill, Medical Publishing Division; 2012.

12. Low A. Shared decision-making: helping your patients decide. Can Pharm J. 2011;144:S23.

CHAPTER 39

Planning Patient Care Services

John Shaske, *BSc(Pharm), ACPR, RPh*

Learning Objectives

- Identify key stakeholders and participants associated with delivering patient care services.
- Examine the financial viability, payment options and willingness of payers to pay for the service.
- Identify appropriate populations aligned with services.
- Develop a plan to implement a patient care service that considers patient needs, financial viability and sustainability.

KEY STAKEHOLDERS

As pharmacy practice evolves with new developments in the health care industry, pharmacists are confronted with the dilemma of how best to adapt their business model so it remains viable and sustainable. The transition to providing patient care services represents just such a challenge. Can a pharmacy deliver these services and remain profitable or even improve profitability?

The first task is to determine the key stakeholders in this enterprise. The stakeholder concept was first used in a 1963 internal memorandum at the Stanford Research Institute. It defined stakeholders as, "those groups without whose support the organization would cease to exist."[1] In medication management services, the key stakeholders are the patient, the physician, the rest of the patient's health care team and the payers (e.g., third-party payers, insurance companies, provincial health and drug plan administrators).

IDENTIFY APPROPRIATE POPULATIONS

Conduct a needs assessment to identify appropriate populations and define the target audience, identify and define the needs the service will meet and determine if there is a sufficient market (see Chapter 38: Developing Patient Care Services). Ensure there is not already a service that is being offered locally that would be difficult to compete with, especially services being delivered by a hospital or community centre that receives funding.

CONSIDER POTENTIAL BARRIERS

Transitioning a pharmacy business from a product-focused enterprise to a patient care practice requires a diligent planning process that will help save considerable time and resources during the implementation phase. There are many obstacles and barriers that need to be recognized, and a transition plan begins with identifying and determining ways to address them. Preconceptions and attitudes represent significant hurdles to attaining the objective. The solution is to commit to training, planning and analysis. Tackling these issues results in tangible drains on energy and time; this must be planned for, recorded and tracked as part of the startup costs. Experience has shown that there can be a temporary increase in the cost of doing business of up to 25% during the conversion process. Plan to involve experts who can reduce the costs and time of implementation and will likely be more effective than having an internal manager or staff attempting to overcome barriers and transition difficulties.

Implementing patient care services involves risk-taking and requires an innovative mindset and good planning. One of the initial steps is to define vision and mission statements for the program and its services and then engage the staff, public, colleagues and other practitioners with this message. Someone with the authority and knowledge will need to take the lead in planning the service and be prepared to be a trailblazer. Regulating bodies or professional associations cannot be relied upon to make the first move in driving the provision of patient care services; it must come from the practising pharmacists and pharmacies.

The safety and health care of patients remain the top priorities. Attention to drug-related issues within the practice must be supported by assigning time and resources to staying abreast of new learning programs, training staff and communicating with other health care professionals.[2]

Have a plan of how to achieve the following:

- Have pharmacists and all staff fully used in delivering the new services.
- Communicate with the local community as a whole about the existence of the new services. Local physicians, nurses, dentists and other health care practitioners are crucial in spreading the word about the expanded services being offered. Do not overlook local businesses, Chambers of Commerce and community associations.
- Improve the clinical skills of the pharmacists on staff. Patient volume is needed to develop these skills. Start with a few patients per day to get into the habit of conducting medication management reviews; increase this number gradually as you become more proficient.

Tools to help staff and a tailored working environment are important elements for the successful delivery of a patient care service. Mandated patient care documentation requires computer hardware, journals and reference texts to support the learning curve. Patient traffic flow should be directed by appropriate signage. Internal posters should explain the new services, dispel confusion and prompt patients to inquire. Provide semi-private stations for the pharmacists to engage patients in medication management interviews at intake and private consultation rooms for longer consultations.

The physical environment would ideally reflect that of an office, not a store. The proper environment aids patients in changing their preconceptions about pharmacy practice from one of dispensing to one of professional health care. Depending on the patient care service provided, the space may need counters, wet stations, medical equipment, furniture, telephones, computers and cash registers housed in a clean, uncluttered office-style environment. The space must be workable and comfortable for staff and patients and have a logical layout enabling good traffic flow.

FINANCIAL VIABILITY

After identifying the steps and planning for what needs to be done to implement patient care services, determine the viability of those services by adding up the costs to start delivery and the ongoing expenses, then compare them with the expected revenue. Be prepared to invest at least one or two years developing the patient care services model into a full-time practice. As the number of patients absorbed into the practice increases, the timeline shortens—more patients represent greater viability, and returns on the initial startup investment will be seen.

A minimum of 10 to 15 patients per day is needed to be viable.[2] That encompasses new patients as well as follow-up encounters with established patients. On an annual basis, this translates into about 4,000 encounters or approximately a practice or 1,500 to 2,000 patients. Building a practice to that level takes time and hard work while the community is being educated and made aware of the services, resulting in referrals and other sources of patients.

The most effective way to expand a service is to provide the care and allow the patients themselves to market it through word of mouth and reputation. This is how most medical services become successful. Providing excellent care for all patients leads to healthy commerce[3] (see Section XI: Marketing, Promotion and Customer Service).

The primary source of professional referrals will come from physicians, nurses and other health care service providers. Being located in a clinic or hospital setting will speed up recruitment of patients. Referrals are just another form of word-of-mouth recommendation, and because it comes from another health care professional, it is a very efficient means to building a patient base. However, do not try to build a practice solely around professional referrals as they can be spotty and unpredictable. Always maintain a broadly based patient recruitment plan using all tools available.

Professional referrals come with several mutual expectations if the system is to work successfully for all parties. A referral comes with the expectation that the favour will be reciprocated. Be prepared to act in kind whenever possible. On occasion, time-consuming, complicated cases will come from physician referrals; be prepared to spend the time and energy servicing these patients and assisting the referring physicians. Serving a high volume of patients requires an efficiently run organization, and the time pharmacists spend with each patient needs to be prioritized and allocated well. It is acceptable to reschedule a patient for a more in-depth discussion at a later time if other priorities are more pressing. Prepare an explanation that communicates the importance of the patient's issues and that appropriate time to resolve them is important, while considering the patient's expectations and needs.

REMUNERATION

Getting paid for patient care services is crucial to viability, just as it is for physicians and dentists. To date, medication management services are not being consistently paid for by government agencies. Until medication management is standardized as a billable service for pharmacists, other approaches to acquiring payment must be pursued. This may include assessing whether a patient has a third-party payer or insurance plan that may reimburse the patient for approved pharmacist-delivered services. The revenue sources will be difficult to plan for but need to be identified. Some research into potential sources of revenue to fund the expenses related to the service will help with planning the financial viability of delivering the service.

PAYMENT MECHANISMS

With delivery of patient care services as the main objective for the pharmacy practice, fair payment for direct patient services is mandatory for sustainability. The pharmacist needs to be dedicated to the provision of these services and the generation of revenue, delegating other activities to staff members (including administration responsibilities). This is just efficient allocation of resources, and ensuring the pharmacists are performing pharmacist-required duties results in the right service value for the salary paid.

Consider the characteristics of the service and devise the best possible structure and mechanism for payment. This will assist in establishing an understanding of the fee structure and clearly identify that these services are separate from the provision of drug products and dispensing. Patient care services need to be seen and evaluated independently of drug products, and the services should be self-sustaining once the implementation period has expired.

Consideration needs to be given to reimbursement for everything the pharmacist works on regardless of duration, complexity of the task and location of service delivery (e.g., pharmacy, hospital, clinic, long-term care). After all, pharmacists deserve compensation for their work and the business needs to generate sufficient revenue to cover costs and provide a return on the investment.

Three payment mechanisms fit the objectives just described: the fee-for-service system, the capitation method and the Resource Based Relative Value Scale System (RBRVS) approach.[4]

REIMBURSEMENT IN CANADA

Approaches to reimbursement for patient care services delivered by pharmacists are in a state of development. A perfect system has yet to be put into practice, especially since the pharmacists' scope of practice in Canada is steadily expanding.[5]

Shortly after the introduction of MedsCheck, the medication review program in Ontario, most provinces/territories in Canada began offering government reimbursement for medication review services.[6,7] (Although medication reviews performed by the pharmacist are recognized in Québec, the patient is required to pay for the service and is not reimbursed by the government.) Reimbursement models continue to be developed and whatever method will be introduced next, it is felt that as consumer demand for the service increases, there will be increasing willingness for third-party payers and others to offer reimbursement when the benefits and improved health care outcomes are seen as being associated with patient care services. Governments have come to better understand the role pharmacists can play in achieving the triple aim objectives of better care, better health and better value.[8]

MONITORING AND INDICATORS

There are two general indicator categories for measuring the service's success: job performance and financial milestones. Job performance evaluations may include tracking total number of encounters, total number of paid encounters, pharmacists' performance in conducting their duties, measuring patient satisfaction and measuring health outcomes. Financial milestone evaluations should target the costs to deliver the service compared to the revenue generated. For example, with dispensing it may be costs to prepare prescriptions, total cost of prescription, percentage of gross profit that goes to salary, percentage of gross profit to rent or percentage of gross profit to all other expenses required to fill a prescription. For a patient care service, financial milestones are more difficult to define since targeting the cost to deliver a service is more variable and is highly dependent on the pharmacist involved as well as the individual patient needs at the time. Nevertheless, financial milestone evaluations should be carried out. Financial targets are usually set by the owner and reflect his/her personal and financial goals (see Section IV: Financial Management for Your Practice).

Plan a structured process:[9]

- Set measureable objectives/goals.
- Set deadlines.
- Look for well-informed or experienced people who can join the team or offer assistance.
- Examine the logistics of what you have planned, looking at the priorities and sequence.
- Determine targets to measure against (may be very individual; e.g., industry standards versus highest financial gain).
- Assign tasks so there is clarity on who is following up on what and when.

To monitor progress, a means of tracking performance is needed. Although this is individual to the service being planned, an experienced service provider or specialist can help develop individualized performance indicators that make sense with the service you are delivering (see Chapter 41: Evaluating Patient Care Services).

Delivering patient care services requires planning and thorough consideration of the stakeholders, target service population, financial viability and reliable measures to track progress. Putting together a plan of who best to involve, identifying barriers and preparing solutions are as important as ensuring the sustainability of the service, which includes recognizing potential sources of payment before taking action. Taking action before a good plan is developed can lead to wasted effort and inefficient expenditures. Carefully consider what is needed and plan accordingly before moving on to implementation.

RESOURCES AND SUGGESTED READINGS

Cipolle RJ, Strand LM, Morley PC. *Pharmaceutical care practice: the clinician's guide.* 2nd ed. New York, NY: McGraw-Hill; 2004.
Houle SKD, Grindrod KA, Chatterley T, et al. Paying pharmacists for patient care: systematic review of remunerated pharmacy clinical care services. Can Pharm J (Ott). 2014;147(4):209–32. http://dx.doi.org/10.1177/1715163514536678. Medline:25360148

REFERENCES

1. Freeman RE, Reed DL. Stockholders and stakeholders: a new perspective on corporate governance. Calif Manage Rev. 1983;25(3):88–106. http://dx.doi.org/10.2307/41165018.
2. Hepler CD, Strand LM. Opportunities and responsibilities in pharmaceutical care. Am J Hosp Pharm. 1990;47(3):533–43. Medline:2316538
3. Shaske J. *Making business sense of clinical services.* Toronto: Rogers Publishing; 2014, Available: www.canadianhealthcare-network.ca/pharmacists/discussions/blogs/outcomes-matter/making-business-sense-of-clinical-services-26547 [cited 2014 Nov. 23].
4. Cipolle RJ, Strand LM, Morley PC. *Pharmaceutical care practice: the clinician's guide.* 2nd ed. New York, NY: McGraw-Hill; 2004.

5. Canadian Pharmacists Association. Summary of pharmacists' expanded scope of practice across Canada. Available: www. pharmacists.ca/cpha-ca/assets/File/pharmacy-in-canada/ExpandedScopeChartEN.pdf (accessed July 31, 2014).

6. Canadian Pharmacists Association. Pharmacists' medication management services environmental scan of activities across Canada. Available: http://blueprintforpharmacy.ca/docs/kt-tools/canada-environmental-scan-of-pharmacy-services---cpha-october-2013---final.pdf (accessed Sept. 11, 2014).

7. Ontario Ministry of Health and Long-Term Care. MedsCheck. Available: www.health.gov.on.ca/en/pro/programs/drugs/medscheck/medscheck_original.aspx (accessed Aug. 5, 2014).

8. Canadian Pharmacists Association. Our way forward: optimizing drug therapy outcomes for Canadians through patient-centred care. Available: www.blueprintforpharmacy.ca/docs/pdfs/blueprint-priorities---our-way-forward-2013---june-2013.pdf (accessed July 31, 2014).

9. Shaske J. How I transformed a drug distribution pharmacy into a clinical pharmacy entailing redesign of the pharmacy environment. Presented at Professional Development Weekend. Vancouver, BC: PDW; 2014.

CHAPTER 40

Implementing Patient Care Services

John Shaske, *BSc(Pharm), ACPR, RPh*

Learning Objectives

- Identify real and perceived barriers to implementing patient care services.
- Develop tactics to overcome barriers and shortcomings in delivering patient care services.
- Set milestones for a developing patient care service.
- Develop an implementation plan for patient care services.
- Identify appropriate documentation tools and describe the importance of documentation.

BARRIERS TO PATIENT CARE SERVICES

Chapter 39: Planning Patient Care Services outlined the many considerations and planning for the adoption of patient care services in a pharmacy practice. The tasks and challenges of implementing this plan constitute the main focus of this chapter. Maintaining an innovative and creative mindset is an essential quality throughout this process; combating ingrained habits and perceptions of what pharmacy practice constitutes is an ongoing challenge. Moving away from being product focused to a patient-centred practice while ensuring business continuity must have a purposeful and well-planned approach. Implementing a new service also requires a high level of determination.

Once the plan for delivering the patient care service is created, moving to identifying the real and perceived barriers to implementation takes priority (see Chapter 10: Change Management). Currently at most pharmacies, a significant part of the pharmacist's day is still devoted to drug preparation and distribution. This is partly the result of pharmacies still using the old dispensing business model. It remains a challenge even for those embarking on the new methods and creating new models of delivery of patient care services as well.[1] Addressing the following most common barriers to implementation will help alleviate impediments to successfully establishing the services that have been planned:

- pharmacists resistant to change
- pharmacists' perceived lack of skills in developing patient care services and unwillingness to make the changes necessary to develop the skills and business procedures required
- unwillingness of major organizations to change (e.g., government, chain drug stores, supermarket pharmacies)
- low expectations and lack of awareness of pharmacist capabilities among the general public
- lack of human resources available for the provision of suitable patient care services
- lack of a proper physical work environment for pharmacists to meet the needs of providing the service (e.g., semi-private work spaces at intake, private consultation rooms)
- lack of a suitable reimbursement model or ability to generate sufficient revenue

OVERCOMING BUSINESS SHORTCOMINGS

Most barriers are problems that are within the power of the pharmacist and manager to change. Attitudes and lack of skills can be adjusted through education; public expectations can be altered through marketing and communications; staff shortcomings can be rectified through training and hiring; and tailoring the physical environment merely requires some interior design adjustments. Reimbursement or generating revenue from these services is potentially the most challenging barrier to conquer, some of which requires changes in government policy.

Despite the range of barriers to implementation, the single most important tool in helping overcome them is a good business plan (see Chapter 53: Business Planning to Business Plan). A business plan can be created for a patient care service as it can be developed for a new pharmacy and will do the following:

- Communicate clearly to everyone involved with the pharmacy the vision and mission of the service. It lets the most important people involved in the endeavour, the staff, know what is expected of them.
- Help change the culture of the organization. By educating, encouraging and motivating staff to envision how their roles will evolve and grow, they will come to understand that their talents will be expanded and skills updated.
- Help guide the marketing and communications program in the task of educating the public and current patients on what to expect from their pharmacy and pharmacist.
- Give guidance in tracking both financial results and measuring patient outcomes.
- Provide steps or a process to manage the necessary changes.

MILESTONES AND MONITORING PROGRESS

As with any journey, it is important to know if one is on course. Chapter 16: Financial Ratios: Putting the Numbers to Work discusses the financial aspects in a pharmacy and guides the manager to identify and assess important indicators and milestones to judge performance. Assessing the financial ratios and where the service lies in reaching the milestones should be conducted on a monthly basis (or more frequently if volumes are high). In addition, all the statistics collected regarding the demographics of the patients receiving care must be collected and evaluated. This includes statistics for the number of drug therapy problems (DTPs) solved, the number of drug therapy regimens that have been changed, the number of patients to whom the services have been provided and some measure or projection of the impact of the services such as the number of physician visits saved, hospital admissions avoided and emergency department visits prevented. These patient care statistics are important because they measure what has been done and how well. The service will have specific measures that are associated with its delivery and the key is to identify measurements that represent what benefit the patient receives, how well the service is being delivered and the outcomes being achieved. DTPs should be followed up and identified as resolved, stable, improved, no change, worse or expired. When implementing the patient care service, ensure there is a process to analyze how the patient is progressing with his/her particular care plan, resolution of DTPs and that a schedule or timeline is in place to reassess the patient's situation. It is not only possible, but likely that pharmacist-delivered patient care services will improve outcomes and simultaneously can help offer savings to patients and the health care system.[2]

There is no universally accepted optimal speed for implementing patient care services. If one moves too fast, there is a risk of leaving staff and the general public behind, leading to frustration and poor performance. If one moves too slowly, there is a risk of losing momentum and the interest of the stakeholders. To help avoid these pitfalls, the following example schedule can provide some guidance.

DAY ONE

Set a day to start offering the new services. This comes after completion of the vision and mission statement, adjustment of staff roles, training, acquisition of primary resources (e.g., computers, documentation system, software), renovations (e.g., semi-private intake stations, private consultation rooms) and understanding of workflow processes. Internal traffic flow signage, brochures and posters explaining the new services should be posted within the pharmacy. (Communication prevents misunderstanding, confusion and a poor patient experience.)

The first day becomes the benchmark against which the pharmacy's progress is measured. This applies to both service delivery and financial performance gauged against initial objectives.

As a start, aim for an attainable first objective; for example, provide the patient care service to a minimum of two new patients each day. Meet with staff on a daily basis at this stage to discuss progress as well as issues that may have emerged. Identify these issues early and work collectively to resolve these in an open and realistic manner.

Preparing an implementation checklist for use on the first day helps to cover all the new changes that may not be normally considered. For example:

- Is the area where the patient meets the pharmacist well signed, clean and professional?
- Are the pharmacist's greetings patient-focused?
- Is there a waiting area consistent with other professional operations such as an accountant's or dentist's office?
- Does the workflow emanate from pharmacist to staff, to task engagement and completion?
- Do staff answer the phone professionally?
- Does the patient always come first?
- Does the pharmacy meet the needs of the patient, including educational materials?
- Is the lighting sufficient?

DAILY

Identify the signs that will identify whether or not patients have a positive therapeutic experience, one that they would value and return for repeat service. These markers may be expressed in the gratitude the patient expresses and/or their willingness to pay.

WEEKLY

During the implementation phase, focus on some items weekly to ensure good communication with staff and manage the new implementation of the patient care service. Hold full staff meetings weekly on top of brief daily updates. Staff input is crucial to success; it keeps morale high during the transition period, makes them feel part of the team and allows the manager to demonstrate leadership. Check with staff regarding how patients are responding to the new service, review patient documentation for accuracy and devise solutions for problems identified. Make sure the staff are educated on identified weaknesses in the system and are properly informed of problems. They should be given the required support to develop solutions and handle issues (e.g., assign appropriate support roles and allocate corresponding resources).

MONTHLY

Include a monthly evaluation of progress to date that contains concrete data on activities that can easily be extracted and reported from the documentation system. For example, evaluate the number of patients receiving the service, the age distribution, the most common indications for drug therapy and the number and types of DTPs identified and resolved. Include a summary of outcomes; this could be the number of drug therapy regimens that have been changed, as well as the number of unnecessary physician visits, nursing home admissions or hospitalizations that have been prevented. This data provides the essential feedback for evaluating progress and making changes.[2]

MANAGING THE IMPLEMENTATION

Regular delivery of patient-centred services in a pharmacy environment is still so new that there is not a solid base of examples available for study and analysis. Observing and learning from other patient care practitioners, such as physicians, dentists and veterinarians, will help further understanding of what may be required to establish a successful service. Identify how these practices deliver customer service, ensure satisfaction of their clients and increase their client numbers. Implementing a change in practice requires an organized approach that is tailored to tackle the needs of the patient and service delivered in a standardized fashion. Create a policy and procedures manual to standardize the service and workflow. Roles and responsibilities should be clearly defined, and each staff member must be clear on where they fit in the delivery of the service and what critical steps must be taken to ensure a high level of customer service and satisfy customer needs as well as expectations. What is communicated to the patient is as important as how it is communicated, and clear direction should be provided to staff to ensure a positive experience by the patient.

All staff members, including personnel not involved in assisting patients, should be trained and aware to communicate details about the patient care services available in the pharmacy and direct clients to the pharmacist. A practice management system will help accomplish an efficient delivery of services and engage all of the staff. This is a system that will attract the patient to the service all the way through to receiving and paying for the service.

The practice management system needs to encompass the following:[2]
- a clear understanding of the vision and mission statements of the patient care service
- all resources required to support delivery (e.g., documentation system, human resources, monetary support, physical changes, reporting system, policy and procedure documents)
- evaluation methods including short-term indicators (e.g., patient experience/satisfaction) and long-term indicators (e.g., overall quality and effectiveness)
- payment mechanisms representing value of the service to the patient and society

The following are key elements for successful implementation:[2]
- leader must be properly prepared and have a business plan
- services are understood well enough to explain to others
- team of highly qualified practitioners who are like-minded and supportive
- an understanding that change takes time and a commitment to building the practice over one to two years, then a lifetime for growth
- an expectation that education for personnel and patients will be ongoing
- new patients recruited through referrals from other health care professionals and patients
- incorporation of all developed associated revenue streams to ensure sustainability
- a marketing plan or approach that recognizes importance of providing high-quality care
- communication skills that include empathy, listening, managing conflict when required, ensuring technical content of explanations can be understood by the receiver and asking questions in a manner that facilitates meaningful answers

The practice management system is responsible for assigning the responsibilities of support staff to facilitate the patient care process, including patient flow, workflow and meeting any other needs of the patient. Questions concerning hours of operation, access to services, eligibility for services, costs, billing procedures, scheduling and other general information are the responsibility of support staff. Defining areas of responsibility and structure of workflow will prove indispensable as the practice expands, avoiding breakdowns and bottlenecks in the system. This is where an experienced management consultant can be invaluable (see Section VI: Operations). Ensure the most appropriate personnel are allocated to the right tasks. Pharmacists should be used in areas where their skills are required and can be leveraged to help patients and drive the positive patient experience. Non-pharmacist support staff should be focused on all roles that do not require a licensed pharmacist.

DOCUMENTATION

The provision of patient care services adds a new level of responsibility for the pharmacist. Reasonably comprehensive documentation of all action between the pharmacist and the patient is required. Three major categories of information must be documented: the data used to make the decisions that fall within the pharmacist's scope of responsibility, the decisions made for and with the patient and the actual outcomes that result from those decisions.

Documenting patient care services requires the step-by-step recording of the complete care process. The documentation not only must be useful to the practitioner but needs to serve as the primary information resource for the patient, the patient's family, the patient's professional health care team and those who manage and evaluate the services provided. Documentation is also a requirement put forward by the pharmacist licensing bodies in each province/territory, and regulations vary across Canada. Particularly with the provision of new patient care services, incorporating new or expanded scopes of practice, detailed and comprehensive documentation is often necessary.

The following are key concepts of documentation:[2]

- Document all patient care according to ethical, professional and legal guidelines to protect the pharmacist and pharmacy in cases of ambiguity.
- An electronic health record (EHR) is the basis for documenting medication management services and communicating action plans to all health care professionals involved.
- The data needed to manage, improve and justify the service is found in the documentation. (Some jurisdictions have certain documentation requirements for reimbursement.)
- Government guidelines and regulatory bodies require electronic documentation that generates data to help improve patient care and population health policies.

When choosing documentation tools and software, focus on the information that needs to be captured for delivering care, following up, monitoring progress, reimbursement and decision making. Some metrics will be derived from the documentation system, and the tools and software used must be evaluated to ensure they are capable of delivering this data. Documentation software that can synchronize data from other sources such as laboratory networks or physicians' electronic medical record (EMR) can save data entry time and simplify processes. The evolution of the universal EHR continues, and each province/territory is at different stages of connectivity and synchronization. The choice of documentation software should be made after weighing current and future documentation needs against expandability, new features about to be released and costs.

The documentation system must output a care plan, which is the core of pharmaceutical or medication management services. It is the most important output in the provision of quality patient care. The capacity to integrate individual patient data from relevant clinical evidence involving groups or populations with similar characteristics to make management, protocol, therapeutic, staffing and staff development decisions is essential to the implementation of a quality patient care service.

The shift from product-focused care to patient-centred care is occurring in pharmacies in Canada. There are many obstacles and barriers that have made it difficult to implement sustainable patient care services. By collecting the right information, recognizing where common obstacles exist, careful planning, setting milestones and monitoring progress, a successful and sustainable patient care service can be implemented. Often, the key elements that are easily overlooked include integrating all staff, both pharmacy and non-pharmacy staff onsite, and having good communications and documentation tools to actively manage the pharmacy practice in the delivery of care to patients.

RESOURCES AND SUGGESTED READINGS

Bradford V. *The total service medical practice: 17 steps to satisfying your internal and external customers*. Chicago: Irwin Professional Publishing; 1997.

Isetts BJ, Buffington DE, and the Pharmacist Services Technical Advisory Coalition. CPT code-change proposal: national data on pharmacists' medication therapy management services. J Am Pharm Assoc (2003). 2007;47(4):491–5. http://dx.doi.org/10.1331/JAPhA.2007.07013. Medline:17616495

Joseph SR. Developing a marketing plan. In: *Marketing the physician practice*. Chicago: American Medical Association; 2000.

McDonough RP, Doucette WR. Dynamics of pharmaceutical care: developing collaborative working relations between pharmacists and physicians. J Am Pharm Assoc. 2001;41(5):682–92.

Strand LM, Cipolle RJ, Morley PC, et al. The impact of pharmaceutical care practice on the practitioner and the patient in the ambulatory practice setting: twenty-five years of experience. Curr Pharm Des. 2004;10(31):3987–4001. http://dx.doi.org/10.2174/1381612043382576. Medline:15579084

REFERENCES

1. Canadian Pharmacists Association. Our way forward: optimizing drug therapy outcomes for Canadians through patient-centred care. Available: http://blueprintforpharmacy.ca/docs/pdfs/blueprint-priorities---our-way-forward-2013---june-2013.pdf (accessed Aug. 31, 2014).

2. Cipolle RJ, Strand L, Morley P. *Pharmaceutical care practice: the patient-centered approach to medication management*. 3rd ed. New York: McGraw-Hill, Medical Publishing Division; 2012.

CHAPTER 41

Evaluating Patient Care Services

Carlo A. Marra, *BSc(Pharm), ACPR, PharmD, PhD, FCSHP; Professor and Dean, School of Pharmacy, Memorial University of Newfoundland*

Nicole W. Tsao, *BSc(Biol), BSc(Pharm), MScPharm; Faculty of Pharmaceutical Sciences, University of British Columbia*

Learning Objectives

- Define evaluation.
- Discuss why it is important to evaluate patient care services.
- Develop an evaluation plan to assess if the patient care service is meeting patients' needs.
- Apply the SMART criteria to develop success indicators for the evaluation.
- Describe the importance of engaging stakeholders.
- Compare the three different methods of evaluation.
- Propose a plan to disseminate the evaluation findings.

This chapter starts with an overview of what evaluation is and the importance of performing evaluations for patient care services implemented in a pharmacy. Key concepts[1-3] from frameworks used in program evaluation sciences will be introduced and adapted to provide a more practical approach to evaluation. The purpose of this chapter is to build knowledge and skill in the area of evaluation of patient-centred care services and to provide guidance on the process of developing an evaluation plan, carrying out the evaluation and disseminating the findings. Last, using the results of the evaluation to help make a decision to identify the success of the service and develop a contingency plan or exit strategy for the case of abandoning a "failed" service will be discussed.

WHAT IS EVALUATION?

A commonly used definition of evaluation is, "the systematic collection of information about the activities, characteristics, and outcomes of program, services, policy, or processes, in order to make judgments about the program/process, improve effectiveness, and/or inform decisions about future development."[4]

WHY IS EVALUATION OF PHARMACY SERVICES IMPORTANT?

With the expansion of the role of pharmacists over the last several decades, increasing empha-sis is being placed on evaluation of new initiatives and services they provide.[5,6] To determine whether a particular strategy or new service is working, or will work, to address a need, accu-rate, credible and timely information is needed to inform decisions made within the context in which pharmacists are working.[2] Evaluations also serve to inform decisions about discontinuing services or changing established processes.[2] A key part of evaluation is the incorporation of con-textual knowledge to inform local decisions. In some contexts, the evaluation serves to inform local policy makers or funders of new pharmacy services so policy decisions and funding of the services can occur.

> "It is important to evaluate all outcomes so you can justify the services you are being paid for to all stakeholders and to reflect on each aspect of the operation from clinical services to finance and marketing and see what you are doing well and what needs to change and improve. Without all aspects of outcomes being measured there is no justification from third party payers to maintain funding. With no measurement of our performance we will never know where we need to improve our performance and take the necessary steps to make sure that improvement occurs." – John Shaske, Owner, Howe Sound Pharmacy

DEVELOPING AN EVALUATION PLAN

Before starting to develop an evaluation plan, ensure objectives, target group and success indica-tors have been defined for the patient care service. These are critical aspects that need to be well described. There are generally two types of objectives: implementation objectives, which relate to the *process* of carrying out the service, and outcome objectives, which relate to the *result* of the service.[3]

Depending on the patient care service, the target patient group could be very broad and gen-eral, such as all patients at the pharmacy, or could be focused on a specific group, such as individ-uals with type 2 diabetes or those taking an anti-hypertensive medication. To determine whether the objectives of the patient care service have been achieved, one needs to set measurable indi-cators of success—pre-determined criteria to indicate whether the service was successful or not with respect to meeting the needs for which it was established.[3] It is useful to refer to the SMART criteria when setting indicators. The SMART criteria state that an indicator should be specific, measurable, attainable, realistic and time-sensitive[3] (see Chapter 6: The Foundations of Building a Successful Strategic Plan).

Consider a patient care service with the outcome objective of improving medication adherence for pharmacy patients who take anti-hypertensive medications. If the baseline adherence rates are not known for the patients in the pharmacy before starting the service, it is helpful to refer to literature and prior research to help inform on the success indicators. Based on literature, the typical adherence rate for anti-hypertensive medications is around 60%;[7] thus, a SMART suc-cess indicator for this service might be to achieve an adherence rate of 70% for anti-hypertensive medications after one year of providing the service. Success indicators are referred to at the end of the evaluation to inform decisions about continuing or stopping a service and can also be used for continuous monitoring throughout the future lifespan of the service.

Once these details have been fully described for the patient care service, the initial step of evaluation planning is to *determine the purpose of the evaluation*. There are several types of evaluations and each has the purpose of evaluating a different stage of the service:
- proof-of-concept evaluation: evaluates the conceptual model of the service
- implementation evaluation: determines whether the new service has been implemented according to plan
- process evaluation: evaluates the early operation of the service
- outcome evaluation: determines the effect or impact of the new service and makes a judgment of its relative worth[1,8]

The most common purpose is to make a judgment about the worth or merit of a program or service,[2] which is mainly an outcome evaluation. Specifically, the purpose of determining the worth or merit of a new patient care service at the pharmacy will help to inform decisions on whether to continue it as is, fund it, develop it further, expand it to other locations or perhaps to discontinue it.

Based on the purpose of the evaluation, one can set out to *engage the relevant stakeholders*. Stakeholders are individuals or groups who have an interest in the evaluation, which may or may not differ from the stakeholders who have an interest in the service itself (e.g., patients may be a stakeholder of the services, but not necessarily a stakeholder of the evaluation). Evaluation stakeholders are the users of the information generated by the evaluation; this could include funders, local government, local policy makers, other health care providers, staff members, management, directors, Board of Directors or shareholders of an organization. Involving stakeholders early in the evaluation planning facilitates support and buy-in for the evaluation. It also increases the likelihood that the results and recommendations of the evaluation will be acted upon. As such, taking the time to understand stakeholders' interests and expectations will ensure the relevance and usefulness of the evaluation. Much frustration can be avoided by knowing ahead of time what the stakeholders' expectations are with regard to how often they will be consulted and the extent of their role in deciding the fate of the service after the evaluation is completed.

When all the preparatory work is underway, it is time to *select the method of evaluation*. When choosing the method of evaluation, it is important to consider the financial and human resources available, the timeline and the expertise required to carry out the evaluation. In certain circumstances, there may be desire to involve external research or evaluation experts, or apply for external funding to conduct the evaluation.

There are three basic types of research designs that can be applied in evaluations: experimental design, quasi-experimental design and non-experimental design. Experimental and quasi-experimental designs are similar in that there is a treatment group (who receives the service of interest) and a comparison group (who does not receive the treatment or service of interest); however, the experimental design employs random assignment of patients to the respective groups, whereas the quasi-experimental design typically involves naturally formed groups of users and non-users. These designs can be robust, but it is not always feasible, ethically or practically, to use them.[1]

A practical approach to patient care service evaluation is to use a non-experimental, or observational, design. This type of design allows easy integration of multiple sources of data collection, both quantitative and qualitative.[9] The use of multiple sources of information, called triangulation, is a best practice in conducting evaluations.[9,10]

Data collection is one of the most important parts of the evaluation since without data, there is nothing to evaluate. There are many things to consider about data collection, including what data to collect, how it will be collected and by whom and when. The what and the how go hand in hand; a good model to follow is the ECHO model for evaluation of economic, clinical and humanistic outcomes.[11] The ECHO model provides a comprehensive assessment of the most important aspects in an outcome evaluation. The economic aspect would include data on costs of providing the patient care service (e.g., staff wages, medical supplies), cost savings to the health care system from providing the service (e.g., laboratory tests saved, emergency department visits avoided) and revenue generated from the service (e.g., patient payment out of pocket, over-the-counter items sold) to name a few. The clinical aspect would include data on health outcomes as a result of the patient care service that could include, for example, blood glucose levels and HbA1c for a service targeting individuals with type 2 diabetes, or blood pressure control and adherence for a service targeting individuals taking anti-hypertensive medications. The humanistic aspect refers to patients' quality of life and satisfaction from receiving the patient care service.

Quantitative methods of data collection involve direct measurements, surveys or routinely collected administrative data sets, and qualitative methods can involve focus groups or interviews. Depending on what data are being collected, it usually makes logical sense to use either a quantitative method or a qualitative method. For instance, blood glucose data would be collected via direct measurement (quantitative), whereas patient satisfaction could be collected via focus group discussions or interviews (qualitative). It may be helpful to develop a protocol for who collects which data and when to ensure systematic collection of information. When developing this protocol, be sure to consider the resources, how often the data will be collected and over how long of a period, as well as the burden on the patients involved to provide the data being requested.

When all the needed data are obtained, the next steps are essentially to *analyze the data, interpret the results* and *disseminate the findings*. Qualitative data are usually analyzed and summarized by identifying the predominant themes and then providing quotes to support those themes. For quantitative data, simple summary statistics can be easily analyzed with commonly used computer software, or if more sophisticated analyses are required, consider eliciting help from a qualified individual such as a researcher or statistician. Using these findings, determine whether the patient care service has achieved the objectives that were set out. Have the success indicators been met? Perhaps some have been met but not others. This is the point where the previously defined success indicators and objective thresholds set can be used for making decisions on the fate of the service moving forward. The last step is to formulate a dissemination plan for the findings to the stakeholders. This could be done in a variety of ways via meetings, presentations or reports; the goal is to use the information to make judgments about the service, improve effectiveness and/or inform decisions about future developments. One possible outcome is a decision to abandon the patient care service altogether. It may bode well to consider some contingency plans, with specific decisions and actions based on pre-determined thresholds and objective measurements, in the event this occurs. Given that pharmacists' foremost responsibility is to patient care, contemplate how to provide a seamless transition for the patients who will no longer receive the patient care service and develop a communication plan to convey the changes to them.

It is a successful new initiative if most of the success indicators have been met or can be met with some changes to the patient care service provided. The stakeholders should be pleased, and there should be positive impact made on patients' health. Once the necessary skills to evaluate patient care services have been developed, consider applying these skills as ongoing monitoring or as continuous quality improvement (see Chapter 28: Medication Incidents and Quality Improvement). For both a new evaluation and ongoing monitoring, there needs to be an evaluation plan with clearly defined purpose, objectives and success indicators. Engage the appropriate stakeholders, determine the method of data collection and analysis and have a dissemination plan for the findings.

Case Study: PhINDMORE (Pharmacist Innovative Drug Therapy Management, Outcomes, Resource Use and Economics)

The PhINDMORE study was funded by the Canadian Foundation for Pharmacy and involved a one-year evaluation of medication management provided by a single pharmacy, Howe Sound Pharmacy, in Gibsons, British Columbia.

An example of an implementation objective of the medication management service provided was *to assess drug therapy problems at the point of prescription intake by all pharmacists*. This objective was directly related to the *process* of carrying out the service. An outcome objective was *identified drug therapy problems will be resolved through interventions made by pharmacists in collaboration with other health care professionals*. This objective was directly related to the *result* of the service. The patient population of interest for the medication management service was broad and included all patients being serviced at the pharmacy.

The PhINDMORE study was an outcomes evaluation, with the purpose of determining the economic and clinical outcomes of the medication management service. Stakeholders included the owners of Howe Sound Pharmacy, funders (Canadian Foundation for Pharmacy) and local government. An observational evaluation was conducted and electronic data collection via e-patient charts was used. The following economic data was collected: cost of providing medication management, physician office visits avoided, emergency department visits avoided and hospitalizations avoided. The following clinical data was also collected: number of drug therapy problems identified, classifications of drug therapy problems identified, goals of therapy, actions taken to resolve problems and status of problem resolution after a pre-specified time period. The analysis was completed by a team of researchers at the Faculty of Pharmaceutical Sciences, University of British Columbia. Results were disseminated via a presentation at the Canadian Pharmacists Association annual meeting.[12] At time of writing, the medication management service is still being provided to patients at Howe Sound Pharmacy.

RESOURCES AND SUGGESTED READINGS

Canadian Evaluation Society. Program evaluation standards. Available: http://evaluationcanada.ca/site.cgi?s=6&ss=10&_lang=en (accessed Dec. 1, 2014).

Centres for Disease Control and Prevention. Communities of practice resource kit. SMART objectives template. Available: www.cdc.gov/phcommunities/docs/evaluate_smart_objectives_template.doc (accessed Dec. 1, 2014).

Frechtling J, Sharp L. *User-friendly handbook for mixed methods evaluations.* Arlington, VA: National Science Foundation; 1997. Available: www.nsf.gov/pubs/1997/nsf97153/start.htm [cited Dec. 1, 2014].

Public Health Research, Education and Development Program, Sudbury, Ontario. Annotated inventory of evaluation tools and resources. Available: www.phred-redsp.on.ca/Inventory.htm (accessed Dec. 1, 2014).

Western Michigan University evaluation center checklists. Available: www.wmich.edu/evalctr/checklists/ (accessed Dec. 1, 2014).

REFERENCES

1. Centers for Disease Control and Prevention. A framework for program evaluation. Available: www.cdc.gov/EVAL/framework/ (accessed Sept. 1, 2014).

2. Canadian Institutes of Health Research. A guide to evaluation in health research. Available: www.cihr-irsc.gc.ca/e/45336. html (accessed Sept. 1, 2014).

3. Public Health Ontario. Evaluating health promotion programs. Available: www.publichealthontario.ca/en/eRepository/ Evaluating_health_promotion_programs_2012.pdf (accessed Dec. 1, 2014).

4. Patton MQ. *Utilization-focused evaluation*. 3rd ed. California: Sage Publications; 1997.

5. Perez A, Doloresco F, Hoffman JM, et al, and the American College of Clinical Pharmacy. ACCP: economic evaluations of clinical pharmacy services: 2001–2005. Pharmacotherapy. 2009;29(1):128. http://dx.doi.org/10.1592/phco.29.1.128. Medline:19113803

6. Nkansah N, Mostovetsky O, Yu C, et al. Effect of outpatient pharmacists' non-dispensing roles on patient outcomes and prescribing patterns. Cochrane Database Syst Rev. 2010;(7):CD000336. Medline:20614422

7. Stewart K, George J, Mc Namara KP, et al. A multifaceted pharmacist intervention to improve antihypertensive adherence: a cluster-randomized, controlled trial (HAPPy trial). J Clin Pharm Ther. 2014;39(5):527–34. http://dx.doi.org/10.1111/jcpt.12185. Medline:24943987

8. Hollander MJ, Miller JA, Kadlec H. Evaluation of healthcare services: asking the right questions to develop new policy and program-relevant knowledge for decision-making. Healthc Q. 2010;13(4):40–7. http://dx.doi.org/10.12927/hcq.2013.21997. Medline:24953808

9. Creswell JW, Fetters MD, Ivankova NV. Designing a mixed methods study in primary care. Ann Fam Med. 2004;2(1):7–12. http://dx.doi.org/10.1370/afm.104. Medline:15053277

10. Frechtling J, Sharp L. User-friendly handbook for mixed methods evaluations. Arlington, VA: National Science Foundation; 1997. Available: www.nsf.gov/pubs/1997/nsf97153/start.htm [cited Dec. 1, 2014].

11. Kozma CM, Reeder CE, Schulz RM. Economic, clinical, and humanistic outcomes: a planning model for pharmacoeconomic research. Clin Ther. 1993;15(6):1121–32, discussion 1120. Medline:8111809

12. Tsao NW, Shaske J. PhINDMORE: Pharmacist Innovative Drug Therapy Management, Outcomes, Resource Use, and Economics. Canadian Pharmacists Association Annual Conference; June 1, 2014; Saskatoon, SK.

X. ORGANIZATIONAL, BUSINESS AND PROFESSIONAL COMMUNICATIONS

CHAPTER 42

An Introduction to Pharmacist Communications, Communication Models and Theories

Lisa M. Guirguis, *BSc Pharm, MSc, PhD; Associate Professor, Faculty of Pharmacy and Pharmaceutical Sciences, University of Alberta*

Learning Objectives

- Review basic purposes of communication.
- Understand why it is important for pharmacists to have strong communication skills from both a patient and business perspective.
- Explore the communication process model.
- Investigate various communication channels.
- Gain an appreciation for communication barriers and facilitators.
- Explore communication models in pharmacy.

BASIC PURPOSES OF COMMUNICATION

While not one theory can be said to be applicable for all forms of communication, understanding and appreciating different communication models and theories can help one become a better communicator. Just because an opinion has been stated or an email sent, it does not mean communication has occurred. Communication is the process that occurs when information is transmitted and understood between two or more people. Communication has many functions including the transmission of information and means for connection in society. To communicate and be heard is necessary to people's health and well-being, not just useful words on how to take a medication effectively, but to be recognized as a part of society.

Communication is more than the words and ideas people wish to share; the process of communication portrays who they are to the world. Many people have experienced saying something out loud and being surprised by the emotion conveyed. This is because the process of communicating helps to clarify thought and create meaning. The purpose of writing is not only to *record* what a person knows, but the process of writing helps to *illuminate* what the person knows. Similarly, it is through the process of talking through a problem with a friend that someone finds a solution. The friend may say very little, but the process of communicating can help a person find answers that could not be identified before.

WHY IT IS IMPORTANT FOR PHARMACISTS TO DEVELOP STRONG COMMUNICATION SKILLS

Some lucky people are born natural communicators and have strong communication skills. Others can develop effective communications skills. There is strong evidence that communication skills can be taught in medication and pharmacy training. The real question is, why take time to develop these skills?

More than one in nine emergency department visits are due to drug-related problems.[1] Pharmacists have the privileged role of providing important medication and health information to patients. Information must be shared in such a way that all patients understand how to safely use their medications. Pharmacists have a tremendous role to help fill this gap. Still, the importance of communication does not end there.

Communication itself has a therapeutic role. While the research is not available in pharmacy yet, the medication literature has established that the quality of a physician's communication skills has an independent impact on patient health including emotional health, symptom resolution, function, physiologic measures (e.g., blood pressure and blood glucose level) and pain control.[2] Following that evidence, strong communication skills in pharmacy help to build patient relationships that may also have positive physical and psychological impact on patient health. Strong communication skills also allow pharmacists to gather a more thorough medication history by being attentive to patient cues, asking inviting questions and building trust with the patient. The resulting patient history increases the opportunity to identify and solve problems for patients.

Communication skills affect patient satisfaction with pharmacy services.[3] Patients who are satisfied are more likely to build relationships and remain loyal to one pharmacy. This makes for both good patient health and strong business for pharmacists.

Pharmacists can realize other tangible benefits. Communication skills such as listening and empathy have been shown in physicians to reduce malpractice lawsuits.[4] One could extrapolate that this would be similar for pharmacists. Strong communications can reduce friction with patients, colleagues, staff and other health care professionals, creating a more positive work environment. As the professional scope of practice evolves, pharmacists must effectively communicate the business case to stakeholders, including bank managers, accountants and pharmacy owners, on why they should invest in services as well as consider new strategies for patient engagement. All of these can increase pharmacists' effectiveness and support career satisfaction.

The question in the current educational literature is not about teaching communications skills, but how to incorporate communication teaching into patient care and management processes.[5] Skills should not be taught in isolation but in conjunction with teaching on patient care and management with realistic experiences.

EXPLORE THE COMMUNICATION PROCESS MODEL

A basic understanding of the communication process model can help people understand how to improve their communication skills. Table 1 has two examples of a typical situation in a

Table 1. The Communication Process Model – Patient Conversation

Conversation 1: Transmission	Conversation 2: Transaction
Pharmacist: This antibiotic, amoxicillin, is effective for most infections in the head and chest.	Pharmacist: I see you have an antibiotic, amoxicillin. What type of infection do you have?
Patient: [nods]	Patient: The doc called and I have strep throat.
Pharmacist: Please take one pill three times a day. It is best to space it out while you are awake. If you get an upset stomach, please take with some food, like a snack or even milk. This antibiotic can take up to three days to start working.	Pharmacist: Amoxicillin can help take care of that. Are you familiar with how to take it?
Patient: Uh huh.	Patient: Yep, three a day with breakfast, afternoon and bed plus food helps my stomach for the first few days until I get used to it.
Pharmacist: Please make sure you take the entire 10 days even though you might feel better sooner. This can help prevent your infection from coming back. Also, if you don't kill all the bugs by taking all 10 days, the medication might not work next time.	Pharmacist: Right. You've done this before. Were you able to finish all the pills last time?
Patient: 'kay.	Patient: I had strep last month and I felt better in a few days, so no, I didn't. Pharmacist: You might be less likely to get strep again if you finish all the pills, even if it takes a few extra days. Patient: I like that idea. I will give it a try.

pharmacy. Both conversations are between a pharmacist and a patient who is picking up a prescription for amoxicillin for strep throat. In both scenarios, the pharmacist provides information about the medication, but the conversations are quite different. The Communication Process Model can explain the difference in the conversations found in Tables 1 and 2. In conversation 1, the pharmacist uses the *transmission model* and is focused on providing the information in a one-way direction to the patient. Unless the patient is motivated to interrupt the pharmacist, the pharmacist will continue to provide the required information. In conversation 2, the pharmacist is demonstrating a *transaction model* of communication where the conversation is a two-way street where the message is sent, received by the patient and feedback is provided before the pharmacist moves to providing the next information. In the transactional model, patient and pharmacist are aware of the communication context, both present and past.[6] The pharmacist and patient each have prior pharmacy experience, which guides them on how the conversation will proceed, yet the content of the current conversation also informs the interaction.

The same information is covered in both interactions with one exception. In conversation 1, the pharmacist mentions that not taking the antibiotics may cause bacterial resistance; however, in conversation 2 this information is not necessary as the patient appears personally motivated to finish the antibiotic to prevent reoccurrence. In order for this to occur, the pharmacist in conversation 2 uncovered the patient's prior medication use and prior experiences and then used this information to tailor the conversation.

Table 2. The Communication Process Model – Promoting Pharmacy Smoking Cessation Services

Conversation 3: Transmission	Conversation 4: Transaction
Pharmacist: I would like to tell you about our smoking cessation service.	Pharmacist: I'd like to see if our Stop Smoking Now program might be of help to you.
Business Owner: [nods]	Business Owner: [nods]
Pharmacist: Our Stop Smoking Now program combines pharmacist coaching, medications and nicotine replacement to help your employees quit smoking. We offer six sessions over a six-month time period with a combination of group and individual meetings.	Pharmacist: Are you concerned about employees' sick days? Why?
Business Owner: Uh huh.	Business Owner: Yep, sick days are a big cost to me and my employees seem to be taking more and more days each year.
Pharmacist: The sessions are customized to your employees and tailored to their needs. First, we offer a general overview with compelling reasons to quit. We find that about 10% of smokers may be willing to try quitting. Our pharmacists will then meet with them one-on-one to explore benefits and set goals. I think we can really help your employees.	Pharmacist: I hear it can be expensive. Our program has helped six other companies reduce sick days by 10%.
Business Owner: It's my busy season right now and I can't spare the time. Maybe later.	Business Owner: Impressive. Still, how long does it last? Won't everyone just start smoking again? Pharmacist: You are right that relapse is common. That's why we offer the program free for any relapse within 18 months. Business Owner: I like that idea. Tell me a bit more about your program. I think it might help me out, especially as the busy season is here.

The same skills can be applied in organizational communication (see Table 2). In business, a pharmacist may present a business plan on the provision of a new smoking cessation service to a local business owner using the transmission mode whereby the pharmacist prepares and delivers information about the program as in conversation 3. The pharmacist may also prepare an interactive discussion that engages the owner in sharing concerns and insights on this model as in conversation 4, which may in turn increase likelihood of acceptance.

Shah and Chewning reviewed the pharmacy literature to identify the use of transmission and transaction models in research on patient-pharmacist communication.[6] They found that approximately half of the studies used the transmission model with the pharmacist providing the information, 40% partially used the transactional model by looking at how the information was conveyed to patients and 10% fully used the transactional model by looking at pharmacist and patient contributions to the conversation.[6] A literature review of pharmacist communication styles in their management roles is not available; however, it is likely that pharmacists may continue to use a transmission mode if this is their dominant communication style.

A third, less commonly used, model is the *ritual model* in which individuals communicate using shared patterns. For example, the most common response to, "How are you doing?" is "Fine." This is often stated even when an individual is not doing well. In pharmacy, there are common ritual phrases that are used. Examples include, "Have you had this before?" or "Any questions?" to which the patient replies yes or no in an automatic fashion.[6] The risk of ritualistic communication is that true experiences may be left behind. On the managerial side, pharmacists often have communication rituals as well. When presented with ideals for new workflow or patient care roles, pharmacists often say, "No, we do not have time for that," before they even consider the potential benefits of a new service. A manager needs to be aware of the ritualistic "no" and be prepared to open dialogue before introducing new ideas.

With the advent of social media and Web 2.0, public transactional communication is more the norm now. Even as recently at the early 2000s, the majority of news was received in transmission mode via websites, radio, television or newspapers. The audience could respond via formal letters or telephone calls, but their participation was limited. Currently, it is common to engage in responding to and passing on news through social media and becoming a part of the story. This fundamental change in communication from a transmission to transaction response to events will have implications for communication with pharmacists. Patients, accountants, lawyers, bank managers, loan officers, city officials (e.g., economic development office) and politicians will expect to engage with pharmacists in two-way dialogue about the implications of new business/ practice models.

INVESTIGATE COMMUNICATION CHANNELS

A communication channel is the mode by which a message is transmitted from one person to another. Examples include in person, fax, telephone, video, written and electronic communication such as text messaging. Often, the choice of communication channels is obvious such as talking with the person one-on-one when physically together in the same place. Other times, a channel must be consciously selected and this choice can influence the success of the message. For example, a community pharmacist has options when contacting a physician to recommend a change in medication therapy. A pharmacist could fax a written recommendation or telephone the physician if the situation is more urgent or requires a discussion. Pharmacists might find that the phone calls result in a higher level of acceptance though the trade-off is more time spent in reaching the physician and greater risk of a confrontation.

Patient-pharmacist communication is traditionally verbal, either in person or on the phone. Yet in today's world, many patients may conduct a significant part of their communication via email or text. Due to privacy concerns, email and text are not commonly used as communication channels in health care. Though examples are available of pharmacists using video conferencing and remote dispensing kiosks,[7] it is not clear what impact these have on the patient relationships or medication-related outcomes. Electronic communication has been more widely accepted for some elements of pharmacy practice. Patients often order refills online or via a smart phone app[8]; however, these systems are designed for one-way transmission of information from patient to pharmacist. A novel communication channel is remote patient monitoring whereby patients' devices such as blood pressure meters, insulin pumps or smart pill vials communicate monitoring data directly to the pharmacist.[8] This information can then trigger the pharmacist to contact the patient as needed. New business models such as these are needed to understand the financial implications of these emerging communication channels.

Another relatively new channel for interprofessional communication is the electronic health record (EHR). Currently, this system (available in many provinces/territories) allows pharmacists, physicians, nurses and other hospital staff to view elements such as medication history, hospital discharges and laboratory values (dependent upon provincial policies). Future uses may allow pharmacists and physicians to communicate about patients as part of the medical record. To learn more about electronic health records, please refer to Canada Health Infoway, a national organization charged with supporting the development and integration of health care systems information in Canada.

COMMUNICATION MODELS IN PHARMACY

In pharmacy, there have been several patient care models such as counselling, pharmaceutical care, medication therapy management and most recently, patient care. While these models include elements of pharmacist communication that are outlined in most pharmacotherapy or patient care texts, they are not comparable to the specific skills frameworks outlined in the physician communication models such as Calgary Cambridge,[9] Four Habits[10] and a model for shared decision making in clinical practice.[11] Two specific skills that have been promoted are the WWHAM and the Three Prime Questions. WWHAM is a mnemonic for what information to gather in non-prescription consults: who is the patient, what are the symptoms, how long have the symptoms been present, action taken and medication being taken.[12] The Three Prime Questions outlines three questions that assess the patients' knowledge and experience with medications. They are three open-ended questions about purpose, directions and monitoring.[13] While pharmacists are encouraged to tailor their own questions, typical examples of questions are as follows: What is this medication used for? How are you going to take it? How will you know it is working? Pharmacist-specific communication texts by Berger,[14] Rantucci[15] and Beardsley, Kimberlin and Tindall[16] provide pharmacist-specific communication skills for exploring medication adherence and taking medication histories.

Evidence-based pharmacy-specific communication models are emerging and may warrant attention in the future. The Alberta College of Pharmacists employs the Chat, Check and Chart model that integrates the three prime questions into routine patient care in community pharmacies.[17] The Canadian Pharmacists Association (CPhA) and the Blueprint for Pharmacy funded the development of the Connect and CARE model that examines practical skills for community pharmacists to develop patient-pharmacist relationships.[18] Finally, Guirguis and Johnson are exploring the application of vital behaviours for pharmacist-patient engagement in community pharmacy practice.[19]

Management communication requires similar skills to those in patient care. When proposing a practice change idea, training new staff or negotiating a new contract, it is beneficial to open a dialogue and take time to explore the understanding of the other party to effectively adapt the message. Sharing concerns or objections early in a new venture helps with anticipating issues and designing mitigation strategies. Furthermore, the public, other health care providers and business partners often view pharmacy as a consumer good, believing it is the patient's role to seek out pharmacy services, negating pharmacists' role to assessment medication appropriateness for public safety.

Perceptions of paternalistic communication may also occur and stifle forward movement in the pharmacy profession. Some pharmacists may feel managers dictate how to practise pharmacy, managers may feel owners are the ones directing practice and in turn, owners may feel constrained by the standards of practice or government policies. An awareness of this cascade of paternalism may help identify opportunities for improvements at each level.

GAIN AN APPRECIATION FOR COMMUNICATION BARRIERS AND FACILITATORS

Many people have been to a restaurant that was too noisy to allow for easy conversation or had a lecture from a novice instructor who was too nervous to make eye contact. To fully understand messages, the restaurant noise would have to be reduced or the instructor's confidence increased. Similarly, in pharmacy practice, identifying barriers helps pharmacists remove or develop strategies to minimize their impact on conversations with patients.

Physical barriers to patient-pharmacist communication include factors such as ambient noise levels, pharmacy layout and lighting.[20] Community pharmacies offer limited privacy despite visual barriers such as walls between consult windows.[21] One study of 282 pharmacist-patient consultations found most were audible at 2 metres and just over half at 4.5 metres.[22] Drive-through pharmacies may have the potential to offer additional privacy and convenience to patients, but an observation of more than 2,000 interactions showed patients using a drive-through window received less information than those who went into the pharmacy.[23] While individual pharmacists may have suggestions for improvements, it may be hard for individuals to change the physical layout of the pharmacy. Still, pharmacists can change the placement of computers or displays to improve eye contact with patients. A small change may have a profound impact on a pharmacist's ability to engage with patients.

Most pharmacists identify time and money as the two most frequent practice barriers to patient communication. Pharmacists, similar to other health care professionals, state they have insufficient time with patients. Research has consistently shown that pharmacists spend more time on technical dispensing than on communication and other patient care activities.[24] As the majority of pharmacists are employees and reimbursement for prescription and services is directed to the pharmacy, more money may not always represent financial gain for the individual pharmacist and, therefore, is not likely a motivator. Money may be intertwined with time; potential increase in reimbursement for the pharmacy may allow for improved staffing and, subsequently, more time with patients.

Interestingly, one study found that while pharmacists named time as the barrier to an intervention, that intervention only took seconds per patient. When explored further, the barrier was the challenge of changing routines without a clear understanding of benefit.[25] Pharmacists sometimes have options of reducing technical work to focus on patients. On the other hand, effective communication skills can help pharmacists to effectively use the time they currently have with patients.

Pharmacists have identified themselves as barriers to effective communication; to be a bit more specific, pharmacists have named their beliefs, lack of self-confidence and routines as barriers.[26] Pharmacists who believe that patient interactions are a part of their jobs are more likely to make time for these activities. Self-confidence (i.e., self-efficacy) is the best predictor of pharmacist behaviour with respect to patient engagement. Pharmacists have frequently stated they lack confidence in their skill to engage in patient interactions.[27] Finally, pharmacists have established routines to keep their patients safe while working in a fast-paced environment, and it takes a conscious effort to alter routines. To facilitate change, pharmacists have identified strategies to start with small focused changes such as asking one new question at new prescriptions, working with others in the pharmacy, keeping it simple and personalizing their approaches.[17]

Patients with communication barriers such as physical disabilities or severe mental health issues are more likely to a have an emergency department visit due to a medication problem.[1] Other patient challenges include low health literacy or not speaking the same language as the pharmacist (see Chapter 44: Communicating with Your Patients and Across Cultures).

Patients generally have low expectation for pharmacists' roles. Research suggests patients perceive that pharmacists' roles are to provide information on medication directions, side effects and adverse events and were less familiar with more in-depth communication.[28–30] In fact, patients who incidentally include policy makers, accountants and lawyers are not familiar with the pharmacist in a proactive or patient-centred role.[31,32] Provincial associations and colleges have begun campaigns to improve public awareness of pharmacist services. Individual pharmacists have the role of delivering on those services with strong communication skills to ensure patients have consistent positive experiences with pharmacists and increase their expectations for future pharmacy services. In the new pharmacy environment, patient care services are the new revenue streams. As patient expectations for services increase, pharmacists will facilitate the shift to a patient-centred, as opposed to a tangible product-centred, business model. The business and patient care models have overlapped.

Awareness of communication barriers, models and channels are a foundation to help build communication knowledge and skills. It is highly unlikely that patients knowingly take their pharmacy business to a location with a transactional style without any physical or practice barriers. However, in the crowded pharmacy marketplace, patients will gravitate toward pharmacists who listen and respond to their concerns. Similarly, two-way communication models can help pharmacists effectively share new practice ideas and business models with pharmacy staff, business people and other health care providers, as well as handle their concerns and potential objections.

REFERENCES

1. Samoy LJ, Zed PJ, Wilbur K, et al. Drug-related hospitalizations in a tertiary care internal medicine service of a Canadian hospital: a prospective study. Pharmacotherapy. 2006;26(11):1578–86. http://dx.doi.org/10.1592/phco.26.11.1578. Medline:17064202

2. Stewart MA. Effective physician-patient communication and health outcomes: a review. CMAJ. 1995;152(9):1423–33. Medline:7728691

3. Paluck EC, Green LW, Frankish CJ, et al. Assessment of communication barriers in community pharmacies. Eval Health Prof. 2003;26(4):380–403. http://dx.doi.org/10.1177/0163278703258104. Medline:14631610

4. Levinson W, Roter DL, Mullooly JP, et al. Physician-patient communication. The relationship with malpractice claims among primary care physicians and surgeons. JAMA. 1997;277(7):553–9. http://dx.doi.org/10.1001/jama.1997.03540310051034. Medline:9032162

5. Skelton JR. Everything you were afraid to ask about communication skills. Br J Gen Pract. 2005;55(510):40–6. Medline:15667765

6. Shah B, Chewning B. Conceptualizing and measuring pharmacist-patient communication: a review of published studies. Res Social Adm Pharm. 2006;2(2):153–85. http://dx.doi.org/10.1016/j.sapharm.2006.05.001. Medline:17138507

7. Notes section. Automated medication dispensary with remote pharmacist counselling moves into the marketplace. Can Pharm J. 2009;142(1):13. http://dx.doi.org/10.3821/1913-701X-142.1.13.

8. Bartolini EZ, Hubbard T. Community pharmacies meet mobile technologies: a whole new world of opportunity. US Pharm. 2013;38(8):43–50.

9. Kurtz S, Silverman J, Benson J, et al. Marrying content and process in clinical method teaching: enhancing the Calgary -Cambridge guides. Acad Med. 2003;78(8):802–9. http://dx.doi.org/10.1097/00001888-200308000-00011. Medline:12915371

10. Frankel RM, Stein T. Getting the most out of the clinical encounter: the four habits model. Perm J. 1999;3(3):79–88.

11. Elwyn G, Frosch D, Thomson R, et al. Shared decision making: a model for clinical practice. J Gen Intern Med. 2012;27(10):1361–7. http://dx.doi.org/10.1007/s11606-012-2077-6. Medline:22618581

12. Watson MC, Bond CM, and the Grampian Evidence Based Community Pharmacy Guidelines Group. Evidence-based guide- lines for non-prescription treatment of vulvovaginal candidiasis (VVC). Pharm World Sci. 2003;25(4):129–34. http://dx.doi. org/10.1023/A:1024819515862. Medline:12964489

13. Smith CP, Christensen DB. Identification and clarification of drug therapy problems by Indian health service pharmacists. Ann Pharmacother. 1996;30(2):119–24. Medline:8835041

14. Berger BA. Communication skills for pharmacists: Building relationships, improving care. 3rd ed. Washington, DC: American Pharmaceutical Association; 2009.

15. Rantucci MJ. Pharmacists talking with patients: A guide to patient counseling. 2nd ed. Philadelphia: Lippincott Williams & Wilkins; 2007.

16. Beardsley RS, Kimberlin CL, Tindall WN. Communication skills in pharmacy practice. 5th ed. Philadelphia: Lippincott, Williams & Wilkins; 2007.

17. Guirguis LM, Lee S. Patient assessment and documentation integrated in community practice: chat, check and chart. J Am Pharm Assoc. 2012;52(6):e241–51. http://dx.doi.org/10.1331/JAPhA.2012.12097.

18. Guirguis LM, Johnson S, Emberley P. Pharmacists Connect and CARE: Transforming pharmacy customers into patients. Can Pharm J (Ott). 2014;147(3):149–53. http://dx.doi.org/10.1177/1715163514530098. Medline:24847366

19. Pharmacist Patient Engagement Initiative. Vital behaviours for patient engagement. Available: www.ppei.org/vital -behaviours (accessed Nov. 17, 2014).

20. Grissinger M. Physical environments that promote safe medication use. P T. 2012;37(7):377–8. Medline:22876099

21. Mobach MP. Counter design influences the privacy of patients in health care. Soc Sci Med. 2009;68(6):1000–5. http://dx.doi. org/10.1016/j.socscimed.2008.12.002. Medline:19152994

22. Bednarczyk RA, Nadeau JA, Davis CF, et al. Privacy in the pharmacy environment: analysis of observations from inside the pharmacy. J Am Pharm Assoc (2003). 2010;50(3):362–7. http://dx.doi.org/10.1331/JAPhA.2010.09001. Medline:20452909

23. Odukoya OK, Chui MA, Pu J. Factors influencing quality of patient interaction at community pharmacy drive-through and walk-in counselling areas. Int J Pharm Pract. 2014;22(4):246–56. http://dx.doi.org/10.1111/ijpp.12073. Medline:24164213

24. Davies JE, Barber N, Taylor D. What do community pharmacists do? Results from a work sampling study in London. Int J Pharm Pract. 2014;22(5):309–18. http://dx.doi.org/10.1111/ijpp.12083. Medline:24423212

25. Cvijovic K, Boon H, Jaeger W, et al. Pharmacists' participation in research: a case of trying to find the time. Int J Pharm Pract. 2010;18(6):377–83. http://dx.doi.org/10.1111/j.2042-7174.2010.00067.x. Medline:21054599

26. Guirguis LM. Mixed methods evaluation: pharmacists' experiences and beliefs toward an interactive communication approach to patient interactions. Patient Educ Couns. 2011;83(3):432–42. http://dx.doi.org/10.1016/j.pec.2011.04.038. Medline:21632196

27. Makowsky MJ, Guirguis LM, Hughes CA, et al. Factors influencing pharmacists' adoption of prescribing: qualitative appli- cation of the diffusion of innovations theory. Implement Sci. 2013;8(1):109. http://dx.doi.org/10.1186/1748-5908-8-109. Medline:24034176

28. Krueger JL, Hermansen-Kobulnicky CJ. Patient perspective of medication information desired and barriers to asking pharmacists questions. J Am Pharm Assoc (2003). 2011;51(4):510–9. http://dx.doi.org/10.1331/JAPhA.2011.10069. Medline:21752774

29. Perepelkin J. Public opinion of pharmacists and pharmacist prescribing. Can Pharm J. 2011;144(2):86–93. http://dx.doi. org/10.3821/1913-701X-144.2.86.

30. Naik Panvelkar P, Armour C, Saini B. Community pharmacy-based asthma services: what do patients prefer? J Asthma. 2010;47(10):1085–93. http://dx.doi.org/10.3109/02770903.2010.514638. Medline:21039206

31. McMillan SS, Kelly F, Adem S, et al. Consumer and carer views of Australian community pharmacy practice: awareness, experi- ences and expectations. J Pharm Health Ser Res. 2014;5(1):29–36. http://dx.doi.org/10.1111/jphs.12043.

32. Gidman W, Cowley J. A qualitative exploration of opinions on the community pharmacists' role amongst the general public in Scotland. Int J Pharm Pract. 2013;21(5):288–96. http://dx.doi.org/10.1111/ijpp.12008. Medline:23418884

CHAPTER 43

Communicating with Pharmacy Employees

Jason Perepelkin, *BA, BComm, MSc, PhD; Assistant Professor of Social and Administrative Pharmacy, University of Saskatchewan*

Learning Objectives

- Consider how communicating with another pharmacist differs from how one communicates with other members of the pharmacy team.
- Examine the role of feedback in a pharmacy team setting.
- Discuss how multigenerational differences among pharmacy employees can affect communication.

How individuals communicate with others, whether as a professional or with friends and family, is affected by the process of communication, the medium/methods used, the environment in which the communication occurs and other factors. When examining communication among the pharmacy team, there are many additional considerations to be made as this team is likely made up of individuals with diverse backgrounds, whether culturally (see Chapter 44: Communicating with Your Patients and Across Cultures), where one's formal education was received, or the generation to which they belong.

Managers will communicate with their employees for a variety of reasons including to relay information (knowledge management), coordinate activities, create and maintain records and send effective messages. Another key task of a manager's role is to provide feedback to employees to encourage or guide learning and motivate employees. By providing feedback to employees, one can adjust the way in which the employees practise, as well as reinforce aspects that an employee does well. If there are no formal mechanisms for managers to communicate with and provide feedback for employees, informal communication and feedback will likely occur, but it is more likely to take on a negative connotation.

Feedback received about one's behaviour, whether positive or negative, is important for managers and pharmacists, as well as other members of the pharmacy team, to have a productive, enjoyable practice. There are four levels and three types or forms of feedback.[1]

LEVELS OF FEEDBACK

Feedback can focus on an individual or group centring on a specific task or procedure. *Task and procedural* feedback centres on how effectively and appropriately the individual or group performed on a given task or procedure.[1] For example, how did an individual or group perform when conducting a diabetes management clinic for patients who have been newly diagnosed with Type 2 diabetes? The focus is on whether the procedure used was the appropriate one for the given task, in this case the diabetes management clinic.

The second level is *relational* feedback and focuses on the interpersonal dynamics within a group, centring on how well members of a group get along while completing a task.[1] Building on the previous example, this type of feedback would be how members of the pharmacy team worked together when planning for and conducting the diabetes management clinic.

With *individual* feedback, the focus is on a specific individual within a group.[1] For example, did the Certified Diabetes Educator pharmacist provide useful skills and work well with others as a member of the team conducting the diabetes management clinic?

The final level is *group* feedback and focuses on how well the group as a whole is performing.[1] In assessing whether the group achieved the goals for the clinic, a manager may provide feedback to the entire group and use that feedback, and the feedback he/she receives from that session, to assess whether the team should remain as is or be changed.

TYPES OR FORMS OF FEEDBACK

Building on the four levels of feedback highlighted, there are three types or forms of feedback. The first is *descriptive* feedback, which identifies or describes how a person communicates.[1] For example, a manager may say that a co-worker was quiet while communicating with a patient and was difficult to hear. This is a description of the co-worker's communication with a patient.

The second type is *evaluative* feedback.[1] It focuses on evaluating how an individual communicates. For example, building on the previous descriptive feedback, the manager may say that the co-worker was very thorough when counselling a patient and the quiet voice, while hard to hear, created a relaxed environment for the patient.

The final type is *prescriptive*, or feedback that on top of being descriptive and evaluative also provides advice about how one should behave or communicate or how one can improve communication skills.[1] Building on the examples, the manager may advise the co-worker to speak louder to ensure the patient can hear and ask the co-worker to try to look the patient in the eyes more often and not just focus on the prescription vial when counselling on a new medication.

The key in any feedback with regard to communication is to ensure that it is not viewed as a negative process, but rather a process in which people can learn and grow their communication skills. When people take the objective structured clinical exams (OSCE), they receive feedback on how the entire session went, not to be negative but to let them know where they did well and where they can improve.

THE JOHARI WINDOW

The Johari Window model improves an individual's communication skills through identifying one's capabilities and limitations.[2]

Window 1 is the open area in which information about a person is known both to that person and to others.[2] For instance, at an office party, the manager reveals to co-workers that the manager does not drink alcohol due to health reasons; the manager is open about this and communicates it so that others know the reason.

Window 2 refers to a blind area in which others know information about someone that the person is either unaware of or does unknowingly.[2] As an example, colleagues know that a particular individual is a close talker—that this individual unconsciously stands too close to people while in conversation with others. Depending on the level of comfort with this individual, one may want to make the person aware of it explicitly (stating it face-to-face) or implicitly, perhaps by sending the person a YouTube clip of the Seinfeld episode ("Raincoats") when Elaine's new boyfriend is a close talker.

Window 3 is the hidden area in which someone has likes and dislikes that the person is unwilling to share with others.[2] This area includes values, beliefs, fears and past experiences that the person would not wish to reveal. It is not that the person will never reveal something in this area, but chooses not to reveal it.

Window 4, the last windowpane, is the unknown. It is also an area of potential growth or self-actualization.[2] It represents all the things people have never tried, participated in or experienced. For example, someone may have a fear of public speaking, like many people, and prefer not to talk in front of a group of people at all costs; however, colleagues encourage the person to try presenting on smoking cessation at a local retirement community.

As one grows as an individual and practitioner, it will be easier to increase the open area (Window 1) and reduce Windows 2 to 4.[2] By seeking feedback from colleagues, they will be more likely to help by providing feedback that will improve communication skills, whether it is with colleagues, patients, other health care professionals or even in someone's personal life. Fostering an open communication environment and providing constructive feedback can increase the morale and productivity of employees.

Figure 43.1

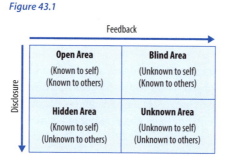

The Johari Window[2]

COMMUNICATION BARRIERS

Communication channels are the means by which messages are transmitted (see Chapter 42: An Introduction to Pharmacist Communications, Communication Models and Theories). It is key to examine barriers that may arise and/or are present when communicating with pharmacy employees. Generally, there are two main forms of barriers to consider: environmental and personal barriers.

Environmental barriers exist due to the characteristics of the organization (e.g., community pharmacy, hospital pharmacy, primary care site) and the environment itself. For example, in a community pharmacy, it is not uncommon for communication to occur among colleagues solely based on the log book, in which messages are written and shared. While this may help communicate some information, patient care can be quite complex, and simply writing down a note for others to read—not even considering whether they will or will not read it—can lead to errors. However, it may not be feasible to have regular staff/team meetings, so as some may say it's better than nothing!

When considering environmental barriers that may exist in hospital practice, the size of the department and the health region as a whole can mean that information is transmitted but may not be received and, therefore, communication does not occur. This is complicated further when considering hospital pharmacists working on different wards in a hospital and the need to communicate with colleagues down in the pharmacy, as well as with other members of the care team and the patient.

Personal barriers exist due to the nature of the individual and one's interaction with others, and not just colleagues but interactions with anyone, including family and friends. For example, one may be having a bad day where nothing seems to go right, and that mental drain can cause personal barriers to rise and exacerbate the problem.

All is not lost when it comes to environmental and personal barriers; following are five ways they can be overcome. First, give time and attention to help facilitate communication. If employees know there are formal mechanisms in place for communication and feedback, they are more likely to be engaged in the organization and even if personal barriers are in place, it is less likely that they will be detrimental.

Another way to overcome barriers is to encourage free flow of communication; in essence, allow communication to happen among all team members. This leads directly into the next method, which is to reduce the number of links through which a message has to be communicated. As the number of times a message is communicated increases, so too is the increased likelihood that the original intended message differs from the one communicated at the end.

Following the reduction in links, removing the power/status barrier among employees can encourage communication and remove barriers. The final way to overcome barriers is to consider the message and its importance. Multiple channels may have to be used to ensure a message is received. For example, if a pharmacist needs to communicate about a patient that is on a complex drug regime, simply writing a note in a log book is not likely to convey the message properly; therefore, it is best that the pharmacist uses multiple channels to communicate—perhaps a phone call to a colleague, an email or if possible, visiting a colleague to discuss the patient face-to-face.

MULTIGENERATIONAL COMMUNICATION

An area of communication that may be missed by some is that of communicating with colleagues of a different generation. While most people understand language barriers and even cultural barriers, communicating with colleagues of a different generation can result in miscommunication that can lead to other issues, such as misinterpreted feedback, not completing a prescription check, etc.

Chances are that pharmacists will work with colleagues from two to three generations that are different from their own. Because of the life events and experiences of colleagues from different generations, the methods of communication used may differ. The following four generations exist in the workforce currently: Traditionalists, Baby Boomers, Generation X and Generation Y (or Millennials).[3-5] It is important to keep in mind that the characteristics of the individuals within these generations are generalized and, as such, some may not fit nicely into one generation despite their birth date.

While many have exited the workforce, Traditionalists are still practising across Canada. Traditionalists are those born between 1922 and 1945 and are known to have a strong sense of duty, sacrifice and loyalty toward people, institutions and governments.[4,5] As a result, they are more likely to have remained with one employer over their career and believe promotion and recognition come from the length of time one has committed to an organization.[4,5]

Baby Boomers are the second generation currently in the workforce and were born between 1946 and 1964. A large percentage of the population falls within this generation, especially as they begin to retire and require more health care.[4,5] In essence, Baby Boomers are in control as they run government and organizations and are managers and CEOs; they tend to believe in teamwork and relationship building, and many are skeptical of technology.[4,5] Many can be described as workaholics and measure work ethic on how many hours one works.

The third generation, those born between 1965 and 1980, are Generation X. This generation tends to be skeptical of authority and as a result, are cautious with their commitments.[4,5] Generation X tends to be more self-reliant than previous generations and prefers to have options available as opposed to sticking with one employer; control of their time, flexibility and freedom are important. Generation X is the first generation to embrace technology and use it to control various aspects of their life, such as communicating with friends and family, keeping track of their work schedules, etc.[3-5]

The fourth generation is Generation Y, also referred to as the Millennials—those born after 1980.[3-5] This generation is very comfortable with technology—a quick look around a classroom shows this generation embraces it. Generation Y tends to value altruism and has positive can-do attitudes, but expects positive reinforcement from employers. They enjoy being around others, connecting with peers and the material comforts in life.[3-5] As well, Generation Y is the first generation in which individuals will not just take any job; they will spend time searching for an employer that can offer them what they are looking for to have a fulfilling job. Also, Generation Y is more likely to work less than full time and take breaks from their jobs to travel.[3-5]

Communicating with pharmacy employees is not a simple, common-sense endeavour. One needs to consider how to communicate with pharmacy team members and the important role feedback plays in nurturing the team. The Johari Window examines how one may improve personal communication skills, while communication barriers are also aspects to consider in communicating a message. Furthermore, with four generations of pharmacists currently in the workforce, understanding and appreciating the differences of each generation can help one better communicate with colleagues.

RESOURCES AND SUGGESTED READINGS

Borkowski N. ed. Organizational behavior in health care. Jones & Bartlett Learning; 2009.

Brooker C. Pharmacy staff hampered by poor management feedback. March 14, 2012. Available: www.pharmacynews.com.au/news/latest-news/pharmacy-staff-hampered-by-poor-management-feedback (accessed Sept. 18, 2014).

Canadian Pharmacists Association. Leading pharmacy through change management: a toolkit for assessing and supporting practice change. July 2012. Available: http://blueprintforpharmacy.ca/docs/kt-tools/managers-toolkit-form_final2a---august-2012.pdf (accessed Sept. 18, 2014).

Guo KL. Workplace communication. In: Organizational behavior in health care. Borkowski N., ed. Jones & Bartlett Learning; 2009. p. 71–101.

Legas M, Howard Sims C. Leveraging generational diversity in today's workplace. Online Journal for Workforce Education and Development. 2012;5(3):1.

Pozen RC. The delicate art of giving feedback. Harvard Business Review Blog Network. March 28, 2013. Available: http://blogs.hbr.org/2013/03/the-delicate-art-of-giving-fee/ (accessed Sept. 18, 2014).

White L, Klinner C. Service quality in community pharmacy: an exploration of determinants. Res Social Adm Pharm. 2012;8(2):122–32. http://dx.doi.org/10.1016/j.sapharm.2011.01.002. Medline:21511541

REFERENCES

1. Keyton J. Communicating in groups: Building relationships for group effectiveness. Oxford University Press; 2006.

2. Luft J, Ingham H. The Johari Window: A graphic model for interpersonal relations. University of California Western Training Lab. *Development, August* (1955).

3. Lester SW, Standifer RL, Schultz NJ, et al. Actual versus perceived generational differences at work: an empirical examination. J Leadersh Organ Stud. 2012;19(3):341–54. http://dx.doi.org/10.1177/1548051812442747.

4. McNamara SA. Incorporating generational diversity. AORN J. 2005;81(6):1149–52. http://dx.doi.org/10.1016/S0001-2092(06)60377-3. Medline:16047984

5. Galt V. Young, old, in-between: Can they all get along? Globe & Mail. (2009). Available: www.theglobeandmail.com/report-on-business/young-old-in-between-can-they-all-get-along/article17996595/ (accessed Sept. 29, 2014).

CHAPTER 44

Communicating with Your Patients and Across Cultures

Kyle John Wilby, *BSP, ACPR, PharmD; Assistant Professor, College of Pharmacy, Qatar University*

Zubin Austin, *BScPhm, MBA, MISc, PhD; Professor, Leslie Dan Faculty of Pharmacy, University of Toronto*

Learning Objectives

- Discuss the practical importance and ethical implications of cultural competence in pharmacy practice.
- Apply the iceberg model of cross-cultural competence to pharmacy practice.
- Discuss the importance of effective verbal and non-verbal communication in managing cultural differences in pharmacy practice.
- Describe Hall's model of high- and low-context cultures.
- Reflect upon cultural assumptions, stereotypes and biases that may affect cross-cultural communication and patient care.

Over the past 30 years, Canadian society has become increasingly diverse and inclusive, benefiting from the significant contributions of new Canadians, Aboriginal peoples and members of the lesbian/gay/bisexual/transgender (LGBT) communities.[1]

The evolving nature of Canadian society is reflected in pharmacy practice. Pharmacists, among other professions, work not only with increasingly diverse patients but also with increasingly diverse co-workers.[2–4] Although diversity can ultimately enrich each of us as individuals, there may be circumstances where misunderstandings arise and management of cultural differences (either with staff or patients) may be necessary. Diversity is also known to create racial/ethnic disparity in health care.[5] While the topic of cultural competency is one that could require a textbook of its own, this chapter provides a general overview of major concepts and gives readers strategies regarding management considerations when facing diversity in the workplace.

Communication is becoming increasingly complex as diversity continues to change the demographics of Canadian society. Twenty years ago, it may have been sufficient to provide patients with short verbal counselling points and a handout of important information. However, factors such as language, ethnicity, verbal and non-verbal communication may affect acceptance of the message in modern times.[6,7] Without recognizing and attempting to understand these differences, pharmacists risk destabilizing trust with patients that could ultimately lead to poor patient outcomes.[5,8] The same holds true for relationships with colleagues, staff and other health care professionals. Without establishment and maintenance of trusting relationships, which largely depend on both verbal and non-verbal communication, productivity may decrease, collaboration may be inhibited and patient care may suffer.

A common theme in the literature related to management of cultural difference relates to the importance of self-reflection, self-awareness and self-management.[8] In many cases, human beings may subconsciously perceive "difference" as threatening and, consequently, respond by shunning, ignoring or devaluing the other.[9] In the past, well-intentioned attempts to deal with this response have included development of checklists or algorithms designed to guide behaviour without challenging or reflecting upon the underlying thinking and beliefs that may be producing these responses.[10] Today, there is greater recognition that diversity is not an external issue to be managed or controlled but instead a socialized response to difference that results in subconscious or unconscious emotional reactions that must first be understood before being adapted.[11]

ICEBERG OF CROSS-CULTURAL COMPETENCE

Culture has been described as an iceberg (see Figure 44.1).[12–14] Using this metaphor, only 10% of culture is actually visible at any time while the remainder lies hidden and out of view. Attributes of visible culture are things actually perceived through our senses: the foods we eat, the clothes

Figure 44.1

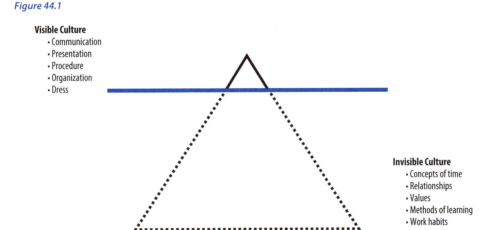

Iceberg Model for Describing the Visible and Non-visible Attributes of Culture (used with permission of Lionel Laroche, PhD)

we wear, the words and gestures we use to communicate, sports we support, etc. The invisible parts of culture may include work habits, our sense of time consciousness, our beliefs about hier-archies and titles, decision-making processes, notion of logic and validity, handling of emotions, religion, etc.

The iceberg model of culture is very relevant to pharmacy practice. When patients present in all types of care settings, practitioners are only aware of a few cultural factors (e.g., language, skin colour, demeanour) that could affect the patients' interpretation of the interaction. For exam-ple, when counselling patients on potential adverse effects of medications, underlying cultural beliefs may put patients at risk of misinterpretation and non-adherence. Many cultural groups also have a mistrust of Western medicine and not addressing it may put patients at risk of harm and negligent care.[15] Pharmacists must be diligent in their dealings with all patients and ensure that opportunities are created for reflection, feedback and advocacy. Pharmacy managers (both community and institutional) have a responsibility to assess population demographics and pro-vide training and support to staff members relating to recognition and effective problem-solving skills when encountering culturally diverse patients.

One particular area of interest for pharmacists is the provision of medications to patients fol-lowing halal, kosher and vegetarian diets.[16] Drug products or excipients may be derived from or contain products from animal sources, including pork. Consumption of these products is not acceptable to many patients worldwide who identify with particular religious beliefs or follow dietary restrictions. Although some products may now be reformulated in acceptable forms, patients may risk non-adherence by actively avoiding them based on previous knowledge.[17] Therefore, open communication between pharmacists and patients with active inquiry regarding dietary constraints is necessary for optimization of care.

CULTURE AND COMMUNICATION

Culture is transmitted in many ways, not the least of which include the verbal and non-verbal communication that occurs in interpersonal settings.[12] The face one presents to others will be, in part, shaped by the multiple cultural groups one belongs to and the prescribed norms of each. Anthropologists have studied communication norms within cultures and noted that even within individual cultures there exist significant variations in what is defined as culturally appropriate.[18] Laroche has described facets of culture that manifest in communication.[12] Many of these are relevant to pharmacy practice and are summarized next.

BOUNDARIES AND PERSONAL SPACE

Everyone has a safety zone. Only those with whom one is truly intimate may cross that zone; those who enter the personal bubble uninvited are frequently felt to be rude, intimidating, hos-tile or a threat. In some cultures, physical closeness may be a norm indicating warmth, interest and psychological connectedness. When those from close cultures interact inappropriately with those from more distant cultures, the emotional feeling of threat that arises may be intellectually translated as discomfort or irritation and eventually, the belief that the other person is different. Conversely, when those from distant cultures interact with those from closer cultures, the emo-tional feeling of aloofness, disinterest or superiority may arise, leading the individual to believe that the other person cannot be trusted.

In relation to boundaries, culture may influence pharmacist-patient interactions in the presence of other people. This is especially true when discussing sensitive topics such as women's health (including contraception), men's health or certain infectious diseases. For example, a female Middle Eastern patient may be averse to speaking about contraception in the presence of her husband or significant other.[19] While the same may be true for other patients, pharmacists should be acutely aware of boundaries and acknowledge both verbal and non-verbal feedback received during counselling sessions.

GESTURES AND BODY LANGUAGE
Personal physical contact, gesticulation, posture and stance all trigger strong emotional responses that may serve to bring people closer or cause them to feel threatened or hostile. In large part, gestures and body language are culturally influenced and socialized behaviours. As with boundaries and personal space, the initial emotional response to non-verbal cues perceived as culturally different may lead to erroneous attributions and stereotyped judgments about others and vice versa.

SENSE OF HUMOUR
Few things bind individuals together more than a shared sense of humour. An inside joke shared among friends signals inclusion, acceptance and membership. Humour, however, is extraordinarily influenced by culture: references to television shows, movie stars, musicians and local celebrities are important parts of what passes for funny in Canada. Individuals who have not had access to that common background may consequently be left out of jokes and unable to participate in banter. This inability marks them as different or outsiders, which may ultimately lead to the judgment that they are boring, uninterested, aloof or diffident. Recognizing the way in which humour shapes social interactions, and the cultural foundation of that humour, should prevent people from drawing sweeping conclusions about others simply because they do not laugh at certain jokes.

DIFFERENT FORMS OF ENGLISH
One need not travel too far in the world to realize how many different variants of spoken English exist. Even within Canada and among Canadian-born and Canadian-educated individuals, considerable regional variation in phraseology exists and subconsciously, people may react or respond to this variation by framing it as inferior or superior, rather than simply different. This may be further compounded in situations where English is not a first, second or even third language. Native English speakers may forget that the language, while somewhat easy to learn to a certain level of use, can be frustratingly complex to master in its entire nuance.

Consider the difference between the words *situation, problem, concern* and *issue*. Semantically, these are all quite similar, yet nuanced speakers of Canadian English immediately recognize that there is hierarchy of emotional significance associated with these terms. When people say they have a problem, it is likely to sound more alarming than if there is only an issue. Similarly, the nuanced differences between *mistake, error* and *boo-boo* may not be immediately clear to someone who speaks English as a third language. Recognizing that fluent Canadian English speakers subconsciously transmit emotion through specific word choices allows one to fit in and be recognized as "us" rather than "them."

The examples noted here are merely illustrative of a broad literature that helps people understand and appreciate the myriad of ways in which culture shapes communication, interpretation and perception. Managing cultural diversity within a professional context requires pharmacists first and foremost to recognize their own preconceptions, stereotypes and biases. When individuals understand their responses to others as being culturally conditioned and subconsciously driven, they are then in a better position to avoid fear or hostility responses and instead regard diversity as simply difference, not a threat.

UNDERSTANDING CULTURAL CONTEXTS

In 1976, Hall proposed that cultures could be characterized according to differences in communication styles by assessing the degree of non-verbal context used in communication.[20] For example, a low-context culture is one that relies on explicit messages (usually verbal) to convey information. Alternatively, a high-context culture is less reliant on the message itself and emphasizes non-verbal communication, preconceived opinions and pre-programmed information to convey meaning. When people from high- and low-context cultures communicate, risk of miscommunication exists due to perceiving the alternative style as threatening.

Japanese, Arab and African cultures are commonly described as high context, whereas North American, Scandinavian and German cultures are described as low context. Consequently, an Arab may perceive the directness of verbal communication from a North American as threatening or insensitive. A North American, however, may become easily frustrated if a colleague from a high-context culture does not readily "get to the point." This discrepancy can easily lead to detrimental effects for pharmacists with patients, colleagues and other health care professionals.

Consider the following scenario: A community pharmacy manager attached to a physician's clinic is required to facilitate and maintain collaborative professional relationships between staff and the clinic employees. The majority of the staff is North American and operates within low-context culture, demonstrated by direct verbal communication with fewer non-verbal cues. However, the clinic has recently recruited five new physicians that operate within high-context cultures and feel threatened when approached directly by staff. Consequently, there is a deterioration of the relationship between the pharmacy and the physician's clinic.

This is not an uncommon situation, especially with the changing demographic profile of physicians, nurses and other health care professionals. It calls for pharmacy managers to have heightened awareness so they can recognize context as an important factor to consider when implementing programs and strategic plans that require effective communication with culturally diverse stakeholders. By doing so, communication may be easier facilitated and unnecessary conflict avoided.

To overcome cultural barriers to communication in pharmacy practice, reflecting upon one's own responses to diversity and truly wanting to engage with another person will frequently result in the best, most authentic outcomes.[21] At the best of times and in monocultural situations, interpersonal communication is complex, nuanced and difficult to navigate. When cultural differences are introduced, the situation may be further complicated. Avoid the temptation of assuming that in situation "x," response "y" should work; communication is rarely that formulaic or simple.

Consider the following scenario: A pharmacist is the owner/manager of a successful pharmacy in a suburban community. Over the past decade, the community has seen significant change, with waves of new Canadians moving in and enlivening the neighbourhood. The pharmacist and pharmacy staff have made specific outreach to ensure all these new Canadians—who, after all, will be new patients and customers—feel welcome. The practice includes multilingual counselling leaflets and links to immigrant settlement agencies, hired multilingual staff, hosted holiday parties and developed other supports. During this time, the response from these new communities has been positive and the business has grown.

One of the long-time staff members, Bob, is a well-respected pharmacist and the owner/manager's friend. Bob and his husband Dave grew up in this community and have lived here their whole lives. When others in the neighbourhood first felt threatened by a surge of new Canadians moving in, Bob and Dave went out of their way to welcome them. Recently, some of these new Canadians have raised concerns about Bob, not in terms of his professionalism or competence, but because of his lifestyle and his marriage to Dave. The owner/manager learns that at least 10 customers have actually shifted their business to another pharmacy because they say they do not "agree" with Bob, even though they like him as a person and respect him as a pharmacist. One customer even tells the owner/manager that unless something is "done" about Bob, other customers may do the same thing.

A situation like this requires reflection. For some the answer is simple: bigotry is bigotry no matter the source and suggesting that Bob is "the problem" is discriminatory. Instead, the owner/manager and the pharmacy staff should seek to help these new Canadians better understand what it means to live in a diverse community and recognize that the sort of unacceptable behaviour they are demonstrating is exactly what Bob and his husband fought against years earlier. For others, there may actually be sympathy and tacit agreement with these perspectives; it is one thing to "tolerate" or "accept" this type of diversity, but quite another to embrace it so fully. Despite well-established and enshrined legal rights and a rapidly changing social consensus, some Canadian-born and -educated individuals may also share these views about Bob.

In this situation, honest and respectful communication will be required. The owner/manager clarifying support for Bob, both as a pharmacist and as a person who has contributed much to the community, is essential. The focus of any conversation should revolve around Bob's ability as a pharmacist, as changing the views of patients is likely unachievable and out of context for the practice. Disrespect to employees or patients must not be tolerated, and workplaces should implement policies and procedures to abide by if presented with similar scenarios. Pharmacy owners and managers should also be encouraged to report incidents to professional organizations to facilitate united approaches for resolution.

Intercultural communication affords many opportunities to broaden personal horizons and engage with people who can enrich lives significantly. In some cases, conflict and disagreement may occur, in which case honest self-reflection and authentic communication become imperative. False attempts to create win-win conditions are transparent and may serve to alienate everyone. Remember, everyone has personal cultural norms and values. The balancing act required to foster mutual respect and acceptance can be challenging, but the reality is there are few other options. For as long as human beings have lived collectively in societies, they have had to deal with diversity. While the accent, complexion or tone of that diversity may evolve over time, the same principles continue to apply: honest self-reflection produces authentic engagement and communication, not oversimplified checklists of dos and don'ts.

REFERENCES

1. Statistics Canada. Immigration and ethnocultural diversity in Canada. Ottawa: Statistics Canada, 2011. Available: http://www12.statcan.gc.ca/nhs-enm/2011/as-sa/99-010 x/99 010 x2011001-eng.cfm (accessed Jan. 31, 2015).

2. Hofstede G, Hofstede GJ. Culture and organizations: software of the mind. New York: McGraw-Hill; 2004.

3. Trompenaars A, Woolliams P. Business across cultures. Mankato, MN: Capstone Press; 2004.

4. Management Committee. Moving forward: pharmacy human resources for the future. Final report. Ottawa: Canadian Pharmacists Association; 2008.

5. Betancourt JR, Green AR, Carrillo JE, et al. Defining cultural competence: a practical framework for addressing racial/ethnic disparities in health and health care. Public Health Rep. 2003;118(4):293–302. http://dx.doi.org/10.1016/S0033 -3549(04)50253-4. Medline:12815076

6. Watermeyer J, Penn C. "Tell me so I know you understand": pharmacists' verification of patients' comprehension of antiretroviral dosage instruction in a cross-cultural context. Pat Educ Counsel. 2009;79(2):205–13. http://dx.doi.org/10.1016/j.pec.2008.09.009.

7. Axtell RE. Essential do's and taboos. New York, NY: John Wiley and Sons; 2007.

8. Zweber A. Cultural competence in pharmacy practice. Am J Pharm Educ. 2002;66:172–6.

9. Burgess DJ, Warren J, Phelan S, et al. Stereotype threat and health disparities: what medical educators and future physicians need to know. J Gen Intern Med. 2010;25(S2 Suppl 2):S169–77. http://dx.doi.org/10.1007/s11606-009-1221-4. Medline:20352514

10. Good TD. Self-assessment checklist for personnel providing primary health care services. Washington: Georgetown University; 2002. Available: http://nccc.georgetown.edu/documents/checklist_PHC.html [cited May 8, 2014].

11. Campinha-Bacote J. Many faces: addressing diversity in health care. Online J Issues Nurs. 2003;8(1):3. Medline:12729453

12. Laroche L. (2008). Managing cultural differences. produced for the Ontario Regulators for Access Consortium. Available: www.regulatorsforaccess.ca/docs/ManagingCulturalDifferencesEnglish.pdf (accessed May 4, 2014).

13. Hanley J. Beyond the tip of the iceberg: five stages toward cultural competence. Reaching Today's Youth. 1999;9:9–12.

14. Weaver GR. Understanding and coping with cross-cultural adjustment stress. In: Paige RM, editor. Cross-cultural orientation: new conceptualizations and applications. Lanham: University Press of America; 1986.

15. Betancourt JR. Cultural competence and medical education: many names, many perspectives, one goal. Acad Med. 2006;81(6):499–501. http://dx.doi.org/10.1097/01.ACM.0000225211.77088.cb. Medline:16728795

16. Daher M, Chaar B, Saini B. Impact of patients' religious and spiritual beliefs in pharmacy: from the perspective of the pharmacist. Res Social Admin Pharm. 2014. http://dx.doi.org/10.1016/j.sapharm.2014.05.004. Medline:24954186

17. Smith KM, Hoesli TM. Effects of religious and personal beliefs on medication regimen design. Orthopedics. 2011;34(4):292–5. http://dx.doi.org/10.3928/01477447-20110228-17. Medline:21469616

18. Kleinman A. Patients and healers in the context of culture: an exploration of the borderland between anthropology, medicine, and psychiatry. Berkley: University of California Press; 1980.

19. Habibzadeh F. Contraception in the Middle East. Lancet. 2012;380:1. Available: http://middleeast.thelancet.com/sites/middleeast.thelancet.com/files/september12_middleeasted_0.pdf (accessed Jan. 30, 2015).

20. Hall ET. Beyond culture. New York: Anchor Books; 1976.

21. Bazaldua OV, Sias J. Cultural competence: a pharmacy perspective. J Pharm Pract. 2004;17(3):160–6. http://dx.doi.org/10.1177/0897190004264812.

CHAPTER 45

Communicating with Other Health Care Professionals

Jason Perepelkin, BA, BComm, MSc, PhD; Assistant Professor of Social and Administrative Pharmacy, University of Saskatchewan

---

Learning Objectives

- Understand that proper communication among health care professionals can enhance patient care.
- Discuss the importance of understanding the role of the pharmacist and other health care team members.
- Recognize the differences between multidisciplinary and interdisciplinary teams.
- Highlight characteristics of successful teamwork, as well as common barriers to interprofessional communication.
- Explore the role of communication in a pharmacist successfully integrating into existing primary care teams.
- Appreciate how looking to industries outside of health care for methods of improving communication may be beneficial.

As the drug and drug therapy experts, pharmacists interact with a variety of health care professionals (HCPs). However, a pharmacist's level of knowledge and experience in patient care is different from a nurse or physician. There are strategies to consider when communicating with other HCPs to achieve improved health care outcomes for patients.

The complexity of health care delivery requires a health care team (HCT) to be a cohesive and a highly efficient functioning unit. Clear and thoughtful communication between team members is an essential element of any team. It has been suggested the main root cause of preventable adverse events that result in serious injury or death is inadequate communication among HCPs or between HCPs and patients/families.[1] Teamwork has many important features, but open communication is a key feature, if not the main feature, of any successful professional team.

Successful communication can only occur when each team member has an understanding of the roles of everyone associated with the team and when there is a clear decision-making process.

It is the role of each individual HCP to, when appropriate, communicate and impart knowledge and skills to improve the care of patients and, ultimately, improve patient outcomes.

As discussed in Chapter 42: An Introduction to Pharmacist Communications, Communication Models and Theories, communication is not a simple process. It involves complex interactions among individuals and can consist of verbal and/or non-verbal communication. When HCPs interact and communicate on patient health care, there is an added complexity to the communication process.

HEALTH CARE TEAMS

In pharmacy practice, especially in the institutional environment of a hospital or primary care centre, pharmacists are part of an interdisciplinary team. It is important to understand the differences between multidisciplinary and interdisciplinary teams. Multidisciplinary teams involve many members of the HCT, but the team does not usually function as a team together; rather, consultations with the patient are done individually, with members of the team meeting to discuss the patient case after interacting with the patient.[2] Interdisciplinary teams involve all members of the team coming together, including the patient; this allows all members of the team to discuss the patient case and arrive at a care plan together.[2]

When practising in the community pharmacy environment, and due to the nature of that environment, it is likely that being separated from other HCPs results in a pharmacist being a member of a multidisciplinary team. While it may be ideal to be co-located with other members of the patient's circle of care, when communicating with a patient in a community pharmacy, one still needs to ensure all the necessary information is available to make professional decisions regarding whether or not the prescribed therapy is appropriate.

One cannot assume a physician or nurse who interacted with the patient earlier has communicated all the necessary information about the therapy prescribed. Therefore, it is important to have a conversation with patients to get a better sense of what they know about their diagnosis and treatment regime. (It may be good to review the communication process discussed in Chapter 42: An Introduction to Pharmacist Communications, Communication Models and Theories.)

Despite being co-located, communication barriers and miscommunication can, and do, occur within an interdisciplinary team. Failure in communication among members of the patient care team may result in patient harm.[3] While many universities across Canada have initiated some form of interdisciplinary education leading to a better understanding of the scope of practice of other HCPs, how best to communicate within an interdisciplinary team is often missing. Furthermore, many HCPs are used to poor communications with other HCPs, and this culture negatively affects patient care.[4]

From the patients' perspective, they are likely to find it easier to communicate with an interdisciplinary team, where various HCPs are present, as opposed to providing what may be interpreted as the same information to each HCP as is the case in a multidisciplinary team.[4]

In a literature review of successful teamwork, O'Daniel and Rosenstein[4] found many components of success relied upon proper communication:

- open communication
- non-punitive environment

- clear and known roles and tasks for team members
- appropriate balance of member participation
- acknowledgement and dealing with conflict
- clear specifications of authority and accountability
- agreed-upon decision-making procedures
- regular and routine communication to share information
- method to evaluate outcomes and revise as necessary

Furthermore, O'Daniel and Rosenstein[4] identified some common barriers to interprofessional communication, including the following:
- personal values and expectations
- hierarchy
- personality differences
- culture and ethnicity
- historical rivalries among HCPs
- semantic differences with regard to language used
- differences in schedules and professional routines
- variation in requirements, regulations and norms of professional education
- differences in accountability, payment and rewards
- concerns regarding clinical responsibility

In their review of articles pertaining to integrating pharmacists into primary care teams, Jorgenson and colleagues,[5] after feedback from expert reviewers, came up with 10 recommendations to successfully integrate into existing primary care teams. Half of the recommendations speak to ways to enhance communication between pharmacists and other HCPs:[5]
- Educate the primary care team about the pharmacist role.
- Educate yourself about the roles of other members (or potential members) of the primary care team.
- Ensure that you are highly visible and accessible to the team.
- Make sure to seek regular feedback from members of the team.
- Develop and maintain professional relationships.

Similar to many of the recommendations made by Jorgenson and colleagues,[5] communication plays a vital role among the six competency domains for effective interprofessional teams as identified by the Canadian Interprofessional Health Collaborative: interprofessional communication, patient-client-family-community-centred care, role clarification, team functioning, collaborative leadership and interprofessional conflict resolution.[6]

In looking to other industries for ways to improve patient care, in the early 1990s health care administrators started to look at the aviation industry.[7] Upon studying errors, the aviation industry found that most errors within the industry were the result of poor communication and coordination, as opposed to individual mistakes.[8] The breakdown of the team was most often the result of the hierarchy in place, where team members below the captain were not to be questioned. When applied to health care, many similarities emerge with placing the physician at the top of the hierarchy.

Recently, Schwartz and Hobbs[9] highlighted the use of implementing the principles of crew resource management (CRM) in training entry-to-practice pharmacists. The module was developed to better prepare students for practice and integration into HCT, and also to provide the tools and confidence to speak up or challenge a situation/individual when justified.[9] In particular, five potentially hazardous attitudes displayed by members of the HCT may negatively impact decision making and, likely, clinical outcomes:[9]

1. "Don't tell or question me."
2. "Do it STAT—no need to double-check."
3. "It won't happen to me; I do this all the time."
4. "I'm highly skilled and I can do it."
5. "What's the use?"

As a result of HCT members exhibiting attitudes 1 to 4, many times the result is resorting to attitude 5: "What's the use?"[9] While one wants to respect the professional decision making and expertise of all team members, if it is known that taking a given course of action, especially with drug therapy, may result in suboptimal outcomes, then one must also communicate one's professional opinion. Human error is a part of practice, yet effective team communication can help to reduce the chances of error and, ultimately, improve patient safety.

Morris and Matthews[10] highlighted the communication challenges that can occur when practising in rural locations. The foundation of a well-functioning interprofessional team is communication. "If you can't communicate, there is no team."[10] This communication also extends to formal channels, such as charting, as well as informal channels, such as hallway conversations. Not only does proper communication improve the functioning of interprofessional teams, it also is a method for professional growth as there is a greater appreciation for members of the team.[10] With varying schedules having the potential to hinder interprofessional teams, Morris and Matthews[10] highlighted that appropriate and timely communication can be an effective solution. This can extend into communication with the pharmacy team itself when practising in an environment where there is little to no overlap; ensuring appropriate and timely communication occurs with members of the team, the functioning of that team will be enhanced.

As highlighted throughout this chapter, communication is key to interprofessional teams functioning properly and competently.[11] Furthermore, "If teams are the foundation of health care delivery, then communication is the cement which holds teams together."[12] If there is a failure to communicate, there is a failure as a team. Communicating in a respectful fashion helps to facilitate the connectedness of team members due to its ability to illustrate uniform power among members of the team and encourages shared decision making, responsibility and authority.[13,14]

REFERENCES

1. Meeting the Joint Commission's 2007 national patient safety goals. Oakbrook Terrace, IL: Joint Commission Resources; 2006.

2. Jessup RL. Interdisciplinary versus multidisciplinary care teams: do we understand the difference? Aust Health Rev. 2007;31(3):330–1. http://dx.doi.org/10.1071/AH070330. Medline:17669052

3. Leonard M, Graham S, Bonacum D. The human factor: the critical importance of effective teamwork and communication in providing safe care. Qual Saf Health Care. 2004;13(Suppl 1):i85–90. http://dx.doi.org/10.1136/qshc.2004.010033. Medline:15465961

4. O'Daniel M, Rosenstein AH, and the Professional Communication and Team Collaboration. Hughes RG, editor. Patient safety and quality: an evidence-based handbook for nurses. Rockville, MD. US: Agency for Healthcare Research and Quality; 2008. Available: www.ncbi.nlm.nih.gov/books/NBK2637/ [cited 2014 Dec. 13].

5. Jorgenson D, Dalton D, Farrell B, et al. Guidelines for pharmacists integrating into primary care teams. Can Pharm J (Ott). 2013;146(6):342–52. http://dx.doi.org/10.1177/1715163513504528. Medline:24228050

6. Canadian Interprofessional Health Collaborative. A national interprofessional competency framework. 2010.

7. Helmreich RL. On error management: lessons from aviation. BMJ. 2000;320(7237):781–5. http://dx.doi.org/10.1136/bmj.320.7237.781. Medline:10720367

8. Oriol MD. Crew resource management: applications in healthcare organizations. J Nurs Adm. 2006;36(9):402–6. http://dx.doi.org/10.1097/00005110-200609000-00006. Medline:16969251

9. Schwartz MD, Hobbs WH. Teaching aviation crew resource management in a pharmacy curriculum. Am J Pharm Educ. 2014;78(3):66. http://dx.doi.org/10.5688/ajpe78366. Medline:24761027

10. Morris D, Matthews J. Communication, respect, and leadership: interprofessional collaboration in hospitals of rural Ontario. Can J Diet Pract Res. 2014;75(4):173–9. http://dx.doi.org/10.3148/cjdpr-2014-020.

11. MacDonald MB, Bally JM, Ferguson LM, et al. Knowledge of the professional role of others: a key interprofessional competency. Nurse Educ Pract. 2010;10(4):238–42. http://dx.doi.org/10.1016/j.nepr.2009.11.012. Medline:20308019

12. Poole MS, Real K. Groups and teams in health care: communication and effectiveness. Handbook of health communication (2003): 369–402.

13. Selle KM, Salamon K, Boarman R, et al. Providing interprofessional learning through interdisciplinary collaboration: the role of "modelling". J Interprof Care. 2008;22(1):85–92. http://dx.doi.org/10.1080/13561820701714755. Medline:18202988

14. Solomon P, Salfi J. Evaluation of an interprofessional education communication skills initiative. Educ Health (Abingdon). 2011;24(2):616. Medline:22081661

CHAPTER 46

Advocacy and Strategic Communications

Jeff Morrison, *MA; Director of Government Relations and Public Affairs, Canadian Pharmacists Association*

Learning Objectives

- Discuss the importance of advocacy and strategic communications to pharmacists.
- Explore ways pharmacists can advocate for patients, the profession and the health care system.
- Highlight some strategies that pharmacists can use to support advocacy and strategic communications.
- Underscore the importance of partnerships in advocacy and strategic communications.
- Examine some successful advocacy initiatives in pharmacy.

WHAT ARE ADVOCACY AND STRATEGIC COMMUNICATIONS AND WHY ARE THEY IMPORTANT FOR PHARMACISTS?

It is a fundamental principle of democratic systems that citizens have the right to speak out and voice their opinions on issues of public interest. Without such public engagement and public accountability, governments would be left to pursue whatever policies they wished, without consideration of the broader public's views or interests, or even without consideration of minority views. This act of speaking out and attempting to influence the course of public policy or public initiatives is referred to as advocacy. Advocacy is as core a principle to democracy as is voting or a free press.

It could be argued that advocacy is perhaps even more important and relevant in sectors, industries and/or professions that are heavily regulated by governments, which includes the health care sector, and which therefore also includes pharmacy. There is a long list of laws, policies and regulations that governments at all levels develop that directly affect the health care sector and, by extension, pharmacy. As professionals who work in the health care system and who see the effect of these laws, policies and regulations on a daily basis, pharmacists, like other health care providers, are in a unique position to speak out and share their opinions and evidence on the impact of these policies.

There are many ways in which individuals or organizations can influence and change the course of public policy. Ultimately, though, an individual or organization will have to evaluate the amount of effort (including time, money, human resources, etc.) that can be devoted to a particular cause and how long the effort and/or initiative can be sustained. However, individuals or organizations with the right plan and passion for their cause will always, at a minimum, introduce a new perspective or add a voice to the issue, which is always a valuable addition to any public policy discussion.

ADVOCATING AT DIFFERENT LEVELS

There are many different kinds of advocacy, with different perspectives and different scopes. This is especially true in health care, given the fact that it involves multiple stakeholders in both the public and even the private sector. For pharmacists, the following levels represent the most common kinds of advocacy in which they would engage:

ADVOCACY AND STRATEGIC COMMUNICATIONS ON BEHALF OF PATIENTS

Patients should be at the centre of health care and, as such, it is logical that for most health care providers, any experience they may have in advocacy will be conducted on behalf of patients, either individually or collectively. Health care providers are in a unique position to change or challenge public policies that directly impact the people they serve.

- patients individually: There is a complex mix of public policies that affect different kinds of patient populations under different health care scenarios. For instance, if one considers public medication insurance plans, there are different plans for Aboriginal peoples, seniors, low-income populations, refugee claimants and patients with rare diseases. It is in the best interest of the health care provider (and the patient) for individual patients to be able to access these programs effectively. When they cannot, it is often left to the health care provider to advocate on the patient's behalf to ensure that problems are effectively addressed.
- patients collectively: Just as providers expect that individually, patients will receive effective service from public plans and policies, so too do they expect that public policies will best meet the needs of their patients collectively. When providers encounter issues with public policies that may place the care of patients at risk, many providers feel an obligation to speak out on the issue or problem that has been identified. For instance, when the federal government announced in 2012 that it would cut back on the health care services it provided for refugee claimants, many health care providers spoke out and advocated against these cuts since they placed the health of that entire population at risk.

ADVOCACY AND STRATEGIC COMMUNICATIONS ON BEHALF OF THE OVERALL PROFESSION

As a profession, pharmacists, like other health care providers, are subject to a long list of public policy regulations and legislation. It is only logical that members of these professions will want to have a say in the evolution and direction of those policies that affect them directly in their day-to-day careers. Expanded scope of service for pharmacists, compensation for services and means of interaction with other health care providers are just a few examples of issues for which individual pharmacists have communicated their views on behalf of the entire profession.

ADVOCACY AND STRATEGIC COMMUNICATIONS WITH RESPECT TO THE HEALTH CARE SYSTEM

Each health care professional, whether a pharmacist, physician, nurse, occupational therapist and so forth, works within a broader health care system. Canada's health care system (or more aptly, individual provincial/territorial systems) is a complex system that has much room for improvement. Health care professionals can provide a unique perspective to advocate for changes that will improve the overall health care system provincially/territorially, nationally and even internationally.

STRATEGIES TO SUPPORT ADVOCACY AND STRATEGIC COMMUNICATIONS

It is one thing to acknowledge that health care providers have a role to speak out and advocate for public policy changes. It is another to know how to communicate strategically to influence and create policy change. There is no one correct or perfect way to influence or advocate a particular position; the individual needs to evaluate the environment and situation and determine the best strategic approach to effectively communicate the position. Although creativity plays a role, there are some standard tools and strategies that can be employed to effectively advocate a position.

JOINING A LIKE-MINDED ASSOCIATION/ORGANIZATION

A person may wish to advocate for a particular issue but simply does not have the time or resources to do so. This is where joining a professional association to advocate on the individual's behalf is useful. By joining associations such as the Canadian Pharmacists Association (CPhA), the Canadian Society of Hospital Pharmacists (CSHP) or a provincial association, individuals have the opportunity to ask their association to communicate and advocate for their particular positions.

PETITIONS

Launching a petition is a good way to broaden the scope of advocacy efforts to allow people to add their voice in support of a cause. Although old-fashioned paper petitions are still valid, new online petition tools (such as change.org) allow for easy dissemination and tracking of petitions, including through social media.

MEDIA EVENT/NEWS RELEASES

There is likely no better way to communicate a message/position to as wide an audience as possible than through the media. Elevating a message so the general public is informed has many advantages: it generates additional support for a position from a wider audience, and it often forces decision makers to respond to the message. Media coverage can often be generated through the use of written press releases, organizing a news conference or contacting individual journalists.

SETTING UP MEETINGS WITH RELEVANT OFFICIALS

The most direct route to successful advocacy is to meet with the individuals, groups and/or organizations who can create the change being sought. This typically means meeting with politicians, regulatory bodies, associations, legislative committees, senior bureaucrats or whichever other body can make the decision that is being advocated. It is important at these meetings to be very clear with respect to the proposed "ask," and the justification for the request—many people in meetings spend too much time focusing on the problem and not enough on the solution.

HUMAN IMPACT STORIES

Decision makers tend to react strongly to human impact stories—those anecdotes that illustrate in human terms the impact that a particular policy is having on real people. Human impact stories can serve as powerful examples to strengthen the message about the need for change with regard to a particular policy.

INFLUENCE ELECTIONS

Elections, and particularly election campaigns, are an excellent opportunity to ask prospective politicians to commit to a particular policy. Obviously, people should vote for the candidate that best aligns with their interests. Individuals who are passionate about public policy change should also consider putting their name forward as candidates.

IMPORTANCE OF PARTNERSHIPS

One element of advocacy that is often overlooked is the importance of partnerships with key stakeholders. Although any individual can initiate and lead an advocacy effort, it is more effective and less resource-intensive to involve other like-minded stakeholders and partners in the effort.

Partners can contribute additional resources, ideas and perspectives and can add additional credibility to an effort. The latter point is important. One of the challenges that groups or individuals have in advocating a certain position is they are often seen as acting in self-interest; it is believed the rationale for the position is to further the personal interest of the individual or group making the intervention. By adding partners to an effort, it is more difficult to label a particular organization as acting solely in self-interest; the advocacy objective is now one that is shared by other interests. For example, if someone were to advocate for lower post-secondary tuition rates, it would be useful to have non-student organizations speaking out on behalf of the issue, as student organizations may be seen as being motivated purely by self-interest. Faculty members, business groups and anti-poverty groups could be potential partners who would bring an unbiased perspective to the issue, and for whom it would be difficult to argue that they are influenced solely by self-interest.

EXAMPLES OF SUCCESSFUL ADVOCACY INITIATIVES IN PHARMACY

The pharmacy profession has realized several advocacy accomplishments over the past several years. The following represent just a few of the ways in which pharmacists have managed to influence and change public policy.

EXPANDING PHARMACIST-PROVIDED SERVICES

Since early 2010, almost every province/territory has witnessed an expansion in the regulated scope of practice that they allow their pharmacists to perform. This dramatic shift in what services pharmacists can legally provide is the result of many years of effort on the part of pharmacists advocating to provincial governments, particularly on the part of provincial pharmacy associations. Several different tactics have been used to achieve this expansion of service, including evidence-based reports, meetings with key politicians and legislative bodies, media interventions and external stakeholder support.

ADDRESSING THE NUMBER OF INTERNATIONAL PHARMACY GRADUATES ARRIVING IN CANADA

In early 2011, the Pharmacy Examining Board of Canada (PEBC) began raising concerns about the increasing numbers of International Pharmacy Graduates (IPGs) applying to Canada at a time when the pharmacist labour market was softening. PEBC arranged meetings with Citizenship and Immigration Canada and Human Resources and Social Development Canada about this situation. Upon receiving the evidence provided by PEBC, the federal government agreed to first cut the number of IPGs allowed into Canada per year and then by 2013, the federal government removed pharmacists from the list of priority professions to come to Canada.

INCLUDING PHARMACISTS AS RECOGNIZED "HEALTH PRACTITIONERS" UNDER THE EXCISE TAX ACT

In 2012, the federal government announced that it would include pharmacists in the list of recognized "health practitioners" under the Excise Tax Act, thereby making all fees charged for any pharmacist-provided service GST-exempt. This change was brought about following a written request by CPhA, a meeting with key Department of Finance officials and expressions of support from all 10 provincial pharmacy associations.

DRUG SHORTAGES

When drug shortages witnessed a dramatic increase in 2010, CPhA undertook several advocacy initiatives to address the problem. A survey of Canadian pharmacists was conducted to get more information on the scope and extent of the problem. A report was issued with specific recommendations on how to address drug shortages. A coalition was created bringing together manufacturers, government, wholesalers, chain drug stores and other health care professions to advocate for solutions, including the creation of a new national drug shortages reporting system that launched in 2011. Media releases were issued to bring the issue to the attention of Canadians at large. Representations were made to the federal government to implement policies to address shortages, and meetings were held at an international level to discuss solutions to the problem from that level. Several of the recommendations and ideas that came out from those discussions were eventually adopted, and several public policies have been changed.

Like every other Canadian, pharmacists have the constitutional right to speak out on public policy issues. Given their unique background and perspective, and particularly given their trust level among Canadians, individual pharmacists have the potential to advocate for a range of issues that they deem important. By using some of the approaches suggested in this chapter, those efforts can be amplified with a greater likelihood of success.

RESOURCES AND SUGGESTED READINGS

Bradley-Baker LR, Murphy NL. Leadership development of student pharmacists. Am J Pharm Educ. 2013;77(10):219. www.ncbi. nlm.nih.gov/pmc/articles/PMC3872938/. http://dx.doi.org/10.5688/ajpe7710219. Medline:24371344

Culhane P. A strategic approach to government relations. Available: www.csae.com/Resources/ArticlesTools/View/ArticleId/1289/A-Strategic-Approach-to-Government-Relations (accessed Nov. 17, 2014).

Fox L, Helweg P. Advocacy strategies for civil society: a conceptual framework and practitioners guide. Available: www.innonet. org/resources/files/Advocacy_Strategies_for_Civil_Society.pdf (accessed Nov. 17, 2014).

Williams H. Helping getting advocacy right Available: www.csae.com/Resources/ArticlesTools/View/ArticleId/1794/Helping-Get-Advocacy-Right (accessed Nov. 17, 2014).

CHAPTER 47

Introduction to Marketing and Key Concepts

Jason Perepelkin, *BA, BComm, MSc, PhD; Assistant Professor of Social and Administrative Pharmacy, University of Saskatchewan*

Learning Objectives

- Define and introduce marketing and its role in general.
- Discuss why marketing is important for pharmacists and highlight some common misconceptions about marketing.
- Examine core marketplace concepts.
- Visit the right principle as it pertains to marketing.
- Identify the marketing mix (4 Ps – product, price, place, promotion).
- Explore the exchange, distribution and facilitating functions of marketing.
- Differentiate between transactional and relationship marketing.
- Define marketing myopia.

If someone asks a person what comes to mind when the word *marketing* is said, it will likely be an image of advertising or those telemarketers who always seem to call at the most inopportune time. While advertising, and yes, even telemarketers, are part of marketing, it is much more. Marketing has been discussed and practised for centuries, but it was only in the 20th century when marketing began to form as a discipline,[1] including the study of marketing theory and thought.

While marketing methods can be used to market products that have a negative impact on one's health (e.g., tobacco products), it can also be used for positive aspects, such as campaigns to reduce the use of tobacco products (e.g., Partnership to Assist with Cessation of Tobacco—PACT—in Saskatchewan).

MARKETING CONCEPT

The marketing concept involves determining the needs and/or wants of a targeted group (in pharmacy, patients). As a result, one must explicitly consider the patient's perspective, with the focus on targeted patients. The ultimate goal of the marketing concept in pharmacy is patient satisfaction.

TARGET MARKET

In marketing, one focuses on the target market: the set of actual and potential buyers of a product (good and/or service). This group of people shares a need or want that can be satisfied through exchange relationships. To identify a target market, one should use market segmentation, which is the process of dividing the total market into groups of members who share similar characteristics.

For example, one may identify all current patients at a pharmacy who are taking at least one diabetic medication; from that point, the group can be divided into all patients taking at least one diabetic medication who are also on an anti-hypertensive medication and are over the age of 65. By segmenting individuals into a defined target market, their needs and wants will be better served, as opposed to trying to be all things to all people. Variables to consider in making decisions about a target market include the size and growth potential of the segment, how accessible the segment is, the nature of the market, the nature/focus of the organization and the financial implications of targeting a given market.

IMPORTANCE OF MARKETING FOR PHARMACISTS

Health care in general, and in pharmacy practice in particular, continues to evolve as patient needs and wants change. While many of these changes, such as increased scope of practice, have benefited stakeholders, sometimes these changes do not always benefit the patient. For instance, many in society have come to expect fast, efficient service in many facets of life. Being fast in dispensing medications may not be in the best interest of the patient. Pharmacists have a choice; they can sit by idly allowing others to dictate practice, or they can work to affect change in the profession for the benefit of their patients, themselves and the health care system as a whole. Marketing allows for the recognition of what pharmacists can do. As well, patients do not always know what they want or need, and it is the obligation of pharmacists to help patients understand how to improve their health care outcomes.

COMMON MISCONCEPTIONS ABOUT MARKETING

One major misconception is that marketing is inherently bad.[2] While marketing has been used in negative ways, there are many examples of it being used for positive outcomes. As an example, marketing has been used to educate women on the benefits of folic acid supplements for those who may become pregnant or are pregnant, and to inform men when they should start having regular prostate examinations. Some feel that marketing is simply advertising. While advertising, whether for profit or for behaviour change, is a core component of marketing, there is much more to it.

With Canadians having a universal health care system (Medicare), some feel that health care professionals, including pharmacists, do not need to market. While some of the final decisions in an organization are left to senior executives to make, the individual frontline pharmacist can and does utilize marketing concepts in practice. As well, the argument that employee/staff pharmacists do not need to market, or that only community pharmacists need to market, is misguided. For example, if a pharmacist fails to educate a patient receiving a prescription for an antibiotic on the importance of taking all the medication and not to stop when their symptoms are gone, and does not fully understand why someone would not be adherent, then the pharmacist is not practising to the level expected. Marketing for pharmacists is about understanding patients and how to communicate with them.

CORE MARKETPLACE CONCEPTS

NEEDS, WANTS AND DEMANDS

Patients have needs, wants and demands. Need is a state of felt deprivation; needs are basic human requirements, including physical, social and individual.[3] A want is a desire for a specific satisfier of a deeper need; thus, needs become wants and these wants are shaped by culture and individual personality.[3] For example, someone may want fish and chips to satisfy their hunger, while the next person may want butter chicken and rice. A demand is a want that is backed by an ability to pay.[3] An example of a demand is that one person may want to buy a Lexus but only have the ability to pay for a Toyota.

MARKET OFFERINGS

Market offerings are the products, services and/or goods an organization offers. There are some pharmacies that offer a complete range of prescription and over-the-counter (OTC) medications, while others may focus specifically on providing compounded prescription and OTC medications. Some pharmacies may be generalists in providing counselling services to patients, while others may focus on specific conditions, such as hormone replacement therapy. The key is to identify what market offerings best serve the wants and needs of the target market, and at the same time remembering not to try to be all things to all people.

VALUE AND SATISFACTION

Patients look for value and satisfaction in exchanges with the pharmacist/pharmacy. For example, if a pharmacy charges a premium price for services, then the value the patient attaches to that service is likely to be higher than a pharmacy offering a discounted price for services. Value and satisfaction are not the same to every person, so it is best to first understand what the target market values and what would satisfy their wants and needs.

EXCHANGE AND RELATIONSHIPS

In order for the process of marketing to occur, there must be an exchange or the potential for an exchange to occur. Without some sort of relationship where an exchange of something of value (for all involved) takes place, needs or wants cannot be satisfied.

MARKETS

Leading directly from exchange and relationships, markets then become (or then are) all actual and potential patients with similar demands that can be fulfilled through an exchange relationship. As described above, segment markets into smaller target markets to better serve patients.

THE RIGHT PRINCIPLE

When practising the right principle, the aim is to get the right products to the right people at the right place at the right time at the right price using the right promotional strategies.[4]

THE MARKETING MIX – 4 PS

The marketing mix is commonly referred to as the 4 Ps of marketing: product, price, place and promotion.

PRODUCT

A product refers to the good (tangible), service (intangible) or a combination of the two that is offered by a person or organization. For example, in community pharmacy, the distribution function involves providing both a good (medication) and a service (professional medication counselling). Hospital pharmacists may provide the good, but many times it is their advanced drug and drug therapy knowledge (service) that is the product they provide.

PRICE

When one considers price it is easy to simply focus on the financial costs. However, one must also consider the non-financial costs involved in the transaction, such as the personal cost of the time it takes to wait for a prescription to be filled.

PLACE

It is common to consider the place as being the pharmacy. However, one should consider all aspects of distribution. For example, if a pharmacist or manager wants to offer a blood pressure clinic for seniors, the first thought may be to offer it in the counselling room of a pharmacy, or in the front store after hours. In considering place (distribution) in a broader sense, also consider where it would be best to provide that product or service. Would it be more convenient to offer it at a retirement home, where the pharmacist goes to the patients, instead of having them individually come to the pharmacy?

PROMOTION

Promotion is the aspect of marketing that most people commonly think of as being synonymous with marketing; however, promotion is what one uses to communicate with the target audience once the product, price and place have been decided on. Building on the example of the blood pressure clinic for seniors, it would probably be better to post flyers at the retirement home and include bag stuffers for patients at the pharmacy than to hire a keen pharmacy student to place flyers on cars and start a Facebook page.

EXCHANGE, DISTRIBUTION AND FACILITATING FUNCTIONS OF MARKETING

Exchange functions are activities associated with understanding why and what people buy, and activities associated with selling them the appropriate good or service. For example, in Canada it is recommended people take a vitamin D supplement in the winter months due to the inability to take in enough from the sun. To ensure exchange can occur, where the patient seeks out and finds vitamin D tablets, the pharmacy makes sure to order enough product for the winter months. However, orders for many products to be shipped in the fall must be placed months ahead of time, so suppliers of vitamin D tablets must also facilitate the exchange function with retailers (pharmacies).

Distribution functions are activities associated with transporting and storing goods, services and ideas. Obviously, services cannot be stored, but distribution does relate to the transporting of goods and even service providers to the patient. For example, a community pharmacy would find it near impossible to have enough product (goods) in stock that would be needed in the dispensary for one month; as a result, there are wholesalers that allow pharmacies to order products on an as-needed basis, and many times these products are delivered the day after ordering.

Facilitating functions are the activities that make the exchange function easier to perform. For example, many wholesalers will not require payment from a pharmacy when they receive product from the wholesaler. Instead, the wholesaler facilitates the exchange by invoicing the pharmacy for the product delivered, often with conditions such as, "payment must be made within 30 days of delivery or a fee and/or interest will be charged." Community pharmacies may even facilitate the exchange function with patients by allowing them to have a charge account at the pharmacy with the expectation that it be paid off at the end of each month.

TRANSACTIONAL VERSUS RELATIONSHIP MARKETING

There are two forms of marketing that encompass most ways marketing occurs: transactional and relationship. In transactional marketing, each exchange/interaction is viewed as an isolated and unrelated event, whereas relationship marketing views each exchange as a series of transactions over time, each transaction building upon the previous (see Chapter 49: Loyalty, Consumer Behaviour and Evaluation).

MARKETING MYOPIA

Something to keep in mind is marketing myopia. In 1960, Levitt said organizations can lose sight of what matters when they do not consider the end user of a product—the customer. This phenomenon was called marketing myopia.[5] (As a reminder, myopia is nearsightedness—having a narrow view of something, a lack of foresight or discernment.[6]) In the case of pharmacy, it would refer to focusing on what the pharmacy or pharmacist wants to provide and not considering what the patient needs and wants. More recently, there has been an extension of marketing myopia to the "new marketing myopia" that comes from three related phenomena: a single-minded focus on the patient while disregarding other stakeholders; a narrow definition of the patient and his/her needs; and a failure to recognize the changing nature of practice that requires addressing multiple stakeholders.[7]

SUMMARY OF THE ROLE OF MARKETING IN PHARMACY PRACTICE

When the term is applied broadly, pharmacists are involved in marketing every day. The key is to harness the marketing tools available to better utilize one's therapeutic knowledge and expertise to practice to one's potential and better meet the needs and wants of patients and the health care system as a whole.

RESOURCES AND SUGGESTED READINGS

Berkowitz EN. Essentials of health care marketing. 3rd ed., Jones & Bartlett Learning; 2011.

Holdford D. Marketing for pharmacists: providing and promoting professional services. 2nd ed. Washington, DC: American Pharmacists Association; 2007. p. 138–49.

Isetts, BJ, Schommer, JC, Westberg, SM, et al. Evaluation of a consumer-generated marketing plan for medication therapy management services. Innovations in Pharmacy, 3(1), Article 66, 2012.

Kotler P, Hayes T, Bloom PN. Marketing professional services. 2nd ed., Prentice Hall Press; 2002.

Perepelkin J. Why pharmacists should not think of marketing as a dirty word. Can Pharm J (Ott). 2014;147(1):15–9. http://dx.doi.org/10.1177/1715163513513866. Medline:24494011

Review HB. HBR's 10 must reads on strategic marketing (with featured article "Marketing myopia," by Theodore Levitt). Harvard Business School Press; 2013.

Tootelian DH, Rolston LW, Negrete MJ. Consumer receptiveness to non-traditional roles for community pharmacists. Health Mark Q. 2005;23(1):43–56. http://dx.doi.org/10.1300/J026v23n01_04. Medline:16891256

Wood, KD, Offenberger, M, Mehta, BH, Rodis, JL. Community pharmacy marketing: strategies for success. Innovations in Pharmacy, 2(3), Article 48.

REFERENCES

1. Shaw EH, Jones DGB. A history of schools of marketing thought. Mark Theory. 2005;5(3):239–81. http://dx.doi.org/10.1177/1470593105054898.

2. Bonaguro JA, Miaoulis G. Marketing: a tool for health education planning. Health Educ. 1983;14(1):6–11. Medline:6443899

3. Holdford DA. Marketing for pharmacists. 2nd ed., American Pharmacists Association; 2007.

4. Burke RR. Retail shoppability: a measure of the world's best stores. Future Retail Now. 2005;40:206–19.

5. Levitt T. Marketing myopia. 1960. Harv Bus Rev. 2004;82(7-8):138-49. Medline:15252891

6. Merriam-Webster. Myopia. Available: www.merriam-webster.com/dictionary/myopia (accessed June 30, 2014).

7. Smith NC, Drumwright ME, Gentile MC. The new marketing myopia. J Public Policy Mark. 2010;29(1):4–11. http://dx.doi.org/10.1509/jppm.29.1.4.

CHAPTER 48

Unique Characteristics of Products as Services

Jason Perepelkin, *BA, BComm, MSc, PhD; Assistant Professor of Social and Administrative Pharmacy, University of Saskatchewan*

Learning Objectives

- Describe the difference between a product as a tangible good versus an intangible service.
- Understand unique characteristics of services: lack of ownership, intangibility, inseparability, perishability and heterogeneity.
- Describe strategies for marketing services.
- Understand the challenges in assessing services: search, experience and credence attributes.

CHARACTERISTICS UNIQUE TO SERVICES

Many unique aspects become apparent when considering products as services. This chapter examines unique characteristics of services and gives consideration to how to improve service performance. While pharmacists provide a distribution function in dispensing tangible drug products, pharmacists provide professional services, not medications.

As defined by Kotler and Bloom,[1] services are, "any activity or benefit that one party can offer to another that is essentially intangible and does not result in the ownership of anything. Its production may or may not be tied to a physical product."

The Marketing Mix consists of the 4 Ps of marketing: product, price, place and promotion (see Chapter 47: Introduction to Marketing and Key Concepts). When a product is examined, it may be tangible (a good) or intangible (a service or idea) or a combination. This area is especially important to pharmacists as the most prominent products pharmacists provide are, in fact, professional services that may accompany a tangible good.

Four criteria that characterize a product as a service are its intangibility, heterogeneity, inseparability (of production and consumption) and its influence by the customer. The intangible nature of services is that the actions or events that constitute a service cannot be seen, held or touched. While a pharmacist may see, hold or touch a patient (e.g., when taking a blood pressure reading or while injecting a patient with the flu vaccine), the actual action or event itself is not tangible.

Services are heterogeneous, meaning that no two service experiences are alike. Service quality depends on uncontrollable factors (e.g., mood of the patient, how busy the pharmacy is, other people in the pharmacy) that influence the service provision. As a result, no matter how much one prepares, it is not possible to deliver a service the exact same way each time. This may result in providing a service that was not planned. However, being prepared and confident in one's knowledge and skills makes one better equipped to handle these uncontrollable factors.

When offering a service, its production and consumption are inseparable. The pharmacist, as the service provider, cannot provide the service without the patient consuming it. Unlike tangible products, services cannot be saved, returned or resold. Once a service is delivered, it is lost. Due to the unique nature of services, it is difficult to synchronize supply and demand. Therefore, forecasting resources (e.g., pharmacists, technicians) also increases in difficulty. What is occurring today, as the profession changes from product-centred (tangible) to service-centred, makes the ability to provide professional services (e.g., medication reviews) difficult due to a shift in thinking and planning. The final characteristic is that the patient participates in, and influences, the service. This may be the case when the pharmacist is providing the service, but it can also be influenced by what others have said about their service encounters and experiences; for instance, word-of-mouth information a patient has been given by another patient.

PHARMACY AS A SERVICE PROFESSION

When patients visit a pharmacy, they may feel they are coming in for a tangible good (medication), but in reality they are actually seeking the benefits that good can provide. However, if the good is not assessed by the pharmacist to ensure it is safe, effective and the best treatment for the patients, then the therapeutic benefits may not be obtained or indeed, an adverse outcome may occur.

What cannot be forgotten is that most services in the practice of pharmacy usually involve tangible goods. For example, when people get the oil changed in their car, they are paying for the oil and filter, but also for the expertise of the oil change technician. Similarly in pharmacy, there are professional fees attached to dispensing medications, outside of markups, that remunerate the pharmacy for the service component of providing medications.

The professional value-added services pharmacists provide enrich the usefulness of tangible goods. Services are routines or ancillary activities that benefit others. These services can be complementary to a tangible good, or they may be the only product provided. For example, when a prescription is dispensed in a community pharmacy, there is the assumption, by regulators and other stakeholders, that the medication is accompanied by the professional service (counselling) of a pharmacist.

As the scope of practice for pharmacists increases across Canada, opportunities to provide a product that is strictly a service are also increasing. For example, pharmacists are being remunerated for providing comprehensive medication reviews that may, at times, result in a reduction in the number of medications a patient is required to take regularly. Another example is the Medication Assessment Centre (MAC) at the University of Saskatchewan and the University of British

Columbia that does not dispense any medications, but works with patients and health care professionals to obtain optimal drug therapy. (See www.usask.ca/pharmacist for more information on MAC.) However, despite the need for product offerings that are purely intangible services, the reality for most pharmacists is that the provision of services will usually be in combination with the provision of a medication.

CHALLENGES IN MARKETING SERVICES

There are bound to be challenges when trying to market services. For one, it is difficult to promote the value of a service. This is amplified by the fact that pharmacists, as professionals, provide a service that the general public may not fully appreciate nor understand. As a result, one needs to consider how to inform other pharmacy stakeholders (e.g., other health care professionals, politicians, administrators) of the value pharmacists provide to patients and the health care system as a whole.

Furthermore, services in general are difficult to evaluate, but when it is the professional services provided by a pharmacist, patients have little knowledge to truly assess the service; therefore, patients tend to evaluate pharmacist services on other aspects, such as if the pharmacist was friendly, if they have to wait long, did they experience an adverse drug event, etc.[2] While these aspects will invariably impact one's evaluation of a pharmacist-provided service, there are many other aspects of which the patient may never be aware.

Services by nature are invisible. For example, while patients may see the pharmacist talking on the phone or typing something into the computer, they are not fully aware of what the pharmacist may be doing unless it is explained to them. Someone may feel the pharmacist is simply checking Facebook or talking with a friend, when in fact the pharmacist entered the prescription into the pharmacy's computer system and noticed the patient has an allergy to sulpha products, so the pharmacist picked up the phone and called the prescribing physician to discuss an alternative drug therapy. Therefore, it is up to individual pharmacists to provide information and education to the patient as to the process that goes on behind the scenes. David Holdford[3] provides a useful resource in his book *Marketing for Pharmacists – Service Blueprint for Dispensing Services* (see Figure 48.1).

Service blueprints illustrate the service process from various actors/people involved in the provision of a service, including the patient, pharmacist (or other health care provider), clerks, etc.[4] Creating a service blueprint in pharmacy is key, especially considering that the public in general does not fully appreciate what pharmacists do and can provide; this underappreciation can be an obstacle in expanding pharmacists' scope of practice. Furthermore, as Holdford & Kennedy[4] highlight, the obstacles to an expanded role for pharmacists are the "result of insufficient planning by service designers and/or poor communication between those designing services and those implementing them." By creating a service blueprint, pharmacists can promote the value of pharmacists in various aspects of health care to patients and other decision makers, such as government and third-party payers. "Blueprints are designed by identifying and mapping a process from the consumer's point of view, mapping employee actions and support activities, and adding visible evidence of service at each consumer action step. Key components of service blueprints are consumer actions, 'onstage' and 'backstage' employee actions, and support processes."[4]

Figure 48.1

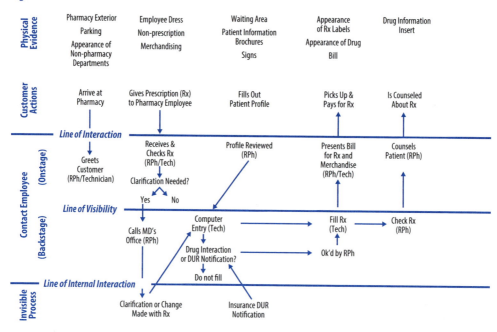

Service Blueprint for Dispensing Services[3] (used with permission)

(Holdford, 2007)

STRATEGIES FOR MARKETING SERVICES

A good place to begin considering what strategies to use in marketing services is with the service blueprint described previously. While services themselves are intangible, one can use tangible cues to showcase the quality of services. For example, appropriate lighting in the pharmacy, a clean waiting room, the dress and appearance of the pharmacist and other staff, how over-the-counter items are arranged on the shelves, etc., are all tangible cues used to portray quality and attention to detail. As well, the patient may walk away with more than the information provided by the pharmacist; they can also take a patient information page or leaflet specific to their concerns or conditions. This shows attention to detail and that the patient is not just a number, but is unique. Is the patient information leaflet specific to the person's gender, age and such, or is it general to anyone taking the medication? Most times, the information leaflet is general in nature and as a result, some patients may disregard the information provided. Think about how far a male patient would read if the first line was, "Do not take this medication if you are pregnant or considering becoming pregnant."

The optimal time for a pharmacist to showcase expertise and the quality of services provided is with each encounter with a patient. Word-of-mouth promotional communication is a very effective way to promote what the pharmacist and the pharmacy can and do provide; simply ask patients to tell others about the service they received if they enjoyed it. Furthermore, identify opinion leaders who could help reach the target market better, but remember, do not just contact them with a request; make sure the relationship is mutually beneficial.

Emphasizing the professional nature of pharmacist services in all interactions with patients and other stakeholders is advised. Being able to show them how pharmacists use critical thinking to assess what options would be worth exploring with the patient will benefit relationships long term and emphasize expertise and training. For example, if a pharmacist is a Certified Diabetes Educator (CDE), make sure patients know what makes a CDE pharmacist special. If the target market is not aware of what the pharmacist can provide them, then having that expertise and credential will be a missed opportunity for the pharmacist and the patient.

Branding is used to establish and maintain images and ideas in the mind of a target market. As defined by the American Marketing Association[5] a brand is a "name, term, design, symbol, or any other feature that identifies one seller's good or service as distinct from those of other sellers." The stronger a brand is, both a pharmacist's personal brand and that of the pharmacy, the less likely patients will look for other service providers. Brands can be strengthened by practising relationship marketing, which is treating each interaction as one in a series of interactions. (When practising transactional marketing, each interaction is viewed as an isolated event, with no expectation of future exchanges.) Therefore, while money or time may be lost during one exchange with a patient/customer, over time that effort will be rewarded long term when practising relationship marketing.

CHALLENGES OF ASSESSING SERVICES

Patients will have difficulty in evaluating many aspects of the professional services provided by pharmacists, just as pharmacists may have difficulty evaluating the services of an accountant or lawyer. There are three attributes for assessing a product: search, experience and credence.[6] While all three may be present in both goods and services, assessing goods tends to fall into search and experience attributes, whereas assessing services tends to fall into experience and credence attributes.

When a product is a good, there are search attributes that one can use to assess the product offering; one can see, feel, touch, taste a good before a purchase decision. Experience attributes can also be used when evaluating a good, but unlike search attributes that can occur before consumption, they occur during and after the consumption of the good. For example, one may reserve a car to rent in Italy that, online, states will hold five adults and five large suitcases, covering the search attributes. When one arrives to pick up the car and it will only hold four adults, at best, and one suitcase, then the experience attributes are quite different than what one was expecting when conducting the search.

When assessing services, there are experience and credence attributes used to assess, to the best of one's ability, the service. For experience attributes, one can only assess and evaluate the product during and after the service provision; pharmacists can help increase positive assessment of experience attributes by explaining to patients why they are doing what they are doing. There are also the experience attributes of a professional service that one uses to assess the service, such as the time spent by the service provider, the appearance of the service provider and the environment in which the encounter is taking place.

Credence attributes cannot be evaluated confidently even immediately after consumption because many times the service is provided by an expert or professional. As a result, consumers tend to rely on a credible source that provides them with a sense of confidence in the credence attributes. For example, each province has a regulatory body that regulates self-regulating professions such as pharmacy, nursing, medicine, dentistry, law, accounting, etc. There may also be alternative forms of assessment that take place; the CBC program *Marketplace* has done many assessments of various consumer concerns across Canada. In particular, in one episode, "Money Where Your Mouth Is" (originally aired October 19, 2012),[7] the show focused on dentists, the services they recommended and the costs associated with the service. The results of the research conducted for the show showed a wide variation in recommended services and costs, but also recognized that many times there is no black-and-white answer; there are shades of grey.[7]

Product attributes affect the ease of evaluation by patients. When a product is a good, it tends to be easy to evaluate; when a product is a service, it is difficult to evaluate. One must recognize that goods and services are not mutually exclusive, and there is a scale that ranges from strictly a good (e.g., a bag of chips) to strictly a service (e.g., laser eye surgery), with a mix in between (e.g., restaurant meal).

SUMMARY OF UNIQUE CHARACTERISTICS OF PRODUCTS AS SERVICES

When a product is a service, there are many unique aspects to consider in designing services. Patients will assess the product offering using search, experience and credence attributes. Being aware of the credence attributes inherent in providing professional pharmacist services can help pharmacists' patients, and other stakeholders, assess their service quality.

RESOURCES AND SUGGESTED READINGS

Berkowitz EN. Essentials of health care marketing. 3rd ed., Jones & Bartlett Learning; 2011.

Doucette WR, McDonough RP. Beyond the 4Ps: using relationship marketing to build value and demand for pharmacy services. J Am Pharm Assoc (Wash). 2002;42(2):183–93, quiz 193–4. http://dx.doi.org/10.1331/108658002763508470. Medline:11926661

Galetzka M, Verhoeven JW, Pruyn ATH. Service validity and service reliability of search, experience and credence services: A scenario study. Int J Serv Ind Manage. 2006;17(3):271–83. http://dx.doi.org/10.1108/09564230610667113.

Isetts, BJ, Schommer, JC, Westberg, SM, et al. (2012). Evaluation of a consumer-generated marketing plan for medication therapy management services. Innovations in Pharmacy, 3(1), Article 66.

Kotler P, Hayes T, Bloom PN. Marketing professional services. 2nd ed., Prentice Hall Press; 2002.

Perepelkin J. Public opinion of pharmacists and pharmacist prescribing. Canadian Pharmacists Journal. 2011;144(2):86–93. http://dx.doi.org/10.3821/1913-701X-144.2.86.

Perepelkin J. Why pharmacists should not think of marketing as a dirty word. Can Pharm J (Ott). 2014;147(1):15–9. http://dx.doi.org/10.1177/1715163513513866. Medline:24494011

Perepelkin J, Di Zhang D. Brand personality and customer trust in community pharmacies. International Journal of Pharmaceutical and Healthcare Marketing. 2011;5(3):175–93. http://dx.doi.org/10.1108/17506121111172194.

Wood, KD, Offenberger, M, Mehta, BH, Rodis, JL. (2011). Community pharmacy marketing: strategies for success. Innovations in Pharmacy, 2(3), Article 48.

Zeithaml VA, Berry LL, Parasuraman A. The nature and determinants of customer expectations of service. J Acad Mark Sci. 1993;21(1):1–12. http://dx.doi.org/10.1177/0092070393211001.

REFERENCES

1. Kotler P, Bloom PN. Marketing professional services. Englewood Cliffs, NJ: Prentice-Hall; 1984.
2. Sen, Mulchand Shambhulal. Patients' satisfaction towards health care services. Available at SSRN 1473782 (2009).
3. Holdford DA. Marketing for pharmacists. 2nd ed., American Pharmacists Association; 2007.

4. Holdford DA, Kennedy DT. The service blueprint as a tool for designing innovative pharmaceutical services. J Am Pharm Assoc (Wash). 1999;39(4):545–52, quiz 584–5. Medline:10467821

5. American Marketing Association. Dictionary: Brand. Available: www.ama.org/RESOURCES/Pages/Dictionary.aspx?dLetter=B (accessed Aug. 13, 2014).

6. Zeithaml VA. How consumer evaluation processes differ between goods and services. In: Marketing of services. Donnelly JH, George WR, eds. Chicago: American Marketing Association, 1981; 25–32.

7. Canadian Broadcasting Corporation. (2012). Money where your mouth is. Marketplace. Originally broadcast Oct. 19, 2012. Available: www.cbc.ca/marketplace/episodes/2012-2013/money-where-your-mouth-is (accessed Aug. 14, 2014).

CHAPTER 49

Loyalty, Consumer Behaviour and Evaluation

Michael Boivin, *Rph.; Pharmacist Consultant, CommPharm Consulting Inc., Barrie, ON*

Learning Objectives

- Explore consumer behaviour and its implication for pharmacy practice.
- Discuss the consumer buying process.
- Discuss the role of loyalty in pharmacy practice and customer relationship management.
- Define marketing myopia and discuss its implications.
- Examine the role of value and satisfaction.
- Discuss a new product lifecycle.
- Discuss the importance of building demand for services at the same time as creating supply.
- Identify common forms of evaluation.

WHY CHOOSE ONE PHARMACY PROVIDER OVER ANOTHER?

In the ultracompetitive retail pharmacy environment, a question commonly asked is, "Why do clients frequent one pharmacy over others in a marketplace?" There are factors that will initially drive a client to a pharmacy, another set that will lead to client retention and another that will lead to client defection. To understand this process, it is important to first understand consumer behaviour and the buying process.

Highly successful pharmacy practices have the ability to attract and retain their clients. This is most commonly done through relationships that increase client value, loyalty and satisfaction. This chapter explores customer behaviour, some key marketing definitions and how these relate to growing a retail pharmacy.

CONSUMER BEHAVIOUR AND THE STAGES OF THE BUYING PROCESS

Consumer behaviour is the sum of the actions a person takes in purchasing and using products and services, including the mental and social processes that precede and follow these actions. Businesses need to understand the following:

- Why do consumers make the purchases they make?
- What factors influence consumer purchases?
- What factors in society are impacting current and future purchases?

There are five stages in the consumer buying process:[1]

1. problem recognition
2. information search
3. alternative evaluation
4. purchase decision
5. post-purchase behaviour

Problem recognition is the difference between people's desired state and their current state. It must be a big enough difference to trigger a person to consider a way to address this. Another way of looking at it is people having a need that by addressing it, will help move them to a desired state. In pharmacy terms, this could be simply realizing they are out of a medication and need a refill (e.g., the desired state is having enough medication to take), or could be influenced by marketing such as letting clients know they should really receive an influenza immunization (introducing a need—protection from influenza) and a method to address the need (receiving the vaccine).

Information search involves the consumer searching for information to clarify available options. This search for a solution for the problem is based on internal and external information. Internal information is based on a consumer's memory and comes from previous experiences with the problem or need, particular products/services that have been used in the past and an opinion of this experience. External information is based on information received from friends, family and other resources, and formal marketing and selling by the retailer, provider or manufacturer.

In pharmacy practice, it is important that the client is aware of the products and services provided by the retail pharmacy. Without this awareness, it is unlikely clients will consider pharmacy products or services as a solution to a problem or to address a need.

Alternative evaluation occurs after the information is collected and the consumer evaluates the different alternatives available, determines the most suitable option for the need and chooses the one considered the best. To do so, the consumer will evaluate the attributes of the product or service based on two criteria:

- objective characteristics (such as the features and functionality of the product or service)
- subjective characteristics (perception and perceived value of the brand by the consumer)

Based on this evaluation, the consumer will narrow down the potential products to the one that best fits current needs.

Purchase decision is done after the consumer has evaluated all the different solutions to the underlying problem/need. During this phase, the consumer will determine from whom to purchase the product or service, when to buy or, indeed, to not follow through with the purchase. The from whom and when of the purchase are influence by the factors in Table 1.

With so many pharmacy providers available, it is important to identify and market differentiators between different competitors. This will help to influence where the consumer purchases the product or service.

Table 1. The From Whom and When Influencers

From Whom to Buy	When to Buy
Terms of sale	Store atmosphere
Past experience buying from the seller	Time pressure
Return policy	A sale on the item (reduced cost)
Location	Quality of the shopping experience
Cost compared to other providers	

Post-purchase behaviour occurs once the consumer has purchased the product or service and has reflected on the overall experience. The consumer will compare it to expectations and will be satisfied or dissatisfied with the purchase. This consumer satisfaction (discussed later in this chapter) affects the following:

- consumer value perceptions
- consumer communications
- repeat-purchase behaviour (loyalty)

TRANSACTIONAL VERSUS RELATIONSHIP MARKETING[2]

A key traditional marketing principle is transactional marketing. With this strategy, the supplier of a product or service is very interested in persuading the client to choose and subsequently buy their product or service. Once the sale is made, the supplier will likely be more interested in seeking a new customer to purchase their goods or services versus focusing time and effort on previous purchasers. It is believed that the best way to grow a business is through the constant flow of new clients.

Relationship marketing is the core of pharmacy marketing. In this model, supplying organizations are not only interested in making the sale but also in establishing, developing and maintaining relationships with clients. The goal is to develop long-term relationships with clients that could not be easily duplicated by competitors and become a point of competitive differentiation.

Relationship marketing is similar to patient-centred care, in which the goal is to develop a long-term relationship with individuals to understand their needs and deliver products and services to meet their needs. A core goal of this type of management is to develop loyalty to the pharmacy and brand.

LOYALTY

Loyalty is commonly viewed as a deeply held commitment to repurchase or re-patronize a preferred product or service provider in the future. Loyalty can be measured by not only the client's

> **Key Definition**
>
> Marketing myopia is a concept originally defined by Theodore Levitt in 1960 that transformed marketing.[3] He argued that that many companies incorrectly take a shortsighted approach to marketing, viewing it as a tool to sell products/services. Instead, he argued that companies should look at marketing from the client's point of view. For pharmacy, this is a crucial component of the patient-centred care model where the focus is on the delivery of products/services that address the health care needs of the patient.

commitment to repurchase, but also by attitudes toward the brand or establishment. The attitude is

Table 2. Types of Loyalty[4]

Type of Loyalty	Repeat Purchase	Attitude	Notes
True	High	High	Most-preferred category Clients have positive feelings about the product/service and are frequent purchasers – "Raving Fan" Cannot be complacent with this group or they can change loyalty categories
Spurious	High	Low	Repeat purchase is high but there is no positive attitude These clients are commonly attracted by promotions but can easily be swayed by promotions from competitors
Latent	Low	High	People want to purchase the products/services but there are barriers to using them (e.g., location, hours of operation, cost)
Absence of loyalty	Low	Low	Worst category The products/services are undifferentiated from other competitors'

commonly referred to in terms of seeing the product/service in favour or disfavour and it could be referred to as likes or dislikes.

Attitude and the repeat purchases can divide client loyalty based on different categories: true, spurious, latent and absence of any loyalty (see Table 2).

Loyalty is an important concept for a retail pharmacy. Loyalty plays a role in retaining clients as they are less likely to be influenced by the offerings of competitors. The economic benefits of customer loyalty often explain why one competitor is more profitable than another. Two important concepts that drive loyalty are value and satisfaction.

CUSTOMER VALUE

Customer value is the client's evaluation of the differences between all the benefits and costs of the product. The benefits are a bundle of positive factors they can expect from a given product or service. Total customer benefit then becomes the summation of the following:

- product value
- services value
- personnel value
- image value

Product or service cost should be looked at beyond monetary price alone. The price a customer pays for a service contains both direct costs (monetary price) and indirect costs (time, energy, psychic costs). This bundle of transaction costs is one the client can expect to incur when evaluating, obtaining and using the product or service. Total customer price for a product or service is the summation of the following:

- direct costs (price for product and service)
- indirect costs (customer's time, energy and psychic costs for obtaining the product or service)

Many pharmacists focus strictly on the pricing of products or services as the sole factor to increase customer value. What is interesting with this equation is that the total customer value can be higher for a higher-priced product/service. This is done by either increasing the customer

Figure 49.1

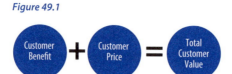

Total Customer Value[5]

benefit through optimizing service and delivery or reducing other costs such as time (e.g., wait time for a prescription) or energy (e.g., convenience) costs for a client.

CUSTOMER SATISFACTION

Customer satisfaction is the match between customer expectations of the product/services and the actual performance of the product/service. The customer's expectation is influenced based on the customer's past buying experience, the opinions of friends/family, what competitors deliver and what the marketer/seller promises. The relationships between expectation and delivery and customer satisfaction are outlined next:

- Expectation < actual product or service value (the service/product far exceeds expectation) leads to a delighted and very satisfied customer.
- Expectation < actual product or service value leads to customer satisfaction.
- Expectation > actual product or service value leads to customer dissatisfaction.

Customer satisfaction[6] is a very important concept for pharmacy-expanded services. It is important to not oversell and underdeliver as this can lead to client dissatisfaction. Pharmacists should not grossly "undersell" as this would decrease the overall demand for the service. It is important to clearly explain what the service/product will deliver and ensure the quality of the service best matches or slightly exceeds client expectations.

The Effects of Customer Dissatisfaction[7]

Many businesses do not understand the full impact of customer satisfaction on their business. It is important to remember in a highly competitive pharmacy environment that clients have a choice to purchase pharmacy service from many different providers. Dissatisfied customers will not purchase products/services from the disappointing pharmacy in the future and will commonly do the following:

- Dissatisfied customers will share their negative experience with other current and potential clients of the pharmacy. (One dissatisfied client can lead to the loss of 2 to 10 other clients.)
- Dissatisfied customers will never share the reason for leaving; they will just start using a competitive service.

CUSTOMER RELATIONSHIP MANAGEMENT

It costs much more to acquire a new client than to retain a current customer. On average, a company can expect to lose a portion of its clients in a given year. Focusing on reducing this defection rate can have a significant impact on profitability. One way of doing this is through customer relationship management.

Customer relationship management (CRM)[8] is a strategy for understanding clients and their needs to optimize the interactions with them. It is used to create stronger relationships with former, current and prospective clients while maximizing your marketing and customer service.

In the CRM framework, a business identifies and differentiates its clients, assesses their touch points with the business and customizes the experience based on the different client. A customer touch point is any encounter the client has with the business. This could include every interaction with the pharmacy staff, front store staff or even through the pharmacy website and social media.

An important aspect with a CRM framework is to identify clients based on their needs and their value to the company. The goal is to identify the business's top 20% clients. This top 20% are believed to account for 80% of the sales of the business and the majority of the profitability.[9] The remaining 80% of the clients contribute significantly less to the sales, and the bottom clients can actually cause negative profitability to the business (meaning the cost to deliver the service to these clients costs the business more than the products or services they purchase).[9]

There are several programs that can help with CRM for business owners to consider. In pharmacy practice, using the data in the dispensary system and point-of-sale (POS) system can help to identify the top clients but also provide insight into their needs (e.g., health conditions) and potential opportunities for future sales. One key factor that affects pharmacies versus other types of businesses is the privacy requirements and legislations. It is important for pharmacists to ensure this is addressed based on national and provincial/territorial standards when designing a CRM system.

> **Business Tip**
>
> It is common for business owners to focus a large portion of time on managing the bottom 20% to 30% of clients. By doing this, they are directing their resources away from the most profitable clients to clients that do not have a significant impact on their bottom line. Worse case is this could lead to dissatisfaction among the top clients and cause them to move to a competitor. It is important to remember that not all clients are created equal, but all clients should be treated fairly.

INTRODUCING A NEW PHARMACY PRODUCT OR SERVICE – LIFECYCLE

Introducing a new pharmacy product or service does not automatically lead to high sales at launch. This can be frustrating for pharmacists as they are hoping a new service will instantly lead to a surge in revenue. One business concept that is important to consider when introducing a product or service is the product lifecycle.

> **Key Definition**
>
> Disruptive innovation is a term coined by Harvard business professor Clayton Christensen. With disruptive innovations, new competitors of a product or service take root initially in simple applications at the bottom of the market and then relentlessly move up the market to displace established competitors.[10] A great example is cell phones, which have displaced the use of established fixed line telephony due to cost reduction and convenience. The key question is how will pharmacy-expanded services disrupt the current market of established health care services?

The majority of new products or services have a lifecycle (see Figure 49.2). This lifecycle will normally progress through recognized stages. Each stage is different and requires changes in marketing strategies and planning. For example, when introducing a new product, the marketing and sales are focused on increasing awareness, where a mature product could have marketing addressed at how the product addresses new consumer needs or problems. Table 3 reviews some features of a lifecycle, and Table 4 reviews the different stages of the product lifecycle.

Figure 49.2

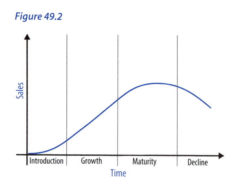

The Product Lifecycle[11]

Table 3. General Principles of a Good or Service Lifecycle[12]

Products have a finite lifespan. This lifespan can vary tremendously from several weeks/months to decades.
The typical product lifecycle curve, as reflected in the sales history of a product, is "S" shaped until it eventually levels off. It is at this point that market maturity occurs and when the maturity phase has run its course, a period of decline follows.
In general terms, the stages in the lifecycle are known as introduction, growth, maturity and decline (see Figure 49.2).
The lifecycle of a product may be prolonged by finding new uses or new users for the product or by getting present users to increase the amount they use.
During its passage through the lifecycle, the average profitability per unit of the product sold at first increases and then eventually begins to decline.

Table 4. The Four Stages of the Product Lifecycle[13]

Introduction	Losses or low profits are common during this stage; investment is required to make the product or to develop the service. Sales are low and promotion costs are relatively high. During the introduction phase, the product or service will appeal to clients that would classify themselves as "innovators" or "early adopters."
Growth	Less promotion is required compared to the introduction stage. (Consumers are aware of the product/service.) Sales are expanding during this stage. There is a decrease in promotion, and higher sales lead to an increase in profit. During this phase, it is common to see new competitors entering the marketplace. During the growth stage, it is common to offer the product or service for newly identified consumer problems or needs. This phase appeals to the consumers who identify themselves as "early majority."

Table 4. (Continued)

Maturity	At this point, there is a decline in the rate of sales growth. This could be due to an overcapacity of the product or service in the industry.
	It is a stage in which profits decline.
	During this stage, firms implement frequent price reductions and increase advertising and consumer promotions.
	It is common to invest again in the product or service to determine if there are new features or aspects that could be introduced to enhance it.
	While the well-established competitors do well, the weaker competitors may quit the market.
	This phase appeals to the consumers who identify themselves as "late majority."
Decline	Sales of most products eventually start to decline for one or more reasons.
	This could be due to a switch in consumer behaviour, the introduction of a new product or service that better addresses the need or overcapacity in the market.
	Prices will normally drop at this stage to attract a declining number of consumers and addressing slower sales.
	Consideration must be made to drop the product or service and to look for new products or services at an earlier point in their lifecycle.
	This phase appeals to the consumers who identify themselves as "laggards."

NEW PHARMACY SERVICES – BUILDING DEMAND WHILE CREATING SUPPLY

Many pharmacists become frustrated when they offer a service in their pharmacy and realize it is not actively used by patients. This frequently discourages them from adding new services in their pharmacy practice.

If pharmacists reviewed the consumer purchasing behaviour model and product lifecycle, they would understand why this occurs. Clients will purchase services and products based on a perceived need or problem. Even if they have a need or problem that could be addressed by a pharmacy service, without knowing about the service, they do not have this information available when they identify a solution to their need. In other words, they are not even aware the pharmacist service can address the need or problem.

When launching a new product or service, it is important to create demand as well as supply. By informing clients of an underlying problem or a potential need and how the product or service can fit this need, the new product or service would be considered. This also provides a key aspect of marketing and sales: it is important to focus on what the product or service will do for a client and what problem or need it will address versus focusing on what the service actually is.

> **Marketing Tip**
>
> When marketing a new product or service to a client, look at it from the client's perspective. Sales and marketing efforts should be able to answer the client's key question: "What's in it for me?" Remember, being too close to the product/service can create a bias and could make it more difficult to market from the client's perspective.

EVALUATING THE CUSTOMER EXPERIENCE

Every successful business must objectively evaluate its strategies and determine if the products and services offered are leading to an increase in sales and profitability. Careful evaluation allows for owners to modify the offerings to best fit client needs and ensure they are providing the best possible customer experience.

As mentioned earlier, the technology in most community pharmacies can be used to provide data on the purchasing behaviours of top clients. By using the data provided by the pharmacy dispensary system and POS system, owners can identify key clients, key information regarding these clients (e.g., demographic information, buying patterns, disease information and history of purchases, including new products and services). This data can be used to tailor pharmacy offerings to address the needs of these top clients.

Another approach to consider is to evaluate current offerings and customer experience through the use of interviews with clients. By discussing their key needs and problems, owners can tailor current and future offerings to reflect their needs. This can also be done with client surveys and even mystery shoppers. By identifying potential weaknesses in their business and offerings, owners can ensure they are delivering the quality of services required to build pharmacy loyalty.

By constantly adapting and improving the products and services and customer experience, the pharmacy owner increases their probability of growing the business in the future by being constantly able to fill the needs of the clients it serves.

KEY LEARNING CONCEPTS

- By clearly understanding the process in which consumers purchase products, the pharmacist will have insight into how to effectively market and sell current and future product and service offerings.
- Relationship marketing focuses on developing a long-term relationship with clients to continually meet their needs.
- Loyalty is crucial for the maintenance of the pharmacy's patient base and this is strongly influenced by client satisfaction and customer value.
- Customer relationship management is a strategy for understanding clients and their needs to optimize the interactions with them.
- Most products and services follow a lifecycle with clearly defined stages.
- It is important for pharmacy owners to use all available measurement metrics to ensure their product and service offerings are meeting the needs of their clients and they are providing the best overall customer experience.

REFERENCES

1. Brody RP, Cunningham SM. Personality variables and the consumer decision process. J Mark Res. 1968;5(1):50–7. http://dx.doi.org/10.2307/3149793.
2. Baron S, Conway T, Warnaby G. Relationship marketing themes. In: Relationship marketing: a consumer experience approach. London: SAGE Publications Ltd; 2010. Available http://knowledge.sagepub.com/view/relationship-marketing/SAGE.xml, [cited 2014 July 5].
3. Levitt T. Marketing myopia. 1960. Harv Bus Rev. 2004;82(7-8):138–49. Medline:15252891
4. Hawkins D, Mothersbaugh D, Best R. Customer retention and loyalty. In: Consumer behavior: building marketing strategy. 11th ed. Boston: McGraw-Hill/Irwin; 2009.
5. Prasad Naik K. Customer value and satisfaction. Available: www.slideshare.net/Kiranprasad153/customer-value-and-satisfaction-16129717 (accessed Dec. 13, 2014).
6. Fornell C, Johnson MD, Anderson EW, et al. The American customer satisfaction index: nature, purpose, and findings. J Mark. 1996;60(4):7–18. http://dx.doi.org/10.2307/1251898.

7. Hunt HK. Consumer satisfaction, dissatisfaction, and complaining behavior. J Soc Issues. 1991;47(1):107–17. http://dx.doi.org/10.1111/j.1540-4560.1991.tb01814.x.

8. Payne A, Frow P. A strategic framework for customer relationship management. J Mark. 2005;69(4):167–76. http://dx.doi.org/10.1509/jmkg.2005.69.4.167.

9. Lawrence A. Five customer retention tips for entrepreneurs. *Forbes*. Available: www.forbes.com/sites/alexlawrence/2012/11/01/five-customer-retention-tips-for-entrepreneurs/.(accessed July 10, 2014).

10. Christensen C. Disruptive innovation. Available: www.claytonchristensen.com/key-concepts/ (accessed Nov. 30, 2014).

11. Dean J. Pricing policies for new products. Harv Bus Rev. 1950;28:45–53.

12. Levitt T. Exploit the product life cycle. Harv Bus Rev. 1965;43:81–94.

13. Rogers EM. Diffusion of innovations. New York: Free Press; Collier Macmillan, 1983.

CHAPTER 50

Market Segmentation and Strategy

Grant Alexander Wilson, *BComm MSc; PhD Candidate, College of Pharmacy and Nutrition, University of Saskatchewan; Marketing Manager at a genetics company*

Learning Objectives

- Examine the role of environmental scanning in marketing.
- Define what a market is and how it relates to market segmentation.
- Discuss the forms of market segmentation.
- Understand the need to define a target market.
- Explore the distinguishing characteristics of differentiation, cost and niche in establishing a competitive advantage in the market.
- Mass marketing versus segmentation—which one?
- Examine the product lifecycle.

The success of an organization's marketing strategy depends on understanding its environment, market and competitors.

Environmental scanning is the process of monitoring external factors that influence a company, its products and services, its industry and its market. Environmental scanning involves understanding economic, political, social and technological changes that may influence the company.[1]

A market is a set of actual and potential users of a good or service.[1] A market is broadly defined. For example, a new pharmacy's geographic market may be the community where it is located. In the market, buyers can be similar in several ways including age, gender, tastes, preferences, resources, etc. Conversely, buyers can differ in several ways. Buyers can then be categorized or "segmented" based on these similarities and differences.

MARKET SEGMENTATION

Market segmentation involves subdividing a market into user or consumer subsets based on similar behaviours or needs.[2] Market segmentation allows an organization to identify all the kinds of users or consumer groups that can be served. Prior to developing market segments, it is important to understand the user or consumer groups and factors that are important to those users or consumers. Creating market segments enables organizations to develop target markets and, subsequently, marketing strategies.

Before creating market segments, a pharmacy manager must understand the factors that influence a consumer when selecting a pharmacy (e.g., location, parking, product diversity, price, pharmacist-patient relationship, loyalty program, etc.).

Pharmacy managers can segment markets several different ways. For example, a pharmacy manager may wish to segment the market by age. The market segment may include individuals in the community over the age of 65. Segmenting by age is a form of demographic segmentation or segmenting based on demographic information. There are three main forms of market segmentation including demographic, geographic and psychographic. A market can be segmented in a variety of different ways based on demographic, geographic and psychographic information, with no segmentation method being right or wrong. The segmentation method, or methods, should be chosen by the pharmacy manager based on what best describes and defines the segment.

DEMOGRAPHIC SEGMENTATION

Demographic information is quantifiable and definable characteristics of a given population. Demographic segmentation uses demographic information (age, sex, race, marital status, occupation, income, etc.) to define a market segment.[3] An example of a potential demographic segment for a pharmacy is as follows: Males and females aged 55 to 75 with hypertension.

Pharmacists can segment the market based on demographic information either narrowly or broadly, including many or few demographic characteristics. Furthermore, other segmentation methods may be included to further segment a market.

GEOGRAPHIC SEGMENTATION

Geographic segmentation uses geographic information (country, province/territory, city, community, neighbourhood, etc.) to define a market segment.[4] An example of a potential geographic segment for a pharmacy is as follows: Individuals living in the community neighbourhood of Avalon in Saskatoon, Saskatchewan, Canada.

As with demographic segmentation, pharmacists can segment the market based on geographic information either narrowly, broadly or in conjunction with other segmentation methods (e.g., demographic segmentation). An example of a market segment that uses both demographic and geographic information is as follows: Males and females aged 55 to 75 with hypertension living in the community of Avalon in Saskatoon, Saskatchewan, Canada.

PSYCHOGRAPHIC SEGMENTATION

Psychographic segmentation is segmenting the market base on consumer lifestyles (e.g., activities, behaviours, interests, opinions, habits, etc.).[5] An example of a potential psychographic segment for a pharmacy is as follows: Physically active individuals who are concerned about their health and wellness.

Psychographic segmentation can be used solely or with demographic and or geographic information to define a market. An example of a potential market segment based on demographic, geographic and psychographic information is as follows: Males and females aged 55 to 75 with hypertension who are physically active and concerned about their health and wellness, living in the community neighbourhood of Avalon in Saskatoon, Saskatchewan, Canada.

Segmentation methods can be used individually, collectively or in combination. Therefore, pharmacy managers can segment a market in a variety of different ways. Regardless, it is important that the segmentation method is relevant to the practice of pharmacy. Furthermore, elements within the segmentation methods must be relevant to the practice of pharmacy. For example, in the case of a community pharmacy, demographic segmentation based on age and sex may be more relevant than race and marital status, as a pharmacy's store front goods, over-the-counter (OTC) drugs and prescription medications may be more age- and sex-dependent. Further to this example, psychographic segmentation based on activities and behaviours may be more relevant than interests and opinions, as the pharmacy's value-added services, physical location and pharmacist-patient relationship may be more activity- and behaviour-dependent.

TARGET MARKET

Segmenting the market allows organizations to understand similarities and differences by creating subsets of users or consumers. A target market is the segment or subset of the user or consumer group that organizations choose to focus their marketing efforts toward.[6] It is important for organizations to target a market that can be realistically served and strategically aligned with the organizational goals (e.g., maximize sales, profits, market share, etc.). For instance, the previous segmentation examples must be of sufficient size with adequate profit potential to be pursued. Organizations should consider the size, competitiveness, growth opportunity and profitability before targeting a segment and implementing marketing strategies.[6] For example, organizations should investigate the market's size in terms of users or consumers and dollars. Once this is known, organizations should investigate the competitiveness of the market and the potential market share they could obtain. Market share is a percentage of the market served by an organization.[2] After the size and competitiveness of the market is understood, an organization should determine the longevity of the market. Once the size, competitiveness and growth opportunity are determined, an organization has an understanding of the profit potential and value of the market. Furthermore, the organization must have the capability and expertise to serve the segment (e.g., unique hypertension knowledge or services). An organization should evaluate and understand its own strengths and weaknesses to strategically select a target market.

TARGET MARKETING STRATEGIES

Depending on the market, it may only be necessary to define and target a market based on geography. For example, a pharmacy located in a small town with a population of 1,500 people and no competing pharmacy may only need to define its market geographically. Conversely, a pharmacy located in a large city may need to specifically and narrowly define and target its market to succeed financially.

There are four target marketing strategies including mass marketing, segmented marketing, niche marketing and micro marketing (see Figure 50.1).[4]

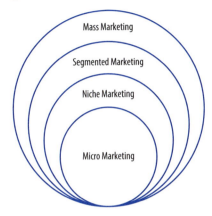

Figure 50.1

Four Target Marketing Strategies[4]

MASS MARKETING

Mass marketing is a marketing strategy that does not target a specific segment but rather the entire market.[4] Mass marketing is often developed for goods or services that appeal to all or to a large number of individuals in the market. An example is the drug acetaminophen. A generic pharmaceutical company may practise mass marketing in hopes of capturing a percentage of the large acetaminophen market. Successful mass marketing depends on effectively communicating something that is appealing to many individuals, thereby selling products in large volumes.[4] Depending on the market size, mass marketing can be costly and require substantial capital to generate sales and gain market share. Mass marketing tends to be difficult for those companies that cannot appeal to a large number of people, thereby not generating sufficient sales volume for survival.

SEGMENTED MARKETING

Segmented marketing is a marketing strategy that targets a specific segment of the market.[4] Strategies are developed to appeal to the chosen segment of the market. For example, if a pharmacy primarily serves a seniors' market, the pharmacy manager may decide to stock more seniors'-oriented products in the store.

NICHE MARKETING

Niche marketing is a marketing strategy that targets a market segment that is less commonly pursued.[4] It requires a clearly defined target market. The goal of niche marketing is to become a large player in a small market rather than a small player in a large market.[1] For example, a pharmacy manager may wish to offer value-added services such as medication therapy management (MTM) to satisfy a niche market composed of patients wanting to improve therapeutic outcomes through education and management.[7]

MICRO MARKETING

Micro marketing is a marketing strategy that targets a small market segment that is narrowly defined.[4] Micro marketing often involves customizing products and services for the individual consumer. For example, a pharmacy manager may wish to offer MTM services, thus creating a niche market. However, micro marketing would entail further developing those MTM services specifically for each patient based on age, health, lifestyle, medications, etc.

Of the four target marketing strategies, mass marketing requires the most broadly defined target market (if at all) and micro marketing requires the most narrowly defined target market.[4] Although each strategy is different, the objective is to create a viable market and a competitive advantage.

COMPETITIVE ADVANTAGE

A competitive advantage exists when an organization's good or service offering is better aligned with the demands of the market than its competitors.[8] A competitive advantage enables the advantaged firm to outperform its competitors. For example, a large pharmacy chain's competitive advantage may be its brand identity, created and maintained by advertising dollars. Natural competitive advantages often exist early in the product lifecycle, as a company may be the only one producing a good or service. Competitive advantages can be sustained throughout the product lifecycle via management (e.g., marketing) or governance (e.g., patents). A patent is an authority to exclude others from creating, using or selling an invention.[9]

Potential competitive advantages can be identified by creating a perceptual map of competitors. A perceptual positioning map shows user or consumer perceptions of organizations based on important dimensions.[4] Figure 50.2 is an example of a positioning map for pharmacies in a small city. Each circle represents a pharmacy's perceived position relative to its competitors based on two metrics (e.g., value-added services and product diversity). The size of the circle represents the pharmacy's market share.

A perceptual map can help determine what user or consumer dimensions are being met and which are not being met. Knowledge gained from a perceptual map can help establish points of differentiation and possibly a competitive advantage.[4] In Figure 50.2, the pharmacies have few

Figure 50.2

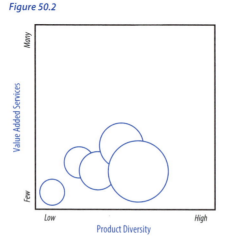

Positioning Map Example 1

value-added services with some product diversity. A pharmacist looking to open a new pharmacy may wish to offer many value-added services with some product diversity (see Figure 50.3).

Continuing with this example, if the pharmacist is able to offer many value-added services with some product diversity, the pharmacy will have points of differentiation among its competitors. However, those points of differentiation have to be relevant and viable to pharmacy patrons in order for a competitive advantage to be established.

PRODUCT LIFECYCLE
The product lifecycle is a set of stages that a product goes through in its lifetime.[5]

CONVENTIONAL PRODUCT LIFECYCLE
The conventional product lifecycle comprises four stages as shown in Figure 50.4.[4,5]

The first stage is introduction.[5] In this stage, a product is first introduced to the market. Oftentimes, if the product is the first of its kind, there is little or no competition. This is known as

Figure 50.3

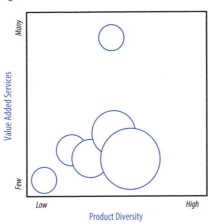

Positioning Map Example 2

Figure 50.4

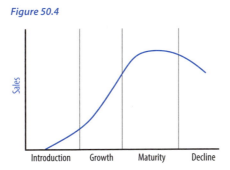

Product Lifecycle[4,5]

first-mover advantage, a form of competitive advantage. At this time, the first sales are generated but profitability has not been reached. The second stage is growth,[5] when sales are gained and most often profitability is reached. In the growth stage, the product becomes well known and faces strong competition, stressing the need for a competitive advantage. In the latter part of the growth stage, competition increases, as other companies market similar products. The third stage of the product lifecycle is maturity,[5] when growth often plateaus. If alternative product uses can be found and marketed, the product lifecycle can be prolonged (see Figure 50.5).[10] If the product lifecycle cannot be extended and there is a product that takes its place, the final stage of the product lifecycle occurs—decline.[5]

The product lifecycle discussed here is the traditional product lifecycle (see Figures 50.4 and 50.5) that applies to conventional products and differs from that of the pharmaceutical lifecycle.

PHARMACEUTICAL PRODUCT LIFECYCLE

The pharmaceutical product lifecycle is also composed of four stages (see Figure 50.6).[10]

The first stage of the pharmaceutical product lifecycle is development.[10] To successfully move through the development stage, a substantial amount of capital is required. Due to the tremendous amount of capital required and risk undertaken, pharmaceutical products are

Figure 50.5

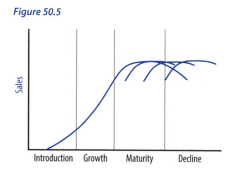

Prolonged Product Lifecycle[10]

Figure 50.6

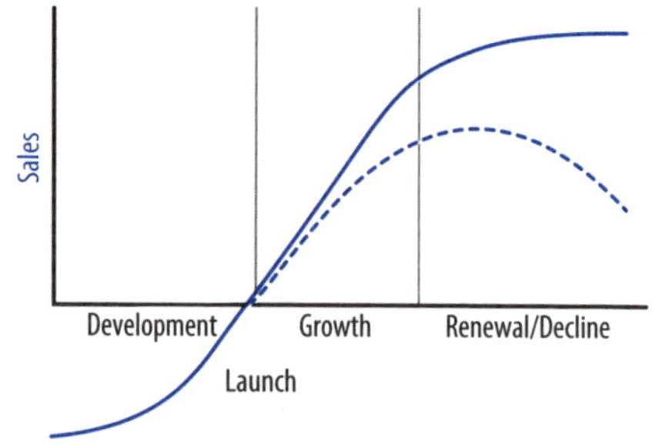

Pharmaceutical Product Lifecycle[10]

patented. The development stage comprises seven substages including basic research, discovery, preclinical testing, phase one clinical, phase two clinical, phase three clinical and regulatory approval.[10] In the basic research substage, companies look to gain an understanding of the disease. In discovery, companies screen anywhere from 5,000 to 10,000 compounds.[10] In the preclinical substage, roughly 250 of the 5,000 to 10,000 compounds enter preclinical testing via computer simulation or animals.[10] In phase one clinical, roughly 5 of the 250 compounds are trialled on 20 to 80 healthy volunteers for the purpose of safety and dose ranging.[10] In phase two clinical, the chosen compounds are trialled on 100 to 300 patient volunteers to determine efficacy.[10] In phase three clinical, the chosen compounds are trialled on 1,000 to 5,000 patient volunteers to determine therapeutic effect.[10] The final substage is regulatory approval.[10]

The second stage of the pharmaceutical product lifecycle is the launch.[10] This stage marks the beginning of sales and revenue. Prior to the launch, all the capital required for development is obtained through investment or borrowing. If a patent is obtained, throughout a pharmaceutical product's launch its competitive advantage is preserved.

The third stage of the pharmaceutical product lifecycle is growth.[10] The pharmaceutical product is introduced globally and sales grow, thereby expanding the market. For example, once a pharmaceutical company receives a Notice of Compliance from Health Canada, it has an exclusive right in the market for a finite period (contingent on when the initial patent was filed). Throughout its patent-protected lifecycle, the pharmaceutical product's competitive advantage is preserved. In the late growth stage, pharmaceutical products come off-patent, often resulting in a plateau of sales and a need for marketing strategies that sustain sales. The term *off-patent* means the pharmaceutical company's exclusive right to create, use or sell a drug has ended.

The final stage of the pharmaceutical lifecycle is renewal or decline.[10] If new growth strategies are introduced, renewal occurs. Continued growth strategies include expanded diagnosis, new indicators, new formulations and product conversion. If no new growth strategies are introduced, decline occurs. For example, when a drug comes off-patent and other companies can legally produce the drug, it may not be financially lucrative for the innovator company to continue to produce the drug.

PRODUCT LIFECYCLE OBJECTIVES
Regardless of the product lifecycle type (conventional or pharmaceutical), the overall objectives are similar. Initially, organizations should focus on having the new good or service adopted by others. After a product is launched, the objective is to grow usage or sales and develop a usage base or market share. As usage or sales plateau, the objective is to devise marketing strategies that expand the good or service's use, postponing its decline.

Practising environmental scanning, understanding the market, segmenting customers, targeting segments that can be effectively served and executing marketing strategies that are based on market intelligence are keys to success throughout any product's lifecycle. Understanding the environment, market and segments enable companies to select a target market and formulate meaningful messages or marketing strategies that are appealing.

REFERENCES

1. Perepelkin J. Marketing strategy. Presented at the University of Saskatchewan. Saskatoon, 2014.

2. American Marketing Association Dictionary. Chicago: The American Marketing Association; 2014. Available: www.ama.org/resources/Pages/Dictionary.aspx?dLetter=M&dLetter=M (accessed April 24, 2014).

3. American Marketing Association Dictionary. Chicago: The American Marketing Association; 2014. Available: www.ama.org/resources/Pages/Dictionary.aspx?dLetter=D (accessed April 24, 2014).

4. Armstrong G, Kotler PR, Cunningham P, et al. Marketing: an introduction. 2nd Canadian ed. Toronto: Pearson; 2006.

5. American Marketing Association Dictionary. Chicago: The American Marketing Association; 2014. Available: www.ama.org/resources/Pages/Dictionary.aspx?dLetter=P (accessed April 24, 2014).

6. American Marketing Association Dictionary. Chicago: The American Marketing Association; 2014. Available: www.ama.org/resources/Pages/Dictionary.aspx?dLetter=T (accessed April 24, 2014).

7. Bluml BM. Definition of medication therapy management: development of professionwide consensus. J Am Pharm Assoc (2003). 2005;45(5):566–72. http://dx.doi.org/10.1331/1544345055001274. Medline:16295641

8. American Marketing Association Dictionary. Chicago: The American Marketing Association; 2014. Available: www.ama.org/resources/Pages/Dictionary.aspx?dLetter=C (accessed April 24, 2014).

9. Oxford Dictionaries [Internet]. Oxford University Press; 2014. Available: http://www.oxforddictionaries.com/definition/english/patent (accessed Aug. 14, 2014).

10. Simon F, Kotler P. Building global biobrands: taking biotechnology top market. New York: Free Press; 2003.

CHAPTER 51

Marketing Communications

Anne Marie Wright; *President, Elements Strategy Inc.* Transforming Healthcare from the Inside Out

---

Learning Objectives

- Understand the difference between marketing and marketing communications.
- Examine the concept of branding and how brands can be used to assist with patient and stakeholder connection.
- Examine the marketing communications planning process.
- Explore various marketing communications vehicles and best practice utilization.

MARKETING VERSUS MARKETING COMMUNICATIONS

Marketing communications is a critical component of the overall marketing plan yet many believe communications covers the entire spectrum of marketing activities. The American Marketing Association defines marketing as, "the activity, set of institutions, and processes for creating, communicating, delivering, and exchanging offerings that have value for customers, clients, partners, and society at large."[1]

Marketing communications, often referred to as MarCom, is a fundamental and complex part of the overall marketing plan and strategy. It is a subset of the marketing plan and loosely defined, represents the messages and media used to communicate with defined target audiences to support the delivery of the marketing plan goals.

Marketing strategy drives the marketing communications strategy. To effectively build a communication plan, it is important to know a product and service inside out, including its unique features and points of competitive differentiation.

Marketing communications is about telling a story, to defined target audiences, in a creative and competitively differentiated way to achieve desired performance.

The 4 Ps of Marketing

Previous chapters explored the 4 Ps of marketing. Marketing communications encompasses promotion, but it is much more and includes advertising, sponsorships, social media, merchandising, community outreach and many more vehicles that are explored in this chapter.

Figure 51.1

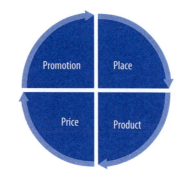

The 4 Ps of Marketing

BUILDING A STRONG BRAND

The global brand-consulting firm Interbrand defines a brand as, "a promise between the company and its constituencies which secures relationships and thus guarantees future loyalty and earnings."[2] Brands are more than just names and logos. A brand is not a product or service, a trademark, the mission or advertising. Brands permeate everything from a company image, investor relations, corporate values, internal communications, marketing directions and initiatives, to technology, business process, training, employee recruitment and engagement. Brands can impact long-term business value creation, growth and cash flow.

In their book *Brand Leadership*, David A. Aaker and Erich Joachimsthaler lay out the principles and model for building brand leadership. Beginning with strategic analysis of the customer, competitors and the strengths and weaknesses of the own organization, a brand identity is created to represent what the brand will stand for. With a clear brand identity, a brand position is then developed to demonstrate the brand's advantage over competitor brands. The brand position is the foundation of the communication plan. With the brand position and brand identity in place, brand building programs, including the marketing communications plan, can then be developed.[3]

TARGET AUDIENCE

Successful communication in the pharmacy market demands a clear definition and understanding of the pharmacy's target audience. It is important to understand who they are, what their most pressing need or issue might be, what attributes of, or benefits from a product or service meets this need or issue, and from where they get their trusted information.

Many potential audiences exist and can generally be grouped into one of two key categories: business to business (B2B) or business to consumer/customer (B2C). A third category, business to government, also exists.

B2B refers to business between companies and audiences that can include other health care professionals such as physicians, payers or disease organizations such as the local diabetes association.

B2C refers to connection between a business and consumers directly. In the pharmacy industry, this connection can also be referred to as business to patient. Many different patient audiences or segments exist such as seniors, young mothers or people with diabetes.

Figure 51.2

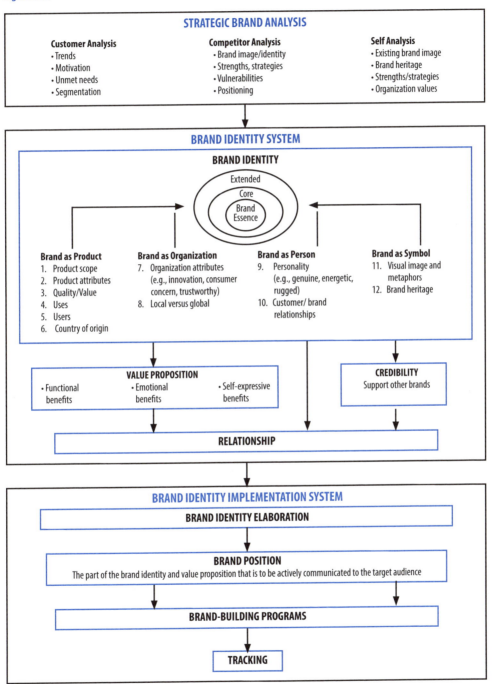

Aaker-Joachimsthaler Brand Identity Planning Model[3]

Depending on the pharmacy environment, the management and prioritization of these potential audiences can be led by different teams or individuals. In a large banner and chain pharmacy, for example, the store-level pharmacist would have responsibility for leading relationship-building activities with their patients while the corporate or head office team would lead all government- or payer-related initiatives. In an independent pharmacy environment, however, the pharmacist store owner would likely have greater involvement over a wider range of target audiences.

BUILDING YOUR PERSONAL BRAND

One of the most important factors for consumers in choosing a pharmacy is the potential relationship that can be established between themselves and their pharmacist. Increasingly, a pharmacist can be a trusted and easily accessed point of care for consumers, particularly in an environment of expanding scope of services.

Personal branding describes the process by which individuals differentiate themselves and stand out from a crowd by identifying and articulating their unique value proposition. For pharmacists, personal branding is important as it can enhance their recognition as knowledgeable experts in their field, establishing reputation and credibility. Developing a personal brand helps pharmacists to grow their networks in a way that interests others.

WHY A MARKETING COMMUNICATIONS PLAN?

The primary goal of marketing communications is to provide information to a target audience in a way that encourages a positive buying response.

A good marketing communications plan requires substantial research, such as that required to have an in-depth understanding of the target audience. Different audiences have different needs and it is important to tailor relevant messages for each target segment. Determine what the goals are for marketing communications activities, what the target audience should know and how best to communicate that information to them. An appropriate budget and schedule for your marketing communications activities will also be needed.

BRINGING THE BRAND ALIVE

Aaker and Joachimsthaler emphasize the importance of brand building programs to bring the brand alive. Marketing communications is a critical brand building program requiring excellent execution that moves beyond the clutter, gets noticed and is remembered, changes perceptions and creates sustainable patient relationships. Excellent execution requires the right communication tools, applied against the right audience, at the right time.[3] (More on this later.)

DEFINING OBJECTIVES: WHAT STAGE IS THE BUSINESS AT TODAY?

If the overall marketing plan is a blueprint for the total marketing effort, marketing communications is a tool to make things happen. Marketing is business planning and strategy—marketing communications is the execution side of selling.

A comprehensive integrated marketing communications plan states specific objectives. For example, an objective might be to increase awareness of a product or service by 25%. The plan's goals should be specific and measurable with some way to determine whether the plan was effective.

Marketing communications plan objectives will be determined by the business stage and needs at a given point in time. For example, if a new pharmacy is being launched, a critical marketing communications objective will be to create awareness. Communicate the brand position or point of difference as part of this awareness building. Once awareness is created, the goal will be to generate trial visits to the pharmacy leading to conversion based on an ability to convince a consumer that the benefit of switching from their current pharmacy is high.

For an established pharmacy, the primary communication goals will be different. Here, the marketing communications goal may be to entrench loyalty by nurturing current and high-value customers.

Continuous assessment and evolution of the marketing and marketing communications plan are necessary. By understanding the business stage and need at a given point in time, different objectives—and subsequently different strategies and tactics—will be required.

DESIGNING A MARKETING COMMUNICATIONS STRATEGY

Once clear objectives are established and the core target audience is identified, a marketing communications strategy can be created. It can take some time as several key process steps are necessary.

- Deciding what to say about the business or service is a first step in this process and is a difficult exercise that should be completed with experts such as communication agencies. Communicating benefits in a compelling and provocative way will draw interest and get the audience's attention.
- Determining budget parameters is a second and important step as it can determine the channels and communication vehicles used to convey your message. This decision can be based on how much the business can afford, a percentage of sales or an assessment of a competitor's spending on communications.

Depending on the market, goals, budget and target audience, some communication channels can be more effective than others. For example, mass advertising to create awareness of a new product or service could be very effective with a broadly defined target audience, whereas a direct mail campaign is likely to be more efficient with a more defined or segmented audience.

- Deciding on the channels is a third step.

An effective marketing communications program should be designed as a continuous improvement process and the effectiveness of the communications mix should be regularly measured and adjusted as necessary.

Figure 51.3

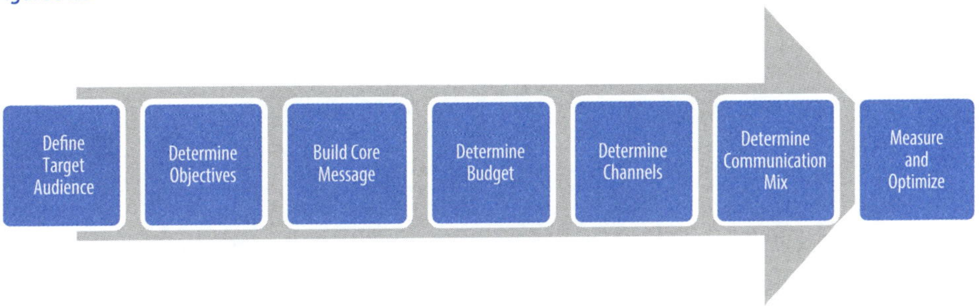

Marketing Communications Strategy Development Process

EXECUTING A MARKETING COMMUNICATIONS STRATEGY AND PLAN

Determine the following to decide on the most relevant and effective communication mix:
- Who is your target audience?
- What is your objective?
- What is your brand message? What do you want to say?
- What budget resources are available?

The following diagram (see Figure 51.4) provides a model through which to assess channel and mix options. In pharmacy, four potential marketing communications channels are possible: external, internal, pharmacist to patient and pharmacist to community. Within each of these channels, there exists a wide range of communication vehicles from which to choose. The communication mix is the combination of these vehicles.

EXTERNAL MARKETING COMMUNICATIONS

External marketing communications can take a variety of forms to deliver messages through a wide array of communication vehicles. Communication vehicles can include broadcast messages such as television and radio advertisements or newspapers and magazines. More advanced marketing communications includes telemarketing and direct mail, as well as public relations.

Fast-growing social media vehicles are increasingly used in the pharmacy industry. Flyers are unique to the retail industry and are used to communicate a broad product message, frequently attached to a price communication. Some flyers incorporate helpful tips, ideas or health content to further engage target audiences along the lines of a magazine.

External communication vehicles are generally used to create awareness of a new product or service and to stay in touch with consumers or patients. These communication vehicles are also widely used to establish an image or a perception about a product or service and the specific

Figure 51.4

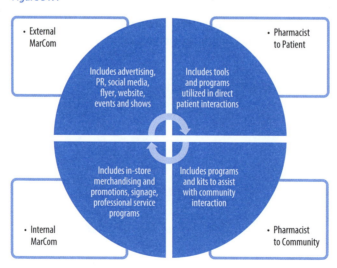

Marketing Communications Model

vehicle is chosen to support the desired image or message, with the desired target audience. For example, a luxury premium-priced women's cosmetic product with multiple product benefits would likely appear in a high-end fashion magazine versus a radio advertisement.

For pharmacy, external marketing communications is also used to invite consumers into the store to meet the pharmacy team with informative and persuasive messaging regarding the services they provide.

INTERNAL MARKETING COMMUNICATIONS

Internal marketing communications vehicles can create opportunities for pharmacy trials and direct interaction with the target consumer. In-store merchandising, announcements and events such as grand openings are all intended to engage a consumer once they are in the store.

Message placement is also an important part of in-store communications. For example, a message in the over-the-counter (OTC) aisle, directing the consumer to speak with the pharmacist regarding a new product, can be very effective. In large format mass merchandise stores, a sign at the front of store can be used to indicate that pharmacy services are available within the store.

Patient disease management programs and clinics are also generally considered to be part of internal marketing communications, primarily because they are critical in driving meaningful interaction between a patient and a pharmacist. For example, a diabetes management program can involve patient screening, device demonstration and consultation on related products and services, all of which assist in establishing a relationship between pharmacists and their patients.

PHARMACIST TO COMMUNITY

Active engagement with the community in which the pharmacy is located can create awareness of a service and lay the foundation for future script capture.

Community outreach in the form of targeted seminars and presentations on various health topics has been used successfully for many years. Planning is an important consideration here; pharmacists need to understand who they want to present to and what and where they want to present. For example, they could reach out to local hospitals, chambers of commerce, seniors' groups and disease associations.

It is common to invest in community-based philanthropy (e.g., sponsorship of youth sport teams and school events) or charitable giving activities as it creates awareness for the pharmacy. Connecting with physicians in the community will also assist in positioning pharmacists for interprofessional collaboration opportunities and establishing them as an integral part of the overall health care team.

PHARMACIST TO PATIENT

Research consistently states that the interactions pharmacists have with patients is the single most important thing they can do. Patients will come back because they have a relationship with their pharmacist and pharmacy team. Trusting relationships are established over time and are defined by simple things such as greeting patients by their name, phoning them to see how they are doing on a new medication, expressing interest in their family and thanking them for using the pharmacy.

It is important to define what type of patient experience to create. Several communication tools are available to assist pharmacists with easy engagement in meaningful conversations. These tools can be used at the pharmacy counter, but also in other parts of the store such as the OTC aisle. Devices such as an iPad with a brief health questionnaire, a pharmacy services brochure, a welcome kit for new patients or simply a business card can facilitate a brief and impactful interaction.

As more pharmacists take advantage of expanded scope of practice opportunities, personal and ongoing interaction with patients will be the single most important marketing communications activity pharmacists can do.

LEARNING SUMMARY

- Marketing communications is a subset of the overall marketing plan.
- The brand position is the foundation of the marketing communications plan.
- Define and understand the target audience.
- Create key messages defined by the brand and target audience.
- Know why a marketing communications plan is needed—what are the specific objectives?
- Based on these objectives, decide on an overall game plan or strategy.
- Choose communication channels and vehicles to align with strategy.
- Constantly assess progress and adjust as necessary.

RESOURCES AND SUGGESTED READINGS

Fill C. Marketing communications: engagements, strategies and practice. New York: Pearson Education LTD; 2005.
Holdford DA. Marketing for pharmacists. Washington, DC: American Pharmaceutical Association; 2003.
Miles L, Mazur L. Conversations with marketing masters. New Jersey: Wiley; 2007.
Ringland G, Young L, editors. Scenarios in marketing: from vision to decision. New Jersey: Wiley; 2006.
Rossiter JR, Bellman S. Marketing communications: theory and applications. Prentice Hall; 2005.
Smith PR, Taylor J. Marketing communications: an integrated approach. London: Kogan Page; 2002.

REFERENCES

1. American Marketing Association website. Available: www.ama.org (accessed Nov. 14, 2014).
2. Interbrand website. Available: www.Interbrand.com (accessed Nov. 14, 2014).
3. Aaker DA, Joachimsthaler E. Brand leadership. The Free Press; 2009.

CHAPTER 52

Social Media Marketing

Kelly A. Grindrod, *BScPharm, PharmD, MSc; Assistant Professor, School of Pharmacy, University of Waterloo*

Learning Objectives

- Summarize the evolving landscape of social media.
- Effectively engage patients through social media by producing or sharing quality information.
- Develop a patient- and client-centred social media marketing strategy for community pharmacy services that accounts for privacy, confidentiality and the needs of the patient.
- Use social media to keep abreast of the latest news and research affecting patient care.

In the last decade, social media has changed how and where people communicate. Social media are Internet-based applications that allow anyone to create, consume, control and connect with information.[1] Facebook, Twitter, YouTube and Wikipedia are all social media platforms that build on emerging digital technologies and networks to allow anyone to easily generate, share and access information.

Social media marketing is about generating awareness and consumer engagement through social media sites. Marketing on social media usually involves developing a message, attracting attention to the message and having people spread the message through their contacts.[2] A 2010 study published in the *Harvard Business Review* found that of 2,100 companies surveyed, 8 in 10 were using or were planning to use social media for marketing.[3] Further, as of 2013, 77% of the Fortune 500 companies were using Twitter, 70% were using Facebook and 69% were using YouTube.[4]

While the adoption of social media has not been as rapid in the health care sector, there is a natural fit between pharmacy and social media. In Canada, there are more than 35,000 licensed pharmacists and almost 9,000 licensed pharmacies.[5] Pharmacists really are one of the most accessible health care professionals, with three-quarters of the profession working in community pharmacies, including small pharmacist-owned dispensaries and large Fortune 500 pharmacy chains.[6]

However, despite being widely accessible in person, almost two-thirds of pharmacists are employed as staff and are likely to be somewhat restricted in how much they can represent their employer online. Further, while there is no direct data on the uptake of social media by Canadian pharmacists, a 2013 survey by the Canadian Medical Association showed that 90% of physicians feel that social media poses professional and legal risks and 40% think social media has little use in the clinical setting.[7] Research on the earliest social media adopters in pharmacy has also found that pharmacist-generated content tends to focus on the experiences of being a pharmacist and is often unprofessional while also being highly critical of patients and other health care professionals.[8]

What seems to be missing from the discussions around social media marketing in health care is that social media may actually provide consumers with a better opportunity to access and understand their own health care. Most people have Internet access, with two-thirds using it to learn about their health and 16% using it to find others with similar health experiences.[9–11] According to a 2012 report from the Health Research Institute at PwC Canada, consumers are also twice as likely to both trust and share information online with a health care provider than they are with a drug company.[12]

At the moment, less than half of Canadians are aware of the scope of services a pharmacist can offer.[13] If consumers go online to find information about a medication-related question or problem, they are apt to find few pharmacists to engage with. Further, the online medication information they find will often be inaccurate and missing critical information on drug interactions and adverse effects.[14–16] As a result, pharmacists interested in social media marketing may find it most rewarding to focus on their own areas of expertise—namely, easy-to-access information about the safe and effective use of medication.

The following information may be useful in planning for the appropriate, effective and meaningful use of social media for marketing for pharmacy. The hope is that pharmacists will be more inclined to promote their own expertise and to contribute to the collective knowledge of medication therapy being produced online.

GETTING STARTED

There are several social media platforms available to help pharmacists market services and share information about medications (see Table 1).

However, before deciding on the best platform, it is important to consider the following questions (see Figure 52.1):

- What am I hoping to achieve with a social media strategy?
- How am I most comfortable representing myself on social media?
- What is my focus or specialty and what can I offer?
- Who is my target audience and how are they using social media?

WHAT AM I HOPING TO ACHIEVE WITH A SOCIAL MEDIA STRATEGY?

Start by writing out the goals of the social media campaign. Is the goal to drive business? Generate awareness of safe medication practices? Promote the profession?

Table 1. A Quick Guide to Social Media Sites[17]

Social media are online platforms that allow anyone to create, consume, control and connect with information. Typical elements include the ability to create a profile; "friend" or follow others to see their activity streams; create content such as text, photos, audio or video; share, tag, rate, comment on or vote on content created by others.

Facebook allows users to connect with friends, share information, photos, videos and website links, and become fans of organizations and companies. More than 1 billion people use it worldwide to upload photos, share links and videos, and to communicate.

A blog is an online journal where users write blog posts to share information or opinions about their lives, areas of expertise or current events. Readers are typically invited to contribute to the discussion by writing their own blog posts or by sharing comments. Publishing platforms include WordPress.com, Blogger.com and Squarespace.com. In many cases, these publishing platforms can be used to create a general website for the pharmacy with different web pages devoted to blogging.

A microblog is similar to a blog, but the posts are brief and often include images or links to other websites. Microblogging platforms include Twitter.com and Tumblr.com.

Twitter is a microblogging service that enables users to post messages of less than 140 characters called tweets. It is often used on a mobile phone.

Professional social networking sites such as LinkedIn and Google+ help users build online networks of colleagues, collaborators and people with similar professional interests. Both sites can be used to drive traffic to your professional identity rather than your personal identity.

Professional landing pages are one-page websites that offer viewers a first glance at a person's expertise. About.me and Expert-File.com both allow users to create simple online summaries of their expertise, often with a focus on public speaking.

A wiki is a website, or collaborative writing platform, where anyone can create or edit content. Wiki stands for "what I know is." The most popular wiki is Wikipedia.com, and RxWiki.com is a pharmacy-specific wiki.

Rating/Review sites allow users to post their own reviews including businesses, service and health care professionals. Rating sites include Yellowpages.ca, Yelp.com and RateMDs.com

Photosharing websites typically allow users to edit, post, store and share photos and short videos online and include Instagram.com and Flickr.com.

Videosharing websites typically allow users to post and share videos publicly or with a small group.

YouTube is the most popular videosharing site with almost 1 billion unique visitors each month. Other platforms include Vine.com, which limits videos to six seconds, and Vimeo.com

Pinterest is a virtual bulletin board launched in 2010 to allow users to gather ideas and images and share collections with other followers. Pinterest has more than 70 million users.

Social bookmarking sites are used to find, aggregate and comment on information online and include Reddit.com, Digg.com and Delicio.us.

Location-based services use a user's location to share information and special deals related to local businesses. Sites include Foursquare.com, Yelp.com and the Places feature on Facebook.

Every social media strategy should have at least one or two clearly defined goals to focus on when identifying the target audience, building the social media profile and measuring success. The goals should also recognize that social media's strengths are openness, shared experiences and user-generated knowledge. Finally, it is important to develop a budget. While much of social media is freely accessible, it can be labour intensive and needs to be regularly managed by qualified personnel.

A growing number of consumers are using mobile devices to choose where to shop by finding local businesses online and then reading about the experiences of other consumers online. In a community where the prevalence of diabetes is high, for example, a local pharmacy may want

Figure 52.1

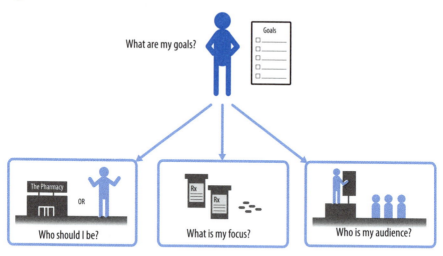

What are my goals?

Goals

The Pharmacy

OR

Who should I be?

Rx

Rx

What is my focus?

Who is my audience?

Considerations for Using Social Media

to use social media to help patients with diabetes implement lifestyle changes. If the pharmacists have a good relationship with some existing patients who have diabetes, they may ask the patients if they would be willing to visit the online rating sites that are popular in their area (e.g., Yelp.com, YellowPages.ca) and leave a favourable review. They could also use Twitter or Facebook to promote a diabetes management service and share regular tips on healthy living that their patients could easily share with each other on their own social media contacts.

HOW AM I MOST COMFORTABLE REPRESENTING MYSELF ON SOCIAL MEDIA?

The second step is for the pharmacist or pharmacy manager or owner to decide if he/she is more comfortable communicating as an individual or as a business.

If the owners, managers or pharmacy staff choose to represent themselves as a business on social media, it will appear as if the business is talking rather than an individual. The advantages to this strategy are that more than one person can manage the pharmacy's social media presence and that the pharmacist will be shielded from overly personal or unprofessional interactions with patients. However, the challenge is that it can be difficult to develop a consistent voice that is both professional and personable when multiple people are sharing the same social media account. Further, because a pharmacist is a person and not a business, the pharmacy may find it difficult to engage the community in meaningful dialogue on health care.

The alternative is for the pharmacist to create a social media presence as a health care professional. The advantage here is that because the pharmacist is a recognized expert on medication therapy, individuals may be inclined to look to the pharmacist's social media accounts as a trusted source of quality information that can be shared within their own contacts and communities. If people develop a relationship with a local pharmacist through social media, they may also be inclined to visit the store when they have a health concern or to direct family or friends to the store.

From a professional perspective, pharmacists could also use social media to connect with colleagues and to keep up to date with industry news or with the ever-expanding medical literature. Pharmacists or pharmacies who offer specialty care could also use social media to develop a provincial/territorial or national reputation or to build relationships with other specialists in the field. Sites such as LinkedIn, Twitter and Google+ are particularly well suited to professional networking.

In Ontario, pharmacist Scott Gavura started a blog called Science-based Pharmacy in 2009 to examine the evidence for commonly held beliefs about medications. He said the blog is, "strongly supportive of pharmacist professionalism and ethical behaviour and strongly critical of using pharmacy as a means to sell products and services that lack credible evidence of effectiveness." Traffic has grown slowly over the years, but with regular posts and with guest posts from other pharmacists, the Science-based Pharmacy blog now gets 1,000 hits each day and has been visited more than one million times. Since starting the blog, Scott has become a recognized opinion leader in evidence-based pharmacy in Canada, been invited to speak on the topic at national conferences and in media interviews, and become a regular contributor to the Science-based Medicine blog, which gets 1 million visits each month.

One final consideration is to plan for negative feedback, trolling any unfavourable reviews online. For example, a patient may choose to tweet about an experience with a pharmacist or to rate the pharmacist on a website such as Yelp.com. Similarly, an anonymous poster may write a negative, offensive or inappropriate comment on a blog post. The easiest way to handle the feedback is to plan for it. For example, in the hospitality industry, many businesses now respond to negative feedback by apologizing and offering to follow up with the customer directly. Many blogging platforms allow comments to be moderated and approved before they are posted.

WHAT IS MY FOCUS OR SPECIALTY AND WHAT CAN I OFFER?

Pharmacists consistently rate among the most honest and ethical professionals.[18] Unlike the social media marketing strategies found outside the health care sector, health care professionals are expected to act at all times with altruism, respect, honesty, integrity, dutifulness, honour, excellence and accountability.[19] These expectations apply even in the arena of social media.

From a patient-centred perspective, social media is likely best suited to helping pharmacists share new, interesting or important information related to medication therapy. The value of easy-to-understand information about health care cannot be underestimated. For individuals to find, understand and appraise online health care information and apply it to a health care problem, they must be not only traditionally literate, but also health literate, information literate, science literate, media literate and computer literate.[20] Considering that health care professionals themselves struggle to navigate the medical literature, the most important thing the pharmacist or pharmacy can offer their audience through social media is practical and accurate information that anyone can understand, even patients with low health literacy.

In Toronto, for example, pharmacist Shelley Diamond has created an excellent website to help patients and health care professionals manage diabetes. The website, www.diabetescarecommunity.ca, includes videos, self-management tools, recipes, a product directory, an online community for people living with or caring for someone with diabetes and a blog written by health care professionals.

In the United States, outpatient pharmacist Dr. Steve Leuck developed the website www.AudibleRx.com to create and share audio recordings of medication information for patients. While the idea came from one of his patients, he was motivated after noticing that many of the patients he encountered needed more information than was being offered by their own pharmacies.[21] Dr. Leuck promotes the recordings through Facebook, Twitter, LinkedIn and his blog, and regularly engages with other health care professionals online to read and review his material.

WHO IS MY TARGET AUDIENCE AND HOW ARE THEY USING SOCIAL MEDIA?

The message and social media platform chosen will be directly tied to what the target audience needs and where they are online. Easy-to-understand information will be valuable to patients but also to other health care providers who may want to share it with their own patients or among their networks. As a result, the target audience may be the pharmacy's own patients or may even extend beyond that network.

Research from the Pew Internet and American Life project in the United States shows that social media use is increasing for all age groups, but adoption is highest for people less than age 50 (see Figure 52.2).[22] While only around half of people aged 45 to 64 are willing to share health information online, 80% of young adults aged 18 to 24 report they are willing to share information about their health online, and 90% are willing to engage with online health activities.[22] A 2011 report from the National Research Corporation also found that Facebook and YouTube are used most by consumers to access information about health.[23]

It is also worth noting that while most social media users will be younger, half of consumers who are online use the Internet to look for health information online on behalf of someone

Figure 52.2

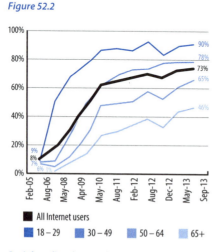

Social media adoption by age group 2005–2013

(used with permission from the Pew Research Center; available: www.pewinternet.org/fact-sheets/social-networking-fact-sheet/)

else,[23] meaning that the audience may extend beyond the people who are actually on the social media platforms. It is becoming more common for family members to show each other a You-Tube video at a family gathering or to share an interesting link through email. The traditional media sources of radio and television are also integrating social media into regular broadcasting. Even on a small scale, if a pharmacy is producing quality content, their own patients could be shown the information on a mobile device while they wait for a prescription in the pharmacy.

PUTTING IT ALL TOGETHER

Once the pharmacist, manager or owner has identified the goals, persona, focus and target audience, the final step is to create the messages. At large companies, social media marketing will often involve teams of communications experts who research and develop high-level strategies and messages. Pharmacists, on the other hand, already have simple and accurate messages they deliver every day to patients. Whether it is tips on non-drug options or information about a new drug or a study, pharmacists spend much of their day sharing information. The key for pharmacists will be to take the high-quality information they are already sharing in day-to-day conversations and adapt it to social media.

Perhaps one of the easiest places to start is with a website. Many established stores will already have a website, especially large chain and banner stores. However, for smaller independently owned businesses, several websites are available to help individuals build their own site for less than $100 per year.

A website can be a simple landing page with basic information about store hours and expertise. A more involved website may offer a profile of the store's staff or a pharmacist-authored blog reviewing new products or emerging research. Similarly, individual pharmacists employed in more restrictive settings may find they want to create a professional landing page through LinkedIn, Google+ or About.me, or they may wish to build a stronger online presence by developing a blog that is clearly separate from their employer's online activities.

Two popular free sites for building websites include Blogger, owned by Google, and Word-Press, owned by Automattic, Inc. Both sites have been available for more than a decade and were originally designed for blogging. Both sites are also easily personalized, with several free and low-cost templates available to users wanting to create professional websites.

There are also multi-network platforms that can help users manage multiple sites such as LinkedIn, Facebook, Twitter and blogs. Hootsuite, for example, allows for scheduling messages, analyzing social media campaigns and exploring the conversations happening in the social media community.

EXAMPLE: A HYPERTENSION CLINIC

A hypertension clinic in a small-town pharmacy offers a simple example of how a social media marketing strategy can be put together.

- What am I hoping to achieve with a social media strategy? Following the approach described previously, a pharmacist could start by identifying the goal, which is to help new and existing patients improve their blood pressure.

- How am I most comfortable representing myself on social media? As the pharmacy is in a small town, the pharmacist may decide to represent the store as a team of pharmacists who are focused on the health of the local community.
- Who is my target audience and how are they using social media? The pharmacist may want to start by identifying the population who is most in need of hypertension management by scanning the pharmacy management system for individuals who are non-adherent to their anti-hypertensive therapy, by contacting a clinician who manages the end-organ complications of hypertension or by asking the local branch of the Heart and Stroke Foundation of Canada. If, for example, the pharmacist finds that the population in greatest need is men over age 60, the pharmacist would know that most men over age 60 spend little time on social media. However, by asking a few patients, the pharmacist may find that many of their target population's adult children are on Facebook.
- What is my focus or specialty and what can I offer? The pharmacy could then develop a Father's Day campaign where the pharmacists help adult children give the gift of life by reducing the risk of heart attack and stroke. For example, the pharmacy could advertise a selection of blood pressure meters, activity trackers and heart-healthy cookbooks. The pharmacy could also promote compliance packaging services, with a focus on adult children who are currently going to their parents' home each week to count out pills.

EXAMPLE: A TRAVEL VACCINE CLINIC

Another example would be a travel vaccines clinic in a bustling pharmacy in a grocery chain.

- What am I hoping to achieve with a social media strategy? If a pharmacist has a particular interest in travel medicine, the goal may be to make travel vaccines more convenient for pharmacy patients and grocery shoppers. The social media goals may be to both raise awareness of the travel vaccine clinic and to keep abreast of the latest travel vaccine news.
- How am I most comfortable representing myself on social media? To promote the travel vaccine service, the pharmacist will likely want to work with the central management and communications teams to identify messages that are consistent with the overall corporate marketing strategy. To keep up to date on travel vaccine news, the pharmacist may find it easier to create personal profiles separate from that of the employer.
- Who is my target audience and how are they using social media? To generate interest in the travel vaccine service, the pharmacist could start by searching patient records to get an idea of the types of patients who have picked up prescriptions for malaria prevention and traveller's diarrhea. If, for example, the bulk of patients appear to be young adults aged 18 to 25 and families in which the parents are aged 35 to 55, the pharmacist could work with the employer to develop a Facebook page to promote the clinic, share information about travel advisories and offer suggestions for packing health care supplies when travelling. To keep up to date, the pharmacist could also start a personal Twitter account to follow the latest news through profiles such as the Government of Canada's Travel Twitter account (@TravelGOC) and the Centers for Disease Control

and Prevention (CDC) travel account (@CDCTravel). The pharmacist could also create a LinkedIn page for other pharmacists and physicians interested in offering travel vaccine services.

- What is my focus or specialty and what can I offer? In this second example, the pharmacist will limit the scope of social media efforts to the prevention of illnesses related to travel.

Social media marketing is as much about the profession as the business. Within the community, the pharmacist is the medication expert and it should be natural that the pharmacist is the medication expert online as well. However, before using the social media space to market a service or a pharmacy, it is very important to ensure the social media profiles are an extension of the pharmacist's and pharmacy's professional identity. Every good strategy will include goals, a pre-determined persona, a focus and a target audience. Regardless of whether one engages as a pharmacist or as a business, whether one is a specialist or generalist, and whether the audience is local or global, an online reputation is about one's professional reputation as much as it is about the reputation of the business. Keep it smart.

REFERENCES

1. Kaplan AM, Haenlein M. Users of the world, unite! The challenges and opportunities of social media. Bus Horiz. 2010;53(1):59–68. http://dx.doi.org/10.1016/j.bushor.2009.09.003.
2. Freebase. Social media marketing (website). Available: www.freebase.com/m/0gpmcb (accessed April 30, 2014).
3. Harvard Business Review Analytic Services. The new conversation: taking social media from talk to action. 2010. Harvard Business Review. Available: https://hbr.org/resources/pdfs/tools/16203_HBR_SAS%20Report_webview.pdf (accessed May 2, 2014).
4. Ganim Barnes N, Lescault AM, Wright S. 2013 Fortune 500 are bullish on social media: big companies get excited about Google+, Instagram, Foursquare and Pinterest. Available: www.umassd.edu/cmr/socialmediaresearch/2013fortune500/ (accessed May 4, 2014).
5. National Association of Pharmacy Regulatory Authorities. National statistics 2012. Available: http://napra.ca/pages/Practice_Resources/National_Statistics.aspx (accessed Nov. 29, 2012).
6. Canadian Institute for Health Information. Pharmacists in Canada. 2010. National and jurisdictional highlights and profiles. Ottawa: CIHI; 2011.
7. Rich P. MDs avoiding social media in droves. Ottawa, ON: Canadian Medical Association; 2014. Available www.cma.ca/En/Pages/MDs-avoiding-social-media-in-droves-poll.aspx , [cited 2014 May 4].
8. Clauson KA, Ekins J, Goncz CE. Use of blogs by pharmacists. Am J Health Syst Pharm. 2010;67(23):2043–8. http://dx.doi.org/10.2146/ajhp100065. Medline:21098377
9. Fox S, Duggan M. Mobile health 2012. Washington DC: Pew Research Center's Internet and American Life Survey; 2012. Available: www.pewinternet.org/~/media//Files/Reports/2012/PIP_MobileHealth2012_FINAL.pdf (accessed Feb. 21, 2013).
10. Statistics Canada, Individual Internet use and e-commerce, The Daily, 12 October 2011.
11. Fox S, Duggan M. Peer-to-peer health care. Washington DC: Pew Research Center's Internet and American Life Survey; 2013.
12. PwC Health Research Institute. Social media "likes" in health care: from marketing to social business. PwC: April 2012. Available: www.pwc.com/us/en/health-industries/publications/health-care-social-media.jhtml (accessed May 2, 2014).
13. Reid I. Pharmacy in Canada survey November 2013 (Sponsored by Pfizer Canada Inc.). Available: www.pfizer.ca/en/media_centre/news_releases/article?year=2013&article=434 (accessed May 5, 2014).
14. Dunne SS, Cummins NM, Hannigan A, et al. Generic medicines: an evaluation of the accuracy and accessibility of information available on the Internet. BMC Med Inform Decis Mak. 2013;13(1):115. http://dx.doi.org/10.1186/1472-6947-13-115. Medline:24099099
15. López Marcos P, Sanz-Valero J. [Presence and adequacy of pharmaceutical preparations in the Spanish edition of Wikipedia]. Aten Primaria. 2013;45(2):101–6. Medline:23159792
16. Kupferberg N, Protus BM. Accuracy and completeness of drug information in Wikipedia: an assessment. J Med Libr Assoc. 2011;99(4):310–3. http://dx.doi.org/10.3163/1536-5050.99.4.010. Medline:22022226
17. Grindrod K, Forgione A, Tsuyuki RT, et al. Pharmacy 2.0: a scoping review of social media use in pharmacy. Res Social Adm Pharm. 2014;10(1):256–70. http://dx.doi.org/10.1016/j.sapharm.2013.05.004. Medline:23810653
18. Gallup honesty and ethics poll. November 2011. Available: www.gallup.com/poll/1654/Honesty-Ethics-Professions.aspx (accessed Nov. 11, 2013).

19. American Board of Internal Medicine Committees on Evaluation of Clinical Competence and Communication Programs. Project professionalism. Philadelphia, PA: Author; 2001. p. 5.

20. Norman CD, Skinner HA. eHealth literacy: essential skills for consumer health in a networked world. J Med Internet Res. 2006;8(2):e9. http://dx.doi.org/10.2196/jmir.8.2.e9. Medline:16867972

21. Poquette J. An interview with Steve Leuck from Audible Rx. The Honest Apothecary. Available: www.thehonestapothecary.com/2013/04/06/an-interview-with-steve-leuck-from-audiblerx/ (accessed May 2, 2014).

22. National Research Corporation ticker survey.

23. Fox S, Duggan M. Health Online 2013. Pew Internet & American Life Project. Available: www.pewinternet.org/2013/01/15/health-online-2013/ (accessed May 2, 2014).

XII. BUSINESS PLANS

CHAPTER 53

Business Planning to Business Plan

Vesna Nguyen, *BSc(Pharm), MBA, PhD*

Bryan Davis, *BSc, MBA*

Learning Objectives

- Understand what a business plan is and who can benefit from a good business plan.
- Define business structures and understand the importance of a shareholder agreement.
- Learn about different business plan models and composition.
- Understand how to integrate management principles and frameworks into the plan, including functional (marketing, human resources management, operations, finance and accounting), business and corporate strategies.
- Understand effective construction and use of financials in the business plan.
- Understand what makes a great business plan (the people, opportunity, context and risk/rewards).

Case Story

Karen is a recent pharmacy graduate and aspiring entrepreneur. She was recently hired as a pharmacist in a national pharmacy in Nova Scotia. Karen is excited to provide patient-centred care and expand the range of pharmacy services provided in her community. The pharmacy manager, Jason, approached her to discuss ways to improve the pharmacy's revenues and offer more value to patients. Karen's excitement grows as she ponders all the potential opportunities. Armed with Jason's business plan from last year, Karen sets out to contemplate the strategic landscape where business meets pharmacy and create a great business plan to support her ideas.

Meanwhile, Anthony has been working for several years as a pharmacist in British Columbia. Anthony's entrepreneurial ambition is to one day start his own pharmacy in his hometown.

WHAT IS A BUSINESS PLAN?

A business plan is a road map of desired future activities; it outlines the what, why, who, where, when and how of a business's operations. Business plans introduce structure and framework. In essence, they are a way to create and record a business idea. It may be improved iteratively to refine the concept and eventually shared with stakeholders.

A business plan is not just for entrepreneurs. It is a tool that can be employed by virtually anyone in business for any scope of project—from starting a new

> A good business plan is designed to prove that there is a unique, compelling and competitive rationale for the proposed business model.
>
> Karen's objective is to comprehensively summarize the extent to which the business can benefit by increasing value for patients. Her intended audience is her manager, Jason, whom she must convince with compelling evidence.
>
> Anthony's objective is to prepare a comprehensive "outward-looking" business plan to eventually present to a loan officer at the bank to finance his pharmacy. Anthony will have to prove that his idea is sound, likely to succeed and considers all risks.

business from scratch to adding new services to an existing business. Business plans vary in both size and formality and can be small or large, formal or informal. The process of business planning is considered more important than the business plan itself—it is a preparation exercise and skill that ensures all aspects of the new venture or project and its potential risks are well thought out. Taking this step strengthens a new venture or project's chances of success. The process of business planning considers the feasibility of the business model and the practicality of setting it in motion.

THE BUSINESS PLANNING TO BUSINESS PLAN PROCESS

Many business processes follow a Plan-Do-Study-Act management model of business process improvements[1] (see Figure 53.1). Like many processes, significant consideration and effort are spent in the planning process before the "doing" phase. A business is an ever-changing evolving entity that

Figure 53.1

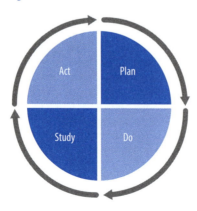

Plan-Do-Study-Act Cycle

(courtesy of The W. Edwards Deming Institute)

requires the planning aspects to be equally dynamic. Further, a business plan is an iterative document that should evolve as the business evolves. The Plan-Do-Study-Act framework can be applied to the process of business planning from inception to the consequent evaluation of the proposed changes. When engaging in business planning, whether proposing a new business or new strategies to an existing business, a change is being proposed. Business planning tries to envision the change, support the need for the proposed change and capture the impact of the change on the current state. The business plan is a communication tool that encapsulates business planning regardless of whether it is limited to internal circulation or shared externally with stakeholders.

Following are the four stages of the Plan-Do-Study-Act model:

- Plan: the stage that results in the creation of the business plan
- Do: the implementation or execution of the business plan (setting the plan in motion)
- Study: an evaluation of the effectiveness of the proposed strategies within the business plan (e.g., How well did you meet your goals?). This stage is an analysis of the effectiveness of the plan.
- Act: where changes are made to the business plan (the iterative process). Based on an evaluation of the plan, an informed decision may be made upon necessary next steps and would restart the entire cycle by engaging in the Plan stage.

PROCESS

Creating a strong business plan integrates three key activities: brainstorming, investigating and researching, and formalizing the business plan (see Figure 53.2).

BRAINSTORMING

Brainstorming is a key stage toward envisioning the dynamics of a business. Osterwalder, Pigneur and Clark's Business Model Generation Canvas[2] is an effective way of illustrating nine important building blocks (see Figure 53.3).

Using a visual "canvas" is appealing as it can be done in a wide range of formats, from paper to whiteboard to electronic, and it is also conducive to brainstorming as a group. For best results, use sticky notes or coloured markers and focus on being creative. Key details of the nine cells are discussed as follows:

Value propositions are central to business planning. What are the customer's problems that the business can solve? What customer needs will be met—ideally in a manner that is better, easier or cheaper—than the competition?

Figure 53.2

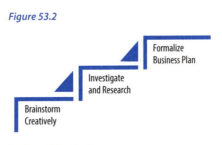

Business Planning Process

Figure 53.3

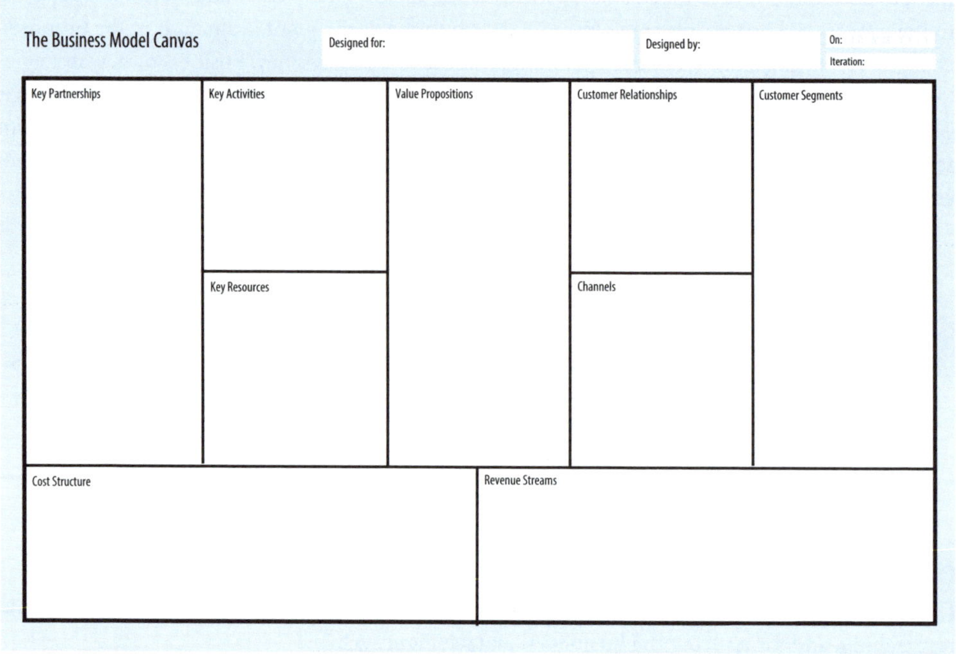

The Business Model Canvas
Designed for: Designed by: On:
                                          Iteration:

Key Partnerships	Key Activities	Value Propositions	Customer Relationships	Customer Segments
Key Resources	Channels
Cost Structure	Revenue Streams

The Business Model Canvas³

Customer segments address who is being served by the business (see Chapter 50: Market Segmentation and Strategy). As described previously, customer segments may be *geographic, demographic* or *psychographic* based on user *benefits, profession, lifestyle, interests, etc.,* or other. There may also be multiple customer segments. Careful consideration of segmentation—and whether or not it is even needed—helps to inform other aspects of the business plan such as the value proposition.

Customer relationships are established and maintained with each of the customer segments that have been identified. Important considerations could include waiting times, personal interaction with the pharmacist and the store layout. For instance, providing pharmacy services or counselling requires a private space.

Focus on Incentives

Retail pharmacies face emerging regulatory challenges in creating customer loyalty and maintaining their competitive advantage. Multiple regulatory bodies across Canada have implemented or supported a ban on rewards tied to the purchase of prescription drugs.

"The colleges argue that the inducements - such as coupons, Air Miles®, Aeroplan® or Shoppers Drug Mart Optimum® rewards - put patient health at risk, damage the relationship between patients and pharmacists, and undermine the profession's reputation." Opponents of the prohibition argue that customers will be shortchanged by the ban. This issue highlights how regulatory pressures can influence the business climate and your competitive advantage, considering the impact on patient safety and business viability.⁴

Incentive programs have played a changing role in pharmacies' customer relationships. Traditionally used to facilitate customer loyalty, incentive programs have been largely phased out at the time of writing. While legal challenges and new evidence make the issue by no means settled, pharmacies will benefit from adopting new and creative ways of maintaining relationships with customers.

> ### Focus on Canada's Anti-Spam Legislation (CASL)[5]
>
> CASL requires businesses to obtain either express "opt-in" or implied consent to send commercial electronic messages that include emails and certain types of social media messages. All electronic marketing messages will need to clearly and prominently identify the sender and provide an unsubscribe mechanism. Organizations that do not comply risk serious penalties, including criminal charges, civil charges and personal liability for company officers and directors, and penalties up to $10 million.

Channels are a business's way of reaching the customer. Pharmacy service-delivery channels are nearly exclusively composed of in-store visits. Communications channels include traditional aspects (print media, signs, radio and telephone books) and newer approaches such as web ads, search engine optimization and social media.

Key partnerships are the alliances and relationships that allow a business to enhance performance or minimize risk. Business Model Generation identifies four types of partnerships:

- *buyer-supplier relationships* to ensure reliable suppliers: A pharmacy may consider partnering with drug intermediaries such as McKesson Canada to undertake vendor managing inventory schemes or companies that provide technology or educational support services such as Pharmacy Access Solutions and Pear Healthcare.

> ### Canadian Competition Act[6]
>
> The Act, Bill C-34, "provides for the general regulation of trade and commerce in respect of conspiracies, trade practices and mergers affecting competition." The Act specifically outs anti-competitive practices such as price fixing, dividing territories or operating areas with competitors to avoid competition and fixing, controlling or preventing the production or supply of a product.

- *joint ventures* to develop new businesses: Is there an opportunity to partner with the local university to support improved training? Could the pharmacist partner with other health care professionals (e.g., physicians, nurses or dieticians) to offer an integrated health care space?
- *strategic alliances* between non-competitors: Such alliances could advance the common good if a pharmacy could ensure prompt and dedicated services to vulnerable populations (e.g., a seniors' assisted-living facility or psychiatric care services) or trending markets (e.g., corporate wellness programs).
- *strategic partnerships* between competitors: While comparatively rare, this includes broad areas of common concern such as regulation and professional standards. The ability to work cooperatively with competitors allows pharmacists to speak with a more unified voice. However, there are clear legal limitations as to the elements that partnerships with competitors may cover.

Business structures

The structure of a business formalizes key relationships. Not explicitly addressed in the Business Model Generation Canvas, this may nevertheless be thought of as a foundational element. The decision about how to structure a business is important as there are advantages and disadvantages to each (see Table 1). Specific needs dictate which of the four primary business structures are optimal: sole proprietorship, partnerships, corporations and cooperatives.[7]

Table 1. Business Structures

Business Structure	Definition	Advantages	Disadvantages
Sole proprietorship	Sole owner of the business	Easy and inexpensive	Assume all risks (liability extends to personal assets)
		Low cost and investment capital to start business	Business income taxable at personal rate (higher personal taxes when profitable)
		Control of decision making	Risk to continuity of business (if owner is absent)
		Personal tax advantages if business performs poorly	Raising capital alone
		Profits directly go to the owner	
Partnership	Two or more persons own the business	Easy to start up	Assume all risks (liability extends to personal assets)
		Combining financial resources by partners	Difficulty in finding suitable partner
		Sharing of profits, management and assets	Potential conflicts as decision making is shared with partner
		Personal tax advantages if business performs poorly	Financially responsible for partner's business decisions
Corporation	Legal entity separate from owners (shareholders)	Limited liability (not personally liable for debts, obligations or acts of corporation)	Highly regulated and greater legal requirements for documentation
		Transferable ownership	Greater expense to incorporate compared to starting sole proprietorship or partnership
		Continuous existence	Potential conflicts between owners (shareholders)
		Separate legal entity	Potential conflicts between shareholders and directors
		Easier to raise capital	
		Some tax advantages to incorporation	
Cooperative	Owned by an association of members	Ownership and control by members	Potential conflicts between members
		Each member has one vote (democratic)	Longer decision-making process
		Limited liability	Requires participation of members
		Profit distribution	Extensive record keeping
			Decreased incentive to invest additional capital

Reproduced with the permission of the Minister of Industry, 2014. Adapted from Canada Business Network[7]

Karen's Perspective on Structures

While Karen often focuses on her pharmacy exclusively, it is part of a larger corporate entity. This means she has input from both her manager, Jason, and corporate directives and policies. She also recognizes that her firm needs to be profitable to support dividend payments to shareholders. Ultimately, any project Karen pursues will have to add value to the corporation to be approved.

Anthony's Perspective on Structures

Anthony has yet to decide if he will pursue a sole proprietorship, partnership or corporate structure. While cooperative structures are compelling, Anthony is planning to invest all his savings into the business—a higher sum than any other investor or partner. As such, he will insist on owning a proportionately larger percentage of the business.

Focus on the Importance of Shareholder Agreements[8]

A shareholder agreement is a contract outlining the relationship between the shareholders of a corporation and lays the foundation of interactions between owners with each other and with the directors of the company. Within the agreement, expectations for each party are set and it outlines how a company is managed and controlled. A shareholder agreement can also further define relationships by outlining management, voting rights, restrictions on new and existing shareholders, financing and the transfer and purchasing of shares. A shareholder agreement is a prudent investment that prevents valuable time and resources being wasted on disputes between shareholders.

Revenue streams are essential for a successful business. Pharmacies will have a host of revenue streams, from dispensing fees, sale of over-the-counter products and pharmacy services.

Cost structure focuses on the most important costs incurred while operating under a particular business model.

Key resources are the assets required to offer the value proposition. They may be physical, financial, intellectual or human. Establishing a location is a critical step, as is staffing. For example, how can Karen balance her staffing levels to recruit and retain the best pharmacists and pharmacy technicians?

Key activities are the actions a business must take to operate successfully. Key activities of this type relate to coming up with new solutions to individual customer problems. The

Focus on Retail Chains and Franchising[9]

Pharmacies are increasingly part of many retailers' strategic plans. In Canada, retailers such as Walmart and Costco join grocers such as Safeway and Save-On to all offer pharmacies on-site. Broadening their businesses is driven by the competitive advantage of being a one-stop shop and also that customers may shop for other goods while in the store. Being part of a large retailer as a pharmacy franchise has several ramifications. The overall health and competitive position of the retail partner must be considered. Furthermore, the appeal to demographic and psychographic populations may be already set.

operations of pharmacies are typically characterized by problem-solving activities, marked by knowledge management and continuous training. That is to say, how can Karen's pharmacy meet an underserved need? Can she adjust her hours and service offerings?

Karen decides that broadening her suite of skills would be a key activity to support her value proposition. Upon getting certified to give injections, Karen provides the St. Francis Xavier hockey team with influenza vaccinations allowing her pharmacy additional revenue.

Karen's Perspective on Franchises

Karen is part of a franchised pharmacy in a large retailer. She sees both the limitations and the benefits. While limitations include reduced operational control and payment of franchise fees, she observes that the steady stream of customers is a net benefit from the brand strength of a large retailer and its ongoing business support.

Anthony's Perspective on Franchises

Anthony also sees the limitations and benefits of being part of a franchise. He plans not to pursue this business model because he values autonomy and flexibility in providing pharmacy services to his patients.

FORMALIZING THE BUSINESS PLAN

Formalizing the business plan involves building on the brainstorming phase—which has ideally gone through several iterations and leveraged outside research and expertise—and writing a compelling narrative. The structure and clarity is important as an exercise in personal diligence, but becomes critical if the business plan is intended for external consumption. Figure 53.4 shows the basic elements.

Each business plan is as unique as the business itself and while several templates exist to help frame the business, they should be used as a starting point to develop a business plan that fits a new venture's specific business. Not all templates include all the basic elements but should include those sections relevant in the evaluation of the business as economically viable, providing value and achieving objectives and outcomes.

Figure 53.4

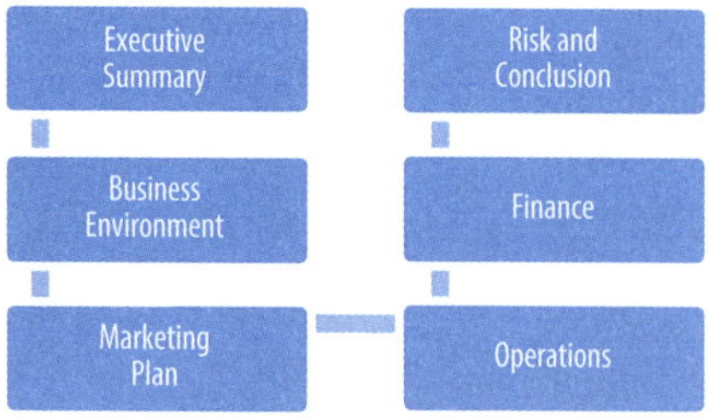

Executive Summary	Risk and Conclusion
Business Environment	Finance
Marketing Plan	Operations

Basic Elements of a Business Plan

Excerpted from the Royal Bank of Canada[10]

Executive summary

The executive summary is an overview of the key points expressed by the business plan and is often considered the most important section. It may be the only part of the plan read, so ensure it is succinct, crisp, neat, compelling and well written. Ideally, the executive summary should be written last, addressing the following recommendations:

- Explain the basics of the business.
- Be interesting! Motivate the reader to continue reading the rest of the plan.
- Be short and concise—no more than two pages long.
- Describe the business concept, competitive advantage, legal structure (e.g., sole proprietorship, corporation; see Chapter 14: Financial Statements and Forms of Business Ownership), the market and personal experience.

> **Principle 1: Define the firm's mission. What does it propose to do, for whom, and how can it do so distinctively?**
>
> One of the key first steps in business planning of a new venture or project is to accurately define it. This permits effective decision making and aligns strategic decisions to the business's mission, vision, key objectives and expected outcomes. In essence, the strategy must fit with what the firm has set out to do. The business concept is a high-level description of the business, in terms of its purpose, unique value, intended target market and goals. One may think of the business concept as an elevator pitch of what the business represents, what makes it special, who may benefit from the organization's offerings and what the firm expects and hopes to achieve.

Business environment

A key component of the business plan is to convey that it has been critically analyzed and realistically assessed for its chances for success. A strengths, weaknesses, opportunities and threats (SWOT) analysis is an effective way to look critically at the business concept (see Chapter 2: Macro-environmental Analysis). The SWOT is populated after thorough analysis of the external and internal environments of an organization (see Chapter 2: Macro-environmental Analysis and Chapter 3: Micro-environmental Analysis). Not only does the SWOT exercise provide an opportunity to strengthen and plan internally, it also conveys diligence of thought and risk management to readers (see Table 2).

Table 2. SWOT Components and Critical Questions[11]

Strengths	Contemplate the strength of the value proposition. Consider what areas the business will excel in. What internal resources exist that are strengths? What advantages are possessed over the competition?
Weaknesses	What are the limitations to the plan? To the industry? What does the business lack (e.g., expertise or access to skills or technology)?
Opportunities	What opportunities in the market exist that could be benefited from?
Threats	What will the competitive response from incumbents be? Who are the existing and potential competitors?

While populating a SWOT, it is essential to conduct a thorough environmental analysis that assesses macro- and micro-environmental forces and trends (see Chapter 2: Macro-environmental Analysis and Chapter 3: Micro-environmental Analysis). A market analysis identifies current marketplace products and services and can highlight the uniqueness of the organization's value proposition and the strength of its industry positioning. A competitor analysis demonstrates an understanding of current and future challenges within the industry and informs business leadership of potential risks to the core business.

Plans and strategies

Break out the key concepts into subcategories. Discuss business, marketing, operational and human resources activities. Please refer to previous chapters for further information on each activity.

Marketing plan

In developing the marketing plan, it is necessary to focus on the core elements, which include defining the value proposition, clarifying the target market and addressing the 4Ps (see Chapter 47: Introduction to Marketing and Key Concepts).

Operations and human resources

This section serves to describe in detail the operations of the firm, including the business structure, the management team, the talents and skills of human resources and logistics of the business. Please refer to previous chapters for further information on leadership (see Chapter 9: Leadership and Management), operations (see Section VI) and human resources management (see Section VIII).

Principle 2: Be informed. Know the competitors and the business environment.

This step involves research and an understanding of internal and external factors that impact the success of the business and the proposed change. The firm does not operate as a silo but is influenced by multiple factors externally, some of which can be controlled, while others cannot. A thorough analysis and understanding of the political, economic, social, technological, legal and environmental factors (see Chapter 2: Macro-environmental Analysis) that can impact the business as well as the impact of the five forces of industry (see Chapter 3: Micro-environmental Analysis) uncover trending threats and opportunities that permit effective strategic planning. Of particular importance in pharmacy is the changing landscape of pharmacy practice and changes within legislation that regulate pharmacy practice and as a whole.

Karen's Perspective on the Business Environment

After a thorough analysis, Karen determines that the surrounding communities are populated by university students and young professionals. Karen adapts the pharmacy business model to attract these customers by extending business hours, adding pharmacy services to increase convenience such as deliveries and promoting the pharmacy through digital marketing strategies.

Anthony's Perspective on the Business Environment

Anthony's analysis has identified that the pharmacy can capitalize on its convenient location near a medical clinic. Anthony focuses his business plan on fostering strong relationships with other health care providers and providing medication management services and patient education workshops for his clientele. Anthony's marketing strategy involves increasing foot traffic from neighbouring clinics to his pharmacy.

Finance

In this section, core financial statements (i.e., a balance sheet, income statement and cash flow statement) are provided. Although most business plans provide *pro forma* or projected financials for the first three to five years of a program, the further the estimation, the less accurate the projection. However, a financial analysis of a business is necessary to understand what are the costs, what are the costs of initial investments and what is the expected profitability. Tools that can be employed to assess the economics of a business have been discussed in previous chapters and include breakeven analysis, sensitivity analysis and multiple financial ratios (see Chapter 14: Financial Statements and Forms of Business Ownership). A financial expert can help prepare this section. Financial projections can be guided by historical company performance, if available, or the use of comparables within the industry for estimations.

Risks and conclusion

A thorough risk analysis of any new business venture or project is critical. Each risk should be viewed through a lens of both consequence and probability; in other words, it assesses the extent of the negative impact of an event and the likelihood that it will happen. Risks should also be envisioned from the perspective of the market/industry, and consumer, where such a multi-lens approach helps to encompass a broader spectrum of risk. Significant risks must have mitigation strategies that may not be perfect but show that the perils and pitfalls that may befall the business

Principle 3: Define the change and justify it.

This step involves describing the proposed change and why it adds value to the business. Here are some questions to ask:

- What change is being proposed and why? Is it a growth strategy? If so, how will it help the business grow (via cost reductions, attracting new customers, addressing an underserved market, etc.)?
- What unique value does the change bring to the business and how does it differ from competitors' offerings?

A key message that should arise from this section is the unique value of the firm's offerings and why the business is a worthwhile investment opportunity.

Principle 4: Design the business with the right people and tools.

It is important to highlight the business's advantages and how the right people will be/have been hired to do the job. The skills and expertise of each key employee or management personnel should be highlighted to demonstrate that the business is built not only on a great idea, but also a sound management team and backed by the personnel to do the job. Describe the firm's competitive advantage and any assets and capabilities that add value to the business, including financial, physical, intangible assets and human resources.

Principle 5: Conservatively estimate the real costs of doing business.

A common pitfall in reporting financials in a business plan is overestimating the financial success of a business. A sound financial analysis demonstrates skill and preparation to external stakeholders such as investors and debtors. Planning, in essence, is a way to assess and mitigate threats and capture current and future opportunities. It is critical to be conservative in estimates of profitability as it reduces the risk of underperforming and underfunding, and demonstrates realism to funding partners.

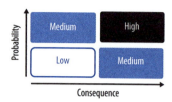

Figure 53.5

Risk Matrix

have been considered and assessed. High risks can be denoted as those of high consequence (e.g., damage, monetary losses, etc.) and whose occurrence are highly likely. Further information on risk management has been provided in previous chapters (see Section V: Risk Management). A simplified example of a risk matrix to visualize and prioritize risks is shown in Figure 53.5. High-impact and high-probability risks should always have a mitigation plan in place.

In this section, contingency planning is provided, in the advent of disasters or those situations requiring emergency responses (see Chapter 26: Contingency Planning) and an exit strategy that encompasses what will happen to the business if key manager(s) exit. Further suggested readings regarding exit strategies are provided at the end of the chapter. A succinct conclusion for your business plan that highlights key messages, goals and objectives should be provided. Supporting documents such as additional financials and timelines may also be included, provided they add value to the business case.

> **Principle 6: Every business has risks, including yours.**
>
> Weaknesses and threats from your SWOT analysis are a good starting point in identifying potential risks. At a minimum, provide a mitigation for each identified threat or weakness. Assessment of risks demonstrates you are prepared and are aware of the challenges to the success of your business.

PUTTING IT ALL TOGETHER

As the business plan nears completion, there are a few more areas to consider:

FOUR PILLARS OF A GREAT BUSINESS PLAN

Sahlman suggests there are four key components to a great business plan:[13]

- people: The right management team and human resources are essential to business success; without them, a great idea can be executed poorly.
- opportunity: Making the business case for the idea as a worthwhile investment involves highlighting opportunities that exist in large markets or those with high growth potential. The market and competitor analyses should highlight the opportunity.
- context: An awareness and understanding of the business as part of a larger ecosystem involving political, legal, social, economic, technological and environmental factors allow one to make more informed decisions, anticipate risks and evolve your business to meet future demands.

- risk/rewards: The greater the potential reward, usually the higher the risks. Identifying and devising appropriate response strategies to risks will help hedge against their negative impacts on the business.

LESS IS MORE

Time is a valuable commodity. Given the speed of business and the inevitably high levels of competition, it is important to concisely and effectively convey the value of the business. A long business plan does not equate to a great business plan. It is a good idea to read other business plans first. Resources containing sample plans and other useful information are provided at the end of the chapter.

EDIT, EDIT, EDIT!

As others only witness the outcome of the business planning process (i.e., the business plan), it is important to ensure the final product is free of errors and polished. Clarity and conciseness are key.

Business planning and the development of a business plan, while time-consuming, are critical investments toward a new venture or project. A business plan is a flexible, dynamic tool that should be adapted and tailored to the business's evolving specific needs and the environment.

Karen's Perspective

Having gone through the process of business planning and developing a business plan, Karen and her pharmacy manager, Jason, identify worthwhile business opportunities and provide the unique, compelling and competitive rationale for their business case.

Anthony's Perspective

After multiple iterations and much research and deep thought, Anthony is ready to put his plan into action. He knows it will not sit on the shelf; it is a living document. He is confident that the rigour and strength will be sufficient to secure funding to let his "Plan" move to a "Do." He is excited to launch his business and have the opportunity to "Study" and "Act" and then repeat the cycle all over again.

RESOURCES AND SUGGESTED READINGS

BUSINESS PLANNING AND BUSINESS PLANS:

Review HB. Creating business plans. Harvard Business Press; 2014.
Schumock GT, Stubbings J. How to develop a business plan for pharmacy services. American College of Clinical Pharmacy; 2007.
Tennent J. The Economist: guide to financial management. Perseus Books Group, 2014.

BUSINESS PLANNING WEBSITES:

Bank of Montreal. Business resources. Available: www.bmo.com/home/small-business/banking/resources/business-resources (accessed Nov. 16, 2014).
Business Development Bank of Canada. How to write an effective business plan. Available: www.bdc.ca/en/advice_centre/articles/Pages/starting_business_plan.aspx (accessed Nov. 16, 2014).
Canada Business Network. Business planning. Available: www.canadabusiness.ca/eng/page/2865/ (accessed Nov. 16, 2014).
CIBC. Your guide to business planning. Available: www.cibc.com/ca/small-business/article-tools/business-planning.html (accessed Nov. 16, 2014).
Royal Bank of Canada. Business resources. Available: www.rbcroyalbank.com/RBC:RnbCjI71JsUAAvCskp8/sme/create-plan/business-plans.html (accessed Nov. 16, 2014).

Scotiabank. Writing a business plan. Available: www.scotiabank.com/ca/en/0,,588,00.html (accessed Nov. 16, 2014).

TD Canada Trust. Business planner. Available: www.tdcanadatrust.com/products-services/small-business/windocs.jsp (accessed Nov. 16, 2014).

EXIT STRATEGIES AND SUCCESSION PLANNING:

Canada Business Network. Succession planning. Available: http://canadabusiness.ca/eng/page/2819/ (accessed Nov. 16, 2014).

REFERENCES

1. The W. Edwards Deming Institute. The PDSA cycle. Available: https://deming.org/theman/theories/pdsacycle (accessed June 18, 2014).

2. Osterwalder A, Pigneur Y. Business model generation: a handbook for visionaries, game changers, and challengers. Hoboken, NJ: John Wiley & Sons, Inc; 2010.

3. Businessmodelgeneration.com. Business model generation canvas. Available: www.businessmodelgeneration.com/canvas/bmc (accessed June 18, 2014).

4. Gautreau M. Drug-free loyalty a sobering reality for pharmacy chains. ShiftCentral, 2014. Available: www.shiftcentral.com/blog/drug-free-loyalty-sobering-reality-pharmacy-chains (accessed June 18, 2014).

5. An act to promote the efficiency and adaptability of the Canadian economy by regulating certain activities that discourage reliance on electronic means of carrying out commercial activities, and to amend the Canadian Radio-television and Telecommunications Commission Act, the Competition Act, the Personal Information Protection and Electronic Document Act and the Telecommunications Act, S.C. 2010, c.23 (2010).

6. Competition Act, R.S.C. 1985, c. C-34 (1985).

7. Industry Canada. Corporation, partnership, or sole proprietorship? Reproduced with the permission of the Minister of Industry, 2014. Available: www.canadabusiness.ca/eng/page/2853/ (accessed Aug. 8, 2014).

8. Bokenfohr M. Shareholders' agreements. Field LLP; 2010. Available: www.fieldlaw.com/articles/MMB_Shareholders Agreements.pdf (accessed June 18, 2014).

9. Gautreau M. Consolidation in Canadian retail space points to the pressures of the times. ShiftCentral; 2013. Available: www.shiftcentral.com/blog/consolidation-canadian-retail-space-points-pressures-times (accessed June 18, 2014).

10. Royal Bank of Canada. Create the plan. Available: www.rbcroyalbank.com/RBC:RnbCjI71JsUAAvCskp8/sme/create-plan/business-plans.html (accessed June 18, 2014).

11. Pickton DW, Wright S. What's SWOT in strategic analysis? Strateg Change. 1998;7(2):101–9. http://dx.doi.org/10.1002/(SICI)1099-1697(199803/04)7:2<101::AID-JSC332>3.0.CO;2-6.

12. Banaitiene N, Banaitis A. Risk management in construction projects. Risk management – current issues and challenges. Available: www.intechopen.com/books/risk-management-current-issues-and-challenges/risk-management-in-construction-projects (accessed Dec. 14, 2014).

13. Sahlman WA. How to write a great business plan. Harv Bus Rev. 1997;75(4):98–108. Medline:10168340

Glossary

4 Ps of marketing: product, price, place, promotion; also known as the marketing mix

Accounting Standards for Private Enterprises (ASPE): a set of standards set by the Canadian Accounting Standards Board (AcSB) that directs private Canadian businesses to use International Financial Reporting Standards (IFRS) for fiscal years beginning Jan. 1, 2011

Accounts payable: an obligation such as amounts owed to creditors for goods and services bought on credit

Accounts receivable: amounts owed to the business by its customers for goods and services sold to them on credit

ACPE: Accreditation Council for Pharmacy Education

AcSB: Canadian Accounting Standards Board

Adjusted Cost Base (ACB): a calculation used to determine the cost of an investment for tax purposes

Administrative Service Only (ASO): an arrangement in which an organization funds its own employee benefit plan, such as a pension plan or health insurance program, but hires an outside firm to perform specific administrative services

Advocacy: the act of speaking out and attempting to influence the course of public policy or public initiatives

Alternative payment plan (APP): a reimbursement model for physicians that can take the form of a salary or capitation, where the physician is paid an annual fee for each patient on the roster regardless of how much attention a patient needs; see also fee for service (FFS)

Angel investor: an investor who provides financial backing for small startups or entrepreneurs

B2B: business to business

B2C: business to consumer

Bad debt: expenses incurred by pharmacy operators as a result of debtors failing to pay their bills

Balance sheet: a financial statement that summarizes a company's assets, liabilities and shareholders' equity at a specific point in time

Best possible medication history (BPMH): a comprehensive list of all prescription, non-prescription and complementary medications the patient is using

Biopharmaceutical product lifecycle: a set of stages a biopharmaceutical product goes through in its lifetime; composed of four stages – development, launch, growth, renewal/decline; see also product lifecycle

Brand: refers to more than just names and logos, products and services, a trademark, the mission and advertising; brands permeate everything from a company image, investor relations, corporate values, internal communications, marketing directions and initiatives to technology, business process, training, employee recruitment and engagement

Brand identity: a feature that distinguishes a product offering from others in the mind of the consumer

Breakeven: the point at which gains equal losses

Business model: a statement of professional pharmacy practice and business goals, the reasons behind believing a person can attain them and the plan to reach those goals

Business plan: a roadmap of desired future activities; outlines the what, why, who, where, when and how of a business's operations; may include an executive summary, business environment, marketing plan, operations, finance, risks and conclusion

Business structures: a business can be set up as a sole proprietorship, partnership, corporation or co-operative

CACDS: Canadian Association of Chain Drug Stores; now known as Neighbourhood Pharmacy Association of Canada

Canada Health Transfer: federal transfer payments provinces/territories receive for publicly funded health care insurance

Canadian Agency for Drugs and Technologies in Health (CADTH): an independent not-for-profit agency funded by the federal and provincial/territorial governments that evaluates the cost and clinical effectiveness of devices and drugs and makes formulary recommendations for the government drug programs

Canadian Institute for Health Information (CIHI): an independent, not-for-profit corporation that aims to contribute to the improvement of the health of Canadians and the health care system by disseminating quality health information

Canadian Pharmacy Services Framework (CPSF): part of the Blueprint for Pharmacy that categorizes services with relation to core dispensing, enhanced medication-related or expanded patient care services

Capital dividend account (CDA): a notional tax account created as a means of tracking these tax-free amounts (capital dividends) for income tax purposes and passing them to shareholders

Capital gains: the profit made after buying an asset at X dollars and selling it at a higher price of Y dollars; the difference between Y and X is the capital gain

Capital requirements: the resources needed for a new entrant into a marketplace

Capital stock: the number of shares authorized for issuance by a company's charter, including both common and preferred stock

Capital structure: the way a corporation finances its assets through some combination of equity and debt

Carriers: a company that offers and/or underwrites insurance policies

Cash flow statement: a summary of the incomings and outgoings of cash in a company over an accounting period

CASL: Canada's Anti-Spam Legislation

CCAPP: Canadian Council for Accreditation of Pharmacy Programs

CCCEP: Canadian Council on Continuing Education in Pharmacy

CCTV: closed-circuit television/security cameras

CDE: Certified Diabetes Educator

CE: continuing education

CEO: chief executive officer, generally the most senior corporate officer (executive) or administrator in charge of managing a for-profit organization

Certificate of Insurance: a document issued by an insurance company/broker that is used to verify the existence of insurance coverage under specific conditions granted to listed individuals

Channels: a business's way of reaching the customer. Pharmacy service-delivery channels are nearly exclusively composed of in-store visits. Communications channels include traditional aspects (print media, signs, radio and telephone books) and newer approaches such as web ads, search engine optimization and social media

CHRP: Certified Human Resources Professional

COGS: cost of goods sold; the price paid for the product, plus any additional costs necessary to get the merchandise into inventory and ready for sale, including shipping and handling

Collateral: something pledged as security to a creditor for repayment of a loan, to be forfeited in the event of a default

Collusion: the illegal practice of price negotiation and agreement between firms

Commodities: undifferentiated goods that are uniform across suppliers

Common area expenses or costs: expenses incurred by tenants attributed to a pro-rata portion of general expenses incurred by the building in which the tenants are housed

Community Pharmacy Incident Reporting system (CPhIR): an anonymous online incident reporting and continuous quality improvement system tool from ISMP Canada

Competitive advantage: an organization has a competitive advantage when its good or service offering is better aligned with the demands of the market than its competitors'

Compounding growth: the returns earned on savings that compound progressively (grow) year after year

Consumer behaviour: the sum of the actions a person takes in purchasing and using products and services, including the mental and social processes that precede and follow these actions

Continuing professional development (CPD): a systematic, self-directed, ongoing and cyclical process where a practitioner reflects on learning needs and goals, plans learning activities to meet needs and goals, implements the learning plan, evaluates success of the plan and documents learning activities in a professional portfolio

Continuous quality improvement (CQI): a management philosophy focused on enhancing various aspects of performance and quality through an ongoing and incremental approach

Corporation: a legal entity that is separate and distinct from its owners. Corporations enjoy most of the rights and responsibilities that an individual possesses; that is, a corporation has the right to enter into contracts, loan and borrow money, sue and be sued, hire employees, own assets and pay taxes.

Cost structure: the most important costs incurred while operating under a particular business model

Council of the Federation (CoF): a group consisting of Canada's 13 provincial/territorial premiers; see also Health Care Innovation Working Group (HCIWG)

CPhA: Canadian Pharmacists Association

CPP: Canada Pension Plan, established in 1966 to provide a basic benefits package for retirees and disabled contributors

Crime Prevention Through Environmental Design (CPTED): a loss prevention concept that states the movement of people, and to a large degree their behaviours, can be influenced by the physical design of a space

CSHP: Canadian Society of Hospital Pharmacists

Current liabilities: a company's debts or obligations that are due within one year. They appear on a company's balance sheet and include short-term debt such as accounts payable.

Current ratio: a financial ratio that measures whether or not a firm has enough resources to pay its debts over the next 12 months. It compares a firm's current assets to its current liabilities and provides an indication of the company's ability to meet short-term debt obligations.

Customer relationship management (CRM): a strategy for understanding clients and their needs in order to optimize interactions with them

Customer satisfaction: the match between customer expectations of the product/service and the actual performance of the product/service

Customer segments: who is being served by the organization or business; see also market segmentation

Debt serving: the cash required for a particular time period to cover the repayment of interest and principal on a debt such as a mortgage payment

Defined-benefit (DB) pension: a type of pension plan in which an employer promises a specified monthly benefit upon retirement that is predetermined by a formula based on the employee's earnings history, tenure of service and age, rather than depending directly on individual investment returns

Defined-contribution (DC) pension: a type of pension plan in which the employer, employee or both make contributions on a regular basis. Individual accounts are set up for participants and benefits are based on the amounts contributed to these accounts (by employer and/or employee) plus any investment earnings on the money in the account. Only employer contributions to the account are guaranteed, not the future benefits.

Demographic segmentation: using quantifiable and definable characteristics of a given population (e.g., age, sex, race, marital status, occupation, income, etc.) to define a market segment

Dividends: payments received from the profits of a company (public or private) in which people have invested, and which distributes some (or all) of its profits to shareholders

DPRA: Drug and Pharmacies Regulation Act (Ontario)

Drug use evaluation (DUE): a structured process to ensure that drugs are being used appropriately in a hospital. It is a form of quality assurance that uses current evidence to develop drug use guidelines that can be implemented in collaboration with prescribers and others on the interdisciplinary team

DTPs: drug therapy problems

EBITDA: earnings before interest, tax, depreciation and amortization; can be used to analyze and compare profitability between companies and industries because it eliminates the effects of financing and accounting decisions

Economies of scale: the ability to minimize the cost for offering a product or service due to increased size, output or scale of operation

EHR: electronic health record

EI: Employment Insurance

EMR: electronic medical record

Entrepreneur: a person who organizes and manages any enterprise, especially a business, usually with considerable initiative and risk in an attempt to make profit

Environmental scanning: the process of monitoring external factors that influence a company, its products and services, its industry and its market

Equity: on a company's balance sheet, the amount of the funds contributed by the owners (the stockholders) plus the retained earnings (or losses). Also referred to as shareholders' equity

Experience curve: operational experience that improves efficiency; relates to cost advantages that can be enjoyed by a firm over time

Extended Reporting Period (ERP): a designated time period after a claims-made insurance policy has expired during which a claim may be made and coverage triggered as if the claim had been made during the policy period

External losses: loss of inventory typically from criminal activity targeted against the business by non-employees; for example, robbery, break and enter and shoplifting are external acts of loss

FDA: Federal Drug Administration (American)

Fee for service (FFS): a reimbursement model for physicians in which they bill provincial/territorial health

insurance plans for each procedure, test or clinical service they provide; see also alternative payment plan (APP)

Financial efficiency: how well dollars invested produce revenues

Financial statements: records that outline the financial activities of a business and are meant to present the financial information as clearly and concisely as possible. Financial statements for businesses usually include income statements, balance sheet, statements of retained earnings and cash flows, as well as other possible statements

Fixed costs: costs that do not change regardless of the quantity of output

Fragmented industry: an industry with a large number of players, where no or few firms possess significant share of the market

GDP: gross domestic product

General liability insurance: insurance policies that protect against bodily injury, property damage, medical expenses, libel, slander, the cost of defending lawsuits and settlement bonds or judgments

Generally Accepted Accounting Principles (GAAP): the common set of accounting principles, standards and procedures that companies use to compile their financial statements. GAAP is a combination of authoritative standards (set by policy boards) and simply the commonly accepted ways of recording and reporting accounting information

Geographic segmentation: using geographic information (e.g., country, province, city, community, neighbourhood, etc.) to define a market segment

Goodwill: an intangible asset that arises as a result of the acquisition of one company by another for a premium value; the value of a company's brand name, solid customer/patient base and good customer/patient relations. Goodwill is considered an intangible asset because it is not a physical asset such as a building or equipment. The goodwill account can be found in the assets portion of a company's balance sheet. It is a factor considered when purchasing an existing pharmacy

Gross margin: a financial metric used to assess a firm's financial health by revealing the proportion of money left over from revenues after accounting for the cost of goods sold and serves as the source for paying additional expenses and future savings (note: for the purposes of this text, gross margin is expressed as an absolute number)

Gross margin return on inventory (GMROI): a ratio that describes a seller's income on every dollar spent on inventory. It is one way to determine how valuable the seller's inventory is, and it describes the relationship between total sales, total profit from total sales and the amount of resources invested in the inventory sold

Gross profit: a financial metric used to assess a firm's financial health by revealing the proportion of money left over from revenues after accounting for the cost of goods sold and serves as the source for paying additional expenses and future savings (note: for the purposes of this text, gross profit is expressed as a percentage)

Group purchasing organizations (GPOs): medication purchase facilitators that utilize the product volumes of a number of member organizations to achieve drug cost savings through economies of scale for multisource products and through volume discounts for single source products from vendors; participation with GPOs is an effective way for hospitals to control acquisition costs of drugs while minimizing the time required to conduct their own contract administration

HCP: health care professional

HCT: health care team

Health Care Innovation Working Group (HCIWG): part of the Council of the Federation that, in addition to seniors' care, has two other focus areas: pharmaceutical drugs and team-based health care delivery models; see also Council of the Federation

Historical analysis: see horizontal analysis

Horizontal analysis: a comparative analysis in which ratios or line items of a company's financial statements are compared over a certain period. For example, a financial comparison that compares this year's results to last year's and is often referred to as a trend analysis or historical analysis; see also trend analysis

Horizontal integration: a strategic merger between larger firms within the industry

Human resources management: a business function within organizations that focuses on the effective management of human capital assets to enable an organization to effectively and efficiently achieve its strategic goals and objectives

Income statement: also known as the profit and loss statement or statement of revenue and expense; a financial statement that measures a company's financial performance over a specific accounting period. The statement provides a summary of how a pharmacy business incurs its revenues and expenses through both operating and non-operating activities. It also shows the net profit or loss incurred over a specific accounting period, typically over a fiscal quarter or year.

Industry concentration: the number of firms possessing the majority of the available market share

Insurance: the transfer of the risk of a loss, from one entity to another, in exchange for payment

Insurer: a person or company that contracts to indemnify another in the event of loss or damage; underwriter

Intangible asset: an asset that is not physical in nature; for example, company intellectual property such as trademarks, copyrights, patents and goodwill

Internal loss: shrink that can be created on purpose or by mistake. Vendors, employees and lack of proper inventory management are all potential sources of internal loss

International Financial Reporting Standards (IFRS): a set of international accounting standards stating how particular types of transactions and other events should be reported in financial statements, issued by the International Accounting Standards Board

Intrapreneurship: project ventures initiated within an existing business

Inventory management: the process of overseeing the constant flow of products in and out of an existing inventory

Inventory turns or inventory turnover ratio: the number of times the inventory is sold in a certain time frame

IPG: international pharmacy graduate

IPP: individual pension plan; a Canadian retirement savings vehicle; typically a one-person maximum defined-benefit pension plan (DB plan) that allows the plan member to accrue retirement income on a tax-deferred basis

ISMP Canada: Institute for Safe Medication Practices Canada

Key resources: the assets required to offer the value proposition

Leverage: the amount of debt used to finance a company's assets with a view to generate returns for the owners of a pharmacy business; often referred to as financial leverage

LGBT: lesbian/gay/bisexual/transsexual

Liabilities: a company's legal debts or obligations that arise during the course of business operations and are typically settled over time through the transfer of economic benefits including cash, goods or services

Liability insurance: a part of the general insurance system of risk financing to protect the purchaser (the "insured") from the risks of liabilities imposed by lawsuits and similar claims

Life insurance: a protection against the loss of income that would result if the insured person died. The named beneficiary receives the proceeds and is thereby safeguarded from the financial impact of the death of the insured.

Liquidity: the degree to which an asset such as inventory and accounts payable can be converted to cash; also a measure of the ability of a pharmacy to pay obligations expected to become due within the next year

Long-term disability (LTD): a type of insurance that pays employees a portion of their salary for a specified period of time when they are forced to be off work with an illness/medical condition; most LTD policies begin to pay benefits when an employee has missed between 30 and 90 days of work

Long-term liabilities: company obligations that extend beyond the current year; typically these include long-term debt such as a mortgage

Loss prevention security: the protection of people (staff), the property (the business and assets) and information (patient information and IT)

Loyalty: a deeply held commitment to re-purchase or re-patronize a preferred product or service provider in the future

LTC: long-term care

Margin: the profit arising from the revenue generated by a business or service, less the sum of all costs and expenses in generating that revenue in a given period; the term is used interchangeably with gross margin

Market: a set of actual and potential buyers of a good or service

Market analysis: a more specific, focused review than an environmental scan that usually includes defining one's customer base and their needs, current gaps in meeting those needs and detailed knowledge of immediate competitors

Market growth: a market's demand for an industry's product/service offerings and an industry's position within a product's lifecycle

Market segmentation: where a market is subdivided into consumer subsets based on similar behaviour or needs (e.g., demographic, geographic, psychographic); see also customer segments

Marketing communications: often referred to as MarCom; a subset of the marketing plan representing the messages and media used to communicate with defined target audiences to support the marketing plan goals

Marketing mix: product, price, place, promotion; also known as the 4 Ps of marketing

Marketing myopia: occurs when organizations lose sight of what matters by not considering the end user of a product

Markup: the percentage added to the cost of the product to enable the wholesaler to cover expenses and make a profit

Mass marketing: a marketing strategy that does not target a specific segment but rather the entire market

MBWA: manage by walking around

Medical Advisory Committee (MAC): the principle policy-making body of the medical staff in a hospital; accountable to and makes recommendations directly to the Board of the hospital; responsible for approving all policies related to patient care and documentation in the health record

Micro marketing: a marketing strategy that targets a small market segment that is narrowly defined

Min/max order points: the minimum amount and maximum amount of stock to have on hand for each individual molecule or drug, as established by a pharmacy operator, to ensure the pharmacy will have adequate stock of each to dispense for prescriptions; the maximum level acts as a control so the inventory does not climb above the determined threshold and negatively affect cash flow

Mission statement: a statement of the reason why the organization exists; it is about the purpose of the organization and should encompass all the goals in one broader statement; a mission statement should state who the market is, what is being offered to them and what makes the offering unique

MMP: methadone maintenance program

MSSA-CAP: Medication Safety Self-Assessment for Community/Ambulatory Pharmacy, a tool from ISMP Canada

NAPRA: National Association of Pharmacy Regulatory Authorities

NDCV: net delivered customer value; the sum of all the benefits provided by the product or service (functional benefits, service, social) minus the sum of all the costs of attaining that product such as finances, energy and time

NDSAC: National Drug Schedules Advisory Committee

Niche marketing: a marketing strategy that targets a market segment that is less commonly pursued

Normalized income before tax: earnings of a pharmacy business adjusted for business expenses attributable to an owner's personal expenses; adjustments can also be made for one-time periodic expenses that are determined to be non-recurring in nature

NVT: new venture template

OAS: Old Age Security program

Occupancy expenses: expenditures required to occupy and maintain the physical space a business inhabits, and usually represents one of the largest expenditures for a pharmacy business; expense items typically include rent, utilities, repairs, maintenance, insurance and any other cost related to the store space occupied

Oligopoly: a situation where the majority of market share is owned by only a few large firms

OSCE: objective structured clinical exams

Owner's equity: the total assets of a business minus its total liabilities; represents the capital available for distribution to shareholders

Partnership: a legal form of business operation between two or more individuals who share management and profits

Patented Medicine Prices Review Board (PMPRB): an independent pseudo-judicial body operating at arm's-length from the federal government

Patient-centred care: the idea that patients are at the centre of services and health care; sometimes referred to as patient-focused care, patient-care management, patient-centred health management, patient-centric care, etc.

PCPA: Pan-Canadian Pricing Alliance, now part of the pan-Canadian Pharmaceutical Alliance

PEBC: Pharmacy Examining Board of Canada

Perpetual inventory system: a method of accounting for inventory that records the purchase and sale of inventory on an item-by-item basis through the use of computerized point-of-sale and pharmacy management computer systems; provides a highly detailed view of changes in inventory and allows for real-time reporting of the amount of inventory in stock

PEST analysis: political, economic, social and technological factors that must be considered when developing marketing and business plans; similar to a SWOT analysis

Pharmacy and Therapeutics Committee (P&T Committee): a subcommittee of a hospital's medical advisory committee (MAC), which is a mandated committee responsible for all aspects of the medication system in a hospital

Pharmacy benefit manager (PBM): most often a third-party administrator (TPA) of prescription drug programs but sometimes can be a service inside of an integrated health care system

PIPEDA: Personal Information Protection Electronic Document Act

POCT: point-of-care testing

Policyholder: the person or entity buying the insurance policy

POS: point of sale

Preferred provider network (PPN): a collection of pharmacies that have a preferred relationship with a given plan sponsor; often the plan sponsor provides members with financial incentives for using preferred providers

Prepaid expenses: an expenditure that is paid for in one accounting period, but for which the underlying asset will not be entirely consumed until a future period

Product: the good (tangible), the service (intangible) or a combination of the two that is offered by a person or organization

Product differentiation: attributes of a product or service that render it unique or differentiated compared to other substitutes in the market that aim to accommodate the same or similar consumer need(s); benefit from product differentiation

Product lifecycle: a set of stages a product goes through in its lifetime – introduction, growth, maturity, decline; see also biopharmaceutical product lifecycle

Product to price performance ratio: involves taking the perspective of a customer in asking, "For what I pay, what benefit(s) do I get?"

Professional liability insurance: insurance that protects professionals such as accountants, lawyers and physicians against negligence and other claims initiated by their clients; required by professionals who have expertise in a specific area because general liability insurance policies do not offer protection against claims arising out of business or professional practices such as negligence, malpractice or misrepresentation

Profit: a financial gain related to the difference between the amount earned and the amount spent buying inventory and, subsequently, operating a pharmacy; the return a company or owner receives for providing value to the customer/patient

Progressive discipline: the formal process of increasingly severe consequences for dealing with issues of misconduct in the workplace

Property insurance: a policy that provides financial reimbursement to the owner or renter of a structure and its contents in the event of damage or theft; can include homeowners insurance, renters insurance, flood insurance and earthquake insurance

Psychographic market segmentation: using consumer lifestyles (e.g., activities, behaviours, interests, opinions, habits, etc.) to define a market segment

QPP: Québec Pension Plan

Quick ratio: an indicator of a company's short-term liquidity; measures a company's ability to meet its short-term obligations with its most liquid assets

Registered retirement savings plan (RRSP): a registered account for savings that can be invested in eligible investment options such as stocks, bonds, mutual funds, real estate income trusts, etc. Each year, a person may contribute up to 18% of income from the previous year, up to a maximum amount determined by the federal government. If one does not contribute the full allowable amount, the difference is carried forward to future years' contributions. Savings grow tax-free until withdrawals begin; see also tax-free savings account (TFSA)

Relationship marketing: a marketing approach that views each exchange as a series of transactions over time, each transaction building upon the previous, unlike transactional marketing; supplying organizations are not only interested in making the sale but also in establishing, developing and maintaining relationships with clients to develop long-term relationships that could not be easily duplicated by competitors and become a point of competitive differentiation

RESP: registered education savings plan

Retail loss prevention: a set of practices and procedures organizations follow to protect their assets and preserve profit

Retained earnings: the portion of a corporation's net income that is kept by the corporation rather than distributed to shareholders as dividends

Return on investment (ROI): the amount of profit or cost saving that will be realized in return for a specific expenditure of money that is usually expressed as a percentage of the original monetary outlay

Revenue streams: where a business acquires its revenue; for a pharmacy, it may be dispensing fees, the sale of over-the-counter products or pharmacy services

Rivalry: the degree of competition or supply that can threaten the size of the market share of an organization

Segmented marketing: a marketing strategy that targets a specific segment of the market

Shareholder agreement: a contract outlining the relationship between the shareholders of a corporation and lays the foundation of interactions between owners with each other and with the directors of the company

Short-term disability (STD): a type of insurance coverage that pays employees a portion of their salary when forced to be off work for a short duration of time with an illness/medical condition; duration can vary, but is often less than 30 consecutive days

S.H.O.T.: screening, hiring, orientation and training

Shrinkage: the difference between recorded inventory and actual inventory on hand; preventable losses; damaged or expired stock needs to be accounted for and will be separated and counted as a loss

Slack: waste in the supply chain of the product or service, whereby upstream suppliers or downstream customers (note this does not necessarily mean the end user) of the venture are inefficient and pass the cost of this inefficiency onto the venture

SMART objectives: objectives should be specific, measurable, action-oriented or attainable, realistic, time-bound/timely/time-sensitive

Social media: Internet-based applications that allow anyone to create, consume, control and connect with information (e.g., Facebook, Twitter, YouTube, Wikipedia); online platforms that allow anyone to create, consume, control and connect with information

Sole proprietor: a form of business ownership in which a person owns 100% of the business and is personally responsible (liable) for its debts and obligations

Specialized inputs: physical supplies or services that cannot be substituted or acquired anywhere else

Stakeholders: people and/or entities that are affected by or can affect the operations and practices of an organization

Stock-keeping unit (SKU): a retail pharmacy's product identification code that helps the item to be tracked for inventory purposes

Stock outs: a situation in which a pharmacy business sells its entire inventory of a certain product or shelf item; the patient or customer is then unable to purchase more product until it becomes available from the supplier or wholesaler

Strategic groups: subgroups of competitors within an industry that generally employ the same strategies and business models to compete

Strategic planning: a continuous exercise in almost every type of organization, from an independent community pharmacy, to a regulatory authority, to a health region; strategic plans allow organizations to review where they have been and to strategize about where they would like to be in the future

Subrogation: a legal right reserved by most insurance carriers to pursue a third party that caused an insurance loss to the insured. This is done as a means of recovering the amount of the claim paid to the insured for the loss. Simply stated, the right of subrogation is the right to pursue someone else's claim

Subrogation agreement: an agreement involving subrogation; pharmacy owners will experience a subrogation when they waive their right to directly pursue a legal claim in return for allowing the owner's insurance company to act on the owner's behalf

Subsequent Entry Biologics (SEBs): generic equivalents of biologic medications

Switching costs: the ease with which a customer may switch from one supplier's product(s) or service(s) to another

SWOT: marketing analysis that considers strengths, weaknesses, opportunities and threats

Tangible assets: assets that have a physical form; includes fixed assets (e.g., buildings and land) and current assets (e.g., inventory and accounts receivable)

Target market: the segment or subset of the consumer group that pharmacy managers choose to target and focus their marketing efforts toward; the set of actual and potential buyers of a product (good and/ or service)

Tax-free capital dividend: a dividend paid to a shareholder upon which no tax is paid, usually associated with a corporate capital dividend account

Tax-free savings account (TFSA): a registered savings account like an RRSP that enables Canadians to invest their savings in investments that can grow tax-free. Unlike RRSPs, TFSAs do not require the payment of taxes upon withdrawals. On the other hand, TFSAs do not generate tax refunds when contributions are made; see also registered retirement savings plan (RRSP)

Technical insolvency: occurs when a pharmacy business is unable to meet its financial obligations

Therapeutic Products Directorate (TPD): the organization through which Health Canada approves and monitors all drugs sold in the country; TPD also administers the Special Access Program, conducts ongoing surveillance on approved drugs, investigates complaints, monitors adverse events and inspects and licenses production sites; when necessary, TPD also manages recalls

Third-party administrator (TPA): an organization that processes pharmacy prescription claims and performs other administrative services in accordance with an employee prescription service contract

Third-party payer (TPP): any company that acts as the payer under coverage provided by an employee prescription drug plan

Time value of money (TVM): a concept in personal financial management that involves knowing the value of a sum of money at different points in time; expressed as an equation composed of present value (PV), future value (FV) and the rate of return (or the discount rate) of (k) over a period of years (t) where $PV = FV/(1+k)^t$

Transactional marketing: a marketing approach that views each exchange/interaction as an isolated and unrelated event, unlike relationship marketing; once a sale is made, the supplier seeks a new customer to purchase the goods or services rather than focusing time and effort on previous purchasers

Trend analysis: an aspect of technical analysis that tries to predict the future key metrics of a pharmacy business based on past data. Trend analysis is based on the idea that what has happened in the past gives various stakeholders an idea of what will happen in the future; see also horizontal analysis

Trial balance: a bookkeeping worksheet in which the balances of all account ledgers are compiled and is available for review by interested parties. A company prepares a trial balance periodically, typically at the end of a reporting period, for the purpose of ensuring the entries in a company's bookkeeping system are mathematically accurate

Umbrella insurance: extra liability insurance designed to help protect a person from major claims and lawsuits; helps protect assets by providing additional liability coverage above the limits of homeowners, auto and boat insurance policies

Union: an organization that represents the interests of the employees in a particular plant, store, office or industry; once certified, the union participates in collective bargaining with management to negotiate the terms and conditions of employment impacting the policies and procedures that govern these employees in the workplace

Value proposition: a concept central to business planning that involves identifying what customer problems the business can solve or what customer needs the business can meet

Wage grid: identifies each job description and wage range within each job description, as well as a time-based wage, which would include a starting wage, a three-month wage and a one-year mark, two-year mark, etc.; this wage grid now becomes the focal point for wage administration

Wages expenses: an expense line item that represents payments made to employees, regardless of whether they are hourly or salaried; may also include payroll tax and other employee benefits paid to the employees

White knight: an individual or company that acquires a business on the verge of being taken over by other forces deemed undesirable by company officials. While the target company does not remain independent, a white knight is viewed as a preferred option to a hostile company completing the takeover. Unlike a hostile takeover, current management typically remains in place in a white knight scenario, and investors receive better compensation for their shares

WHMIS: Workplace Hazardous Materials Information System

Working capital: a measure of a company's efficiency and its short-term financial health; calculated by subtracting current liabilities from current assets

Index